Voice Treatment for Children and Adolescents

Moya L. Andrews

Professor of Speech and Hearing Sciences
Vice Chancellor for Academic Affairs
Dean of the Faculties
Indiana University
Bloomington, Indiana

with

Anne C. Summers
Monroe Couty Schools Corporation
Bloomington, Indiana

with contributions from
Risa L. Nasatir, M.A.
Rahul Shrivastav, M.Sc.

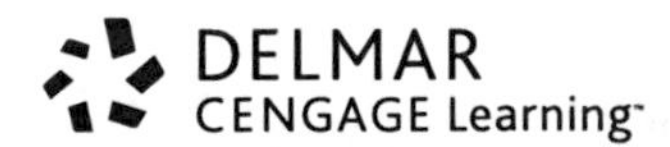

Australia • Brazil • Japan • Korea • Mexico • Singapore • Spain • United Kingdom • United States

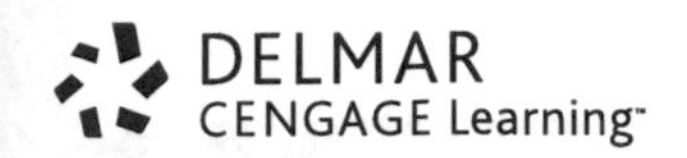

Voice Treatment for Children and Adolescents, Second Edition
Moya L. Andrews, Anne C. Summers

Business Unit Director: William Brottmiller
Acquisitions Editor: Marie Linvill
Developmental Editor: Kristin Banach
Executive Marketing Manager: Dawn Gerrain
Channel Manager: Tara Carter
Executive Production Editor: Barbara Bullock
Production Editor: Sandy Doyle

Library of Congress Control Number: 00–063778

ISBN-13: 978-0-7693-0107-5

ISBN-10: 0-7693-0107-X

Delmar
Executive Woods
5 Maxwell Drive
Clifton Park, NY 12065
USA

Cengage Learning is a leading provider of customized learning solutions with office locations around the globe, including Singapore, the United Kingdom, Australia, Mexico, Brazil, and Japan. Locate your local office at:
international.cengage.com/region

Cengage Learning products are represented in Canada by
Nelson Education, Ltd.

For your lifelong learning solutions, visit **delmar.cengage.com**

Visit our corporate website at **www.cengage.com**

Printed in the United States of America
6 7 8 9 10   17 16 15 14 13

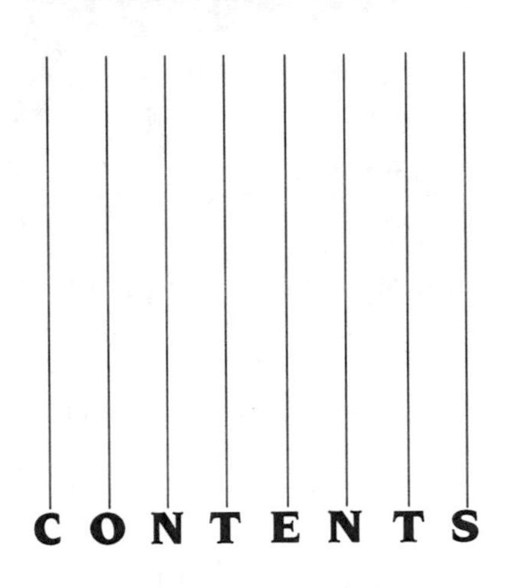

CONTENTS

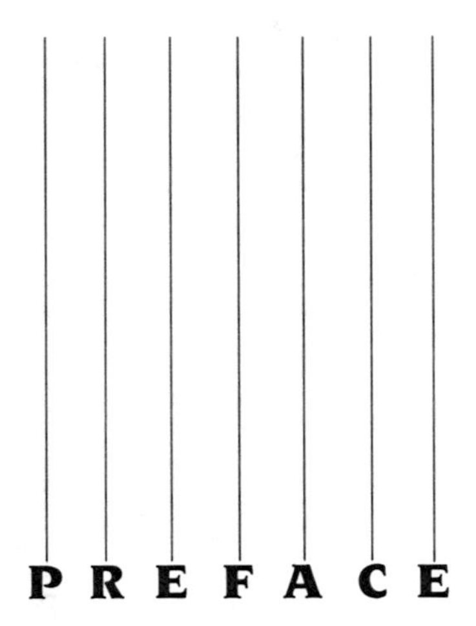

PREFACE

This book brings together in one volume the information that clinicians need to design individualized treatment programs for children of all ages. Information concerning the development of vocal communication from infancy through adolescence, a review of the factors that affect and/or limit development, and strategies to compensate for constraints and maximize vocal learning are presented. This book contains some of the material previously published in *Voice Therapy for Children* and *Voice Therapy for Adolescents.*

Increasingly, speech–language pathologists are emphasizing the importance of early intervention with children who are at risk for communication disorders. It is important to support the emergence of both receptive and expressive voice learning as early as possible and for clinicians to work closely with families of infants who are at risk for voice disorders. The role of the speech–language pathologist working as part of a team in medical settings is addressed in chapter 3, which focuses on the types of intervention typically occurring in intensive care units.

There have been exciting developments in the application of technology in both the assessment and treatment of voice disorders. The various types of instruments that are useful for clinicians working with children are detailed in chapter 9.

The team approach to assessment and treatment is emphasized, and various models of intervention are illustrated for all age levels. This is a resource book for clinicians and for clinicians in training. Rationales for treatment approaches are discussed together with the research literature that supports them. Illustrative materials are presented in the appendices.

The appendices provide examples of materials that can be used with children of all ages and stages of development. Although there are no magic techniques or approaches that can be expected to work with every child, the availability of a range of options to consider is usually helpful for clinicians as they plan individualized treatment plans. Thus, the appendices in this book can be viewed as a resource to assist busy clinicians looking for ideas to stimulate their own thinking and creativity. When we have opportunities to see what other clinicians are doing, we can reflect on the approaches we are currently using, modify them, expand them, and see them in a different context.

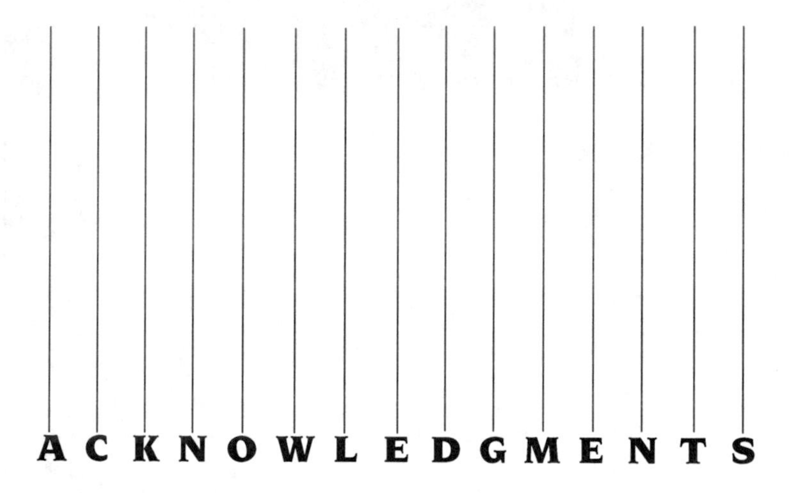

ACKNOWLEDGMENTS

In preparing a comprehensive volume of this type, I have drawn on the published works of many talented people, as well as on ideas that have been generously shared through personal contacts. I have been fortunate to work closely with many fine colleagues in the Department of Speech and Hearing Sciences at Indiana University, Bloomington, as well as in the Monroe County School Corporation. In addition, I have been stimulated by working with many exceptional graduate students and past students from our program. I am indebted to Julia Wood Rademacher, Dr. Jesse Phillips, Dr. John Seward, Dr. Hiroya Yamaguchi, Todd Bohnenkamp, Wen-Hui Su, Rahul Shrivastav, and David Montgomery, who contribute so much to the Indiana University Voice Team.

My collaborators on this volume, Anne Summers, Risa L. Nasatir, and Rahul Shrivastav, are exceptional clinicians and I thank them for sharing their expertise and for their good natures, inspiration, and hard work. Cyndi Connelley, Jerome Dorsey, Joyce Regester, and Christine Savoldi provided exemplary research and secretarial support. Editorial assistance from Delmar Cengage Learning is always superb and I have been fortunate to work on yet another project with Marie Linvill, Kristin Banach, and Sandy Doyle. They have the ability to turn any challenge into a wonderful opportunity.

Finally, I want to thank my family for coping yet again with one of my all-consuming projects with characteristic patience and good will. Stan, Alistair, Jennifer, Hayley and Rebecca provided me with lots of emotional as well as practical support. Anne Summers' family, John, Jill, and Debra also deserve special appreciation.

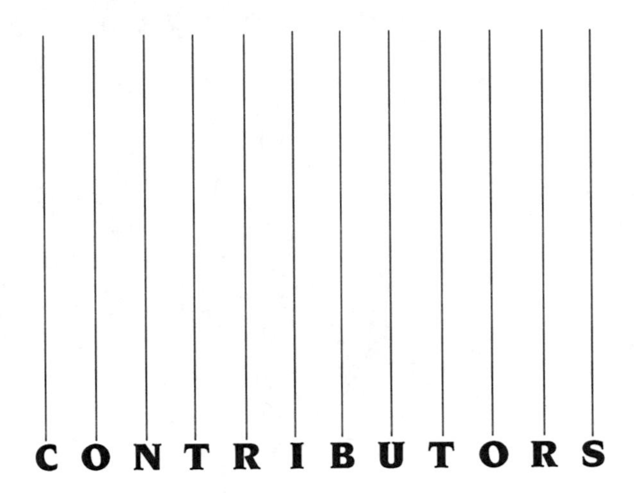

CONTRIBUTORS

Risa L. Nasatir, M.A., CCC-SLP
Lutheran General Hospital
Park Ridge, Illinois

Rahul Shrivastav, M.Sc., CCC-SLP
Speech and Hearing Sciences
Indiana University
Bloomington, Indiana

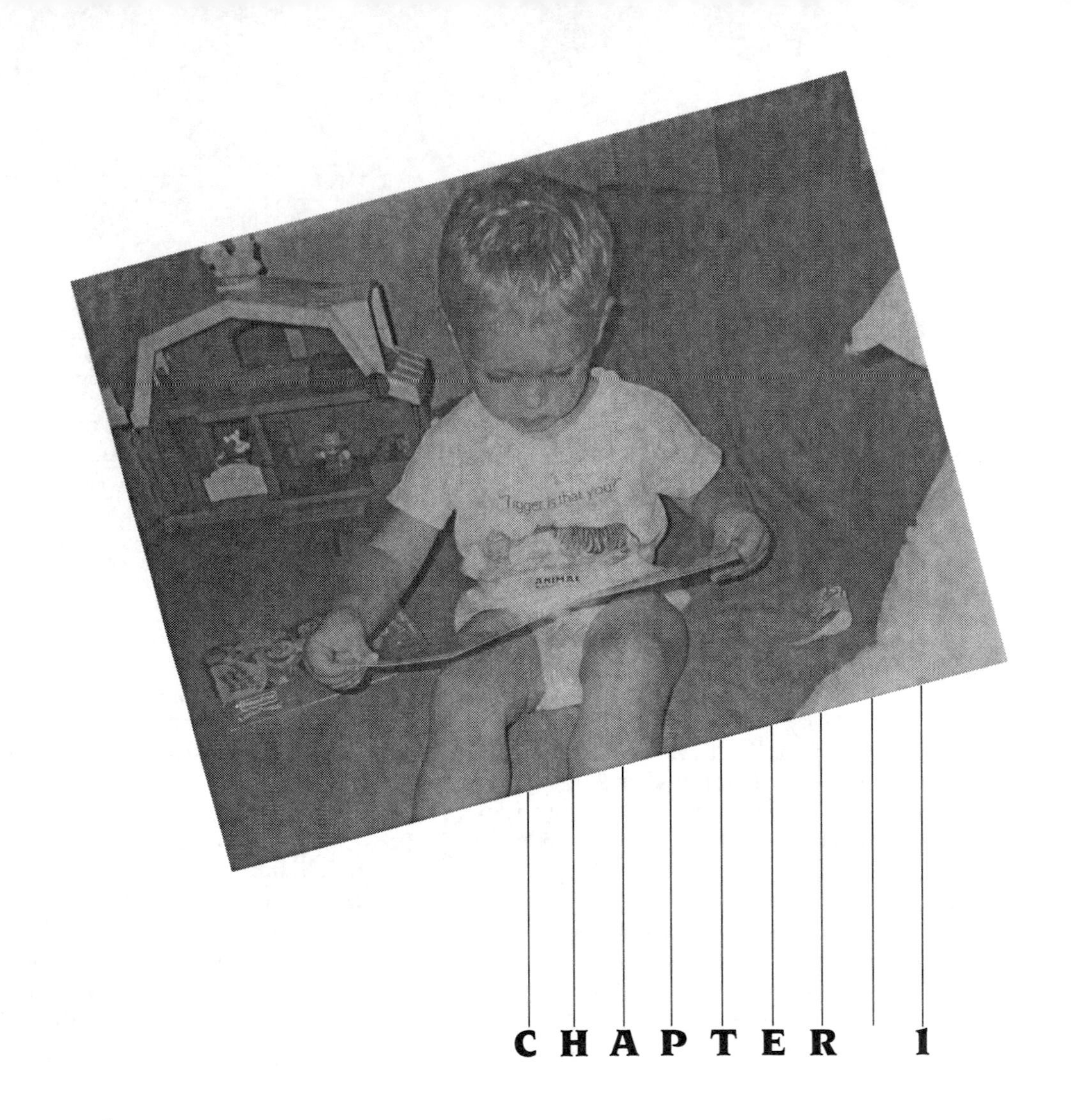

CHAPTER 1

Introduction

"Voice is ephemeral and many factors support it, influence it, and affect perceptions of it."

The human voice is unlike any other sound, yet it is more than just sound. It is the embodiment of the person from whom it springs. It is a defining characteristic of the species. The birth cry is the first affirmation of a new identity and the proof of existence of a new and separate life. It is also the first demonstration of a newborn infant's physical capacity, showing that the respiratory tract is functioning and providing information on the health status of the newborn. It is more than that, however. It is also a means of emotional connection and the first communicative act—the first sign of how the new human being will forge and maintain interpersonal relationships across the entire life span. The voice of the baby proclaims the separation from the mother at birth and evokes joy and awe in all who hear the cry. From that moment, voice will be the vehicle of emotional and intellectual connections that the child makes with an ever-increasing number of people. It will be central to the child's ability to explore and shape the environment, and the voices of others will inform and develop the infant's reality in miraculous ways.

From the moment we are born, voice is not only a defining characteristic of our humanity and membership in our species, it is also a hallmark of our personal identity. It provides information about our gender, age, culture, and personality. Nature and nurture combine to develop voice patterns that are distinctively human, yet personal and individualistic. Frequently, there are strong similarities in the voices of family members. This is attributable not only to similarities in anatomy but also to exposure to similar models and learning opportunities.

Throughout our lives, voices—both our own and those of others—are crucial. Voice is never static. It is, within certain anatomic and physiologic limits, always changing. Voice use is dynamic, and it is an interactive process.

Both listeners and speakers impose constraints on vocal products. To whom we are speaking, as well as who and how we are when we are speaking, affects the voice we hear. Across the life span, our voices change as we change physiologically, intellectually, and emotionally. Our health, our level of fatigue, the environment, and our feelings can cause voice changes from day to day or even moment to moment.

A first step in becoming a clinician who is skilled in voice treatment is the exploration of what voice is and the huge range of voice behaviors that humans can exhibit. Normal or typical vocal behaviors are difficult to define because parameters change. There are different expectations for voices and voice use for infants, toddlers, preschoolers, prepubertal, pubertal, and postpubertal children. Maturation affects anatomy as well as learning. Contexts also exert a powerful influence on decisions concerning what is normal or typical vocal behavior. Both the physical and psychodynamic environments have to be considered. Although screaming may be appropriate for a 5-year-old child on a roller-coaster or a 2-year-old child who has just been given a shot, it may not seem so for a 10-year-old in a classroom. Frequency and consistency of behaviors also have to be considered. An occasional episode of an inappropriate vocal behavior, as extreme as uncontrollable screaming or as mild as throat clearing, may not be significant. Frequent episodes may be viewed differently because of their pattern of occurrence.

Voice, like many intangibles, is affected by the perspective of the evaluator as well as by the structures and functions that influence its production at any given point in time. The vocal product changes, the listeners change, and expectations change. The sound a child emits is fleeting, and for the listener to recall it accurately without recordings is often difficult. We can do an acoustic analysis of a recorded sample and measure the acoustic parameters of the signal, but the results are also subject to human error. Factors such as the quality of the recording equipment, the type of analysis selected, and the skill of the person attempting the analysis must be considered. These aspects will be discussed in a subsequent chapter, as will the factors that affect the perceptual judgments of vocal behavior made with the eye and the ear of evaluators. Evaluation of what is normal or typical about vocal behaviors is still an imperfect process, although there is much in the literature to help us achieve clearer results today than were possible even a few years ago.

The voice we hear, or record for subsequent analysis of its acoustic pattern, is the product that is emitted by a person. The characteristics of the person producing the vocal product are important in the study of voice. The anatomic, physiologic, and neurologic support available and the integrity of the systems obviously shapes the characteristics of the voice that is produced. No single part of the human body is dedicated solely to voice production. Communicative function is an overlaid function. This means that all of the structures used during voice production are designed first of all for other life-supporting purposes. Communication is a secondary, or an additional function superimposed on them. The respiratory system is dedicated to sustaining life, but it secondarily contributes the air supply necessary to produce vocal fold vibrations. The larynx, where voice is produced, is primarily a valve to protect the respiratory tract. Biologically, the vocal folds, with their ability to open and close, are vital to the maintenance of a functioning airway. They close to prevent liquids and foreign bodies from entering the lungs. They work with other protective mechanisms, such as the epiglottis, to close off the respiratory tract during swallowing, for example. The digestive tract and the respiratory tract must always be considered in tandem when we are considering the integrity of structures that support voice production. That is why we talk about the aerodigestive tract.

Air, liquid, and solid food all enter the body through the mouth and proceed into the pharynx before proceeding to their prospective destinations. In the case of breathing, the air proceeds from the pharynx into the respiratory tract. In the case of swallowing, liquids and foods are moved into the esophagus. There is a synchronized interplay of reflexes and actions that allows for the separation and coexistence of these respiratory and digestive systems and functions. They also are influenced significantly by the central, peripheral, and autonomic nervous systems and the integrity of their function. When communication demands are added to the load carried by the respiratory, digestive, and neurologic systems, the exquisitely delicate balance and coordination sometimes can be affected. Adaptations and compensations may occur in one or more systems. Changes in the aerodigestive tract and in sensory and motor functions may be due to the overall health and condition of the person. Systemic chronic illness or congenital or acquired structural variations that inhibit the support of life can, for example, cause such changes. Disruptions may also be due to acute conditions that are more localized, such as irritation of structures, infections, or secretions. Sometimes factors such as thick mucus or swelling of tissues can cause obstruction of the airway. When these conditions exist, the absence of voicing or the observable changes such as disturbances in the quality of the voice, signal the need for immediate medical attention to ensure the viability of the airway to sustain life. Experienced clinicians and physicians can always learn a great deal about airway problems in children by listening to the breathing, crying, and voicing characteristics (Zajac, 1993).

It may be convenient to consider some sort of framework for us to look at voice and the ongoing evolution and development of control over voice behaviors. The sound that is heard can be thought of as the tip of an iceberg. Supporting that sound are many structures and functions that are not easily observed. They are the submerged parts of the iceberg used in our analogy. Yet we must consider and be aware of these parts to understand both typical and atypical voice production.

Anatomy and Physiology and Sensorimotor Integrity

We already have alluded to the importance of structures and functions that support voice production. We know, too, that structures and functions change across time as an individual grows and develops. At birth, there are differences in the stage of development of the structures depending on whether the infant is premature or full term. There may also be congenital abnormalities in the structures and additional challenges placed on the aerodigestive systems attributable to these abnormalities themselves or to systemic illness. Examples include hyaline membrane disease, which prevents the baby's lungs from functioning appropriately, or a fistula in the tracheoesophageal wall, which results in incomplete separation between the trachea (airway) and esophagus (food pipe). In the former, the cry is weak because the air supply needed to set the voice folds in motion is limited. In the latter, liquids from the esophagus leak into the trachea, which leads to the lungs. The cry has a "wet," impeded sound, and the presence of liquids in the airway is also life threatening. These are only two examples of neonatal conditions that need immediate medical or surgical intervention to address the support of life functions. Examples of neurologically based conditions are tracheomalacia and laryngomalacia, which result from immaturity of the muscle tone so that the structures collapse inward, threatening the openness or patency of the airway as the infant breathes. Vocal fold paralysis (Rosin, Handler, Potsic, Wetmore, & Tom, 1990) also results in breathing and voice problems in children and may be unilateral or bilateral. We will discuss other structural deviations in a subsequent chapter.

At this point, however, the importance of the sound of the voice, or the absence of voicing, as a sign of the overall medical condition of the child should be emphasized. The systems that support voice production, the way they function together, and the viability and neurologic integrity of their coexistence is crucial to the overall health of the child. We must understand it fully to understand how it supports or fails to support the child's communicative needs. As voice clinicians, we work closely with physicians and other allied health professionals to obtain this information. In medical settings in which we are part of assessment and treatment teams we are usually engaged in the data gathering process. When we work with children in nonmedical settings, we have the obligation to ensure that we have all of the relevant medical history and that we maintain close communication with other specialists. Below are some areas of interest to voice clinicians regardless of the age of the child with whom they are working. History taking, medical reports, and observation provide us with relevant information concerning the support available for voicing.

Aerodigestive Systems

- Birth information
- Congenital abnormalities
- Acquired abnormalities
- Iatrogenic effects (related to medical treatments)
- Pharmologic effects (medications)
- Medical and health history
- Ventilation or prosthetic devices needed

Neurologic and Sensory Systems

- Congenital deficits
- Central nervous system (motor and sensory)
- Parasympathetic nervous system (cranial nerves)
- Trauma
- Disease

Voice and Voice-Related Behaviors

The sound of the voice is always the voice clinician's focus during both assessment and treatment because it is the actual voice product. As noted earlier, however, voice is ephemeral, and many factors support it, influence it, and affect perceptions of it. Whether it is a reflexive vocalization or an intentional communicative act is also an important consideration. Vegetative or biologically driven sounds, such as coughs to dislodge an irritant or foreign body from the airway, are different from intentional, cognitively mediated vocal messages. Nonetheless, both types of vocalizations tell us that the vocal folds are vibrating and that airflow is driving them. Whether a reflexive sound is elicited or spontaneous is also important. A child may cough only when it is necessary to clear the airway or cough repeatedly in an habitual nonproductive manner. Both behaviors tell us the folds are vibrating. The repetitive cough alerts us to possibilities such as irritation or dryness in the upper respiratory tract, faulty learning, and so on. Reflexes that are elicited (e.g., "show me how you cough") indicate that the sound can be produced at will and that there is cognitive awareness of the instruction and the required response. It may also indicate an emotional willingness on the part of the child to respond to adult requests. When a child withholds sounds with communicative intent (as in the case of electively mute children) but makes sounds during crying, laughing, and coughing, for example, one may conclude that the larynx is capable of making sounds but that emotional factors are constraining vocal communication.

When we think about voice and voice-related behaviors, we are focusing on observable sounds and movements. These are things we can see or hear the child do. They are observable behaviors that can be documented and recorded for future consideration. They are repeatable events, and we can infer that there is some level of anatomic, physiologic and neurologic activity or integrity to support them.

Sometimes respiratory function will be monitored or assisted (e.g., the use of ventilators in infants and children suffering from respiratory distress). This type of monitoring will be described in a later chapter. Here we will review some of the respiratory behaviors that can be observed by a clinician in children of all ages without the use of sophisticated equipment. These signs provide information about underlying structures and function.

Respiratory Behaviors

Appropriate chest movements during inspiration and expiration:

- Breaths per minute (vegetative breathing at rest)
- Quick inhalation, longer exhalation (speech breathing)

- Length of exhalation to sustain connected speech
- Appropriateness of replenishing breaths during speech
- Dyspnea (disordered breathing)
- Stridor (noisy breathing)
- Snoring during sleep
- Habituated mouth breathing
- Control of air flow
- Coordination of airflow and phonation

When breathing is labored or noisy, it suggests that the child is working harder than normal to meet oxygen requirements. Dyspnea (disturbed breathing) may be due to respiratory disease, immaturity, or obstruction. Obstructions may be due to swollen tissues, flaccidity of structures (e.g., laryngomalacia or tracheomalacia), thick or copious secretions, congenital malformations of the aerodigestive tract, or paralysis of the folds. Labored noisy breathing (e.g., snoring) may also be caused by nasopharyngeal obstruction such as swollen tonsils and adenoids. Sleep apnea (periods of arrested breathing) may occur in severe cases of nasopharyngeal obstruction. This is characterized by periods of silence followed by noisy labored inhalation. The child will be a restless sleeper at night and may present a drowsy, pallid demeanor during the day.

It is usually advantageous to obtain endoscopic evaluations of the aerodigestive tracts of medically fragile children. When medical conditions are not severe enough to warrant intrusive evaluations of this type, however, some of the laryngeal behaviors can be inferred from reflexive and phonatory behaviors. Such behaviors may be observed spontaneously or specifically elicited by the clinician.

Laryngeal and Phonatory Activities

- Laughing and crying
- Sighing, grunting, coughing
- Babbling
- Stopping, starting vocalizations
- Prolonging vocalizations
- Imitating sounds, patterns
- Spontaneous words, phrases
- Pitch, loudness, duration changes
- Quality changes in vocalizations
- Onset of vocalizations
- Effort level during vocalizations

We can infer a great deal about the laryngeal adjustments a child is making from the sounds that are emitted spontaneously. We also can experiment with stimulating the child in various ways to ascertain whether the vocal product can be shaped. For example, we can see if a child can imitate repetitive vocal fold closure patterns to observe laryngeal diadochokinesis (ʌ ʌ ʌ ʌ), and we can note whether the airflow can be segmented by observing whether the child can repeat short sighs in an organized sequence of air emission. Similarly, we can observe the child's ability to make velopharyngeal and oral adjustments within the upper respiratory tract. Imitative play can be used to show us Valsalva maneuvers, repetitive nasal and oral sounds, prolonged humming and vowel production, and so forth. We can observe children's ability to imitate sequences of the same and different phonemes, consonant-vowel-consonant (CVC) combinations and pitch, loudness, and duration patterns associated with sound sequences. Thus, we can learn about the potential that exists for speech production, separation of nasal and oral cavities, prosodic variation, and other significant characteristics of emerging resonatory and articulatory control. Of course, our expectations are shaped by our knowledge of what is age appropriate tempered by our awareness of any medical or maturational constraints that may be limiting vocal development in any individual infant or toddler. In the case of older children, we also will observe the effects of physical activity on the vocal product. Does the voice sound the same when the child jumps repeatedly while phonating? In what vocally demanding activities does the child normally engage? What kind of compensatory behaviors appear to be part of the vocal pattern? Are muscle tension, posture, hydration, or allergic reactions possibly implicated in contributing to the way this voice sounds?

Factors Influencing Phonation

- Posture or muscle tension
- Lubrication or secretions
- Compensatory behaviors (e.g., substitutes laryngeal for velopharyngeal valving)
- Endocrinologic factors
- Ability to imitate and modify vocal attempts
- Hydration
- Gastroesophageal reflux
- Allergies; postnasal drip
- Coordination of breathing & swallowing

Balance of Oral and Nasal Resonance

- Supraglottal structures
- Medical conditions or obstructions
- Adjustments of velopharyngeal sphincter
- Oral breath pressure or nasal emission
- Mouth opening or tongue position
- Tone focus (forward versus backward)
- Articulation and projection of sounds

Cognition: Thought Processes Associated With Voice

The central nervous system is essential to all communication, vocal and nonvocal. It is obvious that thought and intent are intrinsic to self-generated utterances and that vocalizations are monitored through both sensory and motor feedback mechanisms. Depending on the child's level of self-awareness and overall maturity, vocal behavior is shaped, to a lesser or greater extent, by cognitive mediation. Matching one's voice to those of others in the immediate environment occurs as part of learning oral communication. Typically, it occurs easily and naturally, so that each child learning language acquires the prosody as well as syntax and semantics of the native linguistic culture. Thus, a child growing up in Mississippi learns a somewhat different set of vocal patterns than does a child in Minnesota. If a child moves to a different American-English linguistic environment during the elementary school years, he or she will adjust vocal patterns relatively easily. A move at an older age may require more conscious effort for linguistic alteration to occur. Conscious awareness plus conscious relearning will be required.

When children have structural, sensory, or motor deficits related to the learning of vocal patterns, more conscious awareness is needed to aid the matching of their own voice patterns to those in their linquistic environment. What other children learn easily may be more of a struggle because of the greater cognitive load imposed for appropriate learning to occur. As has been seen in studies of children with hearing impairment learning oral communication skills, the child's IQ plays a dramatic role in the level of skill that is attained under such circumstances.

When we consider infants and toddlers with impairments that make it difficult for them to learn vocal patterns, we must always be aware of the need for cognitive as well as vocal stimulation. It is also essential that the need to address and compensate for the lack of spontaneous voice and speech rehearsal activities be recognized early. Young children who are medically fragile are limited in their opportunities for peer interactions, spontaneous play, and environmental stimulation and learning. As they grow older, they may need to be specifically taught to focus on and attend to certain distinctive features of oral communication that other children spontaneously acquire without help. Additionally, the parents and caregivers of children with problems need access to information about their child's condition and needs and to be provided with strategies for stimulating vocal communication.

Receptive as well as expressive vocal skills need to be addressed, both with the child and the caregivers. A lot of the learning necessary for talking goes on in the brain itself. Children can be learning to talk (i.e., learning about language, including the vocal suprasegmentals such as pitch, loudness, duration, rate, inflection, nonverbal cues, etc.) without actually saying anything. Silence on the child's part does not imply that no learning is taking place. Modeling and environmental stimulation are essential for receptive learning.

As infants and toddlers grow into preschoolers and school-age children, their "mindfulness" about voice needs to be nourished and expanded to enable them to develop the cognitive and perceptual framework to support increased receptive and expressive voice learning. Clinicians need to ensure that children know the concepts, terminology, and meanings associated with learning about voice, for example.

Cognitive Processes Associated With Voice Learning

- Receptive voice skills (e.g., "You sound like a big boy.")
- Key concepts and terminology (e.g., "Big bears sound loud.")
- Knowledge base and information
- Factors influencing voice (e.g., "Remember to open your mouth.")
- Appropriate self-talk (e.g., "I did it myself.")
- Adjustments to differences in listeners and settings

Psychodynamics: Feelings Affecting Voice

Voice use rarely occurs in a vacuum. For voicing to be truly functional, it is used to effect some change in the person uttering the sound or in those hearing it. Sometimes, however, vocalization is used for catharsis. This occurs primarily when a child loses control and sobs or screams to allow for emotional discharge. However, such outbursts can also have the intent of manipulating listeners. Vocalizations can also be the result of happy feelings or can be methods of self-gratification and stimulation. They may be reflexive or emitted as signals of pain, hunger, fear, or other emotional or biologic states.

Voice forms a connection with one's self and with others. We can protect a fragile self-concept by withholding voice just as we can lash out in anger or fear with our voices. Sometimes we try to shore up our insecurities about ourselves or our environment by making our voices sound loud and bombastic. Sometimes we try to be like others whom we admire or fear by trying to sound like them. At other times, we reject their influence over us by trying to sound completely different or by refusing to interact with them at all. Our voices can be used as tools, weapons, currency, and inducements in different relationships and contexts.

It is safe to say that voice use is a kind of barometer by which others can read how we feel about ourselves and other people in our world. Depending on our skill as a voice user, we reveal varying amounts about our self-concept and our relationships at different times in different situations. Although adults can often protect some or all of their feelings from being known to others some or even most of the time, children are much more transparent. The younger and the more immature a child is, the more easily adults can read his or her emotions through the paralinguistic cues in voice and body language.

Voice clinicians need to observe the way infants, toddlers, and older children use their voices to control their environment, meet their needs, and establish trusting and appropriate peer and adult relationships.

Psychodynamic Aspects of Voice Behavior

- Self-concept and emotional adjustment
- Relationships with significant others
- Penalties and rewards of current voice use
- Insight regarding cause and effect
- Compliance with and resistance to change
- Reading voices of others
- Providing feedback to others
- Seeking feedback from others (questions, pauses, etc.)
- Sharing talking time and listening time
- Adjusting or changing vocalizations to satisfy needs

Summary

From birth, human beings use their voices to understand their reality and connect with the physical and emotional realities of those around them. Failure to develop appropriate voice use carries a heavy penalty in terms of learning the skills needed to establish a personal identity and to develop appropriate coping mechanisms and developmental benchmarks of cognitive and emotional maturity commensurate with chronological age. During assessment and treatment of voice disorders in children, clinicians need to be alert to the fact that although the actual vocal behavior, or lack of it, may be the most observable aspect of the problem, it must not be seen as the totality of the problem. Disturbed or absent voicing and other observable voice-related behaviors are important signs and symptoms, but the precipitating, causative, and maintaining aspects of the disorder are not readily observable. To diagnose and treat the true nature of the problem, clinicians must work as a team with other allied health professionals and with concerned caregivers. It is essential that the anatomic and physiologic support for voicing be examined and that the integrity of the aerodigestive and neurologic and sensory systems be considered. Additionally, the cognitive and psychodynamic dimensions of the voice problem must never be overlooked during assessment and treatment.

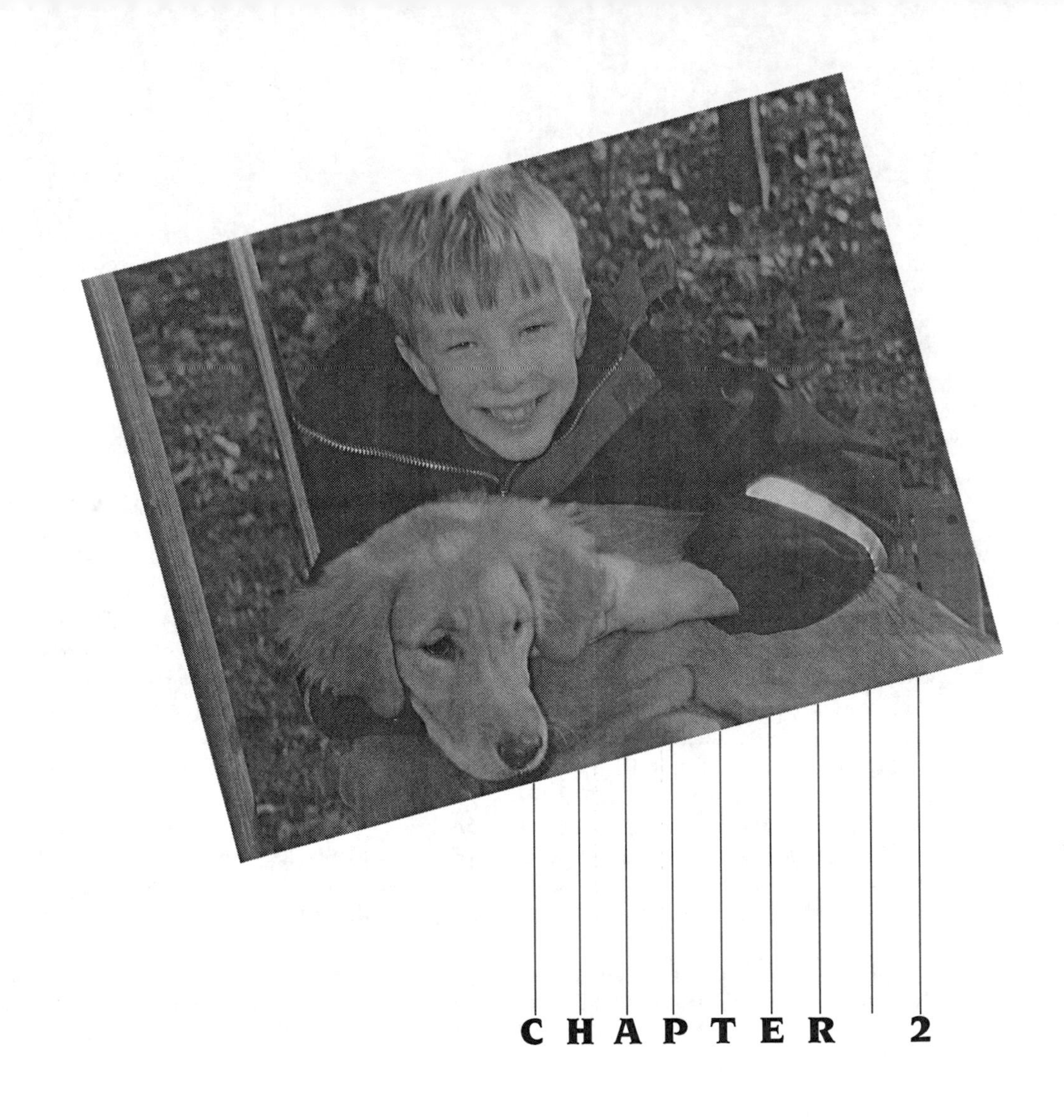

CHAPTER 2

A Clinical Perspective: Infants, Toddlers, and Preschoolers

Before beginning our discussion of the overall development of infants and young children, it may be helpful to review some relevant information about the development of the larynx itself. The infant larynx is different from the adult larynx, and these differences are significant with respect to history taking and intervention planning.

The Larynx

The larynx of the newborn is higher in the neck than it will be at any subsequent time in life. The tip of the epiglottis is at the level of the upper portion of the body of the second cervical vertebra, and the tip of the epiglottis can be in direct contact with the velum. The infant epiglottis is softer than that of the older child and has an omega or U shape. The contact between the epiglottis and the velum (soft palate) and the high position of the infant larynx allows for uninterrupted nasal breathing during nursing and helps avoid aspiration.

Unlike the adult airway, where the glottis is the narrowest portion of the tube, the infant airway is narrowest at the level of the cricoid cartilage, which is the tracheal ring (shaped like a signet ring), which is the base of the larynx. Even slight mucosal swelling can significantly reduce the small lumen (opening) of the infant trachea. Subglottal stenosis (narrowing) of the airway is more common in infants than in older children because of the narrowed lumen at the level of the cricoid. Blahova and Brezovsky (1981) estimated that 1 mg of mucosal swelling in the larynx or trachea of a 12-month-old infant reduces the cross-sectional area of the airway by 50%. Reactive or inflammatory lesions and neoplasms as well as congenital abnormalities may contribute to subglottic stenosis.

The embryonic laryngotracheal tube can be first identified during the 4th week of gestation. The tracheal bronchial tree derives from the fifth and sixth branchial (visceral) arches and arises from the tracheal bronchial groove. A primary lung bud bifurcates into two main bronchi. The tracheobronchial groove is located in the ventromedial aspect of the foregut, caudal to the pharyngeal pouches. Furrows along the lateral aspect of the tracheobronchial groove gradually deepen and eventually unite. This forms the tracheoesophageal septum or wall between the laryngotracheal tube and the esophagus. It is completed by the 5th week of gestation. In the 5th or 6th week of gestation, three tissue masses can be seen around the primordial glottic slit at the bases of the third and fourth branchial arches. The most anterior swelling is the embryonic epiglottis. The two swellings at the bases of the fourth arches are the genesis of the arytenoid cartilages. Until the 8th week, there is a T-shaped opening that is temporarily obscured by the fusion of the swellings. During the 8th week, the thyroid cartilage begins to develop from the fourth branchial arch and the cricoid and arytenoid cartilages are derived from the fifth and sixth arches (this arch disappears during the fetal development). During development of the thyroid, the first sign of the vocal folds appears, drawn out between the arytenoid cartilages and the inner surface of the developing thyroid laminae. Simultaneously, a vestibular sinus that will become the ventricle appears. The hyoid bone is derived mainly from the second branchial arch, which gives rise to the styloid process, stylohyoid ligament, most of the anterior portion of the body of the hyoid, and the lesser cornua of the hyoid bone. The greater cornua and the rest of the body arise from the third arch and the two structures fuse at the midline. About the 10th or 11th week in the life of the embryo, all of the major landmarks of the larynx can be identified. The paired branchial arches have contributed the entoderm for the epithelial lining of the larynx and mesoderm has provided connective tissue, skeletal bones, voluntary muscles, blood and lymph systems, and cartilages for the larynx.

At birth, the infant not only has a smaller sized or miniature version of an adult larynx, but also has a somewhat different mechanism with respect to structure. The first major difference is its relative position in the neck. The laryngotracheal mechanism will descend from its newborn position where the tip of the epiglottis is at the level of the upper portion of the body of the second cervical vertebra. At puberty, there is a marked descent of the larynx relative to the base of the tongue and in some adults it can be as low as the sixth cervical vertebra.

The infant airway is much more vulnerable to obstruction than is the older child's because of the overall differences in size and width and also because the cricoid cartilage is funnel-shaped, making the opening in the airway narrower from side to side in the subglottal portion of the respiratory tract. Additionally, more than 50% of the infant's glottic structure is cartilaginous, whereas almost two thirds is made up of muscle and soft tissue in adults, who have a relative increase in the proportion of the membranous versus cartilaginous parts of the vocal folds. This, along with the lack of stiffness in the cartilaginous support of the infant larynx, may contribute to the condition of laryngomalacia in some infants (Tucker, 1993).

The structure of the vocal folds in infants is also markedly different from that of adults. The lamina propria is very thick, more uniform in structure, and without a vocal ligament, so it is loose and pliable. A vocal ligament begins to appear between the ages of 1 to 4 years, and differentiation of the two layers of elastic and collagenous fibers occurs between 6 and 12 years as the ligament thickens. After puberty, the differentiated three-layer structure of the lamina propria is observed (Colton & Casper, 1996).

Communicative Development

Eye contact is one of the aspects of an infant's behavior that is significant and one that provides us with information about whether the child is beginning to focus on and connect with his caregivers. During the first 3 months of life, infants typically maintain brief periods of eye contact during certain pleasurable activities, such as when the adult is talking to them; preparing to pick them up; and during feeding, cuddling, or rocking activities. When the adult interacts with the infant in a playful way, it is also interesting for the clinician to note whether the child shows varied physical responses when he or she hears different types of vocalization or vocalizations produced with different emotional tones. Physical responses on the part of the child include both small and large motor movements. For example, a child may smile, stop previous movements entirely, widen the eyes, frown, kick, or stop crying. It is also interesting to observe the way children respond to a caregiver's voice when they cannot see her or him. Do they stop crying when they hear the familiar voice, turn their eyes to look for the caregiver, or smile before or after the caregiver comes into view?

Between the ages of 3 and 6 months, we expect smiling in response to voice recognition without visual cues and in interactions where face-to-face contact does not occur. We also look to see if children smile at other familiar people in addition to the primary caregivers. A favorite toy may also elicit smiles, and children smile when they play with toys in solitary situations at this stage. Different adults also may elicit different reactions from a child. Does a child expect and need comfort from the parents and social contact from the grandparents, for example? Does the child lean toward the adult with the toy or the playful sound in his or her voice and stop crying at the sound of a comforting voice? In other words, at this stage, the voice clinician looks for signs of a differentiation in responses to different people, feeling states, and situations.

By 6 to 9 months of age, the child's attitude to familiar and unfamiliar people in the environment has crystallized. One notices more reserve with strangers and a more enthusiastic attitude with familiar people. Gestures and phrases such as "come here" will elicit attempts to lean, roll, or crawl in response to familiar people and stimuli. At this stage, there may be some anxiety in separation from primary caregivers and the signaling of a desire to be involved with familiar people engaged in interesting activities, as if the child wants to be part of the action. The child also may react by crying if a sibling is upset and seems sensitive to the feelings expressed by others in the environment. Facial expressions, laughter, and gestures seem to register with the child as awareness of paralinguistic cues develops. Crying, fussing, withdrawing, and reaching for the primary caregiver often are seen when a stranger attempts to interact with the child, although the child may tolerate a brief time of separation with respect to physical contact with the mother or father. Somewhere between 9 and 12 months, the child begins trying to get and hold the attention of others by vocalizing, moving, or using a specific behavior to elicit a response from others. The clinician should note the ways the child attempts to get attention or uses repetition of certain behaviors to hold attention.

By the time a child is a year old, he or she has begun to demonstrate the social foundations of communicative interactions. He or she uses both gesture and vocalizations to reach out to others, to get and hold their attention, to recapture their attention, and to gain assistance. The child also uses closeness and contact with familiar people to deal with anxieties when facing new people and situations. The child also is gaining confidence in the ability to entertain himself or herself when a caregiver moves out of the immediate line of vision. Imitation of others and vocal reactions as responses to the overtures or greetings of others occur.

One also sees the child's ability to signal that he or she is ready for a change in toys or activities in the 2nd year of life. Stimulus-response rituals, turn-taking routines, more frequent meaningful vocalizations, and the ascendancy of one- and two-word phrases over the gestures that predominated earlier are observed.

The child now seems aware of the fact that he or she has some influence over the behavior of others, pointing to objects on request, giving objects on request, using words and loudness increases to indicate displeasure, and using "no" frequently to protest. The cadence and prosody of adult speech are produced indicating that the child is aware receptively, of the ebb and flow and turn taking in speech patterns of others. The child's "conversations" may be jargon to adult ears, but he or she captures the shapes and rhythms of conversational exchanges, and a number of recognizable words are heard. The child uses words intentionally, plays peekaboo and pattycake, feeds and grooms others during play, hugs his toy friends, leads others to do his or her bidding, uses music makers, communicates the need to have pants changed, dances to music, and likes to push wheel toys. He or she also likes to pretend to do things others do, such as talk on the telephone, and pretend to read and write, or move toy vehicles. When prompted, the child can engage in simple self-care activities, such as combing hair, washing the face, and indicating readiness for a snack. These behaviors show awareness and ability to demonstrate the functional use of objects and items of clothing. The child now plays with a toy in different ways, plays ball, places one object inside another, imitates activities around the house, groups similar objects together, and engages in pretend play. He or she accompanies activities with spontaneous vocalizations.

Between 27 and 30 months, children demonstrate a wide variety of play activities and are selective in their choice of toys and use them appropriately most of the time. At this age, a child plays in a parallel manner alongside other children, talks more while playing, learns to share when prompted, and engages in longer and more elaborate play sequences and rituals. He or she also uses objects creatively to represent other things. By the 3rd year, a child is answering "yes" and "no" questions correctly, follows a three-step command, and identifies parts of an object. He or she is interested in how things work; knows size concepts, colors, and other attributes of objects; and responds to "wh" questions.

By age 3, a child can state his or her first and last name, gender, and recent happenings. A 3-year-old can express physical and emotional states, imitate the voices of characters in stories, do action rhymes, repeat a melody or rhythmic pattern, and delights in interactions and conversations.

Planning Intervention for Infants, Toddlers, and Preschoolers

When considering the form and structure of intervention to stimulate and solidify appropriate vocal patterns in young children, the clinician formulates a treatment plan in consultation with other team members. The approach that is chosen is influenced by the developmental stage and chronological age of the child, by the type of disorder, and by the setting in which the child will be treated.

Infants, toddlers, and preschoolers, especially children who are medically fragile, usually first come to the attention of the speech-language pathologist via a referral from medical personnel. In institutional or home health care settings, the clinician works primarily with the parents and caregivers to educate them about the child's needs and ways that communication can be stimulated and shaped. Although total communication stimulation is the goal, it is important that specific voice-related objectives are included. Some direct behavioral goals will usually be considered, as will indirect intervention that involves goals to change and enhance the support network and the physical and psychosocial environment of the child. The following checklists review the preliminary data-gathering process that takes place before establishing the goals for an intervention program. They provide an overview of areas that may need to be addressed in treatment to build a foundation for developmentally appropriate voicing behaviors.

Anatomy and Physiology

- Referrals and requests for medical reports
- Hearing testing
- Prostheses (e.g., Passy-Muir valve)
- Review of medications and effects
- Consults about medical status and constraints
- Aerodigestive tract data
  - ➢ Swallowing evaluation
  - ➢ Vocal fold visualization
    - → Structure and configurations
    - → Color
    - → Secretions
    - → Innervation
    - → Reactivity
  - ➢ Congenital abnormalities
  - ➢ Infectious conditions
  - ➢ Signs of gastroesophageal reflux disease (GERD)
  - ➢ Lesions
  - ➢ Tone (epiglottis, trachea)

Voice and Voice-Related Behaviors

- Voicing occurring on reflexive behaviors
  - Coughing
  - Sighing
  - Laughing
- Voicing during babbling, cooing, and so forth
- Voicing on intentional communication
- Voicing when stimulated
  - Length of utterance
  - Quality of utterance
  - Cues used to elicit voicing
  - Prolongations, repetitions, and so forth
  - Functional oral mechanism
- Breath support for voicing
  - Length of exhalation phase
  - Replenishing breaths
  - Inhalation pattern (e.g., labored, appropriate)
- Resonance-related behaviors
  - Presence/absence of nasal congestion
  - Produces nasal sounds
  - No direct nasality on oral sounds
  - Imitates humming; vowel prolongations
- Hearing assessment

Cognition

- Parents
  - Parents understand nature of problem
  - Parents provided with written information
  - Parents responsive to suggestions
  - Caregivers responsive to suggestions
- Child
  - Cognitive function relative to development
  - Child's general communication development
  - Receptive language
  - Expressive language
  - Nonverbal behaviors
  - Mean length of utterances (MLU)
  - Phonological development
  - Speech motor skills
- Functional behaviors
  - Ability to follow directions
  - Attention span
  - Ability to listen to a story
  - Takes turns
  - Matches or identifies numbers, shapes, colors
  - Sorts, classifying by color, shape, and size
  - Letter and sound correspondence
  - Imitates patterns (visual; auditory)
  - Names or writes letters of the alphabet
  - Identifies rhyming words
  - Sequences vocal patterns

Psychodynamics

- Parents
  - Patterns of vocal interaction in family
  - Attentiveness to child
  - Level of stimulation provided
- Child
  - Pragmatic levels relative to maturity
  - Prosody relative to emotional state
- Functional behaviors
  - Persistence or misbehavior relative to difficulties
  - Attention to nonverbal behavior of others
  - Understanding of consequences
  - Ability to play alone and with others
  - Attention to the vocal communication of others
  - Strategies to get and hold attention
  - Overtures to other children and group-entry behaviors
  - Use of questions and requests
  - Understanding and following of directions
  - Voice reflects awareness of situation and listener
  - Responsiveness to reinforcement and praise

- ➢ Comfort level in separating from parents
- ➢ Expresses sense of self-worth

After reviewing the child's profile of current assets and liabilities as well as the child's interests and needs, the speech-language pathologist is in a better position to establish treatment priorities and goals. An approach to treatment that suits the child and his or her situation also can be identified. Factors that contribute to the decision-making process include the following:

- Severity of symptoms and signs of the disorder
- Availability of support in the environment
- Need for other professional services
- Strengths the child possesses that can be built upon
- The most pressing needs that must be addressed

The speech–language pathologist then decides whether an indirect, direct, or combined approach to treatment is warranted. If, for example, parents, caregivers, and other professionals are in an optimal position to provide the necessary care and assistance to change the environment and stimulate change in the child, an indirect approach is appropriate and justified. This is frequently the case with infants and toddlers and children who have not reached the point developmentally where they can be active participants in their own rehabilitation. A more systematic approach to structured, direct, one-on-one modification with a clinician will be necessary for children with the potential to benefit from it. In such cases, the indirect approach may also be used in combination with the direct intervention so that maximum benefits occur from additional parent and caregiver support of the treatment plan.

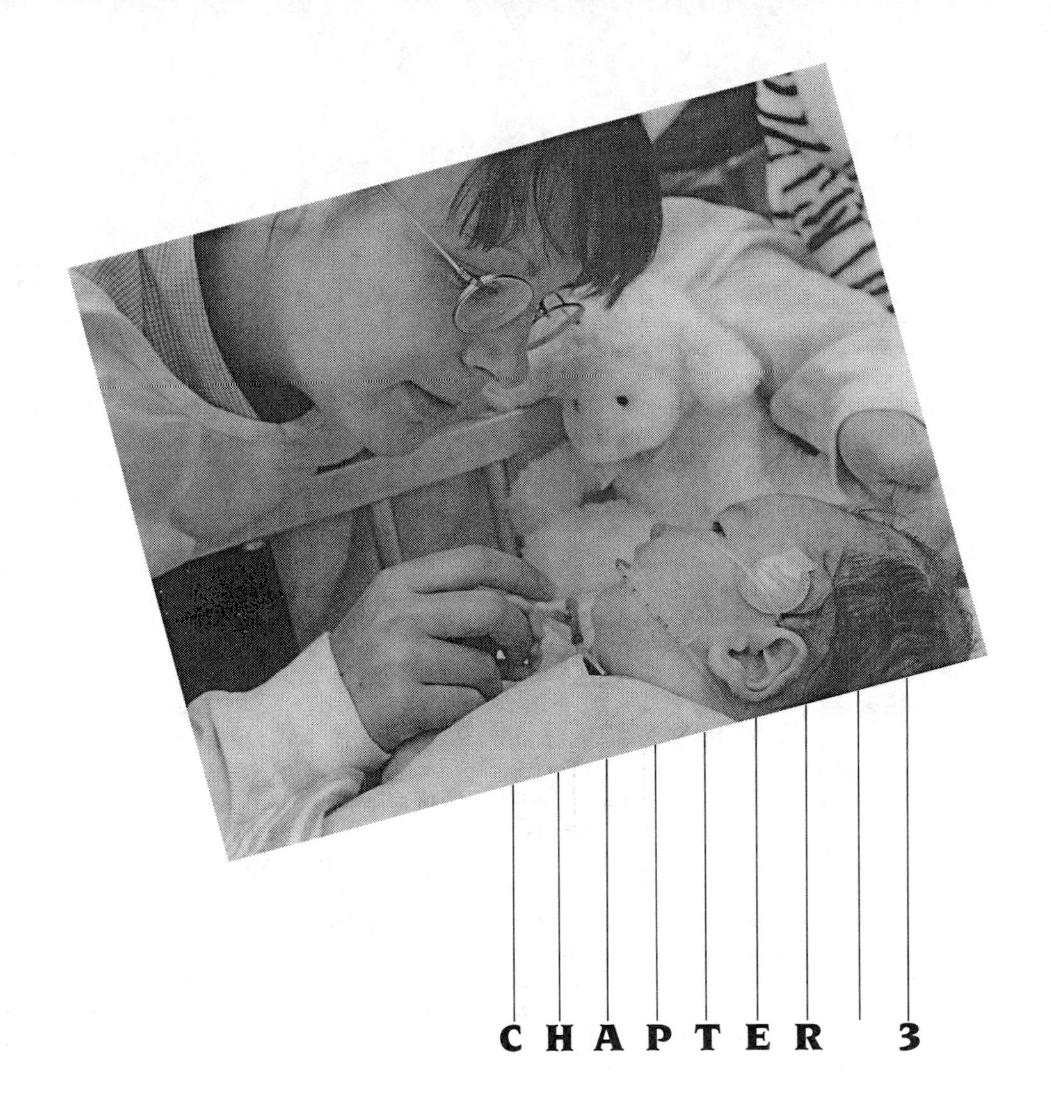

CHAPTER 3

Medically Compromised Infants: A Clinical Perspective

Risa L. Nasatir

In the last chapter we discussed some of the benchmarks of normal communication development in young children. Speech–language pathologists play an important role in assessing and treating children who are at risk for arrested, delayed, or atypical voice production. The range of skills clinicians need to master is influenced by the setting they work in, as well as by the medical, physiologic, and social factors that influence the potential for vocal development in their patients. Medically compromised infants, who are treated in intensive care units in medical facilities, pose unique challenges for the clinician. In addition to information about the medical status of the infants in such settings, clinicians also need to know their role as members of a medically oriented team. Most newborn patients in this type of setting have immature or disordered aerodigestive systems. An understanding of the aerodigestive system, how it develops, and how it can be compromised is therefore important as a basis for understanding the clinician's role.

This chapter provides: (1) a brief overview of the aerodigestive system; (2) a description of voice and voice-related behaviors of the medically fragile child; (3) a discussion of information the clinician needs to know; and (4) a discussion of feelings and psychodynamics associated with voice that are relevant to this population. A list of medical terms and their meanings is provided for reference at the end of the chapter.

Overview of the Aerodigestive System and Its Disorders

A great deal of literature is available regarding introduction of oral feedings and assessment and intervention of oral motor and feeding difficulties. This chapter is not intended to be a complete reference for assessment and treatment of swallowing and voice disorders. Other sources provide assessment formats, treatment strategies, and so on; these are listed in the Recommended Readings at the end of the chapter. All clinicians, however, must have a strong knowledge base in oral motor and feeding difficulties as well as competency in conducting videofluorographic swallow studies, which can be a useful tool in further assessment of swallowing function. The focus of this chapter, however, is to provide information useful when a speech–language pathologist works with medically fragile children. It is by no means all-inclusive but rather a summary of common issues faced in the neonatal and pediatric intensive care units in a medical setting.

The same systems that are used for voice, speech, and language (i.e., respiratory, laryngeal, neurologic) are also necessary for swallowing. As discussed in Chapter 1, the digestive tract must always be considered in tandem with the respiratory tract. Speech–language pathologists' scope of practice includes how speech, language, voice, and swallowing affect the "whole" child and are affected by physical development. We, of course, never begin our assessment and intervention until a child is medically stable.

Children born with precarious medical conditions need special care. In today's largest health institutions, miracles occur every day. Lives are saved due to the excellent care of health professionals, because of research, advanced medical technology, and the support of the patient's families and caregivers. The speech–language pathologist may be consulted immediately after the birth of a child or later when it becomes apparent that voicing and/or swallowing may be at risk. Sometimes parents will ask why a speech clinician is needed when a child cannot even talk yet. We explain that communication is not only words and thoughts, but it also entails crying, eye contact, and facial expressions. These early forms of communication are often delayed or nonexistent in children with complex medical issues. It is our role as speech–language pathologists to assist with precursors of oral communication to improve quality of life.

Embryology of the Aerodigestive System

There are many distinct differences between the anatomy and physiology of the aerodigestive tract of an infant, child, and adult. Differences also exist between a full-term infant (37–40 weeks gestation) and a premature infant. An understanding of the structure and function of the aerodigestive tract is necessary before discussing the relevance of these structures to infant and toddler communication. Let's first review the embryological development of the aerodigestive tract, specifically the vocal tract.

The rudimentary formation of the lung occurs at 4 weeks gestation. The larynx develops at approximately 6 weeks gestation. The epiglottis forms 2 weeks later along with facial features. Harrison (1983) described the fetus as being able to open its mouth and lips and swallow at 13 to 16 weeks gestation. By 16 to 20 weeks gestation, inhalation and exhalation of amniotic fluid takes place as well as the establishment of a sleep–wake cycle and hearing. Between 24 and 28 weeks gestation, the fetus becomes viable. All structures of the lung are complete, but maturation is needed. The fetus is not yet able to produce surfactant, the fatty substance that lines the alveoli of the lungs. It is this substance that prevents the walls of the alveoli from collapsing.

Harrison noted that before the 28th week gestation, the baby is able on occasion to cry out or smile (during sleep). These actions are regarded as the first signs of communication. Non-nutritive sucking (sucking that is not for the purpose of nourishment, i.e., pacifier) occurs at 27 to 28 weeks gestation, but it is sporadic and uncoordinated. It is the first use of oral motor movements. Nutritive sucking (sucking that is used as a means to obtain nourishment) has been reported as early as 29 to 30 weeks gestation but usually occurs between 32 and 33 weeks gestation. Nutritive sucking is immature at this time due to the baby's difficulty coordinating respirations. By 34 weeks gestation, a coordinated nutritive suck is acquired and oral feedings are possible. In the case of the premature infant, the speech–language pathologist is usually consulted anytime after 34 weeks either to fully assess whether introduction of oral feedings is appropriate or to assist with difficulties that have already been encountered with previously started oral feedings. In some medical facilities, oral feedings may be introduced to premature infants as early as 31 weeks for breast feeding and 32 weeks for bottle feeding. Education must be provided to infants' families regarding developmental levels of feeding acquisition. An infant at 32 weeks gestation would not be expected to be a "nutritive" feeder, or full oral feeder, for example, at this stage of development.

Differences Between Preterm and Full-Term Infants

Besides the obvious weight differences between full-term infants and premature infants, there are other differences that are important for clinicians working with this population to consider. We need to remember that term infants have 9 months to mature. The small space that they have occupied in utero forces the hands to move toward the mouth. Therefore, there is time to practice sucking and sucking pads develop. This is not the case with premature infants.

A premature baby at 40 weeks gestation is quite different from a full-term baby. Because a premature baby weighs less, overall development is delayed. According to Morris and Klein (1987), premature babies are also not visually responsive. They may have inconsistent reactions to sight and sounds. Also, the sleep–awake state is disorganized and the preterm infant may not remain

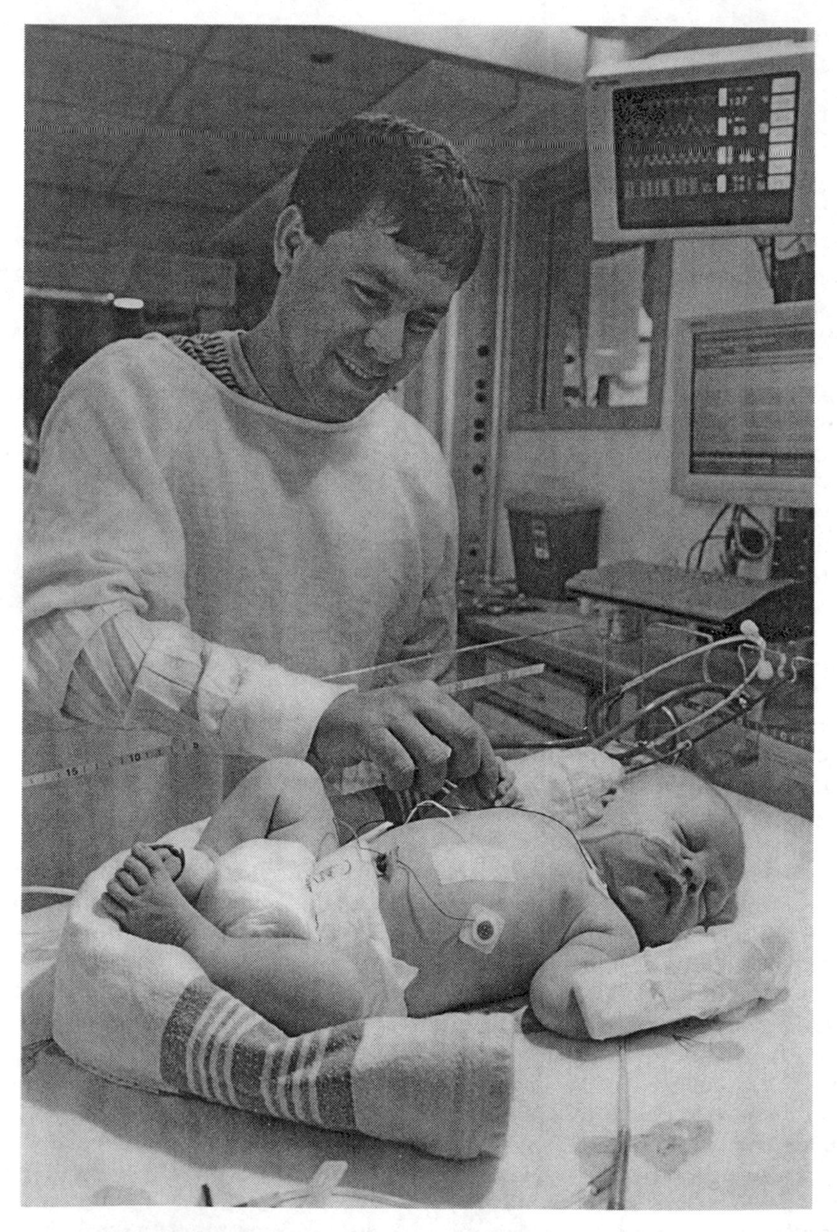

A typical bedside setting in the NICU. (Copyright Todd Hochberg, Advocate Media Center)

alert. They also often have difficulty adjusting to stress. Additional associated medical problems may require long hospitalizations. Premature infants often also become selective at hearing buzzers and noises from the neonatal intensive care environment. In addition, the premature infant often lacks typical daily experiences that their full-term counterparts experience. Any of these factors may predispose the premature infant to be at risk for long-lasting developmental problems.

Morris and Klein explained that preterm infants assume a posture of extension (a position in which the arms are pulled outward from the trunk) because they have had more space in utero and retain that position after birth. The posture may also be related to endotracheal tubes forcing infants to lie flat. Preterm infants are also neurologically immature. When mechanical ventilation is used to support respirations in preterm infants, it is also difficult for caregivers to hold the infant. Therefore, because of the neurologic immaturity, such infants have a much more difficult time calming and organizing.

The sleep state of the infant is also different with prematurity. When this is seen in association with the factors mentioned above, stress for parents and caregivers can occur. The caregiver may not know when the child is hungry or tired, for example, as the infant is unable to communicate needs by giving clear signals. Methods of coping with this stress will be discussed later. Learning about the nonverbal signals of communication given by these infants is an important task for the speech–language pathologist.

The overall appearance and the muscle tone of a preterm infant also differs from full-term infants. Preterm infants are 'floppy." For instance, the heel of the preterm infant can touch the ear. Reflexes are weaker. The grasp reflex is present but not strong enough to allow the infant to be lifted by the grasp. The skin of a preterm infant is translucent. Therefore, all ethnic groups have the same skin color at birth. Skin color develops when the baby is closer to 33–36 weeks gestation. The outer ears are soft. The hair is fine and often there is hair all over the body. Bones of the skull are soft and malleable.

Differences Among the Adult, Pediatric, and Infant Structures and Functions

Changes in structure begin between 3 to 6 months after birth and continue into adulthood. Morris and Klein (1987) list the following changes: (1) The jaw grows downward and forward creating less stiffness; (2) sucking pads diminish; (3) the oral cavity elongates creating more space for movement for the tongue. The tongue begins to cup to prepare to move food throughout the mouth. With more room, more exploratory play is possible: (4) oral sounds are heard; (5) oral breathing is established; (6) a greater separation occurs between the larynx and epiglottis since food must pass over the epiglottis; and (7) sucking, swallowing, and breathing become better coordinated. The structure and function of the adult mouth and pharynx is considerably different from that of an infant.

Differences in Anatomy

According to Morris and Klein (1987), several differences in infant, pediatric, and adult structures are relevant to communication. In infants, the jaw is smaller and retracted. The overall size of the oral cavity is smaller, causing the tongue to appear larger. The tongue, soft palate, cheeks, and epiglottis all touch. Infants lack teeth; however, they have sucking pads, which help maintain cheek stability. The larynx is higher and in closer proximity to the tongue. The eustachian tube is in a horizontal position from the middle ear to the nasopharynx. This horizontal position leads to increased susceptibility to ear infections.

Differences in Physiology

As a result of direct contact with the soft palate, tongue movements are backward and forward versus up and down. Infants are obligate nose breathers. That is, they do not have adequate room to breathe out of the mouth when the tongue, palate, and epiglottis are touching. All sounds are produced through the nasal cavity. In contrast to adults, during the swallow, the infant epiglottis does not move downward.

Physiologic Parameters and Medical Issues

Orientation to Physiologic Parameters: What the Speech–Language Pathologist Should Know

At birth the medical status of an infant, especially a preterm infant, must be assessed quickly so that treatment can be initiated if it is needed. One method of evaluating a newborn's response to the outside world is called the Apgar score. Observations of the newborn's heart rate, respiratory rate, color, tone, and reflexes are ranked on a scale of 0–2 for each category. Scores are recorded at 1 minute and at 5 minutes after birth. Thus, a perfect score would be 10. According to Harrison (1983), a score of 6 or below equates to moderate to severe distress. Although the Apgar scores do not predict children's developmental abilities, they are used to provide initial summaries of a baby's overall condition immediately following birth.

When a speech–language pathologist is assessing or treating medically fragile children, physiologic parameters must always be considered. The most frequently considered physiologic parameters include respiration, heart rate, and oxygen saturation levels. Most of the literature suggests the same physiologic parameters/norms with some slight variation on respiratory rate and heart rate depending on baseline measures (Table 3–1). Clinicians agree that a significant change in values is of greater concern than the actual numbers on a monitor, but familiarization with typical measures is helpful.

Respiration and heart rates are usually read on a cardiorespiratory monitor. This type of monitor gives a visual and numerical display. It will usually alarm when parameters drop or increase out of normal ranges. The child is connected to the monitor by cables or wires that attach to the chest, and the possibility always exists that connections may malfunction. A speech–language pathologist working in a medical setting must be familiar with all types of equipment that are used. For example, intravenous (IV) poles, oxygen tanks, tubing, and pulse oximeters (see below) are common in all hospital settings.

Oxygen saturation levels of capillary blood flow (i.e., how much oxygen is in the blood) are determined by pulse oximetry. Wolf and Glass (1992) described measuring oxygen saturation levels by placing a light sensor probe that can be taped around a finger, toe, hand, or foot to measure the percentage of oxygen in the blood. It can be used to measure changes in saturations during feeding, handling, and play. It can alert caregivers to signs of hypoxia. Reduced oxygen can result in cyanosis (color changes). Thus the readings on the equipment dials as well as careful observation of the infant provide vital information for the clinician.

Clinical observation is just as important for the speech–language pathologist as learning how to read the monitors. For example, an infant may demonstrate a SaO_2 level of 95% but be gasping for air. Although the monitor reading is appropriate, the infant may be in distress. Likewise, an infant may have a saturation level of 60% but have adequate coloring and be breathing easily. This may indicate an error such as a pulse oximeter that is not placed correctly or loose wiring. Conservative practice is always recommended when infants are fragile and physiologic states can change within a matter of seconds.

Table 3–1. Normal vital signs for preterm and full-term infants, children, and adults.

	Preterm Infants	Full-term Infants	Children	Adults
SaO_2	>90%	95%	>91%	>91%
RR	40–70	30–60	20–26	14–20
HR	160–180	120–140	70–150	60–80[1,2]

[1]Arvedson, J.C., & Lefton-Greif, M.A. (1998). *Pediatric videofluoroscopic swallow studies: A professional manual with caregiver guidelines.* San Antonio, TX: Communication Skill Builders, pp. 67–68.

[2]Wolf, L., & Glass, R. (1992). *Feeding and swallowing disorders in infancy.* Tucson, AZ: Therapy Skill Builders, pp. 140–144.

Respiration

Clinicians always need to be alert for changes in respiration. For example, abnormally high or low respiration rates need to be recognized. Tachypnea, or a high rate of respirations, can result in shortness of breath. Children who are tachypneic will have difficulty coordinating respirations with swallowing and aspiration may also occur. Tachypnea also results in reduced breath support for voicing. A high rate of respirations may indicate shallow breathing, which can also result in voicing and swallowing difficulties.

Apnea, or the absence of breathing for more than 15 seconds, may also occur in fragile infants. Wolf and Glass (1992) discussed three types of apnea: central, obstructive, and mixed. In *central apnea,* the diaphragm does not move because signals are not sent from the brainstem. In *obstructive apnea,* respirations are attempted, but air is not passed through the tract due to an obstruction. In *mixed apnea,* an infant may demonstrate both of the above difficulties. Sometimes, children recover spontaneously; at other times, bradycardia (lower than normal heart rate, i.e., 100 times/60 seconds, in infants) and desaturation (oxygen saturation level below 85%) can occur. Other conditions that are relevant to development of a preterm or otherwise fragile infant may also occur. These are reviewed in the following sections. Speech–language pathologists do not diagnose medical conditions, but they do need to be able to read medical charts and understand the effects of certain conditions on overall and communication development.

Heart Rates

Tachycardia refers to an increase in heart rate. *Bradycardia* describes lower than normal heart rates. Tachycardia and bradycardia can occur in isolation or in conjunction with apnea. Children who experience episodes of tachycardia or bradycardia need to be monitored closely. Infants and children who experience changes in heart rate during therapy sessions most likely are not appropriate for speech intervention and need medical clearance prior to further intervention by speech therapy.

Oxygen Desaturation

Oxygen desaturation refers to saturation levels that are lower than 85%. Reduced saturation levels refer to levels ranging from 85% to 91%. Some monitors are set with low levels at 85% (e.g., for children with cardiac difficulties). It is important to check with the nurses and physicians to understand the appropriate saturation levels for each child. Oxygen saturation can increase, for example, when coordinated sucking and swallowing occur. Oxygen saturations levels can also change as a result of

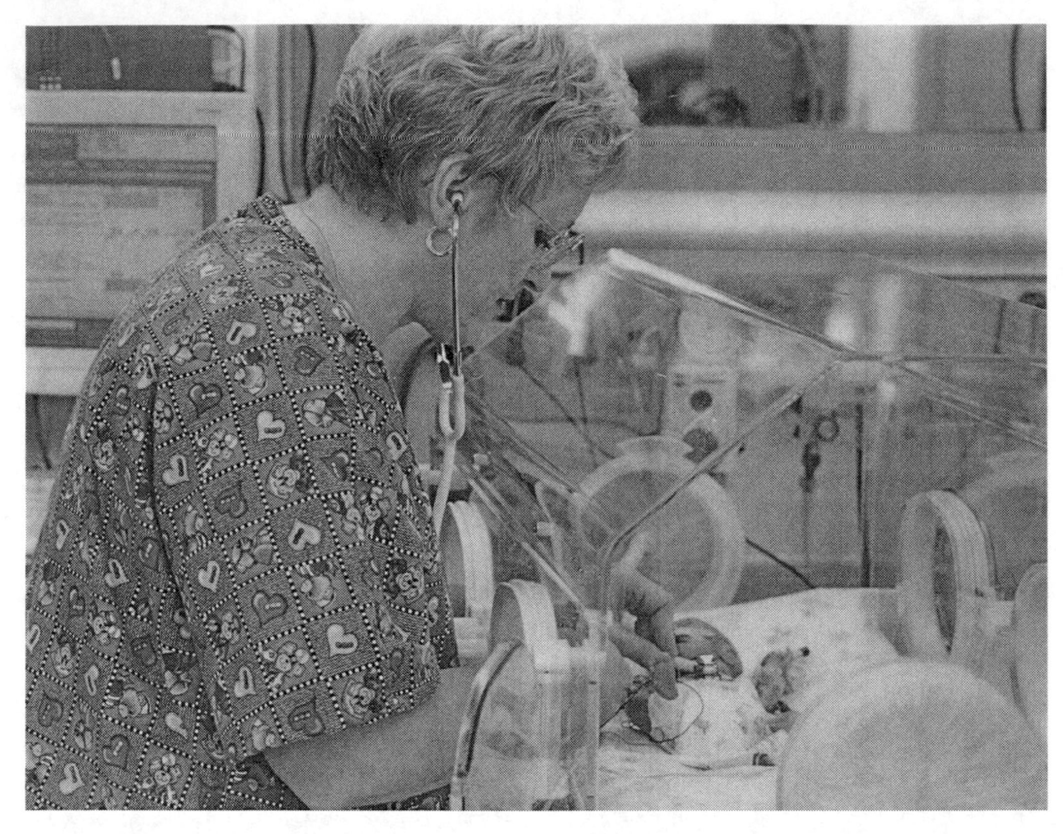

An RN taking vitals on a premature infant. (Copyright Todd Hochberg, Advocate Media Center)

bradycardia, apnea, aspiration, gastroesophageal reflux, or other changes in the child's medical status and may signal distress.

The Speech–Language Pathologist's Role in the Intensive Care Unit

Adequate training is essential for speech–language pathologists before they begin to work with patients in the intensive care unit (ICU). Most hospitals have implemented competency training and will not allow independent treatment of patients without clinicians demonstrating competency. Initially, speech–language pathologists working in ICUs must be certified in CPR. Most hospitals offer courses. Yearly recertification is necessary. A 10- to 12-week practicum in a neonatal and pediatric intensive care unit prior to assignment to such a unit is strongly encouraged. Speech–language pathologists must be familiar with neonatal disorders and have competency prior to providing any type of assessment or treatment. This is usually obtained during hospital practice, preservice orientation, or supervised initiation to the ICU. Besides adequate training clinicians also need the skills to locate information that they need once they are on the job. This is especially critical in the ICU when so much parent education is part of the speech–language pathologist's role. Not only must the speech–language pathologist be adept at locating resources for his or her use, the speech–language pathologist must also be able to locate them for parents. Many parents will try to locate information on the Internet as soon as they have their child's diagnosis and may need the clinician's help in sorting through the information for details that are relevant to their child's situation.

Familiarity and comfort in working with all types of equipment (e.g., monitors/lines) already has been noted as necessary for speech–language pathologists working in an ICU. The neonatal and pediatric ICUs use many different types of equipment with warning alarms, buzzers, and beeps. As a member of a hospital team, the clinician must know which alarms need immediate attention and be able to answer parents' questions about the alarms. Early familiarization with the monitors and ventilators can save unnecessary panic and confusion. One way to learn is to spend some time with the respiratory therapists and nurses on the unit. Extra time spent meeting the other members of the team builds confidence in the other professionals on the unit that the speech–language pathologist is fully trained and prepared to work as part of the team.

At some medical facilities, cross training of professionals is required. For example, respiratory therapists may be trained to feed infants. It is important for every clinician to know the role of each member of the team and how the team functions.

Another crucial step in achieving competency in the ICU is for the clinician to recognize when to get help. For example, if an infant is making an unusual noise when breathing or the color of the face appears different, it is imperative to obtain assistance immediately. In emergencies, it is important to remain calm and to state firmly that assistance is needed immediately. If the facility is equipped with an emergency button, learn where it is and how to use it. Other infants and families are close by and will be disturbed to see a child nearby go into distress. If no one responds, then call loudly for help. Do not leave the infant or child. You may be the only person available and you may need to begin CPR. It is much better to err on the side of caution and to call for help unnecessarily than to take the chance of a life-threatening event occurring. The preceding caution underscores the necessity for thorough preparation and familiarization with equipment, routines, and emergency procedures for all clinicians during orientation to work in medical facilities.

Populations Served

Speech–language pathologists in hospital settings will work with infants, toddlers, and children with congenital abnormalities and acquired abnormalities. In the medical setting speech-language pathologists will receive referrals that range across structural abnormality, pulmonary difficulty, neurologic deficit, gastrointestinal and cardiac disease, and so on. Acquired abnormalities that may affect the aerodigestive system include, but are not limited to, recurrent laryngeal nerve injury, traumatic intubation, shaken baby syndrome, brain injury, failure to thrive, aspiration of foreign bodies, and infection.

In all cases, swallowing, voice, speech, language, cognitive function, and hearing must always be considered. Mandatory hearing screenings are being conducted more frequently in the United States nurseries. If the facility does not mandate routine hearing screenings, the speech–language pathologist must make recommendations. Clinicians must take responsibility to ensure that all

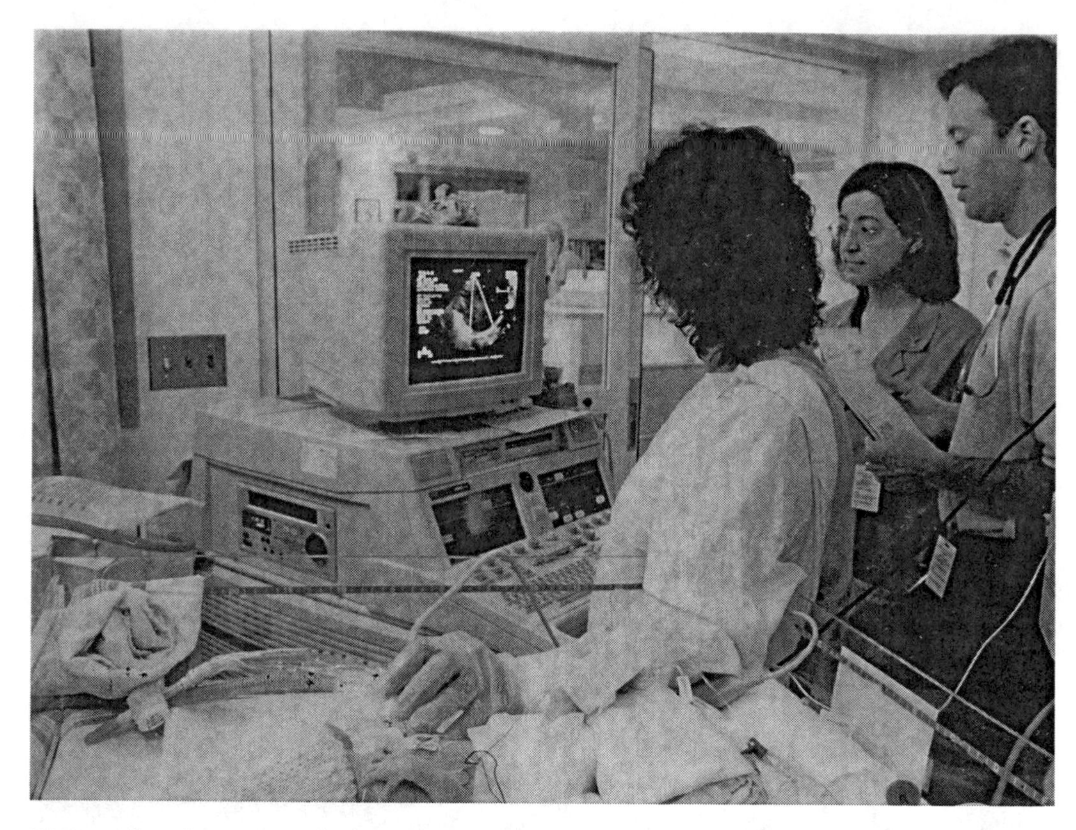

NICU staff performing an ultrasound on an infant. (Copyright Todd Hochberg, Advocate Media Center)

aspects of development pertinent to communication are considered.

Practicing clinicians need to recognize the disorders commonly seen in a medical setting. Clinicians must familiarize themselves with terms noted in medical charts and understand the role a speech–language pathologist plays when working with families and patients with complex conditions. The following is a brief overview of some of the conditions seen in ICUs.

Congenital Abnormalities

A variety of different, syndromes are encountered by a speech–language pathologist working with medically fragile children. Sometimes, genetic syndromes are not diagnosed until sometime after birth when additional medical or developmental problems arise or when a slowing or stopping of maturation occurs. Some infants, however, will present at birth with dysmorphic features. Characteristics of dysmorphic features may include low-set ears, tongue protrusion, asymmetry of facial features, missing digits, distorted or missing auricles, a high-pitched cry or unusual vocal patterns, and unusual head circumference. Referral for further medical and genetic work-up is warranted when these characteristics are noted.

Structural Abnormalities

A variety of conditions that may impinge on vocal development are reviewed below.

Stenosis. Respiratory and vocal characteristics vary with diagnosis. For example, patients diagnosed with subglottic stenosis (i.e., a narrowing of the space below the glottis) may experience labored breathing or wheezing. In severe cases, air is not exchanged and tracheostomy may be necessary. If several emergency oral intubations have taken place, damage to the vocal folds may have also occurred and/or scar tissue may be present.

Respiration Papillomatosis. Respiration papillomatosis, or recurrent respiration papillomatosis (RRP), are multiple benign laryngeal neoplasms that can cause hoarseness, stridor, and/or respiratory distress. Surgical intervention may be necessary to create a patent airway. If hoarseness or stridor is observed at rest or during feeding times, a referral to a pediatric otolaryngologist is appropriate. Multiple surgeries are usually needed because these growths recur. Thus scar tissue may be an iatrogenic effect of surgeries and voice therapy will be needed.

Laryngeal and Glottic Webs. According to Grey, Smith, and Schneider (1996), laryngeal and glottic webs mostly occur in the anterior glottis. Voice problems are usually first noted at birth. Glottic webs that cover less than 35% of glottic airway usually require minimal to no treatment. Webs that have 50% or more involvement of the folds usually require tracheotomy, because the airway is obstructed.

Laryngeal Clefts. Clefts of the larynx also can lead to respiratory difficulties, including stridor, respiratory distress, and often a hoarse vocal quality. Laryngeal clefts may be small (type I), which may result in serious hoarseness and recurrent respiratory tract infections, or severe (types III–IV), which may lead to severe aspiration pneumonia and respiratory failure.

Tracheoesophageal and Esophageal Atresia. If coughing, sputtering, or desaturations are noted during initial feedings, it may be an indication that the infant has a tracheoesophageal fistula (TEF) and/or an esophageal atresia (EA). However, the diagnosis often may not be fully documented. The child may have coughing with feedings for unknown reasons and speech pathology may be consulted for an evaluation. As a result of liquid sitting on top of the vocal folds or in the pharyngeal area, a "wet" sound may be heard with crying. In esophageal atresia, a nasogastric (NG) tube will not be able to be passed if the esophagus is a blind pouch. When oral feedings are introduced, the food has nowhere to go and rises to the top of the esophagus. Aspiration (food or liquid falling through the vocal folds) may then occur from spillover from the esophagus. An esophagram or barium swallow is usually a better diagnostic tool than a videofluoroscopic analysis. Arvedson et al. (2000) reported that TEF/EA is prevalent in babies born to women who demonstrate polyhydramnios during pregnancy. This occurs when a fetus is not able to swallow amniotic fluid.

After a structural abnormality has been identified, the speech–language pathologist plays an important role in establishing an oral stimulation program, providing prespeech and language stimulation, and educating caregivers. Depending on surgical management, a spit fistula may be placed. This consists of an esophagostomy or a "hole" that is created from the esophagus to the neck to allow saliva to drain. Oral or "sham feedings" may be introduced. When sham feedings occur, the baby can experience practice sucking and swallowing; however, the food can drain out of the stoma (the hole in the neck). This allows the child practice feeding without the risk of damage to the esophagus and allows the repaired esophagus time to heal and grow. Pharyngeal skills must be intact, however, and depending on the anatomical structure of the child, aspiration can still occur.

Vocal Fold Paralysis. In unilateral (one side) or bilateral (both sides) vocal fold paralysis, vocal quality may be compromised and voice has been described as hoarse, breathy, strained, or absent/aphonic. Swallowing difficulties may also be present if the folds are in the abducted position. Respiratory distress may be present if the folds are in the adducted position.

Rosin, Handler, Potsic, Wetmore, and Tom (1990) provided perspectives on the etiology and treatment of both unilateral and bilateral vocal fold paralysis in children. They reported vocal fold paralysis can be a result of pulmonary, neurologic, gastrointestinal, and congenital-familial syndromes. Symptoms of vocal fold paralysis include stridor, cyanosis, apnea, feeding difficulties, intercostal retractions, and hoarseness. According to Rosin et al., stridor, cyanosis, and apnea are more frequently seen in children with bilateral vocal fold paralysis (paralysis on both sides). On the other hand, they reported that increased hoarseness and voice changes are more likely to occur with unilateral paralysis. Feeding difficulties and sternal retractions occur equally in bilateral and unilateral paralysis. They further explained that neurological deficits more often lead to bilateral vocal fold paralysis whereas unilateral paralysis occurs most often as a result of trauma or cardiac surgeries.

Left-sided vocal fold paralysis tends to occur more frequently than right-sided paralysis. This is possibly due to the longer course of the recurrent laryngeal nerve on the left. The anatomy of innervation of the larynx differs on the left from the right. Gray, Smith, and Schneider (1996) described the course concisely. Signals begin with the 10th cranial nerve and are sent to the recurrent laryngeal nerve.

> On the right, the recurrent laryngeal nerve passes the larynx and hooks around the subclavian artery to double back toward the larynx. The left recurrent laryngeal nerve comes off the Vagus in the thorax at the level of the Aortic arch and then head back up towards the larynx. On both sides, the recurrent laryngeal nerve ascends in the groove between the trachea/esophagus until it enters the larynx just posterior to the cricothyroid joint. The route of the left recurrent laryngeal nerve predisposes it to many injuries of the thoracic origin. (Gray et al., 1996)

Management of vocal fold paralysis varies. Rosin et al. (1990) reported that 66% of the cases in their study of bilateral vocal cord paralysis (children) required tracheotomy placement, whereas 36% of cases with unilateral paralysis required tracheotomy placement.

Laryngomalacia and Tracheomalacia. "Malacia" means "softening"; therefore, laryngomalacia refers to the lack of tone in the cartilages of the larynx. Tracheomalacia, which is less common, refers to softness of the trachea. If the structures obstruct the airway, this can result in breathing difficulties. Laryngomalacia is diagnosed by an otolaryngologist by fiberoptic endoscopic evaluation. Children may be at high risk for aspiration with oral feedings (especially liquids) as the airway has difficulty maintaining patency. For example, a child may take a breath at the same time that he or she is attempting to swallow. Incoordination may result with possible laryngeal penetration (food or liquid entering the airway) or aspiration (food or liquid going through the level of the vocal folds). It is common for children to outgrow laryngomalacia by approximately 18 months. Severe laryngomalacia and tracheomalacia may have a neurologic etiology; therefore, such infants benefit from a neurology consult. If airway obstruction persists, surgical intervention may be necessary to maintain patency.

Many infants with mild forms of vocal fold paralysis and tracheomalacia at birth manage the first year of life without the need for significant medical intervention. However, frequent follow-up is necessary to ensure that difficulties do not arise. As the child develops and becomes more active, the demand for oxygen exchange increases. This may exacerbate breathing difficulties as a child gets older.

Pulmonary Disorders

Pulmonary disorders may include hyaline membrane disease; gastroesophageal reflux disease (GERD, although this is sometimes categorized under gastrointestinal disorders); and bronchopulmonary dysplasia (BPD). Respiratory distress and failure may occur in association with any of these conditions, and careful evaluation of swallowing is recommended in all children with pulmonary disorders. Patients are at risk if their respiratory systems are stressed by aspiration because their pulmonary status is already fragile. The clinical literature suggests that management of the airway is the number one priority in the treatment of these children. In addition, clinicians must be aware of the risk of fluctuating status. For example, a child may have adequate respirations during one session and may "crash" during another. Therefore, evaluation and intervention by the speech–language pathologist must be planned carefully with an awareness of such possibilities.

Hyaline Membrane Disease. Another name for hyaline membrane disease is infant respiratory distress syndrome or IRDS. Infants with this condition are not able to produce adequate amounts of surfactant. The risk of IRDS decreases with age. Mechanical ventilation is often necessary and recovery may occur when surfactant levels increase as the child matures.

Bronchopulmonary Dysplasia (BPD). *Bronchopulmonary dysplasia* (BPD) is a chronic pulmonary syndrome that occurs with prolonged ventilation, when supplemental oxygen is needed for 28 days or more. Abnormal findings are seen on a chest X-ray. Infants with BPD often experience tachypnea, tachycardia, and chest retractions. Such infants should not be stimulated by feeding or play when respiratory rates are more than 70 beats per minute prior to stimulation or if they increase to more than 80 beats per minute during tasks such as feeding or play. If a child is breathing rapidly following eating, the child's energy may be spent breathing and digestion may be slowed. If delayed emptying of the stomach occurs, increased acid build-up may cause the child to "reflux" the stomach contents into the esophagus. This may result in desaturation and coughing. It is common for infants with BPD to also have this type of "reflux" known as GERD. GERD will be discussed later; however, infants with respiratory problems are prone to GERD. Often infants may demonstrate subtle clinical signs of GERD but they may not have any symptoms. The speech–language pathologist may be the first to note these signs and make the referral to the physician for medical management.

Neurologic Disorders

Neurologic diseases commonly seen in infants and toddlers include seizure disorders, perinatal asphyxia, neural tube deficits, and intracranial hemorrhage.

Seizure Disorders. There are multiple causes of seizures. Four types of seizures occur in infants (subtle, clonic, tonic, and myoclonic) and are not the same as seizures that occur in older children and adults. According to Arvedson et al. (2000), jerkiness can easily be mistaken for a seizure. She distinguishes jerkiness from seizures by noting that no abnormal eye movements occur and that movements cease with passive flexion. Diagnosis of seizures is determined by an EEG. Long-term concerns vary as some children outgrow seizures and other children require long-term anticonvulsant (medication) therapy. There may also be side effects of long-term use of medication as pharmalogic agents may affect swallowing, speech, language, and voice development.

Perinatal Asphyxia (Hypoxic Ischemic Encephalopathy). Seizures are frequently present in children with perinatal asphyxia. This can occur when the umbilical cord is wrapped around the neck of the child, either in utero or during the birthing process, cutting off oxygen supply to the brain. Resuscitation occurs immediately after delivery and some infants respond positively in a matter of minutes. Others demonstrate multisystem failure. Careful observation by the speech–language pathologist is needed to observe any subsequent neurological deficits that may be present. Coordination of treatment with a pediatric neurologist is essential in such cases.

Intracranial Hemorrhage. Intracranial hemorrhages include cortical, cerebellar, brainstem, or intraventricular bleeds. Physicians use routine ultrasound testing to assist in diagnosing and grading an intracranial hemorrhage. All infants less than 1500 grams are usually screened by ultrasound. Hemorrhages are graded according to severity on a scale of I to IV, with IV being most severe and having the poorest prognosis. Severe intracranial hemorrhage may result in hydrocephalus (cerebral spinal fluid on the brain or in the cranial cavity), requiring surgical intervention with a shunt placed to drain the excess fluid from the brain.

Effects of Neurological Deficits. Organization (sensory regulation) of the sensory system is an important task for infants. If they have neurologic deficits, infants have difficulty organizing themselves. Unpredictable patterns of organization can affect sleep–awake states. Inconsistent sleep–awake states in turn can affect feeding abilities. If a child cannot remain organized for feedings, feedings may become unpleasant for both the infant and the caregiver. Feeding aversions later can affect development. It is important to consider this when dealing with children who have possible neurologic involvement.

When neurologic deficits are suspected or confirmed, the speech–language pathologist needs to work to improve the infant's overall organization. This is done in conjunction with physical, occupational, and medical therapies to provide benefit to children whose neurological state of alertness remains inconsistent. Organization may include calming techniques to maximize the child's participation level during therapy. See Table 3–2.

Occupational therapists also provide helpful resources to assist with sensory integration activities. Speech–language pathologists and occupational therapists co-treating a child, to help achieve organization through sensory integration, is usually the optimal approach.

Some children with neurological impairments may have cranial nerve involvement. Asymmetry of the face may be present. Oral motor skills, voice, and swallowing may be affected. Neurologic deficits cross a wide spectrum of skills and behaviors. Long-term sequelae should be considered with this pop-

Table 3–2. Ways to help the child achieve organization.

1. Give the infant time to transition from a sleep state to an awake state. Just as some adults cannot "jump" out of bed and start talking, an infant may not be a "morning" person.
2. Closely monitor the child for any seizure movements or jerkiness. Jerkiness will often cease with passive flexion.
3. Place the infant's arms and hands as close to midline as possible.
4. Swaddling the child with a light blanket may help extremities remain at midline.
5. Firm, slow movements will calm an infant, whereas light, fast stimulation will excite an infant.
6. Limit distractions in the environment: dim the lights, remove extraneous noises, and reduce eye contact.
7. Vertical rocking and firm patting may assist in calming an infant.

ulation as both sensory and motor difficulties can occur. Often development problems are twofold. First, reduced organization and attention make learning time spans short. Second, motor skills may be reduced, affecting overall coordination. Often infants need external support during feeding, including reducing distractions in the room and providing physical support for the cheek and jaw. Later, as the infant becomes a toddler, low stimulation rooms and a supported chair may be needed to increase attention span during treatment.

Gastrointestinal Diseases

Necrotizing Enterocolitis. Necrotizing enterocolitis usually is detected first during 3 to 10 days of life. This condition occurs when bacteria mix with abdominal gas fed by breast milk or formula. It produces large amounts of gas and sometimes feeding intolerance. Abdominal distention is often the first indicator of this problem. Intestinal necrosis can also result in bowel perforations. In such cases surgery may be necessary and mortality can range up to 40% in severe cases (Wolf & Glass, 1993).

Vascular Ring. Stridor or dysphagia may also present in infants and children who have a vascular ring. According to Arvedson et al. (2000), a vascular ring is an anomaly of the aortic arch and its branches. It consists of a ring of vessels around the trachea and esophagus. This may result in a partial obstruction because of the pressure that is exerted. Obstructions can result in reflux, aspiration, or both and can be detected by a barium swallow test. Surgical intervention may be necessary.

Gastroschisis. Another common gastrointestinal disorder is gastroschisis. This is described as an opening in the abdominal wall. Because of the fragility of children with gastrointestinal disorders, nothing can be given by mouth until cleared by the child's medical team. Speech pathologists working with these children should implement an oral motor program to prevent aversion and should continue to provide families with suggestions for appropriate voice and language stimulation.

Gastroesophageal Reflux Disease. As mentioned earlier in this chapter, GERD is common in medically compromised children. GERD may occur independently or as a result of other conditions. It is not a diagnosis but rather a symptom of a primary problem. For example, children with cardiac or pulmonary difficulties often use the majority of their energy for eating, and with reduced endurance, digestion is slowed. When gastric emptying is affected, the food remains in the stomach longer and increased acid buildup occurs. The result can be reflux. Clinical indicators of reflux include one or more of the following:

1. Sour smell in the mouth.
2. Frequent episodes of emesis.
3. Eager to begin eating, but stops shortly thereafter.
4. Crying after or during eating.
5. Arching, irritability after eating.
6. Gagging or coughing after eating.
7. Refusal to eat.
8. Constipation.
9. Apnea/bradycardia/desaturations.
10. Stridor.
11. Sleep disturbances.
12. Weight loss.
13. Hoarse vocal quality.
14. Atonic neck reflex.

Gumpert, Kalach, Dupont, and Contencin (1998) described the history of reflux and voice problems beginning in 1968 when two researchers, Cherry and Margulies, discovered contact ulcerations on three patients who demonstrated GER on barium studies. Gumpert et al. reported that Koufman (1991) found that 20 to 50% of refluxers with voice involvement had complaints of symptoms. According to Gumpert et al. (1998), there are two theories of how GERD causes voice disorders in adults: the vagally mediated reflux theory and the direct acid injury theory. The first theory describes acid lying in the lower esophagus. Repetitive throat clearing and coughing occur, which leads to vocal abuse. In the direct acid injury theory, reflux transfers through the upper esophageal sphincter. Other factors that may contribute to reflux affecting the voice include how well the lower esophageal sphincter is working, how resistant to acid is the lining of the esophagus, and the clearance of acid following reflux. Infants may be especially susceptible to direct acid injury because of the immaturity of the structures.

Extraesophageal Reflux. With increased public awareness concerning GERD, a new term, extraesophageal reflux, is being used in the literature. *Extraesophageal reflux* or EER occurs when acid travels into the pharynx. Up to 30% of the acid esophageal contents may enter the pharynx. According to Arvedson et al. (2000) less than 50% of children demonstrate typical symptoms of reflux. Disrupted sleep is often the primary behavior associated with EER and GERD in young children and voice quality changes are frequently noted by the speech–language pathologist.

Cardiac Disorders

Congenital heart disease is generally classified as acyanotic or cyanotic. In acyanotic diseases, all of the blood is oxygenated. The most common causes include atrial septal defects, ventricle septic defects, and patent ductus arteriosus.

Acyanotic Heart Diseases. ATRIAL SEPTAL DEFECTS (ASD). An *atrial septal defect* (ASD) is characterized by a hole in the wall that separates two sides of the upper portion of the heart. Generally, shortness of breath may occur. Infants fatigue easily, especially during play or feeding times.

VENTRICLE SEPTAL DEFECT (VSD). According to Wolf and Glass (1992), a ventricle septal defect, or VSD, is the most common category of heart defect. VSD consists of a hole in the wall that separates the two sides on the lower portion of the heart. Infants usually demonstrate poor weight gain, high respiratory and heart rates, and irritability.

PATENT DUCTUS ARTERIOSUS (PDA). PDA occurs when a ductus artery (which connects the left pulmonary artery with the descending aorta) remains open after birth. Lower respiratory tract infections may be present. Normally, the patent ductus closes at birth. Infants may demonstrate poor feeding due to increased respiratory rates. In severe cases, ligation as well as mechanical ventilation may be necessary. Communication may be affected.

CYANOTIC HEART DISEASES. Cyanotic heart diseases usually are more serious than acyanotic heart diseases. The most common include Tetralogy of Fallot, transposition of great vessels, and hypoplastic left heart syndrome (Wolf & Glass, 1992).

TETRALOGY OF FALLOT. *Tetralogy of Fallot* consists of the presence of four abnormalities: VSD, pulmonary stenosis, displacement of aorta to the right, and right ventricle hypertrophy. This condition is not usually detected during the neonatal period. Rather, it is noticed at 4 to 6 months when the child is beginning to be more active. Children with this disorder often demonstrate episodes of hypoxia. Episodes consist of rapid breathing, irritability, and cyanosis. Reducing systemic blood return to the heart, as well as pharmalogical intervention, is used to assist with stabilizing the child.

TRANSPOSITION OF GREAT VESSELS. Transposition of great vessels results in abnormal circulation. Heart failure often presents early at 1 to 2 weeks of age. Wolf and Glass (1992) reported this to be the most common form of cyanotic heart disease. Frequent respiratory infections, developmental delays, and clubbing of fingers and toes may occur.

HYPOPLASTIC LEFT HEART SYNDROME. This syndrome presents with an ascending aorta, aortic and mitral valve atresia, and hypoplasia of the left atrium and ventricle. Infants who are affected are extremely fragile during the first few days of life. Symptoms include sudden onset of cyanosis, respiratory distress, and poor feeding. Mortality is high, although new surgical interventions have improved prognosis for these patients.

In general, speech–language pathologists working with patients who have congenital heart disease frequently find that poor endurance affects efficiency of feeding. Organization is typically within functional limits. Eating and play times are usually limited because of the risk of cardiac stress that occurs with lengthy feeding or play times. It is important to limit preparatory exercises or unnecessary stimulation. For example, try not to schedule therapy times after changing or bathing times because these activities may deplete all the child's energy prior to therapy.

Voice deficits can also occur as a result of damage to the recurrent laryngeal nerve during heart surgery. If the recurrent laryngeal nerve is stretched or damaged, vocal fold paralysis may occur. Referral to a pediatric otolaryngologist is necessary if children with heart disease also demonstrate a hoarse cry. Aspiration risks must also be considered at all times with children who may have vocal fold paralysis.

Acquired and Iatrogenic Problems of the Aerodigestive Tract

Acquired and iatrogenic problems in young children can range from mild vocal fold injuries to severe respiratory failure. Strangulation, falls, gunshot wounds, and motor vehicle accidents are some of the laryngeal traumas that cause voice difficulties. Merritt, Bent, and Porubsky (1998) in discussing laryngeal trauma reported that the immature larynx is often protected by the mandibular arch so that problems may not be as severe as they are in adults. They also stated that the increased pliability of the cricothyroid may help reduce the severity of laryngeal fractures in children. The narrow laryngeal tracheal passageway makes establishing a patent airway the most important factor in managing laryngeal injuries, however, and this increases risks of iatrogenic problems.

Pharmacological effects also often occur as side effects of treatment and must be considered. Often the speech–language pathologist must refer the patient to acute medical management when voice and swallowing is affected. For example, if a child has sepsis or infection, that must be addressed prior to intervention for voice and swallowing. Infections such as whooping cough, polyneuritis, diphtheria, rabies, syphilis, tetanus, botulism, tuberculosis, and Guillain-Barré syndrome may cause sequelae in the aerodigestive tract. If a child has a surgical procedure to place a shunt, malfunction may also result. Gray et al. (1996) stated that vocal fold paralysis is occasionally the first indicator of shunt malfunction.

It is important for the speech–language pathologist to recognize the priorities in treatments that patients must receive. If medications affect voice and swallowing but are necessary for a patient's neurologic, respiratory, or cardiac condition, then voice and swallowing therapy must be delayed until the patient is stabilized medically.

The Role of the Speech–Language Pathologist in the NICU and ICU

In addition to knowledge about how to identify the possible voice sequelae of medical problems seen in children in the ICU, the speech–language pathologist must also understand the team approach to intervention in medical settings (see Appendix E). The team may be organized as a multidisciplinary team, an interdisciplinary team, or a transdisciplinary team. Regardless of the organization a facility uses, it is important to remember how vital communication among team members is when treating young patients. Members of the team can include:

- Parents/caregivers
- Primary physician
- RN/nurse practitioner
- Physical therapist
- Occupational therapist
- Speech–language pathologist
- Audiologist
- Social worker
- Dietitian
- Consulting physicians (neurologist, pulmonologist, otolaryngologist, gastroenterologist, etc.)
- Developmental therapist
- Pharmacist
- Chaplain

One way in which team members acquire knowledge of patients' needs is through access to shared information. For example, attendance of the speech–language pathologist at rounds is extremely beneficial. This is where cases are discussed, referrals made, and recommendations shared. Rounds may be held on a daily or weekly basis depending on the operation of the facility.

When the speech–language pathologist is working as part of a team he or she needs to be clear about the following aspects of each case and be able to communicate and document during rounds and conferences:

1. The reason for evaluating the patient;
2. Procedures that are implemented;
3. Findings resulting from procedures implemented;
4. Speech–language pathologist's recommendation;

5. Records of team members consulting on evaluation;
6. The response of family and staff to the treatment plan.

Arvedson et al. (2000) encouraged all clinicians to review treatment options. She and her colleagues emphasized the importance of evaluating the patient's immediate anticipated benefits and risks as well as long-term functional outcomes. The provision of ways to empower and reinforce patients and their family from the start of treatment also assists in compliance with recommendations for treatment.

Voice and Voice-Related Behaviors

Voicing can be classified as both reflexive and intentional. Because children from birth to the toddler years do not have a sophisticated form of communication, careful observation of both reflexive and intentional vocal patterns is crucial. For example, a child may cough repetitively. This reflexive pattern may be the child's way of communicating distress. The behavior may also indicate respiratory difficulties, aspiration, or gastroesophageal reflux, and so on. However, the child may cough intentionally for attention due to a learned pattern of response by caregivers. Coughing may also be a result of a combination of both reflexive and intentional communication. For instance, the child may cough in response to aspiration. When he or she coughed in the past, caregivers frequently responded by holding the infant. The infant may then have adapted coughing as a way to communicate a need to be held. Examples of additional voice-respiratory-related behaviors include hiccups, hoarse vocal quality, strained vocal quality, "gurgly" vocal quality, wheezing, and stridor. Clinicians must not only observe the pattern of occurrence of the behaviors but also analyze the psychosocial aspects of the behaviors.

Respiratory Behaviors

When we consider a child's respiratory behavior we need to observe all of the pertinent aspects that can be observed. How does the child breathe? Is the child orally intubated? Does he have a tracheostomy? Is the child breathing room air but respirations sound noisy and labored? Does the child's nose flare when breathing? Do differences exist between quiet breathing versus active breathing? All of the these factors are significant in the assessment and treatment of voice and swallowing disorders. When an infant has oral intubation, it severely restricts communication. Usually, speech–language pathologists are consulted following extubation. However, they are sometimes contacted to assist in providing education regarding swallowing and voicing to the family and caregivers prior to extubation or during intubation.

With the neonatal population, speech–language pathologists are responsible for providing suggestions about ways to facilitate more pleasurable oral and facial experiences while the child is being orally intubated. Children who require mechanical ventilation often cannot tolerate tactile stimulation, for example. Such children lack oral experiences, and as a result, delayed communication development may occur. By providing early intervention to the caregivers of this population, the speech–language pathologist may reduce the negative consequences of the child's restricted sensory feedback.

Suggestions for providing positive oral experiences are provided in Table 3–3. Prior to any intervention, a doctor's order (prescription) and clearance from nursing staff must be obtained. A handout for parents is presented in Appendix A.

Table 3–3. Providing positive oral and facial experiences for infants who are intubated.

1. Start by providing slow firm movements to an infant's hands when he or she is in a calm relaxed state. Often using a towel or blanket will yield positive results. Skin-to-skin contact often is overstimulating.
2. Continue with slow firm movements from outward in. Move up the child's arms to the neck and eventually to the face. If the child becomes agitated or demonstrates facial grimacing, pull back and start over.
3. Be mindful of overstimulation. Often infants cannot handle tactile stimulation in conjunction with visual or auditory stimulation. Therefore, keep your voice low and minimize distractions.
4. Once you have established trust with touching the infant's face, smile and kiss the childs' cheeks. Encourage stimulation to the cheeks during feeding times in an attempt to establish some oral awareness with feedings.
5. Minimize tape on the face. Switch taping to alternating sides to minimize irritation.
6. Always obtain clearance from the child's nurse prior to providing any type of stimulation. Sometimes, even the slightest disturbance can send a child into distress.
7. Check to see if your facility has a kangaroo program. Nurses specially trained in this type of intervention can assist you in working with a child.

Rationale for Tracheostomy Placement

When a young child's respiratory problems cannot be quickly resolved, a long-term alternative to intubation is needed. Infants and children whose breathing is not stable cannot be extubated (removal of the breathing tube) without another procedure to replace the tube in the upper airway. A tracheotomy is a surgical procedure that is used to create an alternative airway. A hole (stoma) is cut into the neck to the trachea to allow the infant to inhale and exhale directly into the trachea. The tracheostomy is the tube that is placed in the stoma to keep the entrance from closing. If there was no tube to hold the entrance open, the tissues would grow back together.

There are three main reasons for a tracheostomy placement in a medically fragile child.

1. *Upper airway obstructions:* Obstructions consist of nasopharyngeal obstructions, swollen tissues/edema, flaccidity of structures, malformations, and injury or trauma that prevents normal passage of air through the airway.
2. *Prolonged ventilation.*
3. *Pulmonary toileting* (the need to frequently clear secretions because the patient cannot effectively manage the secretions).

Parts of the Tracheostomy Tube

Tracheostomy tubes come in several sizes and are made by several manufacturers. A tracheostomy tube consists of an outer and inner cannula. The flange is the part that holds the inner and outer cannula in place. Besides the inner and outer cannula and the flange, some tracheostomy tubes have a small cuff that is attached around the inner cannula. It lies between the tube and the tracheal wall.

The cuff cushions the tracheostomy tube. It is connected by a thin plastic cord that ends on the outside of the tracheostomy tube with a small balloon. When the balloon is inflated with water or air, the cuff around the inner cannula expands. When it is deflated, a small "leak" of space remains between the trachea and the tracheostomy tube. Cuff inflation is used to prevent secretions from slipping around the tracheostomy tube into the airway. Prolonged use of cuff inflation may cause scarring along the tracheal wall in some patients.

With a deflated or absent cuff, air may reach the mouth and nose by leaking through the space between the tube and the trachea. Although air reaches the mouth and nose, it is not the same amount of air that would reach these cavities with normal mouth or nose breathing. Infants and children have a narrow trachea, and the presence of a cuffed tube in the trachea increases the risk for scarring. Uncuffed tracheostomy tubes reduce the risk of scarring as they allow more room. Thus physicians prefer that children have uncuffed tracheostomy tubes. Uncuffed tubes also allow for some leakage of air through the larynx. If the larynx is functional, some limited vocalization ("leak speech") may occur. Signs of laryngeal inadequacy include:

1. Aphonic or weak cry
2. Absent cough and inaudible laugh
3. Soundless or absent babbling or sound play
4. Inadequate vocal fold closure observed by transnasal laryngoendoscopy when the child is crying
5. Evidence of adequate hearing

A fenestrated tracheostomy tube consists of an inner cannula that has a small hole in the top portion of the inner cannula. This allows air to travel through the hole and may assist with some breathy voicing. Cautious suctioning (removal of secretions through the tracheostomy site via sterile catheter and suction device) must be practiced as the suctioning catheter can perforate other tissues if not placed correctly. In addition, infection can occur around the fenestrated tracheostomy tubing causing further difficulties. Openings in the tubes to facilitate communication have been used by some manufacturers, who have marketed their tubes using the term "Talking Trach."

Advantages of a Tracheostomy Tube

One of the advantages of tracheostomy is that it allows the tubing from the oral intubation to be removed from the face. This allows speech, voicing, and swallowing rehearsal activites and development of oral patterns. In addition, it provides more mobility for the patient. The child can adopt more varied positions with a tracheostomy than with oral intubation. Thus a "trach" is the preferred method for children who must be given help with breathing or mechanical ventilation for longer than a few weeks.

Another advantage to having a tracheostomy is it allows gradual weaning from a mechanical ventilator. For example, the patient may be able to tolerate small amounts of time off the ventilator during the day but require full ventilator support at night. The tracheostomy tube provides flexibility as it can be attached to the ventilator or used with supplemental oxygen with a tracheostomy collar (a flexed tubing device that attaches to the oxygen tank and blows oxygen in the front of the tracheostomy) or used with room air (no supplemental oxygen). A child who must have mechanical ventilation for longer than 6 hours in any 24-hour period is termed "ventilator dependent."

Disadvantages of a Tracheostomy Tube

The major disadvantage of tracheostomy, of course, is the need for an additional surgery. The child must be medically stable to go through the tracheostomy surgery. A second disadvantage to tracheostomy placement is that the tracheostomy tube often "anchors" the larynx, limiting opportunities for laryngeal elevation. If laryngeal elevation is affected, swallowing may be impaired. Therefore, if long-term swallowing difficulties are suspected, some physicians place a gastrostomy tube during surgery. This eliminates the need for an additional surgery later and allows removal of the nasogastric or oral gastric feeding tube.

Tracheostomized patients are at risk for mucous plugs, dislodgment of the tube, and/or infection. Therefore, infants and children with tracheostomy tubes must be monitored carefully at all times. Restraints are not optimal, however, as all children need to learn to explore with their hands; however, a tug on a tube by a curious hand could become a life-threatening situation. Also, as with all stomas (holes), infection can occur. Sterile suctioning and meticulous hygiene should be practiced when clinicians work with patients with tracheostomy. Parent and caregiver training in this aspect of care is also essential in preparation for a child's discharge.

A tracheostomy is sometimes necessary to enable excess secretions to be regularly suctioned. Suctioning poses a disadvantage, as adult patients often describe suctioning as "uncomfortable" during the process. However, following deep suctioning, adult patients report a feeling of relief. When the airway is clear of secretions, breathing is often less labored and therefore more comfortable. Infants and children usually adapt more quickly than adults to the suctioning process, and although suctioning is never enjoyable, it soon becomes a part of a child's routine. However, children are less able to tell the adults about their anxieties and concerns. Clinicians need to talk to parents and caregivers about soothing children before and during the procedure. Models of how to talk to young children about what occurs should be provided.

An infant's sense of taste or smell may be compromised by the tracheostomy placement. Because outside air enters directly at the neck, it does not reach the nose hairs. Nose hairs warm and moisten the air and assist olfaction. If you have tried eating when you have a cold, you noticed reduced taste or smell. This is similar to what a person with a cuffed tracheostomy experiences as no air is reaching the mouth and nose.

Tracheostomy limits a child's ability to explore vocally and therefore extra language and voice stimulation is crucial for these children. Children need to hear the different prosodic patterns of voice as oral and vocal play are often limited. Voicing around the "leak" between the tracheostomy tube and the tracheal wall takes good breath support, something these children have difficulty demonstrating. Thus, emphases on receptive language stimulation and on the maximizing of skills to enhance the intelligibility of the leak speech may be advisable with some children.

Voicing After Tracheostomy

Voicing following a tracheostomy can be accomplished by two approaches: manual occlusion and use of a mechanical valve. An example of a mechanical valve is the Passy-Muir Speaking Valve. (More information can be obtained on the use of this valve by contacting Passy-Muir Inc. at 800–634-5397 or visiting their website at www.passy-muir.com.)

With manual occlusion, a clean gloved finger is placed during exhalation on the tracheostomy site for 1 to 2 seconds at a time. Time is limited to these short spurts because occluding the tracheotomy site inhibits inhalation. With a mechanical valve, the device may be placed directly on the tracheostomy site or in line in cases where the child is on a ventilator. Once the child builds up tolerance to the valve, the valve can be left on (supervised) for increasing lengths of time during waking hours. Either way, infection control must be implemented. The child must inhale through the tracheotomy site and exhale while the tracheostomy is covered either by a finger or by valve action. This allows air to be exhaled through the child's larynx, mouth, or nose. A child with significant upper airway obstruction will not be able to accomplish this, so it is critical that a complete assessment of the child's capacity to use a valve is completed before a valve is fitted. Occasionally, children will discover that, if they drop their chin to cover the tracheostomy stoma, they can make noises. Children must be carefully watched, however, as they can cut off their air intake into the airway. Chin dropping can become a habit that is hard to break and often is dangerous. Giving a child an appropriate form of communication (e.g., manual signs, gestures, pictures, or a speaking valve) is one of the major tasks of a speech–language pathologist. Assessment of the child's status, options, and abilities is critical to the decision-making process.

A child who has had a tracheostomy for his or her entire life views the tracheostomy as a part of the self. The goal of the staff and parents often is to remove the tracheostomy or "get decannulated." This may affect such a child in the same way as having an arm removed. It is scary and he or she may feel like a piece of him- or herself is being removed. One child I worked with truly liked his tracheostomy. His parents had eliminated all negative connotations associated with the tracheostomy and he felt sad when it was removed. Although it was a joyous occasion for his parents and caregivers to have decannulation take place, for this particular child, it was a traumatic day. Naturally, the clinician faced a special challenge in explaining what was happening to the child, what benefits would follow, and accepting his need to mourn his loss as part of the process.

Laryngeal and Pharyngeal Behaviors

When we consider the laryngeal mechanism and the way it functions, we need to assess how changes in a child's medical status affect his or her capacity for phonatory function. Vocal quality, for example, gives the clinician a lot of information. Recent extubation (removal of the breathing tube) can result in a pattern of breathy vocalizations. Wet or gurgly sounds can indicate difficulty with the management of secretions. Coughing, depending on when it occurs, can indicate gastroesophageal reflux, aspiration, or croup. A hoarse vocal quality may indicate vocal fold paralysis or paresis, swelling of the vocal folds, or reflux. Pitch and loudness limitations also provide clues to laryngeal conditions.

Pharyngeal behaviors that are significant include snorting and hiccuping. Additionally, children with croup may sound like they are barking. Any sudden or significant change in phonatory behaviors or atypical quality warrants careful monitoring and consultation with the otolaryngologist and/or pulmonologist.

Balance of Oral and Nasal Resonance

Signs that indicate difficulty with oral and nasal balance are often easily recognizable. Asymmetry of the face can indicate reduced range of motion of the lips, tongue, velum, and jaw. This may affect a child's sucking skills and also his or her swallowing skills. A unilateral facial weakness or paralysis also can indicate a pharyngeal paresis or paralysis on one side. The posture of the mouth can affect coordination of sucking, swallowing, and breathing. If an open mouth posture is observed, the child may be breathing exclusively through the mouth. For example, if a child has any type of nasal obstruction, mouth breathing may be the child's only way to ventilate. This can cause significant difficulty during feedings, specifically with the coordination of sucking, swallowing, and breathing. Voicing may sound hyponasal in patients with choanal atresia or other conditions where the child is unable to breathe through the nose. If the tongue closes off the oral cavity, respiration may also cease. Therefore, the child may compensate by spontaneously pushing the tongue forward to open the airway.

Children with hypotonia (reduced muscle tone) also may demonstrate an open mouth posture. This may give the appearance of a large tongue when, in reality, the tongue is merely lying forward. This tongue posture is often observed in patients with Down syndrome. Drooling may also be a sign of reduced neurologic support for swallowing, poor head posture, and/or oral-motor immaturity, and so on. If resonance sounds muffled or if the tongue or mouth position is atypical, the clinician must consider all possible reasons.

Clefts of the palate, especially submucosal clefts that are undetected, can cause difficulties with oral and nasal balance in the voice. If a child has poor velopharyngeal competence, nasopharyngeal reflux may also result. If it goes untreated, the child may develop frequent colds, infections, and so on. Hypernasality and nasal emission may also occur and the clinician needs to be alert to these signs and try to interpret their significance.

Integrated Behaviors

The crucial point for the clinician to consider is how the respiratory, digestive, laryngeal, and resonance systems work together to support each child in communicating and feeding. We must consider how all of the behaviors together affect the whole child and his level of function, rather than only observing the function of each system in isolation. Attempts to communicate needs and wants and the sounds and movements made tell us a great deal, even before the child can speak using words.

Cognition: Thought Processes Associated With Voice in the Medically Compromised Child

Direct and Indirect Treatment Strategies

The speech–language pathologist is responsible for providing direct and indirect treatment strategies to facilitate optimal development of communication. Direct treatment may include scheduling formal sessions where direct voice stimulation and/or therapy is provided. Indirect therapy may consist of adapting the intensive care environment and providing support and/or education to families and caregivers. Teaching significant adults to talk to the child as they engage in day-to-day activities is also important to the development of receptive language concepts. Frequent talking also allows caregivers to bond with the child and establish emotional connections.

Voice and Language Stimulation During Therapy Sessions

Stimulation from the environment and from significant adults is important for all children. It is especially important for children with special needs. Hospitalized children start off at a severe disadvantage. Lengthy hospitalizations and the need for frequent unpleasant and painful medical procedures leave little time or energy for caregivers to provide and children to respond to voice and language stimulation. For example, a child with an immature respiratory system may be using all of his or her energy to breathe and have little available energy for learning. For children who are fragile, one activity per day may be all they can handle. This places a hospitalized child at significant risk for language, speech, voice, and cognitive delays. The child's physical world

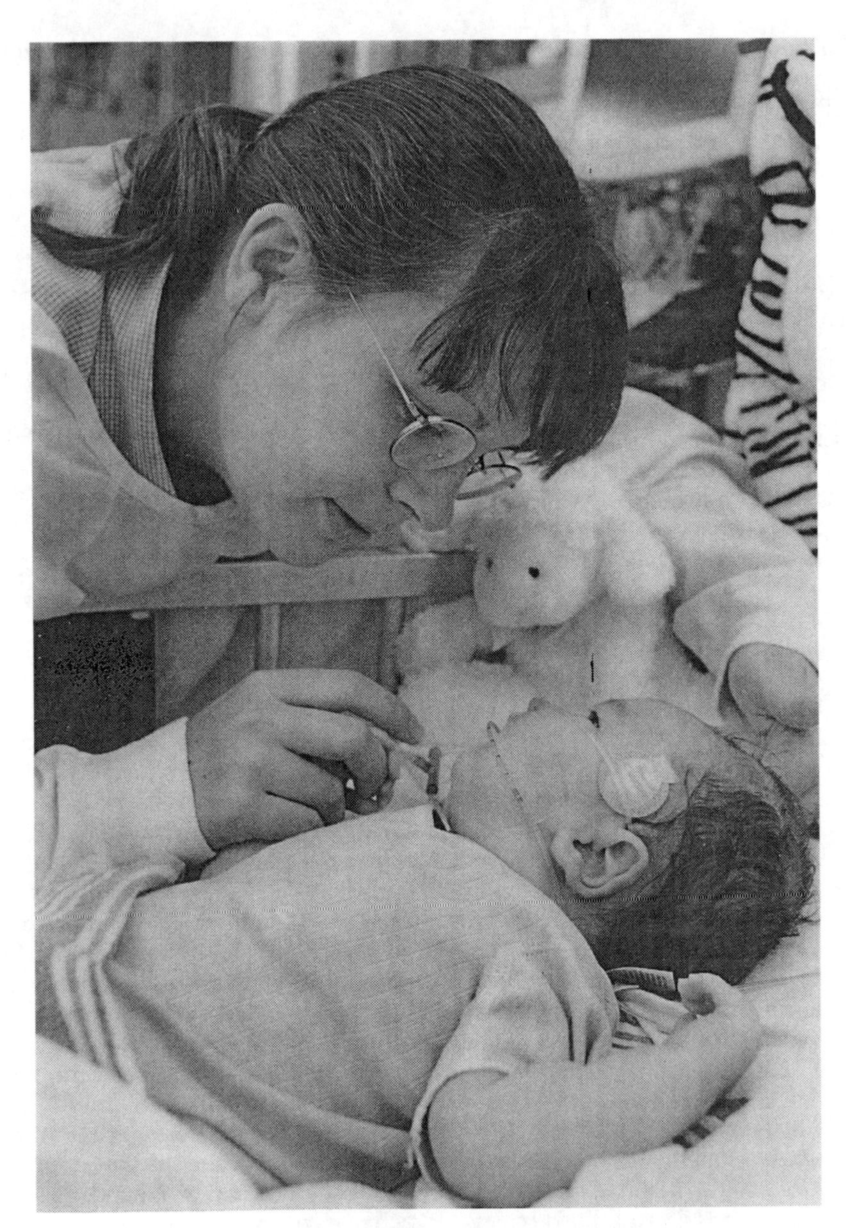

A child's first form of communication. (Copyright Todd Hochberg, Advocate Media Center)

is restricted, vocal play is limited, and typical parental interactions are constrained.

There are several things a clinician can do to facilitate appropriate voice and language stimulation in the least restrictive manner. For example, one way to provide voice and language stimulation is to talk to the child using simple language (1–2 word utterances) during daily events such as bathing. Vocabulary such as body parts and clothing can be introduced and repeated frequently. Even though a child is not yet talking, he or she needs language input. Creative interventions can facilitate effective and efficient programs involving all members of the team, including the child's family. Programs are less effective if only one person works with a child and there is no carryover into the child's daily environment when he or she leaves the hospital.

Because everyday experiences (e.g., going to the grocery store) are not possible in the medical setting, the need for repetitive vocal play, reading, and language stimulation is increased. Reading and singing to children are ways that adults enhance children's language learning. These activities help build receptive concepts, create a bond between caregivers and the infant, and model prosodic voice patterns. Repetition of these activities allows a child to enjoy, predict, and remember oral patterns. Pitch, loudness, and resonance contrasts should also be modeled. The child then begins to associate voice patterns with pleasurable feelings experienced during time spent with adults and soon recognizes varied voice patterns. Even though a child may not be able to vocalize or verbally express what he or she understands, language models provide direct input that builds vocal competence and receptive vocabulary. As mentioned earlier, hearing and vision must also be considered and assessed to ensure that all appropriate sensory channels are available for input. Facial expressions and gestures should be matched to vocal patterns and repeated regularly while eye contact is maintained with the child. The link between feelings and vocalizations needs to be discussed with all significant adults and a set repetoire of patterns can then be repeated consistently (e.g., "what a good baby" accompanied by smiling, holding, stroking, and a warm positive vocal quality).

Adapt the Intensive Care Environment

Initially, the clinician's task is to establish effective rapport with family members and caregivers. Providing a warm interpersonal environment as well as honest communication will assist the clinician in developing the trusting relationships that are essential in providing good quality care. It is important to be consistent with families. For example, coordinating with other hospital staff members to ensure that families are not given conflicting information is necessary. For lengthy conversations, it is helpful to talk with families in a quiet room to ease the stress of being at the child's bedside. This helps focus attention and leads to better listening as the family can concentrate on their questions rather than being distracted by the status of their child.

Provide Support for Families and Caregivers

Help families formulate questions for the team and help team members to provide models for parents. Help prioritize goals for caregivers and family members. Explain the active role that staff and families can play during daily activities to help stimulate the child's development. For example, teach caregivers to label body parts during bathtime. Encourage parents to talk and sing during play hours. Help staff teach the child the concepts "night" and "day" by covering the cribs and dimming the lights at night. Often children in the intensive care unit do not know the difference between night and day, because it is always light, and the same types of noises are always occurring around them. Provide parents with examples of phrases they can murmur softly to their child to express their farewells as they leave in the evening. This can be contrasted with the spontaneous joy of greeting the child in the morning when the child is rested.

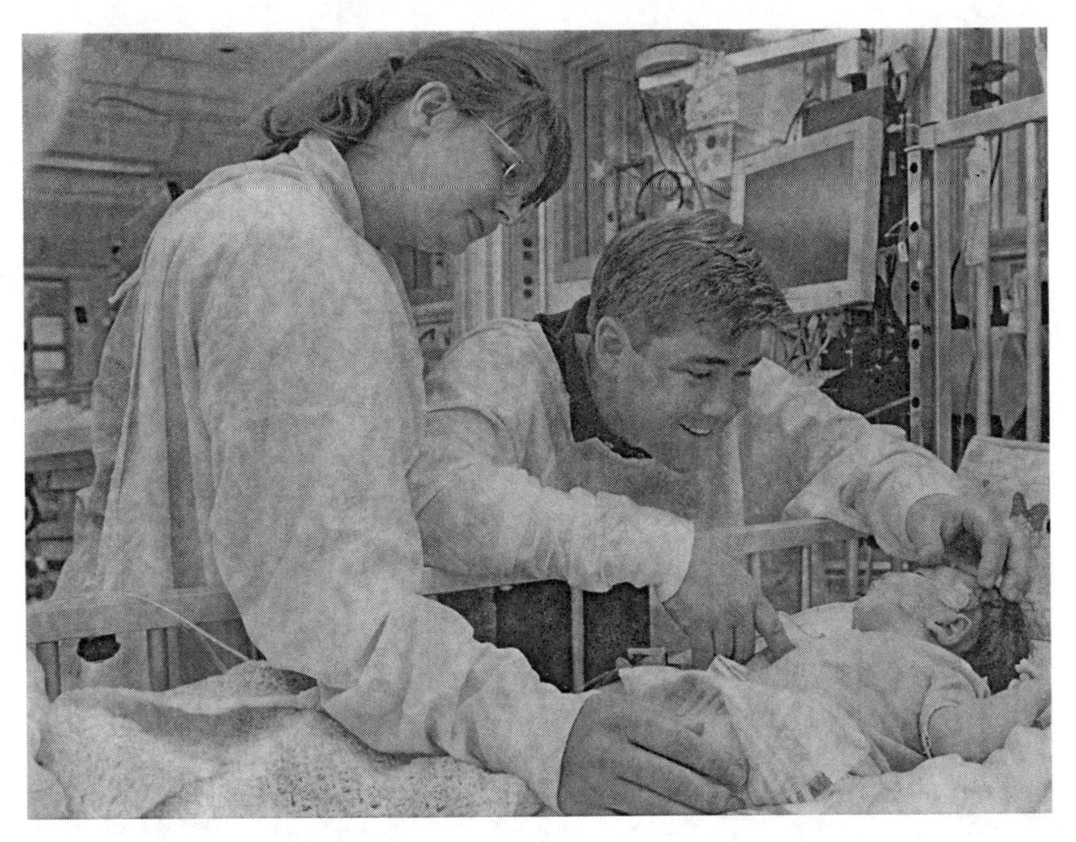

Playtime in the NICU. (Copyright Todd Hochberg, Advocate Media Center)

The speech–language pathologist must also be aware of ways to facilitate the most focused type of intervention strategies in relation not only to communication but also to feeding. For example, it may be too overwhelming for an infant to be fed by his mother while his toddler sibling is demanding attention. Help the family set up strategies so that all members can be involved, but at the appropriate time (e.g., eliminating distractions such as television, dimming lights, and giving the sibling a special snack or toy to enjoy during the patient's feeding time).

Eliminate Negative Oral Experiences

Medically fragile infants and toddlers have to cope with a variety of negative experiences. Emesis (regurgitation), congestion, reflux, respiratory difficulties, pain from needle sticks, dislodged IV, and other unpleasant events recur in the lives of medically fragile infants. Lack of oral stimulation may cause oral aversions. Negative oral experiences may deter oral motor, speech, and voice development. Eliminating or minimizing even a few of these negative experiences can improve the overall state of the child and "talking" children through unavoidable experiences can provide emotional support. Saying "mommy is here" may be a reassuring way for a mother to remind her child that a comforting presence is in the room when the child is experiencing discomfort and cannot be picked up.

Reducing negative oral experiences is obviously a high priority. Oral feeding tubes and oral intubation tubes need to be removed as soon as they can be and the use of tape on the face should be monitored. When nasal gastric tubes are used, a small amount of tape is necessary to hold the tube in place. If a conscious effort to be gentle is made by those in charge of application and removal of the tape, it can make a difference to the child. One solution is to alternate tape and NG placement between different sides of the face and nose. This allows the skin on the face and nares to "breathe" and irritation is minimized. Stroking the child's hands while the nurse applies or removes tape is something a parent can be encouraged to do, as this helps not only the child but also the parent to deal with anxious and helpless feelings.

Oral, nasal, and tracheal suctioning also presents challenges. All children dislike having their faces wiped. It is not pleasant to have a catheter placed down the airway. On the other hand, if a child is drowning in secretions, discomfort and respiratory distress may occur, so suctioning is an important aspect of treatment for many young patients.

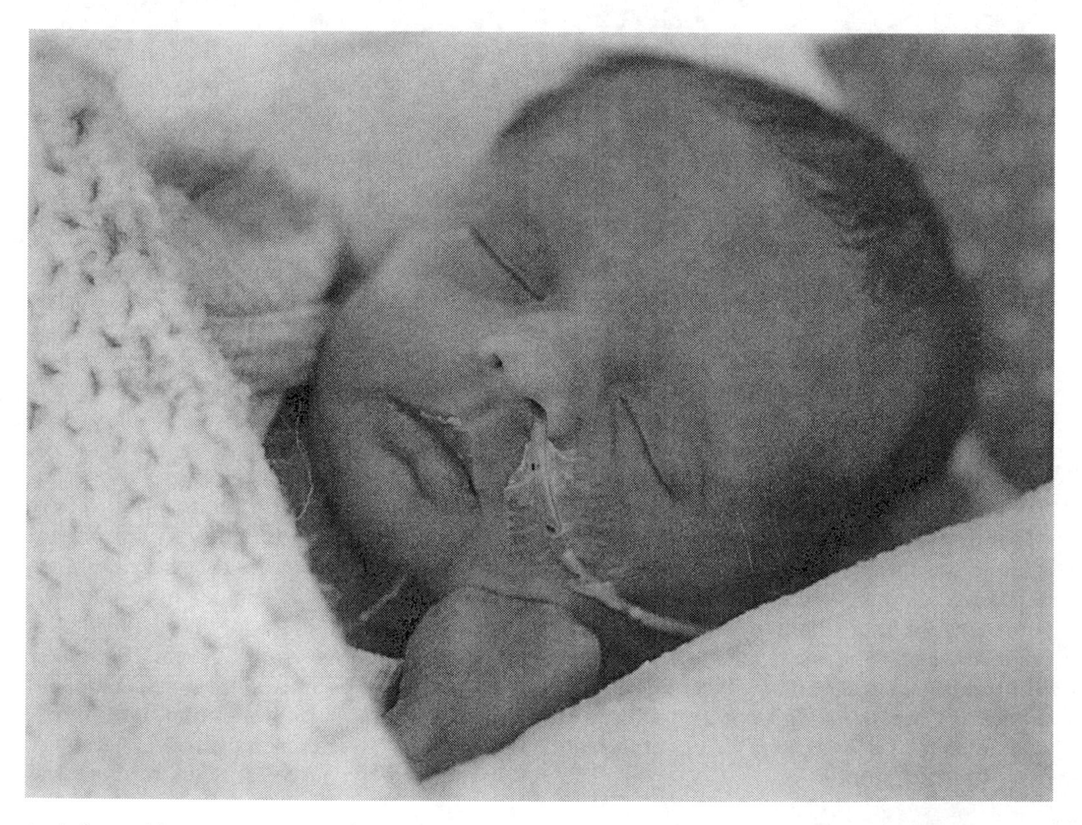

An infant with a nasogastric tube. (Copyright Todd Hochberg, Advocate Media Center)

While the suctioning is in progress, comforting talking may help the child feel secure and expressions of relief and pleasure, coupled with cuddling the child, may help the patient and the parent experience pleasure together at the conclusion of the procedure.

If emesis occurs frequently, children may start to associate any type of oral stimulation with vomiting. Subsequently, they may become "afraid" to place anything in the mouth, including nipples, toys, and so on. Oral aversion can develop and also delay the emergence of vocal play. The child's throat may be sore from the acid reflux irritating the mucosa of the vocal folds. Reflux may also make eating and talking uncomfortable. To prevent orally aversive behaviors from forming, it is best to focus on oral play when no emesis or gagging is present. For example, if caregivers give a child extra attention every time he or she vomits, the child will start to associate increased attention with this behavior. There is a risk that a child could continue to vomit or gag when oral stimulation is conducted to receive the extra attention or because of a learned response. Therefore, it is important to give a child positive verbal reinforcement when he or she is not gagging or vomiting. The placement of a drop of formula on a child's tongue immediately after vomiting may also give the child a pleasant taste after the bitterness of acid from emesis.

Forced feeding can also turn the pleasant experience of feeding into a very unpleasant one. Satter (1987) stressed that it may be helpful to tell parents to remember that they are responsible for providing the food, but are not responsible for how much the child eats. Children of all ages may be inconsistent about eating. The child's current medical and emotional status will impact the ability to eat, speak, socialize, and play. Understanding that there will be good and bad days helps the clinician and the family. The clinician can help by reviewing the child's overall development and the factors affecting it with family members. Additionally, the speech–language pathologist must be sensitive about when to push or hold back with therapy to reduce the probability of the child's development of a negative attitude. By spending time explaining to the family that the child's feelings are more important than pushing the child too hard on a bad day, the clinician can turn an apparent failure into a teaching moment.

Helping caregivers and parents deal with their own as well as their child's stress is also an important goal for the speech–language pathologist during intervention with a medically fragile infant. It is usually helpful to explain that, if one is tense when holding a baby, the baby will sense the tension and may become tense and irritable too. This is something that the clinician may need to repeat over time. Praising the parents when they are relaxed and reinforcing them for caring so much about how they can help are examples of ways in which the clinician reassures anxious family members.

Not only is it important for staff members to remain calm and reassuring but it is crucial for parents to be reassured so they are not fearful when they are with their child. Assist them by finding the calmest area for them to work with their child. Sometimes facilities will have a "safe place" for the child where all uncomfortable medical experiences are prohibited. If the child is able to leave his or her crib, this may provide an excellent opportunity for teaching in a different quiet, stress-free environment. The clinician should always try to help parents feel that they have done the right thing and that the child has benefited by their attempts to do it. The more confident an adult can be made to feel, the more a child will benefit. By praising the adult, we encourage behavior that will help them bond with the child as positively as they can in the circumstances.

Establishing oral and vocal awareness in nonoral feeders during tube feedings allows the clinician to encourage meta-cognitive

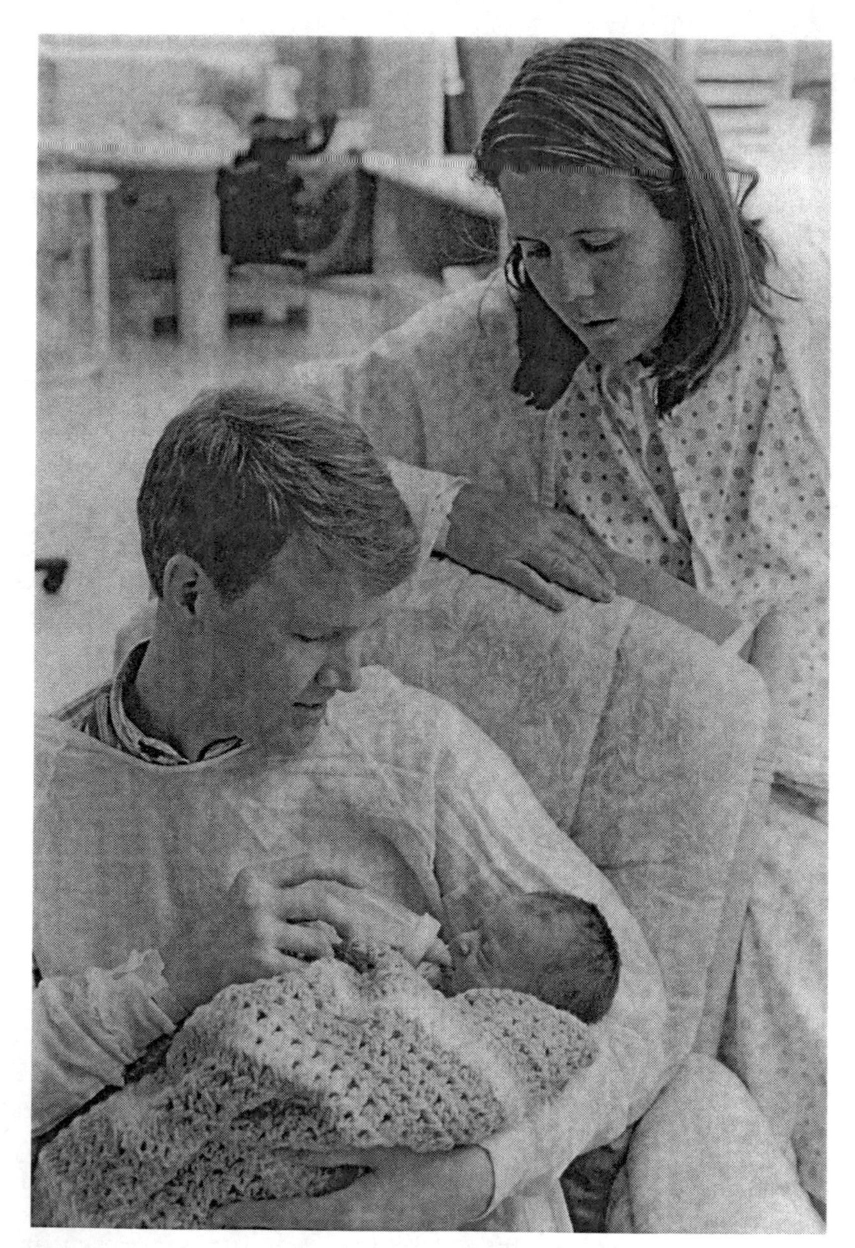

Feeding time with Mom and Dad. (Copyright Todd Hochberg, Advocate Media Center)

development of voice and swallowing. As the baby is becoming satiated via the tube feedings, he or she is learning to use the lips, tongue, and in some cases the swallowing mechanism. This creates an association between the notion of satiety and oral movements. It can also be accomplished by using pacifiers or other forms of non-nutritive sucking. Water or drops of formula via nipple also can be used, provided the child does not have a history of aspiration.

Psychodynamics: Feelings Associated With Voice in the Medically Compromised Child

Vocalizations communicate various meanings. Cooing, screaming, shrieking, and crying all consist of voicing but communicate very different feelings and attempts to meet needs and wants. It is important for caregivers to interpret and reinforce a child's nonverbal communication as well as the vocalizations that are used. The speech-language clinician helps parents learn by drawing attention to salient examples and by praising caregivers when they "read" the child's cues in a sensitive way. For example, by saying, "Look how well you understood that he wanted you to pick him up."

Descriptions of a child's physiological state in conjunction with voice behaviors can provide insight for others about a child's needs and wants. For example, reduced eye contact while crying can signal the child is overstimulated. Body movement can indicate that a child is uncomfortable or needs additional support. Children who have gastroesophageal reflux may arch after feedings. In addition, they may demonstrate a hoarse cry. On the other hand, a positive response to touch may communicate feelings of contentment. Describe and model how rhythmical patting may be noted as helpful for a crying baby to calm down and begin cooing. By helping parents make these kinds of connections, the clinician assists the parent-child relationship to develop in a more satisfying way for all concerned. On occasion, it may even be necessary to help anxious parents to write out examples of things they might do and say to their child in particular situations. Planning in advance may seem artificial, but it may provide necessary structure for frightened adults who are overwhelmed.

The Passy-Muir Speaking Valve

If a child with a functional larynx and a tracheostomy cannot vocalize, a speaking valve is sometimes fitted. The Passy-Muir Speaking Valve is a one-way valve that allows children to inhale through the tracheostomy and exhale through the mouth and nose. It allows air to vibrate the vocal folds and the air stream to exit through the mouth and nose, so that the child can talk. For children, use of this valve provides opportunities for vocal exploration and auditory feedback. Engleman and Turnage-Carrier (1997) studied charts retrospectively to examine evidence of tolerance of the Passy-Muir valve in infants and children 2 years of age and younger. Of the 29 children studied, 83% tolerated the valve, and 75% of those children vocalized on the first trial. Another 21% produced vocalization on a subsequent trial. The results of this study indicate that the speaking valve is safe for use in infants as young as 13 days when the child is fitted in a monitored setting us-ing appropriate guidelines. It reinforces the child's use of voice for communication. As the child associates the use of the valve with creating voice, the person placing the valve gives positive reinforcement. The child then soon associates positive feelings with using the valve and hopefully will vocalize when that person reappears. Cause and effect can be established as reoccurrence occurs.

Facilitation of communication also affects the child's relationship with the professional and caregivers. When a Passy-Muir valve is fitted, it may be the first time a parent or caregiver has heard the child's voice. This can be an emotional and rewarding session for the clinician and for the family members. Although the majority of the time, children's reaction to the valve is positive, it may occasionally be negative. Some children may not tolerate the placement. Then disappointment also may occur and family members may not fully understand the reasons for temporary or permanent discontinuation unless it is carefully explained to them. Therefore, it is crucial to help families through counseling and by the provision of alternative methods of communication. Gestures, signs, pictures, and other forms of communication can be encouraged either as substitutes or in association with the Passy-Muir Speaking Valve or other voicing aids.

It is usually difficult for parents to deal with the social and emotional components of having a child who may not talk or cannot use his or her voice at all. Support must be provided within as well as outside the medical setting. With information widely available on the Internet, it is important to provide credible resources for families. Some parents will want support in finding information for themselves; others will want information provided for them by a clinician. All will benefit from discussing the research and references with the speech–language pathologist so that they are knowledgeable about their child's needs and resources that fit those needs.

Parents and caregivers need concrete ways to intentionally provide means to create positive emotional connections. The clinician must demonstrate empathy (placing yourself in someone's shoes), rather than sympathy (i.e., pity). Different levels of support and education for families are needed at different times during a child's course of treatment. For instance, explaining the entire early intervention process will not assist a parent if his or her child just had an episode of respiratory distress. Prioritizing and practicing good timing will help the clinician reduce the need for repeating information and will help family members become advocates for their children.

Before a child is released from a medical setting, the clinician should arrange for follow-up services. Dobres et al. (1990) studied 731 children referred to otolaryngologists and found that subglottic stenosis, laryngomalacia, vocal paralysis, and papillomatosis represented 53% of the diagnoses in their population. Specialized skills are needed by clinicians working with children with these and other organically based voice disorders. Although a speech–language pathologist is not the decision maker in specific areas such as nutrition or medical management, when referrals and recommendations are made, the clinician discusses the reasons for management decisions with the family. Because the speech–language pathologist is a specialist in communication, he or she plays a vital role in coordinating and interpreting the way information is used by other team members and is understood by the parents, caregivers, and family members.

Summary

In this chapter we reviewed some of the types of aerodigestive problems that affect children's medical status and potential to thrive. We also noted behaviors and skills related to the acquisition of vocal patterns. We discussed the problems that are caused by anatomic and neurologic deficits and how the speech–language pathologist functions as part of the team treating newborns and young children in medical settings. We saw how some respiratory difficulties can be so severe that a tracheotomy may be needed to ensure an unobstructed airway. We also discussed how the clinician must educate caregivers and family members to become active participants in the children's learning to develop voicing and oral communication. Throughout we stressed the psychodynamic aspects of communication and the challenges faced by the medically complex patients and their caregivers.

Acknowledgments

My thanks and appreciation are extended to my family, friends, and colleagues who gave generously of their time and support in writing this chapter. For professional contributions, my thanks to Barb Klein, Allison Hoffman, and Penny Huddleston, and to Marion Mito for use of her resources. Thank you to Steve Schneider for his assistance in updating my computer skills into the 21st century and to Todd Hochberg, photographer at Advocate Lutheran General Hospital in Park Ridge, Illinois, for his exquisite photography. A special thank you is reserved for Dr. Moya Andrews who shared her professional knowledge and guidance and to Jennifer Larrabee who was my mentor and clinical fellowship supervisor and graciously taught me "the ropes." And finally, a most important thank you to Lonnie, my husband, for love, encouragement, humor, and extraordinary patience throughout this rewarding experience.

Terminology*

Anomaly: a malformation of a part of the body.

Airway: the path air travels from the atmosphere to and from the alveoli; in anesthesia or resuscitation, a mechanical device used to keep the passages of the upper respiratory tract open for the passage of air.

Anastomosis: the surgical union of parts, especially hollow tubular parts

Anoxia: literally means "without oxygen."

Apgar score: a score ranging from 0–10 indicating a baby's physical condition immediately following birth.

Apnea: complete cessation of respiration.

Asphyxia: lack of proper oxygen and blood flow. At birth, an Apgar score of 5 or lower indicates asphyxia.

Aspiration: 1. Breathing a foreign substance such as meconium, formula, or stomach contents into the lungs; may cause aspiration pneumonia. 2. withdrawal of material from the body by suctioning.

Atresia: congenital absence or closure of a normal body opening.

Bagging: pumping air and/or oxygen into the lungs by compressing a bag attached to a mask that covers the mouth and nose.

b.i.d.: abbreviation for the Latin words meaning "twice a day."

Bradycardia: a slow heart beat characterized by a pulse rate under 60 beats per minute in an adult; in an infant, below 100 beats per minute.

Bronchopulmonary dysplasia: abnormal development of tissue of the lungs and bronchioles caused by the ventilator, and abnormal respiratory function.

CHARGE association: congenital anomaly which includes *c*olobomatous malformation, *h*eart defect, *a*tresia choanae, *r*etarded growth, *g*enital anomalies, and *e*ar anomalies.

COPD (chronic obstructive pulmonary disease): a general term describing disorders that result in chronic airflow obstruction of the lungs.

*Definitions compiled from *The Premature Baby Book,* by Helen Harrison, 1978. New York: St. Martin's Press; *Voicing! Communication Approaches for Tracheostomized and Ventilator Dependent Patients,* by M. Mason, A. Jerome-Ebel, and P. Romey, 1994. Newport Beach, CA: *Voicing!* Inc.; and *Medical Topics in Speech–Language Pathology: The Role of the SLP in the NICU,* a course presentation by Jennifer L. Larrabee, 1996.

CPAP (continuous positive airway pressure): provision of pressurized air to the airways and alveoli throughout the respiratory cycle when the patient is breathing spontaneously.

Cyanosis: a blue or dusky color of the skin caused by a lack of oxygen.

Decannulation: removal of a tracheostomy or endotracheal tube.

Decannulation plug: a button that attaches to the outer cannula of a fenestrated tracheostomy tube when the inner cannula has been removed; it blocks airflow through the tracheostomy tube and directs breathing through the nose and mouth.

Dry swallows: swallowing without taking food or liquid into the mouth; refers to swallowing saliva.

Endotracheal tube (ET tube): a thin plastic tube inserted into the trachea to allow delivery of air and/or oxygen to the lungs.

Gastrostomy tube (G-tube): a feeding tube surgically inserted directly into the stomach.

Gavage feeding: feedings through a tube passed through the nose or mouth and into the stomach.

Hyaline membrane disease (HMD or RDS): respiratory distress that affects premature babies. It is caused by a lack of surfactant, the substance that keeps the lungs' air sacs from collapsing.

Hypoxia: lack of sufficient oxygen.

Intubation: the process of passing a tube through the mouth or nose into the trachea.

Laryngomalacia: softening of the tissue of the larynx.

Leak: expired air that escapes past a tracheostomy tube, either room air or during ventilation, and passes through the glottis and allows vocalization.

Meconium aspiration: the inhaling by the baby of meconium-strained amniotic fluid. Serious respiratory problems may result.

Nasal CPAP: continuous positive airway pressure administered to an infant through nasal prongs.

NG tube: a small flexible tube inserted through the nose or mouth, down the esophagus, and into the stomach.

NPO: abbreviation for the Latin words *non per os*, meaning "nothing by mouth."

Otolaryngologist: a physician who specializes in disorders of the ear, nose, and throat.

Patent ductus arteriosus (PDA): an abnormal condition, common in premature infants, in which the ductus—the fetal blood vessel connecting the aorta and the pulmonary artery—fails to close after birth.

Patent: open, clear.

Penetration: entry of material into an unprotected airway.

Pierre Robin syndrome: unusual smallness of the jaw combined with cleft palate, downward displacement of the tongue, and an absent gag reflex.

Positive end expiratory pressure (PEEP): application of positive pressure to the airways and alveoli during expiration when the patient is breathing with a mechanical ventilator. Maintains a small amount of air in the lungs, preventing complete emptying on exhalation to avoid airway collapse.

Pulmonary hypertension: increased pressure within the pulmonary circulation.

RDS: respiratory distress syndrome.

Stent: a mold formed from a resinous compound that is used to hold a surgical graft in place.

Stridor: abnormal, harsh, high-pitched sounds that occur during respiratory difficulty or obstructed respiration.

Subglottic: beneath the glottis.

Suctioning: procedure in which a small catheter is placed into the tracheostomy tube to remove accumulated secretion from the tube and lungs.

Tachycardia: an abnormally fast heart rate. In an infant, above 160 beats per minute; in an adult, over 100 beats per minute.

Tachypnea: an abnormally fast breathing rate. In an infant, above 60 breaths per minute; in an adult, over 20 beats per minute.

Tracheal stoma: an opening in the neck that forms as an additional path for airflow to the lung, usually bypassing the mouth and nose.

Tracheoesophageal fistula: an opening between the trachea and esophagus.

Tracheomalacia: softening of the trachea and/or larynx.

Tracheostomy: an artificial opening in the trachea that facilitates the passage of air or removal of secretions.

Tracheotomy: the surgical operation of cutting an opening in the trachea at the level of the third and fourth tracheal rings.

Treacher Collins syndrome: named for Edward Treacher Collins, a British ophthalmologist. Mandibulofacial dysostosis characterized by hypoplasia of the facial bones; downward sloping of the palpebral tissues; defects of the ear and acrostomia. It occurs in two forms that are thought to be autosomal dominants.

Ventilation: the act of inhaling and exhaling; the movement of gas into and out of the lungs.

Recommended Readings

Andrews, M. (1991). *Voice therapy for children.* San Diego: Delmar Cengage Learning.

Andrews, M. (1995). *Manual of voice treatment: Pediatrics–geriatrics.*San Diego: Delmar Cengage Learning.

Arvedson, J., & Brodsky, L. (1993). *Pediatric swallowing and feeding: Assessment and management.* San Diego: Delmar Cengage Learning.

Burklow, K., Phelps, A., Schultz, J., McConnell, K., & Rudolph, C. (1998). Classifying complex pediatric feeding disorders. *Journal of Pediatric Gastroenterology and Nutrition, 27,* 143–147.

Charkins, H. (1996). *Children with facial difference: A parent's guide.* Bethesda, MD: Woodbine House.

Groher, M. (1997). *Dysphagia: Diagnosis and management* (3rd ed.). Stoneham, MA: Butterworth-Heinemann.

Kertoy, M., Guest, C., Quart, E., & Lieh-Lai, M. (1999). Speech and phonological characteristics of individual children with a history of tracheostomy. *Journal of Speech, Language and Hearing Research, 42,* 621–635.

Mathew O. P. (1988). Regulation of breathing pattern during feeding-role of suck, swallow and nutrients. In O. P. Mathew (Ed.), *Respiratory function of the upper airway.* New York: Marcel Dekker.

Morris, S. E. (1989). Development of oral-motor skills in the neurologically impaired child receiving non-oral feedings. *Dysphagia, 3,* 135–154.

Moungthong, G., & Holinger, L. (1997). Laryngotracheoesophageal clefts. *Annals of Otology, Rhinology and Laryngology, 106,* 12.

Nash, M. (1998). Swallowing problems in the tracheotomized patient. *Otolaryngologic Clinics of North America, 21,* 701–710.

Rosenthal, S., Sheppard, J., & Lotze, M. (Eds.). (1995). *Dysphagia and the child with developmental disabilities: Medical, clinical, and family interventions.* San Diego: Delmar Cengage Learning.

Rosing, H., & Peek, S. H. G. (1999). Swallowing and speech in infants following tracheotomy. *Acta Otorhinolaryngologica Belgica, 53,* 59–63.

Wilson, S. L., Thach, B. T., Brouillette, R. T., & Abu-Osbu, Y. K. (1980). Upper airway patency in the human infant: Influence of airway pressure and posture. *Journal of Applied Physiology, 48,* 500–504.

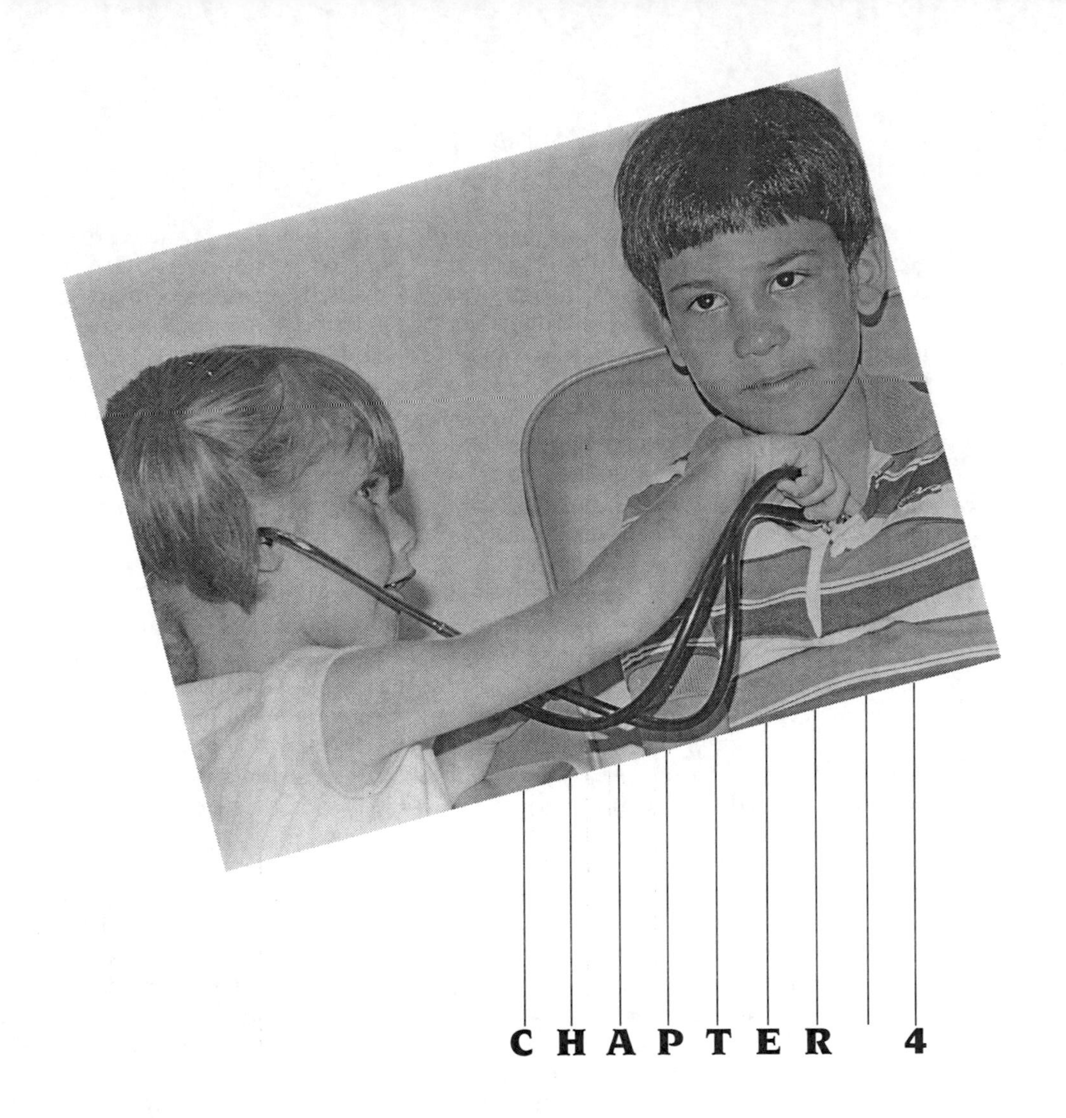

CHAPTER 4

A Clinical Perspective: The School-Age Child

Predictable voice changes related to age and gender occur during the maturation process. In addition to the normal vocal changes that occur throughout the life cycle, short-term and intermittent changes result from varied conditions and situations. For example, a voice may sound different first thing in the morning than it does at night. It may change in response to the weather, the seasons of the year, the amount and kind of use, overall fatigue, and one's feelings. A tremendous variety in vocal behavior falls within the normal range.

Individuals develop idiosyncratic ways of using their voices to express themselves, to initiate and maintain contact with others, to satisfy needs, and to control their world. Some people do a better job of this than others, and we are all refining our skills throughout life. Voice models influence our early vocal behavior a great deal. At first we imitate the voices of our parents and family members; later, the peer group assumes greater significance. Trial and error and the pattern of reinforcement operating in the home and school environment also have an effect. If children get what they want when they talk loudly, use a whining tone, or keep talking incessantly, they learn to perpetuate those vocal strategies. If their needs are frustrated, they sometimes try harder using the same technique (i.e., talking more loudly), or they may switch and try a different strategy. Families usually have identifiable vocal styles of interacting, as do school classes and most social groups. As children grow older and are exposed to a greater variety of groups and models, most of them learn to adjust their vocal style spontaneously according to the communication context. There are contextual and interpersonal constraints and rules that they learn and internalize.

Deviant Vocal Behavior

We do not know why some children with normal mechanisms habituate unproductive vocal behaviors, even when those strategies are repeatedly unsuccessful. Imitation of poor vocal models and faulty learning undoubtedly contribute in some cases. Other deviant patterns of voice production are the result of either short-term or permanent changes in the vocal mechanism. When the voice problem is related to anatomic or physiologic deviations of the vocal tract, the child frequently attempts to compensate. In some cases, this results in an overlay of additional deviant or even harmful vocal behaviors, and thus the problem becomes more complex and more difficult to evaluate. Unless a voice problem is the direct result of an obvious or severe organic abnormality of the mechanism, and we have specific medical information about the extent of the abnormality, it is perplexing to try to establish a direct cause–effect relationship concerning the etiology of a voice problem. Usually, many factors are operating simultaneously in precipitating and maintaining problems.

An example from our own experience may help illustrate this. We all have had periods in our lives when we kept talking even though our voices were not functioning normally. We may have been suffering from a cold or allergic reaction that caused swelling of our vocal folds and impeded their smooth vibratory pattern during phonation. At such times, we probably used more effort to adduct our swollen folds, coughed and cleared our throat frequently to get rid of the feeling of mucus on our folds, and strained to make ourselves heard. On some occasions, we may also have automatically continued these compensatory behaviors long after the original infection or allergic reaction had subsided. Eventually we could even have caused new irritation or swelling of the folds by continuing to overadduct, strain, talk too loudly, cough, and clear our throat. In other words, we may have eventually abused the voice mechanism by perpetuating behaviors that were no longer appropriate. If this occurred infrequently during our lives or if we quickly became aware of what we were doing and adapted our behavior, no long-term consequences were felt. If we were especially susceptible to upper respiratory tract infections, however, or suffered frequently from allergic reactions affecting the vocal tract, we may have set up a pattern of behavior that put us at risk for vocal problems. Children who are prone to allergic reactions (Frazier, 1978, has said that one in four children are allergic) or children who suffer from frequent infections are especially susceptible to vocal abuse secondary to their primary problem. The intermittent nature of the primary problem and the gradual habituation of the abusive behaviors across time tend to confound the clinical task of early diagnosis and treatment.

The Complexity of the Clinician's Task

The example just cited reminds us of one way in which the adoption of a pattern of compensatory behaviors may lead to a long-term vocal problem that was precipitated by a short-term or intermittent change in the vocal mechanism. This is just one example illustrating the complexity and interrelationship of vocal behaviors. Other symptom patterns are discussed in Chapter 8, which deals with assessment. At this point, however, it is clear that deviant vocal behavior cannot be considered in isolation. Children with voice disorders use their voices in a particular way, and this response pattern may be the result of the interplay of anatomic, physiologic, social, emotional, cognitive, or environmental factors. These children are operating in a context, and that context always needs to be considered. An analysis of the success a child achieves by the use of his or her voice to satisfy basic needs and drives is as important as the analysis of the specific vocal behaviors produced. The child who is not meeting basic needs because of the use of unproductive vocal behaviors can be motivated to change and adapt. One of the challenges of voice therapy with children is the task of analyzing each child's vocal interactions and assessing how well they are working. When children can be helped to understand why certain vocal strategies work for them and others do not, motivation to change is enhanced.

Although we have noted that the child with a voice disorder must be considered in context and that this child's vocal behavior is shaped by many factors, we have not yet discussed the specific task of focusing on the actual sound of the voice. The evaluation of an individual child's voice is difficult because of the transitory nature of voice patterns. In addition, the voice is the fleeting end product of a series of complex physiologic events. The larynx, or sound source, is not visible, and the voice itself is only one aspect of the total message transmitted to a listener. A clinician, listening to the voice of a child, first has to concentrate on separating the vocal patterns from the semantic content of the utterance then to attend to the individual parameters of the sound—pitch, loudness, quality, and timing. Later in this book, we discuss specific diagnostic procedures that are useful in evaluating these individual parameters. Because evaluation is a comparative task, it is helpful to remember that the more children's voices we have listened to, the easier it is for us to have a reliable set of auditory references available as we compare each new voice. This storehouse of experience, in addition to normative data gleaned from the literature, helps provide a context within which we can make judgments concerning what is an appropriate voice with respect to age and gender.

We have discussed the complexity of both normal and deviant vocal behavior and the way in which the human voice is a bridge between the individual and the world. We are aware that the child with a voice problem experiences difficulties not only in using his or her mechanisms effectively but in relating to others within his or her world.

Many clinicians believe that they need special qualities or skills to treat voice problems, yet we know that speech pathologists' skills are not disorder specific. All speech pathologists who understand basic anatomy and physiology and basic principles of programming have the potential to develop effective voice therapy programs for children. Clinicians who have the listening and discrimination skills to evaluate articulation disorders are certainly capable of applying the same skills in voice evaluations. Practice and experience are all that is needed to refine these skills.

A myth that needs to be addressed is that voice disorders are esoteric problems that can be treated only in a medical center. An extension of this idea is that a clinician in a school setting may possibly do harm to a child with a voice problem. Because a child spends most of the day at school, however, the school speech pathologist is in a unique position to coordinate the voice therapy program. The clinician will, of course, insist on a complete medical report and frequently will work as part of a team that includes otolaryngologists, psychologists, and so on. The team approach ensures that the clinician understands the exact nature of the problem and the type and extent of medical treatment provided or projected. But the school clinician is usually able to provide the kind of continuity of treatment and team support that supplements what is available in medical settings. The school environment provides special opportunities for the clinician to shape a child's vocal behavior in direct response to that child's everyday world.

Many of our fears and insecurities concerning voice disorders stem from our eagerness to do our best with these children. Because they represent varied symptom patterns, we are sometimes anxious if we encounter a child who seems different from those with whom we have worked before. Yet this variety can become an asset. It helps us to look at each child as a unique individual. There is certainly nothing mysterious about children with voice disorders. Each is different, but then so is every child.

How Voice Therapy With Children Differs From Therapy With Adults

An adult who enrolls in a voice therapy program usually is aware of the nature of the problem and can describe some of the ways that listeners respond to the voice disorder. Although in some cases the disruption in overall communicative effectiveness may not be understood fully, the adult usually presents with at least a partial understanding of the need for, and possible benefits of, intervention. Thus, in the initial phase of an adult voice therapy program, it usually is not necessary for a clinician to create an awareness of the problem or to demonstrate the need for therapy. The awareness phase of therapy can focus on developing a more complete understanding of the specific characteristics of the disorder and identifying the behaviors to be modified.

Children, on the other hand, particularly those of elementary school age, are frequently unaware that their voices are significantly different from those of their peers. It is not unusual for children with voice disorders to be unable to analyze the complex speech signal. Thus they may not even understand that meaning and feelings are communicated not only through the semantic context of words, but also through the voice used to express those words. Unless listeners' reactions to their voices have been extremely pointed or they have been teased by their peers, children also may not be aware of negative reactions. Therefore, in the beginning of a voice therapy program designed for elementary school children, the clinician frequently must spend considerable time teaching the children about vocal communication in general, and specifically about the characteristics of their own vocal behavior. Creating an awareness of the problem and definition of the possible benefits of therapy is frequently challenging and time consuming. If it is completed successfully, motivation can be enhanced, and momentum through subsequent therapy stages can be increased. It is critical to present the expected outcome of therapy in a way that is relevant to the child's current needs and daily life. Whereas an adult may be able to project that an improvement in voice may lead to increased satisfaction in personal or occupational relationships, a child may not automatically make this connection. Such an abstract generalization of the benefits of changing vocal behavior may seem unimportant to a child. The child's reality is in the present; future benefits or detriments may seem remote from everyday needs. For many children, and probably for most young children, cause–effect relationships need to be explicitly tied to situations that are concrete, current, and meaningful. For example, a young boy may be encouraged to change unproductive vocal behaviors if he can see that a different vocal strategy is more effective in getting what he wants from his parents, siblings, or playground peer group. Therefore, he may first need to be helped to identify what it is that he wants and needs; for instance, he wants to be liked, he wants to be able to persuade others, he wants other people to listen to what he is saying. If he first learns to analyze what he wants to achieve and how he can help or hinder his chances of success by the way he uses his voice in specific situations, he may then be helped to develop a personal rationale for change.

Therefore, one important difference between voice therapy for adults and that for children is the assumptions that we, as clinicians, hold as we approach therapy. Although we can reasonably assume that an adult client recognizes a problem exists, we cannot safely assume that a child understands this. Although we can assume most adults automatically know that an improvement in their voice is related to improvement in other areas of their life, this is not necessarily the case with children. Thus there is a very real difference in the way clinicians approach the task of planning the initial phase of a therapy program for children as opposed to that for adults. It is probably realistic to say that, in all cases, the awareness phase of a therapy program for children will take a longer period of time to accomplish. The relevance of the therapy goals and procedures to the everyday life of the child need to be stated more explicitly and tied to specific situations that are meaningful.

An integral part of the awareness phase of any voice therapy program is the introduction and explanation of descriptive terminology. Again, there are differences in what can be assumed by a clinician. Adults, unless they are intellectually handicapped, generally will have the prerequisite linguistic development to understand the meanings of most terms used in voice therapy. Specialized terminology also can be easily grasped by an adult when a clinician explains or demonstrates. Children in the early elementary school grades, however, may not have the linguistic development necessary for them to understand and use all the terms appropriately. Further discussion of the importance of gearing the language used in voice therapy to the developmental level of the child is found in Chapter 5. But it is important to emphasize here that there are significant differences between the way we communicate with children and adults during voice therapy. We frequently need to teach important linguistic concepts to children during the early stages of the therapy program.

An additional concern when we plan voice therapy programs for children is the importance of the role of the family and other significant adults. Rarely in the case of an adult client do we need to ensure that parents and teachers are actively involved in the therapy process. With the child client, the family's understanding and cooperation are essential. If, for example, the parent does not believe that a problem exists or refuses to cooperate in obtaining a medical examination, the clinician is faced with the additional task of attempting to change the parent's attitude if the child is to be helped. The enlistment of support from parents and teachers and the ongoing need for communication between the clinician and these significant adults are important aspects of voice therapy for children.

Another reason why contact with the child's family is important during the design and implementation of voice therapy programs for children is the part played by voice models. In arriving at an understanding of the factors precipitating or maintaining a child's voice problem, the clinician needs to hear how the parents use their voices. An adult client can tell us if people say he or she sounds "just like" a parent or other family member. The sound of a child's voice or the child's style of vocal interaction is frequently similar to that of a significant person in the environment, but the child may not be aware of this. The clinician working with children assumes a far larger role in the data-gathering process. Direct observation and analysis of the context in which the child operates at home and at school become tasks for the clinician. The child is not usually able to be the reliable informant that the adult client may be. During both assessment and therapy, the clinician works closely with the child's family and with school personnel. In most cases, the team approach is more critical to the success of therapy with children than it is with adults.

The charting of therapy progress is another area to consider in effective voice therapy for children. Task sequences need to be designed and described in a way that fits the developmental stage of the child. Specific concrete examples of the steps to be accomplished in achieving long-term goals need to be clearly laid out. The use of visual aids assumes great importance when a clinician discusses a child's progress. The adult may "know" when he or she is improving. The child needs frequent and tangible evidence of progress across time. Examples of charts and summaries that can help children see the steps to be accomplished can be found in later chapters. It is important to remember how specifically and concretely the behaviors need to be defined for children as they progress through the therapy program. The clinician must reduce complexity and abstractness of tasks so that children can focus on observable and discrete behaviors.

Children are different from adults. They are developing and changing as we work with them. Their development is much more dramatic and dynamic than adult development. Our therapy programs need to be designed with this fact in mind. Although many of the disorders exhibited by children and adults are similar with respect to symptom patterns, treatment approaches for children are different. They need to be designed so that they mesh with the child's developmental stage. Therapy tasks need to be relevant to the child's world, translated into the child's language, and tied to specific, concrete events and situations.

Justification for Intervention: Cost Benefits

Conservative estimates indicate that at least 6 to 9% of elementary school children have voice disorders and yet only about 1% of children on clinicians' caseloads are voice cases (Wilson, 1979). The discrepancy between the incidence percentages and the treatment percentages is puzzling. What is even more puzzling is that, although Wilson's study was completed a long time ago, this difference in the number of children needing services for voice problems and those receiving services still exists today. One possible reason for this discrepancy that is often discussed by clinicians is the difficulty in ensuring that a child is examined by a physician before enrollment in therapy. The recommendation that all voice cases be given a medical examination is certainly sensible and necessary. We know that vocal problems are sometimes symptoms of complex physical or emotional disorders. For example, a hoarse voice is sometimes associated with malnutrition or other health problems that increase susceptibility to upper respiratory tract infections. The possibility that the clinician's detection of vocal problems can, on occasion, result in a child's receiving attention for a major health problem alerts us to the need for accurate voice diagnosis and appropriate medical referrals. The benefits of early identification of children with voice problems are obvious, but there are practical difficulties. Medical examinations cost money, and they may not be covered by insurance. They are not available as part of school services and necessitate that the child's family schedule an examination with a physician. Of course, when a child's voice problem is severe or incapacitating, the question of the need for the medical examination is rarely debatable. Clinicians can be skillful in seeking out agencies and service clubs that may help. School personnel also may assist in helping to offset the expense incurred by families of limited means who are motivated to seek help for their child. The most provoking problems are likely to occur when a family does not perceive the need or does not consider the problem severe enough to warrant the medical expense. In such cases, or when the problem is a subtle one, a clinician is placed in an uncertain position. At such times, clinicians ask themselves such questions as, "How handicapping is the voice problem?" "Should I wait and see if it improves as the child gets older?" "How much time can I afford to spend counseling this

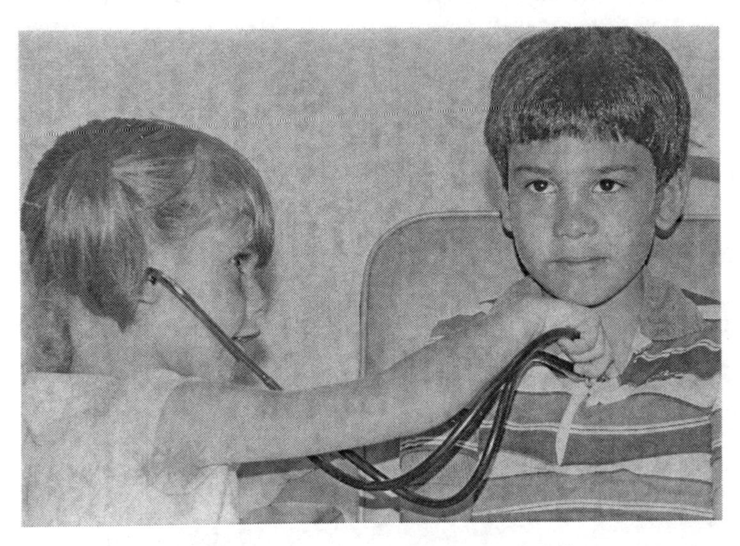

Role-playing a physician's examination is an excellent way to prepare children for a visit to the doctor.

family to persuade them to get help for their child?"

If the child in question has difficulties in addition to the voice problem, there is considerable temptation to assume that the vocal problem may indeed be the least pressing. In a hierarchy of priorities for treatment, there may seem to be other areas that need help first. If the child is presenting vocal problems only and is a high achiever in all other areas of performance, the temptation may be to assume that other strengths will compensate for the vocal symptoms.

Understandably, these reasons for failing to proceed with time-consuming and frustrating attempts to gain parent cooperation may seem attractive to a busy clinician. When a clinician has many children to serve and many parents to counsel, it may not appear to be cost efficient to persevere. Clinical experience suggests, however, that short-term costs may not be the only factor to consider. Chronic voice disorders rarely disappear without treatment. Unlike some developmental disorders of articulation, maturation alone does not seem significantly to affect vocal symptoms. The most striking example of a common and persistent vocal problem is that of vocal abuse, with which a cluster of identifiable vocal symptoms is associated. We are all familiar with the behavior of the child who uses too much effort to talk or talks too much. Such a child habituates a hyperfunctional pattern that in time may result in additive lesions on the vocal folds. Even if, as has sometimes been suggested, the lesions themselves disappear at puberty, the hyperfunctional vocal pattern may continue. Excessive effort and tension during vocalization, inappropriate interpersonal skills, and inefficient respiratory support during speech are liabilities that some children carry with them into high school and adult life.

Habituated maladaptive vocal behavior and styles of vocal interaction do not always disappear spontaneously. Some adults with voice disorders reveal a history of vocal abuse dating back to their elementary school years. Behaviors that have been habituated and over-learned across time are the most difficult to ameliorate. Thus the lack of early intervention may result in costly long-term consequences. The costs will be borne by the child and affect the individual's personal and professional development. They also may impinge on school personnel. The same child may be referred each year for testing. A series of classroom teachers may inquire about what is wrong with the child's voice. The music teacher may complain about and eventually exclude the child from the choir. A child who is a habitually loud or incessant talker may exhibit disruptive behavior throughout his or her school career. In extreme cases, such children are stigmatized as nuisances. A ripple effect occurs, and the fallout eventually obscures the root cause of the problem. Initially, some of these children may have been trying too hard, and so their efforts to communicate were misdirected and inefficient. Some vocal abusers seem especially eager to communicate. Unfortunately, this kind of child can easily become trapped in inappropriate habits that arose from an eagerness to talk and a need to be heard.

As we assess the cost effectiveness of voice programs, we may find ourselves listening to a child's voice problem and asking the question, "Could this child's voice be a liability in life?" Of course, we can neither see into the future nor be sure about the validity of our predictions. But many children will aspire to become professional voice users, for voice use is an important part of a great variety of occupations. Lawyers, ministers, physicians, salespeople, executives, teachers—members of these professions and others depend on their voices. In taking a long-term view of the benefits of effective voice therapy, it is surely important to ensure that children's future options are not restricted. A voice that draws attention to itself and results in negative listener reactions is a significant lifetime handicap, although at times an insidious one.

There is also the importance of the effect of vocal models to be considered. In occupations such as teaching, for example, a person with a voice problem may serve as a model for many children during an active career. It also may be reasonable to assume that the majority of children with voice disorders who do not receive treatment may grow up to be parents with voice disorders.

The Prevention of Voice Disorders in Children

Wilson (1987) found that the incidence of voice disorders reported in various studies ranges from 1% to 23.4%. Powell, Filter, and Williams (1989) screened children aged 6 to 10 years in a rural school division and found 23.9% of their 203 children showed voice deviation. Revaluations in two subsequent years showed that 39.9% of those initially evaluated still had disorders 1 year later; 4 years later the disorders were still present in 38% of the children retested.

Although it is well documented in the literature that a significant number of school-age children have voice disorders (Baynes, 1966; Senturia & Wilson, 1968; Shearer, 1972; Silverman & Zimmer, 1972; Warr-Leeper, McShea, & Leeper, 1979; Wilson, 1979), it also is clear that many of these children do not actaully receive voice therapy. Some of the reasons for this discrepancy between incidence and treatment have been discussed already. Clinicians may not feel as comfortable with voice cases as they do with other kinds of cases because of the nature of their training. There are also problems involved in convincing parents of the importance of seeking help (Baynes, 1966; Cook, Polski & Hanson, 1979; Wilson, 1979) and difficulties involved in obtaining medical examinations. Teachers' awareness of differences in vocal behavior among children also varies significantly and contributes to the quite small number of children that they refer for evaluation and treatment (Diehl & Stinnett, 1959; Wilson, 1979). In addition, as Mowrer (1978) and Nilson and Schneiderman (1983) have suggested, children who have voice problems that do not dramatically affect their academic performance in the classroom may not be considered by their teachers to be eligible for services. As noted in the previous section, the effect of hoarseness and other vocal symptoms is often insidious rather than dramatic but can certainly limit the achievement of full potential.

Education of classroom teachers through personal and public discussion and through in-service programs needs to be vigorously pursued; not only are classroom teachers important in identifying children with difficulties and as models of vocal behavior, but they are a population that is at risk for voice problems. Deal, McClain, and Sudderth (1976) showed that in-service training and direct instruction enhanced teachers' abilities to identify hoarseness and vocal abuse in children. It is likely that teachers who participate in programs of this kind benefit additionally from an increased awareness of vocal hygiene as it applies to their own vocal practices.

Nilson and Schneiderman (1983) reported on a successful educational program to prevent vocal abuse and misuse developed and presented to second and third graders in a public elementary school. The program taught basic information concerning the vocal mechanism, discrimination of voice qualities and identification of abusive and compensatory behaviors. Teachers were asked to remain in their classrooms during the times the program was implemented. They also were tested subsequently, and their awareness of the parameters of voice was compared with that of teachers who had not participated in the program. Results showed a significant difference between teachers who participated and those who did not, thus demonstrating the efficacy of the approach. The teacher participants were positive about the program, supported carryover activities, and receptive to future programs. This report and others dealing with similar activities (Cook et al., 1979; Deal, McClain, & Sudderth, 1976; Blonigen, 1978) emphasize the importance of educating school personnel in the basic principles of vocal hygiene.

One specialist group of teachers that is knowledgeable and concerned about vocal behavior and that provides an additional resource for speech-language pathologists in the schools are the music teachers. In a program conducted in the Monroe County schools in Bloomington, Indiana, it was found that a speech–language pathologist and a music specialist working as a team were considerably more effective in identifying children with vocal abuse, in educating classroom teachers about these problems, and in conferring with parents than when they approached the tasks individually. The advantages of this team approach are that the child's vocal pattern can be described in terms of both speaking and singing and that the two professionals can coordinate a more comprehensive program of intervention. Additional benefits are that vocal screenings and vocal hygiene lessons can be combined with music lessons and choir activities, and increased communication and heightened awareness occurs among all school personnel. In some schools in Monroe County, the interest in working as a team in the area of vocal abuse has resulted in requests that the music teacher and the speech–language pathologist be scheduled to work in the same schools on the same days. In one school, the speech–language pathologist regularly conducts, during choir rehearsal periods, a voice therapy group for children with vocal abuse who are excluded from choir.

The American Speech and Hearing Association statement (1974), and other statements in recent years, encouraged speech–language pathologists to engage in activities to prevent communication disorders in children. Flynn (1983) has presented some specific ideas showing how a philosophy concerning the necessity for prevention can be translated into positive strategies. She mentioned that activities should be designed to reflect Katz, McDonald, and Stuckey's (1972) three levels of preventive activity. Let us consider these three levels and the ways in which speech–language pathologists can initiate activities related to the area of voice. We will review many of Flynn's (1983) suggestions.

The *tertiary level* of preventive activity includes all activities carried out to alleviate existing disorders. We have already seen that much still remains to be accomplished at this level. Specifically, training programs in universities and colleges need to strengthen the preparation provided for students in the area of vocal rehabilitation. Students in training need to be exposed to a greater variety of clinical training experiences with voice cases. More research needs to be completed to increase our understanding of normal and disordered vocal behavior. Testing procedures need to be improved and standardized. Our aim should be to improve our therapeutic skills in the area of voice disorders of children so that we narrow the gap between the incidence and treatment figures.

The *secondary level* involves activities related to early detection. If problems are detected in their early stages, it is reasonable to assume that remediation is quicker and easier. Activities that help teachers and school personnel recognize the early symptoms of vocal problems are significant at this level. Programs that improve collaboration with other specialists (e.g., classroom teachers, otolaryngologists, music teachers) are helpful in this regard.

Nevertheless, it is at the *primary level* of prevention that most work still needs to be done. A focus on primary (before the fact) preventive activity is obviously the most positive and economic approach. The general public, school personnel, parents, and children need to be exposed to information that will heighten awareness of the importance of good vocal hygiene and preventive strategies for voice conservation. Populations who are at risk for vocal problems (e.g., professional voice users, people who suffer from allergic conditions affecting the vocal tract, individuals with a family history of voice problems, cheerleaders) need information that will alert them to their susceptibility. We need to disseminate information in a variety of ways. Materials need to be prepared (articles, pamphlets, films), and programs need to be presented (at in-service training sessions for teachers, during classroom science lessons, at science fairs, at career days, during health lessons, and as part of disability-awareness activities). Specifically, we need to educate ourselves, the general public, and the children we teach by explicitly discussing the importance of vocal health and ways in which vocal health can be jeopardized. Environmental considerations of noise level and pollution; the effects of stress on the vocal mechanism; the structure of the mechanism itself; and common illnesses, injuries, and accidents that affect the voice are other issues that need to be addressed. The creative clinician will find many opportunities to develop and disseminate information relating to the prevention of voice disorders in children.

Susceptibility: Conditions of the Upper Respiratory Tract

We have noted that alterations in the vocal tract that occur as the result of medical conditions can heighten a child's susceptibility. Conditions that occur repeatedly or that result in compensations that are habituated across time are especially significant in precipitating voice problems. Children who experience frequent allergic reactions or upper respiratory tract infections are particularly at risk, especially if their lifestyle includes many vocally demanding activities. Normal reflexive activities, such as coughing and sneezing, if they occur repeatedly because of congestion or irritation, may also become habituated and result in damage to the vocal mechanism. With this in mind, let us consider some of the medical conditions that occur frequently in elementary school children and contribute to susceptibility.

Upper Respiratory Tract Structures

Before turning our attention to the specific conditions that may occur, it may be useful to review some general information concerning the upper respiratory tract.

The entire pathway from the lungs, bronchi, trachea, through the larynx, pharynx, oral cavity, and nasal cavity is continuous and lined throughout with moist mucous membrane. In addition, the pathway to the middle ear, the eustachian tube, is also connected to the respiratory tract, because the eustachian tube opening is located in the nasopharynx. Because of the continuity between structures and the interrelationship that exists, upper respiratory tract conditions tend to spread readily and affect changes throughout the entire pathway.

Infection

The suffix *itis* means redness, heat, and swelling. Words ending in this suffix are frequently used to describe changes in the upper respiratory tract. It is not uncommon for an individual to contract, for example, an infection that attacks the nasal cavities and to experience rhin*itis* or sinus*itis*. If there is a discharge that causes a postnasal drip, the infection and irritation of the tissues may spread and result in pharyng*itis*, laryng*itis*, or maybe even bronch*itis*. Vigorous nose blowing may also force an infection to spread into the eustachian tube and middle ear cavity, resulting in ot*itis* media. The sequence or progression of an infection varies, of course, but the location of the discomfort rarely is confined to one area of the continuous respiratory tract. Swelling of the tissues and an excess of secretions usually accompanies infections. The tonsils, located between the faucial arches on either side of the mouth cavity, and the adenoids in the nasopharynx are frequently affected. These structures are made up of lymphatic tissue, and as part of the body's defense mechanism, they play a role in helping prevent bacteria from invading the system. At times they become enlarged, and when they are infected, we can often see the redness, increased size, and even white flecks of pus on the tonsils when we inspect the mouth cavity of an individual who has tonsill*itis* or adenoid*itis*. When the adenoids are very swollen, they may even press on the eustachian tube opening, causing that opening to be blocked. This prevents free circulation of air into the middle ear. In such cases, or if there is congestion blocking the tube, we say that it is no longer "patent," or open. Enlarged adenoids may also block the nasopharynx to such an extent that the individual has difficulty breathing through the nose and has to resort to relying completely on mouth breathing until the swelling subsides.

There are three kinds of infection: viral, bacterial, and fungal. Frequently, children experience a sore throat as the first symptom of diseases caused by all kinds of infection. A sore throat may be a symptom of a serious bacterial infection, such as bacterium beta hemolytic streptococcus ("strep"). If a sore throat is associated with a high fever, headache, and swollen glands in the neck, it may be due to a strep infection. A diagnosis of strep is based on a throat culture (today more rapid tests for strep are also available). In addition to the throat culture, an examination by a physician is essential for an accurate diagnosis. If a diagnosis of strep or some other bacterium is made, the patient can be treated with antibiotic therapy. This can be administered in injection form or taken orally. If taken orally, it is critical that the patient not stop taking the medication when the symptoms disappear. Medication must be continued as prescribed for the entire period (usually 10 days) advised by the physician. The physician may take another culture at the completion of the full course of antibiotics to ensure that the infection has cleared completely.

Sore throats or other symptoms of the upper respiratory tract that are not caused by a bacterial infection are usually the result of viral infections. Whereas the symptoms of bacterial infections tend to appear suddenly, the symptoms of viral infections usually start slowly. There is often a feverish feeling, loss of appetite, headache, dry cough, and runny nose associated with the onset of a viral infection. One virus that causes frequent sore throats in children and is common during the summertime is herpangina. A child's temperature may soar, and the patient may complain of a reduced energy level and very painful raised sores at the back of the mouth. Symptoms usually disappear by the 4th day.

Although such symptoms as sore throats are common (the most common cause is viral infection), it is important to be vigilant when children complain of such symptoms. A sore throat may reflect something as mild as a common cold or as serious as leukemia, tuberculosis, or infectious mononucleosis. Consequently, any one of the following warning signs warrants a prompt call to a physician: (a) a severe sore throat or one that causes the child to have difficulty swallowing, (b) a sore throat that has persisted longer than a week, (c) a temperature of more than 102° Fahrenheit for children under 8 and 100° for older children, (d) difficulty breathing, (e) soreness accompanied by coughing or hoarseness (f) episodes of similar soreness that have recurred several times in recent weeks, (g) a past history of rheumatic fever. Although all of the above conditions do not necessarily mean that the child has a serious illness, they do suggest that the condition merits medical attention.

We have discussed some of the symptoms and implications of sore throats in detail to provide a framework of reference that may be useful for a speech–language pathologist. During the process of evaluation of children with atypical voices, the clinician needs to consider the length of time children have had problems and the possibility of recurrent infections. Through discussions with the classroom teacher and with parents, the clinician may discover indications that suggest that the child's vocal symptoms may be related to his or her general state of health. As noted, a malnourished child or one with chronic physical problems may experience recurrent upper respiratory infections that are secondary to a more serious health problem. If a clinician suspects that this may be the case, vigorous attempts should be made to persuade the parents to obtain medical help.

Allergies and Asthma

According to the Task Force on Allergic Disorders, allergies are responsible for two million lost school days every year in the United States. This task force issued its 300-page *Allergy Report* summarizing standardized information on the diagnosis and treatment of 13 common allergic conditions, including allergic rhinitis and asthma. It can be accessed at the Web site of the Task Force: *www. aaaai.org*. Dr. Gary S. Rachelefsky, cochair of the Task Force, notes that allergies are serious disorders that should be managed by a physician and not by over-the-counter medications.

Physicians who specialize in the treatment of allergies are highly trained. After completing medical school, those who plan to treat allergies in children complete 3 years training in pediatrics and must then pass the examination given by the American Board of Pediatrics. They then apply to 1 of the 78 U.S. training programs in allergy and immunology for study for another 2 or 3 years. Approximately half of this training is devoted to learning to evaluate, diagnose, and manage disorders involving the immune system. Physicians work with patients who have hay fever, asthma, eczema, hives, and adverse reactions to drugs, foods, or insect bites and stings. They also research the medical literature relevant to their specialty and study nose, throat, and skin reactions and diseases. Thus, these specialists, upon completion of their studies and clinical training, are well qualified and the best medical professionals to provide comprehensive care. In fact, studies have shown that children under the care of an allergist or immunologist make fewer visits to emergency rooms and are better equipped to manage the everyday challenges associated with their allergies and asthma.

Professional groups, such as the American Academy of Allergy, Asthma, and Immunology, the largest professional medical specialty organization representing allergists, clinical immunologists, allied health professionals, and others with a special interest in allergy, are working to raise public awareness and disseminate information (*www. fromcausetocure.com*). They want people to know that more than 50 million Americans suffer from allergies. For some, it is a minor inconvenience; for others, it can lead to disabling or even fatal asthma attacks.

An allergy is a specific immunologic reaction to a normally harmless substance, such as pollen, mold spores, or foods that do not bother most people. Some people may also be sensitive to other substances such as nickel, latex rubber, or insect venom. Scientists now believe that the tendency to develop allergies is inherited.

The immune system acts as a defense against bacteria, viruses, and other harmful substances. When a child is allergic, however, the immune system causes the problem because it treats the allergen as the invader by generating large amounts of immunoglobulin E (or IgE) that is a unique type of antibody. Interestingly, children with allergies have an IgE antibody on their mast cells that can identify each substance to which they are allergic. Once the allergen is encountered, the mast cells release chemicals (histamine, cytokines, and leukotrienes), which act on targeted tissues to cause the allergic reactions.

Voice clinicians need to be knowledgeable about allergens because so many allergic reactions occur in the respiratory tract and may affect the air supply for voicing, the tissues in the larynx itself or the epiglottis, pharynx, mouth, or nasal cavities. Swelling, inflammation, the production of copious secretions and compensatory adjustments of structures, as well as repetitive reflexes such as coughing and sneezing, may be involved. Respiratory, phonatory, resonatory, and articulatory signs and symptoms may be observed in afflicted children. Additionally, even in children with mild allergic reactions of the respiratory tract, there may be a susceptibility to voice disorders if compensatory behaviors lead to abuse or misuse of irritated structures.

It is also important for clinicians to be aware that some children develop asthma if allergens and the chemicals that are released in reaction to them irritate the sensitive lining of airways in the lungs themselves. The airways then become inflamed and narrower, and excess mucus is produced, causing a feeling of tightness in the chest, the sound of wheezing, and frequent coughing. The incidence of asthma is increasing in the United States. Now more than 17 million Americans of all ages have this serious respiratory disease, at least twice the number reported in 1988. The National Institutes of Health report that the greatest increase in asthma has been noted in children of less than 10 years of age where the incidence has increased 72% since 1988. More female and African Americans seem to be victims of asthma than male and white Americans. Experts are trying to identify reasons for this as well as for the dramatic increase in incidence. Most agree that there is probably a genetic predisposition to asthma, but that environmental triggers seem to precipitate attacks.

Dr. William W. Busse, president of the American Academy of Allergy, Asthma, and Immunology, quoted in *The New York Times Magazine* (March 19, 2000) said: "The immune system also may play a major role in setting the stage. One of the great mysteries is why children who have measles and chicken pox and last-born children subject to numerous viral infections passed on to them by older siblings don't develop asthma." It may be that there is some critical point in a child's development when the immune system is activated by having to repel infectious diseases, such as the common childhood diseases of measles and chicken pox. If, for instance, a child does not contract these common diseases, maybe because of vaccinations or even lack of exposure, the immune system is not turned on. Rather, one theory suggests, substances such as animal dander, dust mites, pollen, or environmental pollution and cigarette smoke may turn it on. It has been noted that more children are admitted to emergency rooms in hospitals at times when pollution levels are high. Reactions to environmental allergens seem to play a major role in the subsequent development of asthma because at least 80% of asthma patients are allergic to one or more allergens. Exposure and sensitization to house dust mites has been specifically implicated to the development of severe asthma symptoms in children.

There is also a relationship between physical exercise and asthma. Exercise-induced asthma is a temporary narrowing of the airways in the lungs, and it has been estimated that 80 to 90% of asthma sufferers breathe with difficulty during vigorous exercise (Edelman, 1997). This condition also may occur in children who do not develop symptoms at any other time except when exercising. About half of those with exercise-induced asthma have allergic rhinitis (hay fever).

Recent research indicated that exercise that facilitates muscle tone, a stronger heart, and increased stamina could be safe and beneficial for individuals with asthma. Nonetheless, the American Lung Association recommends that guidance from physicians is needed. The federal government's National Asthma Education and Prevention Program includes specific provisions for managing exercise-induced asthma. It may be that increased demand for oxygen by the heart and other vital organs during physical exertion causes the lungs to work faster, which then makes the airways cooler and dryer. If the airways are chronically inflamed already because of allergy, they are hypersensitive to cool and dry air. The mast cells in the airways then react by releasing chemicals that trigger asthma. Some activities, such as those that involve only brief episodes of exertion, are less disruptive to the airways. Walking and weight training may be less likely to result in exercise-induced asthma then running or soccer, which require deep, rapid breathing for extended periods. Symptoms of exercise-induced asthma may include:

- Wheezing
- Tightness in chest
- Shortness of breath
- Coughs
- Chest congestion
- Feeling winded after exercise
- Feeling out of shape
- Paradoxical vocal fold motion (gasping for air because the laryngeal valve spasms and is not wide open during inhalation)

Guidelines to observe for participation in exercise:

- Consult a qualified physician.
- Carefully select and plan exercise opportunities.
- Avoid cold, dry air (indoors or outdoors).
- Avoid exercise when air pollution indexes are high.
- Avoid exposure to high pollen count.
- Avoid fresh mown grass and dust.
- Avoid strong scents (e.g., people wearing perfume).
- Don't exercise during recovery from a cold.
- Don't exercise during an asthma attack.
- Warm up and cool down to decrease possibility of attacks.
- Drink fluids to keep the air pathways moist.

Caregivers should consult with a physician about the child's exercise regime and medications. Certain prescribed medications taken before periods of exercise can help asthma patients prevent symptoms. For example, individuals who have well-controlled asthma may be advised by their physician to take several puffs of their beta-adrenergic medications 10 to 15 minutes before exercising to open their air passages. Others may be advised to inhale several puffs of antiinflammatories before physical exercise. Although regular exercise is not a cure for asthma, it can be used judiciously to improve overall fitness. According to Dr. Norman H. Edelman (1997) of the American Lung Association, if the child is under the care of a physician who is trained in this specialty, carefully planned management of exercise is possible and can result in less troublesome exercise-induced asthma.

Not only is education important for parents and caregivers, but children's emotional distress about their allergy and asthma attacks can be greatly reduced by educational opportunities provided by allied health professionals and teachers. As children mature and have the cognitive skills to understand basic concepts concerning their breathing and factors that affect it, they need to be taught this information. Knowledge about their condition and how to manage it empowers them to take responsibility, thereby reducing their feelings of insecurity and fear.

Even preschool children can be taught about "easy breathing" versus "hard breathing" and the behavioral characteristics associated with both patterns. Older children can be taught basic anatomy and physiology and ways to avoid triggers that cause severe attacks. Voice clinicians can help them learn the relationships between what they do in reaction to difficult breathing situations and the expected outcome. They can teach children to avoid strenuous use of their voices when their allergies are causing their voice mechanism to be susceptible to irritation and abuse. Compensatory techniques can be defined and compared. For example, a comparison of coping strategies may include:

Good Tricks	Bad Tricks
Stay calm.	Panic or getting frightened.
Take slow, deep breaths.	Take quick, tense breaths.
Tell an adult.	Cry.
Open and relax the throat.	Stiffen and tense the throat.
Ask an adult about medicine.	Have hysterics.
Think about the triggers.	Forget what triggers an attack.
Use self-talk (e.g., I can cope with this).	Think: "I can't get my breath."
Keep a diary of symptoms and times.	Don't think about cause and effect.
Exercise indoors when pollen count is high.	Exercise whenever you like.

Gastroesophageal Reflux

Specialists are less likely to vigorously pursue the cause of hoarseness in children compared with adults. Often it is assumed that a child suffers from phonotrauma, forgoing aggressive exploration of alternative causative factors. This is because malignancies are rare in children, and it is more difficult to complete full laryngoscopic examinations than it is with adult patients. Additionally, some observers believe that children will "grow out of it" or see hoarseness as inconsequential. During the last 2 decades, however, reflux has been found to cause chronic laryngeal symptoms such as cough, sore throat, hoarseness, throat clearing, and globus (the feeling of a lump in the throat). Twenty-four-hour esophageal pH monitoring has increasingly become the gold standard for documenting reflux in adults. Monitoring over a long period of time increases the physician's chances of making accurate diagnoses. Nonetheless, pH monitoring is used infrequently with children who have otolaryngologic disorders, yet pathogenic reflux in children has been implicated in acute laryngitis, recurrent croup, stridor, obstructive sleep apnea, laryngospasm, and cough (Contencin, 1995). Gumpert, Kalach, Dupont, and Contencin (1998a) studied 21 children aged between 2 and 14 with a mean age of 8 who had been hoarse for more than 3 months. All had posterior laryngoscopic findings suggestive of reflux: interarytenoid erythema (redness) and edema (swelling), granuloma or nodule formation, or both. None of these patients were known to have the classic symptoms of reflux: emesis (vomiting), dysphagia, rumination (nonfunctional chewing), belching, choking, gagging, failure to thrive, heartburn, indigestion, sour taste in mouth, cough, or nocturnal awakening. After otolaryngologic exam, the children were transferred to gastroenterology for dual channel pH monitoring. Of the 21 hoarse children, 13 (62%) had pathologic reflux between 0–2% and 62.7%. Most of the documented refluxes occurred when the children were awake. They had frequent diurnal refluxes, ranging from 0.4 to 37.4 refluxes per hour. The median number of refluxes per hour while they were awake was 14.8 compared with 0.9 refluxes per hour when they were asleep. Four children with severe reflux were both supine and upright refluxers, however. In the children with mild to moderate reflux disease, the episodes were frequent but of short duration (i.e., less than 5 minutes). Those children with severe reflux disease had frequent short refluxes but also demonstrated a greater number lasting more than 5 minutes.

Reflux is common in infants and children, with a prevalence in newborns of between 20 to 40% (Heymans, 1996, cited in Gumpert et al., 1998b). Heymans has postulated that it is usually a benign, self-limiting problem in infancy and early childhood but that it can result in serious problems on occasion. The Gumpert et al. study provides evidence that in ear, nose, and throat (ENT) patients, reflux does not present with esophagitis and its symptoms but is a different pattern, often occult and intermittent from day to day. Children in this study appeared to tolerate the pH monitoring remarkably well. Gumpert et al. reported that there is an absence of data in the scientific literature about the effectiveness of antireflux treatments. Most studies have included such measures as raising the head of the bed and antacids. As Kamel et al. (1994) noted, however, it is erroneous to assume that laryngeal manifestations of the disease parallel esophageal manifestations because these two epithelia have different reactions to the exposure to acid. Dejonckere (1999) has suggested that flexible transnasal endoscopes with a small diameter (2.1 mm) are optimally suited for accurate endoscopic diagnosis, especially when combined with video recording and stroboscopy for obtaining laryngeal examinations on children.

Some Reflexive Behaviors

We have reviewed some conditions that can affect the continuous pathway between the nose, mouth, and lungs. When we inhale, the air is filtered by the cilia (hairs) in the nose and warmed and moistened by the mucous membrane that lines the entire passageway down to the lungs. When we exhale, the air travels from the lungs through the bronchi into the trachea (windpipe) and through the valvelike larynx, to be emitted finally through the mouth and nose. The respiratory tract is protected by various reflexive mechanisms, and the primary biologic function of the larynx is to act as a protective valve to prevent foreign bodies from entering the lower airway.

One protective reflex is that sudden glottal closure that occurs when an individual is suddenly plunged into water. This immersion reflex, as it is sometimes described, protects the airway from the entry of water into the lungs. We have all felt the movement of this laryngeal reflex when we have suddenly been jolted downward in an elevator. We also are aware of the sudden closure reflex activated when it is necessary to build up subglottal air pressure preliminary to sudden exertion associated with lifting, pushing, or pulling. When force needs to be exerted, the laryngeal valve closes abruptly to stabilize the thorax to facilitate the necessary action.

Biologic functions of the larynx are of interest to the voice clinician for more than one reason. A diagnostician may check to see if a child who is not phonating can use the larynx for nonspeech functions, for example. A child with aphonia associated with emotional difficulties will usually exhibit appropriate responses during nonspeech activities. In some children with severe central nervous system impairment, however, reflexive behavior may be affected. In addition, the frequency of occurrence of certain reflexes, such as coughing and sneezing, may be helpful in indicating health problems. Coughing and sneezing help rid the respiratory tract of irritating or potentially dangerous substances. When nerve cells in the nose sense an irritating substance, they send a message to the medulla. This part of the brain controls breathing and swallowing. A series of involuntary spasmodic reactions is set into motion. There is a quick, deep inhalation, and the abdominal muscles contract and push against the diaphragm. Then there is a sudden explosive exhalation propelling air through nose and mouth at a rapid speed to expel the irritant. This process is repeated until the irritant is eliminated. Coughing may also be a symptom of underlying respiratory conditions such as allergies and asthma and also of reflux disease.

The Relevance of Respiratory Difficulties to Voice Disorders

During interviews with parents, it is important that the speech–language pathologist ask questions geared specifically to obtaining information concerning a child's history of medical conditions of the respiratory tract and treatment procedures that may have affected the airway. The airway may be obstructed by foreign bodies, excessive mucus, swollen tissues, or congenital deformity. Today, many critically ill children survive a variety of serious illnesses that formerly would have proved fatal because physicians can provide prolonged assistance to breathing. Ventilation is initiated through an endotracheal tube, and because of greater use of this treatment for longer periods of time, there has also been an increase in laryngeal injury. The injury may be temporary and reversible (as is often seen in premature infants treated for respiratory distress in intensive-care units), but the potential for an iatrogenic stenosis of the airway does exist (Henry, Pashley, & Fan, 1983). Injury of the vocal folds and of the subglottal airway can occur, and Noyce (1983) reported that injuries occuring during intubation of the infants may be due to the shape of the infant subglottis. He studied 45 neonatal and infant larynges and found that the subglottal area varied significantly in shape from the vocal folds down to the lower border of the cricoid cartilage. The subglottal area below the vocal folds is elliptical in shape, but this shape changes until it is circular at the lower border of the cricoid cartilage. The size and shape of the endotracheal tube inserted into the airway is therefore an important consideration for physicians dealing with infants. Subglottal injuries can lead to a serious narrowing or stenosis of the airway. When children cannot be intubated successfully, the therapeutic alternative is tracheotomy. This procedure involves the insertion of a tracheostomy tube to allow the patient to be ventilated through a stoma in the anterior neck. This procedure is used frequently in cases where there is progressive glottal injury as a result of intubation or severe obstruction. An example of a condition that is treated by tracheotomy is acute epiglottitis. In this condition, airway obstruction occurs as a result of enlargement of the epiglottis.

Simon, Fowler, and Handler (1983) studied the communication development of 77 children aged 2 months to 7 years with long-term tracheostomies. All were aphonic and consequently deprived of speech experience for extended periods while tracheostomized. Twenty-three were studied postdecannulation. They found that children with long-term tracheostomies can develop speech and language skills commensurate with intellectual functioning despite extended periods of deprivation of babbling. Monitoring and follow-up are important in ensuring identification of later problems in vocal quality and breath support. Direct speech–language therapy for the linguistically mature child, including use of alternative communication modalities, was crucial in decreasing frustration and maximizing skill. The role of the speech–language pathologist in relation to the tracheostomized child has been specifically described by Simon and Handler (1981).

During the history-taking portion of the voice evaluation, the clinician should be alert for indications such as respiratory distress suffered following birth, periods of time in intensive-care units, and surgical and medical procedures that could have affected the laryngeal or tracheal structures. If information given by parents suggests that the child may have been intubated during infancy or childhood, it is important to request a medical report providing details of any possible residual effects on the phonatory system.

As more and more children survive serious illnesses as a result of improved neonatal and pediatric medical care, the clinician's responsibility to obtain the medical history assumes greater importance. We also may be seeing more children with permanent tracheotomies. Most frequently, the tracheotomy is a temporary condition, but occasionally, if an airway obstruction persists (as in the case of malformation of structures or chronic illness), a child may be forced to continue breathing through a tracheostomy tube. Sometimes the tracheotomy will be kept open to suction mucus and secretions from the airway at periodic intervals. In these instances the opening may be closed most of the time, and the child will be able to phonate normally when it is closed. When the child is forced to breathe through the trach tube all of the time because of a long-term problem, medical and educational management is more complex. In such cases, the speech–language pathologist will need accurate information concerning the child's potential for voice usage. If the larynx is normal, the child may be taught to phonate by using a finger to occlude the stoma during exhalation so that phonation may occur. If the child can use a speaking valve, such as the Passy-Muir valve, this option is preferable. If the child exhibits malformation of the laryngeal structures or other conditions that prohibit normal phonation, consultation with the child's physician and a team approach to treatment is necessary. In such cases the use of an artificial larynx, sign language, or an electronic device may be appropriate alternatives to oral communication.

Schoen, Gill, and Wallace (1983) described a program in southeast Los Angeles for healthy school-age children with tracheostomies. These children attended regular public schools and participated in most activities (excluding those in sand and water). Speech–language clinicians worked with teachers, specially trained nurses, and parents. Special in-service training sessions were conducted to teach tracheostomy care. The description of this program development and the protocols that were established provide excellent guidelines for the speech–language clinician faced with the problem of helping a child with a permanent tracheostomy.

The majority of the children we evaluate, however, will suffer from less dramatic medical conditions that may nevertheless be relevant to their vocal symptoms. Children who suffer from allergies and asthma may have periodic partial occlusion of the airway that affects their airflow during phonation. In such instances, the clinician should seek medical information concerning the conditions, the type of medication prescribed, and the possible effect of the condition on phonatory behavior. The effects of excessive mucus, vocal-fold edema, intermittent or persistent irritation that may increase reflexive coughing and sneezing, and dryness of structures related to specific medications taken may be important considerations. Goldstein and Abramson (1983) reported on airway obstruction in the lung that was due to allergy. This is an uncommon pediatric problem where an abnormally viscid mucoid plug, mimicking a foreign body, obstructs the endobronchial airway and must be removed surgically. Frequently, but not always, the patient has a history of asthma. After bronchoscopic removal of the obstruction, a complete allergy evaluation is necessary.

Kero et al. (1983) reported on the treatment of children who had inhaled foreign bodies in the tracheobronchial tree. In the management of foreign bodies, bronchoscopy is the method of choice, but sometimes postural drainage, tracheostomy, and other surgical treatments are needed. Many children experience edema and trauma to the larynx subsequent to the bronchoscopy. There may be quite a long asymptomatic period of months or even years between time of inhalation of a foreign body and development of symptoms. Spasmodic coughing and choking are the most frequent symptoms, and inspiratory stridor may be present as well. Symptoms may subside or recur intermittently. Such examples remind us that if we observe children who appear to have respiratory difficulties that persist, who have trouble phonating when they are engaged in physical exertion that requires additional air expenditure, or who have problems regulating a smooth, even exhalation, we should ensure that a medical referral is made.

Voice symptoms may be residuals of earlier trauma sustained by the laryngeal mechanism, or they may be indications of more comprehensive medical conditions. The clinician frequently will encounter children whose past medical history and present medical management will be critical to a comprehensive evaluation of the voice disorder. An understanding of the significance of medical conditions and treatments affecting respiratory and phonatory function is therefore important for the speech–language clinician who must seek and interpret medical information.

Additionally, persistent or recurrent alternations in the respiratory or phonatory structures (or both) may predispose a child to adopt compensatory behaviors that, if habituated, may be abusive or distracting. When a clinician considers such behaviors as throat clearing, coughing, excessive tension during phonation, it is helpful if he or she is knowledgeable about underlying conditions that may predispose, precipitate, or maintain maladaptive vocal behaviors. Children who suffer from chronic infections, allergies, asthmatic conditions, or reflux may be at risk for developing hyperfunctional patterns of vocal behavior. When voice symptoms occur in association with such conditions, the clinician will need to make sure that medical care is part of the total management program.

Vocal Competence: An Aspect of Communication Competence

There is no evidence that, as a group, children with voice disorders have problems with linguistic competence, and if we suspect that they may have problems in this area, tests are available to help us diagnose their specific difficulty. Another area of competence is more difficult to test formally: the area of communicative competence, or the knowledge of the more social aspects of interpersonal communication. Subsumed under this is the knowledge of the role vocal behavior plays in determining the form and substance of communication messages. Children must learn, for example, when to talk and when to remain silent and when certain kinds of vocalization are appropriate or inappropriate. They learn such rules of communication by observing others, imitating others, through explicit instruction, and by trial and error. Some children have learned these rules better than others. Some children, for example, abuse their voices continually, maybe because they have never learned to adjust their vocal volume to particular situations. Thus, they talk in a quiet library at the same loudness level as they talk on a noisy playground. These children may need specific training to improve this aspect of their communicative competence. Specifically, they need to learn to focus on and interpret the feedback they get from listeners (e.g., words and sentences, eye movements, facial expressions) in face-to-face communication and the purely vocal feedback available during telephone interactions.

Context

The context in which interpersonal communication takes place has at least four dimensions: physical, social, psychological, and temporal (DeVito, 1980). An individual must adjust his or her voice in relation to the concrete, tangible demands of the physical environment in which he or she is operating, as shown in the following examples:

1. The physical demands of an open-air, dusty, noisy playground or football stadium differ from the restrictions of a sickroom, a library, or an art gallery.
2. The social dimension involves a recognition of and adaptation to the status relationships among the speakers, the rules of the games, the roles of the participants, and the general norms of the culture. Children must make adjustments in the vocal behavior required for appropriate responses to a reprimand by the principal in his or her office and an unfair play by a peer on the ballfield.
3. The psychologic dimension consists of aspects such as the amount of emotional involvement or distance possible in a given interaction, the recognition of the degree of formality or informality, or the seriousness or humor involved. The perceived need for friendliness or guardedness in a specific communicative exchange may also be important. A boy may wish to be accepted by a peer group but may misjudge the psychologic effects his group-entry behaviors have on his peers. The vocal behavior demanded by clowning with peers with the teacher out of the room contrasts sharply with a subsequent attempt to convince the teacher that "It wasn't me yelling, it was Juan." A significant change in loudness, level of formality, emotional involvement, and nonverbal behavior would be necessary if the teacher were to be persuaded!
4. The temporal dimension includes the time of day as well as the time in history. How likely is a teacher to respond positively to a denial of a child's culpability if that same child had been active in similar skirmishes all day, or perhaps all semester? Some children are adept at interpreting the temporal aspects during communication and adjusting their behavior accordingly (e.g., "I'd better be careful and talk quietly and nicely, 'cause she's mad about all the noise today"); others are not. They operate in every interaction as if it existed in an isolated present, with no past and no future.

Of course, all four dimensions of context interact, and each is influenced by the other. If, for example, the temperature changes (a physical change) or it is the last afternoon before Christmas vacation (a temporal change), there are probably changes in the social and psychologic dimensions as well.

Field of Experience

The effectiveness of communication is related to the extent that the participants share the same experiences. As children develop increased affective maturity, they realize that in similar situations, everyone does not necessarily feel the same way they do. With increased social awareness comes the insight that people are indeed different in the way they see the world and the way they respond to it. The amount of overlap that exists in experiences and the stage of awareness participants have achieved determines the effectiveness of the communication process. Parents sometimes have difficulty communicating with their children because children do not share the parental experience (DeVito, 1980). Children who transfer from a different school or who come from different cultural backgrounds also encounter difficulties adapting their communicative behavior. Strategies that worked in one classroom or playground environment do not always work in the new context. The child needs time to accumulate some shared experiences before he or she can predict and modify behavior and share a common experiential field. This is why the technique of role playing can be such an effective teaching tool during voice therapy. See Sederholm, McAllister, Dalkvist, and Sundberg (1995), which includes parents' questionnaires that focus on personality profiles associated with vocal behavior problems.

Effect

Communication always has some effect because for every communication act, there is some consequence (DeVito, 1980). Even when an effect is not observed, it is there. As children develop, they become more adept at observing subtle clues that illuminate the effect their communication has on others. At first, they usually attend only to the effect of their words on their listeners. Gradually, they become aware of the paralinguistic features (e.g., loudness, voice quality, eye contact, facial expression). They also learn to interpret their own reactions to these aspects of other people's behavior. Some children may need special assistance in learning to decode the more subtle aspects of the communication process. For helpful ideas on the management of these children, see Nowicki and Duke (1992). It is possible that some children with voice disorders plateau at immature levels in their development of communicative effectiveness. They lack the observational skills to detect that their vocal strategies are not working for them, or they are powerless to modify their habituated vocal behaviors. When this occurs, frustration and tension levels increase. This exacerbates the problem, especially if the voice disorder has a hyperfunctional pattern.

Voice therapy with children often needs to include analyses of communication effectiveness. What is the child trying to achieve in specific interactions? What does he or she want—to be liked, to influence others, to express his feelings, to share his ideas? Once personal goals have been defined, it is easier for a child to understand the reasons for working on changing vocal behavior in therapy.

Ethics

No discussion of communication effectiveness and how an understanding of the communicative act is basic to voice therapy programming would be complete without a consideration of ethics. It is feasible that when the clinician asks, "What did you want when you screamed at the teacher, 'It wasn't me, Miss'?" that the response could well be, "I wanted to con her into blaming Juan." As well as using an unproductive and naive vocal strategy (e.g., defiant yelling), the child is demonstrating unethical behavior. There is an ethical dimension to interpersonal communication: a rightness–wrongness aspect to any act. We cannot always so easily observe the rightness–wrongness of the act itself, but we can speculate concerning intent. Interwoven into the fabric of understanding the effectiveness of communication is the basic consideration of ethical intent. This raises the question of choice. Communication is the art of making choices. When we communicate, we choose—consciously or unconsciously. DeVito (1980) noted some of the ways we choose:

- To talk or not to talk
- To begin with one point or another
- To say certain words
- To be open or to withhold information
- To lie or not to lie
- To consider others' feelings or not
- To maintain a relationship or to terminate it
- To answer questions or not
- To assume the right to choose for another or not

We can learn to predict and control our behaviors only when we know ourselves. Children need to understand the nature of the choices available to them and the ways in which ethical effective interpersonal communication affects their self-esteem, friendships, family relationships, ability to love and be loved, and their ability to resolve conflict and attain personal goals. Such understanding provides a springboard from which they can move into dynamic, motivated behavioral change.

The Relationship of Vocal Competence to Voice Disorders

Many people in our society, both children and adults, are handicapped by inappropriate habits such as excessive talking and insensitivity to their listeners. Many individuals seem to exhibit inappropriate interpersonal communication patterns. Evidence of this is the number of self-help books on the market designed to help improve communication skills. Clinical experience suggests that many children (e.g., some children with learning disabilities, fluency problems, articulation disorders, and voice disorders) also exhibit inappropriate interpersonal communication or pragmatic skills. Nevertheless, we have no research evidence to tell us the extent to which immature or ineffective interpersonal communication strategies affect the development or maintenance of a voice disorder. We do not know the extent of the overlap between the group of children who have problems with interpersonal communication in general and those who have problems with interpersonal communication in the presence of a voice disorder. As we work with children day-by-day, we often suspect, for example, that there may be a causal relationship between immature vocal competence and a child's susceptibility to develop hyperfunctional vocal behavior. But we have no way of knowing whether children with interpersonal problems (e.g., insensitivity to the reactions of others, unsatisfied needs for attention) are more prone to develop vocal symptoms than are other children, nor do we know the extent to which a vocal handicap, once developed, affects a child's self-esteem, acceptance in the peer group, and so on. Research is needed before any definitive statements can be made.

It is certainly possible that a child's communicative competence (especially the level of vocal competence acquired) does have an impact on his or her vocal behavior, however. Common sense and practical experience suggest that this is so. Thus, when we observe a child with a voice problem, we need to be cognizant of what the child is trying to achieve through voice use. In the absence of normative data, we must rely on subjective impression. As we watch and listen to a child, we can observe whether the vocal strategies used seem to be helping or hindering his or her interactions with others. If the child has two problems (i.e., interpersonal and a voice problem), considering and treating both is a valid approach even if we cannot define a clear causal relationship. It may be that a child with a voice disorder needs even better interpersonal skills than other children if the problem is to be understood and the vocal mechanism protected.

Summary

We have described some aspects of interpersonal behavior with special reference to the development of vocal competence. Vocal competence can be seen as underlying vocal behavior. In subsequent sections of this book, we illustrate methods of teaching improved awareness and practice of appropriate vocal interactions.

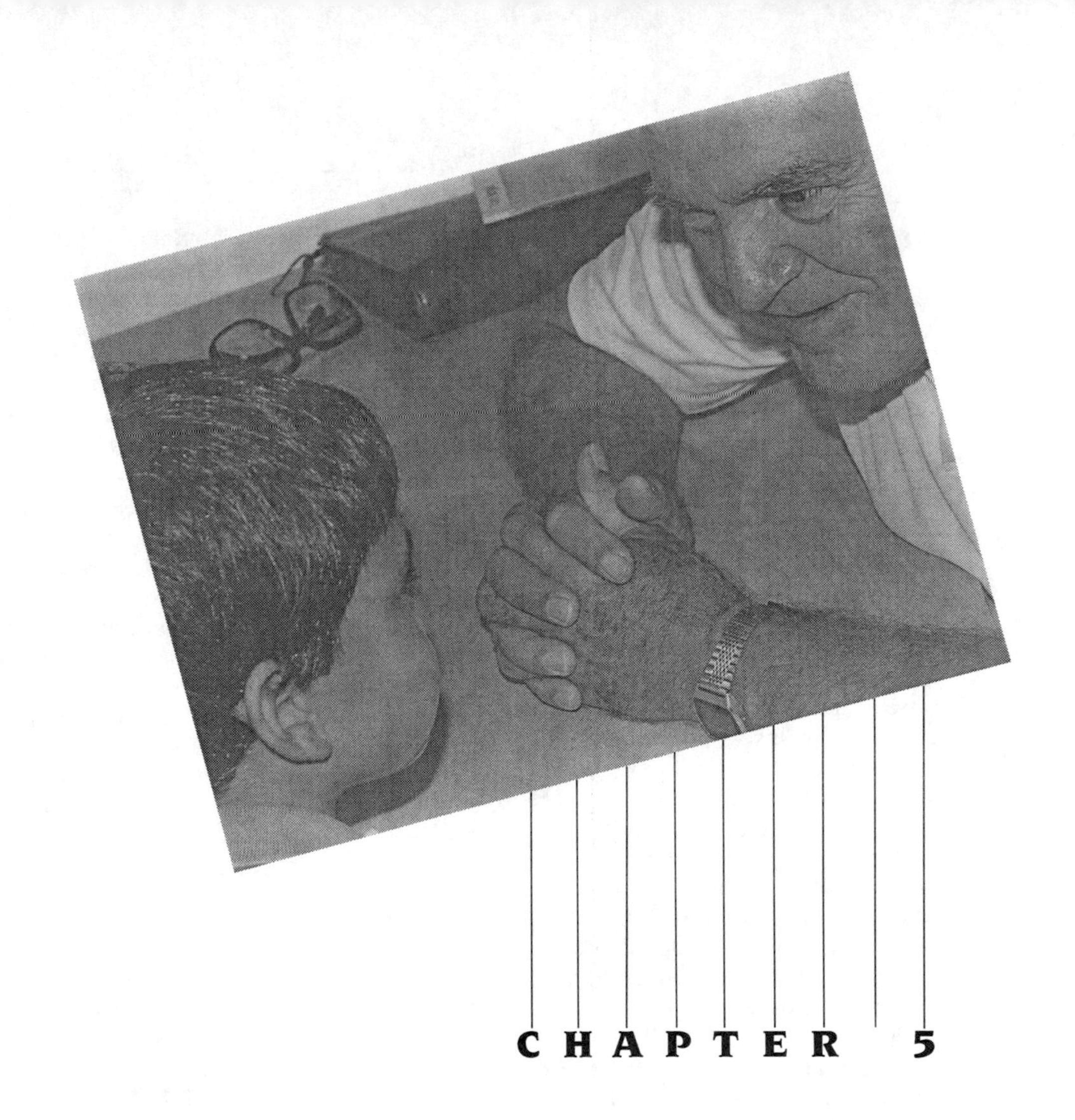

CHAPTER 5

A Developmental Perspective: The School-Age Child

Pitch Characteristics

Age

In his review of the research of age-related changes in fundamental frequency from birth on, Kent (1976) noted that the results he cited support the following generalization: There is a discernible, gradual decline in fundamental frequency (F_0) from age 3 through 11 or 12 years. He concluded that fundamental frequency data may not actually reflect the developmental changes occurring as children grow. He pointed out that what appear to be age-related changes related to maturation may actually be due to the variability in vocalizations and differences in methodology. He also noted the small number of subjects studied in some of the age groups. Discrepancies in the findings reported for children in the 7- to 11-year-old groups in particular prompted Bennett (1983) to collect data on children in this age range using a longitudinal approach. She noted that when she used group rather than individual data to obtain year-to-year comparisons of the same children, both sexes showed a generalized lowering of F_0 over a 3-year period. The largest decrements occurred between the ages of 8 years 2 months and 11 years 2 months. The only exception to the general downward trend from 8 years 2 months to 11 years 2 months was the 1-year period between 9 years 2 months and 10 years 2 months when neither of the group means showed any change. White (1999) presented acoustic evidence of major differences in voice characteristics between boys and girls in Sweden. She posited that the differences she found in formant frequencies can be ascribed, at least in part, by anatomic and morphologic characteristics that differentiate gender even before puberty. Her 11-year-old subjects were asked to produce four sustained spoken and sung vowels. All were experienced choral singers chosen to control for larynx height changes that may be associated with pitch variation in inexperienced singers. Formant frequencies were significantly higher for speech than for singing. Formants were also consistently higher in girls than in boys, suggesting that boys have a longer vocal tract. Also, formant scaling showed vowel-dependent differences between the genders, which suggests nonuniform differences in male and female vocal tract dimensions. These vowel-dependent gender differences were not consistent with data reported on adults. White sought to circumvent the problems with measurement experienced by Eguchi and Hirsh (1969), and Bennett (1983) by including both spoken and sung vowels and a gliding "F" to provide sufficient harmonic energy to resolve the vocal tract resonances of her child subjects during spectrographic analysis.

Gender

Most studies of children's voices before puberty have focused on measures of fundamental frequency (mean F_0). Glaze, Bless, Minlenkovic, and Susser (1988) analyzed /a/ productions of 121 children between the ages of 5 and 11 years and found a mean of 226 Hz for boys and 238 Hz for girls. They concluded that F_0 for both genders decreased as a function of age, height, and weight increases. Hasek, Singh, and Murry (1988) also analyzed F_0 /a/ productions of 15 boys and 15 girls at each age from 5 to 10 years. A decline in F_0 for the entire group they studied was attributed to the change in the boys', but not the girls', voices between the ages of 6 and 8 and 9 and 10 years. Vuorenkoski, Lenko, Tjernlund, Vuorenkoski, and Peerheentupa. (1978) also found that the male F_0 lowers between the ages of 8 and 9 years.

Ferrand and Bloom (1996) hypothesized that representative information about how children of both genders use F_0 in running speech may be obtained by obtaining the voice samples in contextual speech, rather than through the elicitation of isolated vowels. When Ferrard and Bloom (1996) actually studied intonational variables in children's conversational speech, however, they concluded that the mean F_0s were comparable to those reported in prior research. In fact, despite differences in speaking tasks and types of analyses, they found many of the values to be very similar. See Table 5–1 for a comparison of values reported for F_0 in prepubescent children listed with type of task.

It can be seen that there is a discernible decline in boys' mean F_0, but not in girls' F_0, as they approach puberty. Ferrand and Bloom (1996) noted that not only do boys' mean F_0 begin to decrease around the ages of 7–8 years, but that around this time they also begin to restrict their range of intonation whereas girls do not. Ferrand and Bloom argued that because control of intonation patterns seems to be a developmental process that is completed by age 5, that sociocultural reasons may be responsible for declines in rising and falling frequency shifts after age 7–8 years. This reduction in range and variability, emerging in boys but not in girls, seems to be consistent with the vocal behavior of adult models in their environment.

Ferrand and Bloom (1996) cited Crystal (1981), who noted that awareness of prosodic rules develops between the ages of 7 to 10 years and that this may be a critical time in the acquisition of gender specific vocal characteristics related to intonation. Ferrand and Bloom concluded that a combination of F_0-related variables seems to be apparent in the differences between intonation patterns used in spontaneous speech by boys and girls approaching puberty. Physiologic maturation and sociocultural learning from adult models, they believe, seem to impact boys' usage much more than girls' usage at this time.

Ferrand (2000) also studied harmonics-to-noise ratios (HNR) in 80 children with normal speech aged 4, 5, 8, and 10 years. Ten boys and girls at each age level participated in the study. Overall, the HNR values were lower than those of adults. There were also some differences with respect to gender and to the vowels sampled. These findings suggest that children's age, gender, and the vowels used to obtain samples of their voices should be taken into account when samples

Table 5–1. A comparison of values reported for mean fundamental frequency (in Hz) for 5- to 10-year-old children, compared by method of sample elicitation.

	Age (years)	*Girls*	*Boys*	*Task*
Hasek et al. (1980)	5	257.7	247.5	/a/
Hasek et al. (1980)	6	254.3	262.5	/a/
Ferrand & Bloom (1996)	5–6	243.07	256.09	/a/
Hasek et al. (1980)	7	261.7	256.09	/a/
Hasek et al. (1980)	8	264.0	235.6	/a/
Ferrand & Bloom (1996)	7–8	252.7	234.36	spontaneous speech
Hasek et al. (1980)	9	246.7	230.4	/a/
Hasek et al. (1980)	10	253.7	228.9	/a/
Ferrand & Bloom (1996)	9–10	253.81	240.50	spontaneous speech

of children's voices are examined using acoustic measures.

Puberty

Many references in the literature concern the effect of vocal mutation on the pitch characteristics of children's voices. It is not clear when mutational changes occur, especially in boys because there is no dramatic physiologic change signifying the onset of puberty. Physiologists such as Rose Frisch (1975) have described such a salient factor as the amount of body fat in relation to overall body weight, which affects the onset of the menarche in girls. Variability in the onset of puberty itself (Tanner, 1969), in the length of time from its beginning to end, and in the timing of the laryngeal changes that relate to vocal mutation (Kahane, 1975; Klock, 1968) cause practical difficulties for researchers. Wilson (1972) stated that a boy's voice may lower as much as an octave during the period of mutation, and a girl's voice may lower three or four semitones. Huskiness and voice breaks may also be noted. Voice breaks were noted by Fairbanks, Herbert, and Hammond (1949) and by Fairbanks, Wiley, and Lassman (1949) in both boys and girls as young as 7 or 8 years of age. None of Bennett's (1983) 10- or 11-year-old boys showed evidence of changes in their voices. Hollien and Malcik's (1967) data suggest that changes occur between 14 to 18 years of age in boys. Duffy (1970) suggested that girls undergo a form of vocal mutation at the time of the menarche, although the transition from the child to the adult voice probably occurs gradually over a long time. Limited data are available, and the relationship between the onset of menstruation and voice change in girls is not completely understood. Here we are concerned with elementary school children, therefore we probably can assume that most of the changes in children's voices occur after the fifth grade and during the middle school or high school years. Ten- and 11-year-old males, as seen in studies by Bennett (1983), Curry (1940), Hollien and Malcik (1962), and Hollien, Malcik, and Hollien (1965) appear still to exhibit childlike frequency characteristics. It might be important for us to remember, however, that articles in health publications dealing with the onset of puberty in girls refer to the gradual lowering of the age of the onset of menstruation during the 20th century. Frisch (1975) noted that the diet of children in highly developed countries has changed significantly during the last century, and this may have contributed to an increased proportion of body fat, which triggers an earlier onset of puberty. Some girls may begin to enter puberty as young as 8 years of age. Certainly, more information is needed before we fully understand the relationship between puberty and vocal development. Variables such as height and weight, in addition to chronological age, need to be considered carefully because the growth spurt is a signal that puberty has begun.

Experimental Tasks

Variability in results of studies of children's voices may be related to differences in methodology. Especially important may be the way that the vocal behavior is elicited and the kind of sample analyzed. In any discussion of the vocal behavior of young children, one needs to consider carefully the way in which the vocal response is obtained. Young children frequently do not understand an abstract vocal task, and they also may be influenced by the voice of the adult experimenter. Eguchi and Hirsh (1969) had their 7-year-old speakers repeat sentences after the investigator and derived their F_0 values from spectrograms of six vowels occurring in two short sentences. The older children in this study read the sentences, as did the children in the study by Fairbanks,

Wiley, and Lassman (1949). Vuorenkoski et al. (1978) and Hasek et al. (1980) analyzed a single isolated sustained vowel. Bennett (1983) provided a model for her subjects and asked them to say the sentence with a comfortable level of loudness. She noted that F_0 values obtained from a single vowel would probably differ from those in a sentence utterance and that it is difficult to ascertain where, in their vocal range, children produce an isolated vowel. Reading tasks and imitation tasks are probably also likely to result in differences in suprasegmental patterns when compared with spontaneous utterances.

Sorenson (1989) found no gender-related differences in the mean fundamental frequency of male and female preadolescents when he recorded voice samples across a series of reading, speaking, and vowel prolongation tasks. He noted that (i) and (u) have the highest fundamental frequency and that (ae) the lowest among seven prolonged vowels. In both boys and girls, aged 6 to 10 years, spontaneous speech had a significantly lower fundamental frequency than either reading or sustained vowel production. Sustained vowels had the highest fundamental frequency. Hacki and Heitmuller (1999) studied 180 normal children between the ages of 4 and 12 years and determined that the lowering of the habitual or modal pitch during speaking, as well as the entire speaking pitch range, occurred for girls between the ages of 7 and 8 years and for boys between 8 and 9 years. Both boys and girls demonstrated a temporary restriction in minimum vocal intensity between 7 and 8 years. A decrease in the maximum intensity was found for boys between 8 and 9 years and girls between 7 and 8 years. A lowering of the pitch as well as of the intensity of the shouting voice occurs for both genders from 10 years on. The authors hypothesized that girls seemed to enter a stage they called permutation between 7 and 8 years, and boys entered it 1 year later. When Morris (1997) studied 90 boys aged 8 to 10 years, he found no differences between White and African-American children with respect to speaking fundamental frequency. However, the 10-year-old African-American boys exhibited significantly greater variability than younger African-American boys and White boys.

Herzel and Reuter (1997) reported documenting unusual high-pitched vocalizations made by a 9-year-old boy with normal phonation during speech and singing. They asked the boy to produce steady phonation at very high pitch and he was able to produce a whistlelike phonation with a pressed voice and forceful expiration that appeared to be similar to what is termed "whistle register" in the adult soprano voice. The boy produced frequencies that were in the range of 1000 to 1700 Hz, whereas the maximum recorded for normal phonation was 950 Hz. In the transition region between whistle and falsetto frequency jumps, the researchers noted coexisting pitches that they termed "biphonation."

This study draws attention to the methodologic problems concerning the elicitation approaches used during measurement of the upper limits of children's voices. To ascertain the speaking range, accurate measures of the upper and lower limits are crucial. With young children it is difficult to ensure that the tasks and instructions are clear. Visual cues such as steps and slides can be helpful, as can the use of a keyboard to provide an ascending or descending series of notes. Technologic advances have resulted in improved automatic voice range profiling instrumentation. Hacki and Heitmuller (1999) used VRP and elicited speaking samples by asking subjects to tell a story, to count using softest to loudest, to shout "hello, come here" four times and to sustain singing /la/ at minimum and maximum intensity levels. Modal F_0 and modal intensity were determined from the story-telling samples.

When we consider that the subjects participating in the studies mentioned were between 7 and 11 years of age, we also must consider the influence of cognitive development of the younger versus the older children in responding to task instructions. As we see later in this chapter, when we discuss cognitive development, children younger than 8 years of age sometimes respond differently than older children when given instructions concerning vocal performance. For example, a 7-year-old child may not comprehend the instruction "a comfortable loudness level" as completely as a 10-year-old.

Duration of Sustained Vocalizations

Measurements of children's ability to sustain phonation on vowels and voiced and unvoiced consonants have been reported by a number of investigators. The duration of prolonged sounds (i.e., mean phonation time) has been measured by some investigators to ascertain whether an individual has a sufficiently long exhalation to support connected speech. Westlake and Rutherford (1961) reported that whereas normal children could sustain a tone for 20 seconds or longer, their study of children with cerebral palsy led them to hypothesize that a child needs to be able to phonate for a minimum of 10 seconds to speak in phrases of more than two or three words. Clinicians also have traditionally used prolongation tasks to ascertain information about continuity of voicing and to note pitch breaks or variations in voluntary control. Boone (1977) stated that the phonation of /s/ and /z/ provided information about how well an individual sustained exhalation with and without voicing. Eckel and Boone (1981) found that 95% of their adult voice patients with laryngeal pathologies demonstrated s/z ratios in excess of 1:4. They found that individuals with glottal lesions exhibit significantly shorter /z/ durations than did healthy patients, although /s/ durations were of normal length.

Frey (1978) studied preschoolers' prolongations and noted the importance of standardized protocols for testing that ensure young children understand the concept of continuity. She advocated the use of specific concrete materials, visual clues, and models. Michel and Tait (1977) reported average phonation times for elementary school children aged 5, 7, and 9 years. The results of these two studies are summarized in Table 5–2.

Table 5–2. Prolongation of /s/ and /z/ by healthy children.

		/s/		/z/		
Age (Years)	**N**	***Mean in Secs***	**SD**	***Mean in Secs***	**SD**	***Researchers***
3.0–4.8	183	3.7	1.99	4.15	2.08	Frey
5.3–6.6	162	4.56	2.12	5.31	2.94	Frey
3–6	450	4.07	2.52	4.71	2.30	Frey
5	15	8.13	3.25	9.47	2.97	Michel & Tait
7	14	9.79	2.27	13.40	3.83	Michel & Tait
9	24	15.80	7.21	17.20	6.36	Michel & Tait
5–9	53	12.06	6.33	13.95	5.95	Michel & Tait

Note. Data are from Frey, M. J. (1978). *Prolongation of /s/ and /z/ by preschool children.* Unpublished master's thesis, Indiana University; and Michel, J. F. & Tait, N. A. (1977, November 3). *Maximum duration of sustained /s/ and /z/.* Paper presented at American Society of Speech and Hearing meeting, Chicago.

Launder (1971) reported on both boys' and girls' average phonation times for the three vowels /a/, /i/, and /u/ and found that there were no significant differences between the three vowels. The boys' phonation times were longer for all ages (9 through 17), except for the 12-year-olds, where the phonation time was the same for both genders. A summary of some of these data appears in Table 5–3.

Relevant Information on Child Development

As noted earlier, although children may frequently exhibit the same kinds of vocal symptoms as adults, they cannot be treated in exactly the same way. Children are not miniature adults, and strategies that work with adults do not necessarily translate to children. The cognitive, linguistic, social, and emotional developmental level of the child is an important consideration in all therapy planning. We have noted that children are not always aware of the nature of their problem or the effect of their vocal behavior on themselves and others. The abstract quality of the behaviors compounds the difficulty. One of the challenges of voice therapy with children is to reduce the general level of abstractness. We can do this best when we understand the developmental stages that young children go through in acquiring concepts and skills that are relevant to voice therapy.

Cognitive Development

Some of the cognitive skills that a child needs to participate in voice therapy are the same as the skills needed to participate in other learning tasks (i.e., the ability to attend to stimuli, focus on relevant elements, understand instructions, remember, match auditory patterns, and so on). Many associations that are made in voice therapy are especially complex, however, and children do not always make these associations the same way that adults do. For example, in an association between a target voice and the obligatory modifications in the vocal tract, the target response is a fleeting sound that is "heard," the sequence of behavior used to produce the sound may be "felt" in various parts of the mechanism, and visual cues may be minimal. Thus, the child is asked to make a connection between a vocal sound and a kinesthetic awareness of how that sound is produced. We cannot assume that children automatically focus on salient aspects of the behavioral gestalt. Explicit statements, such

Table 5–3. Average durations of sustained vocalizations.

		Average Phonation Time in Seconds	
Age (Years)	*Vocalization*	*Girls*	*Boys*
9	/a/ /i/ /u/	8.8	11.4
10	/a/ /i/ /u/	9.4	10.4
11	/a/ /i/ /u/	11.5	12.8
12	/a/ /i/ /u/	12.2	12.8

Note. Data are from Launer, P. G. (1971). *Maximum phonation time in children.* Unpublished master's thesis, State University of New York, Buffalo.

as "If I feel this, then my voice sounds like that," need to be explained, taught, and reiterated. This kind of explanation usually involves cause–effect relationships. A review of some literature concerning children's development of causative reasoning is helpful.

The early work by Piaget (1928, 1929, 1930) on causality, substantiated later by work done by Inhelder and Piaget (1964), suggests two important aspects of children's development. First, the development of a concrete operational conception of causality stems from the child's egocentric projection of his or her own point of view onto the material world, whereas reversible mental operations remain absent. Egocentric projection leads to the assignment of psychologic or human causes to natural or mechanical phenomena (i.e., precausal thought). Second, the child develops the concept of objective causality, which involves the relationship between two phenomena in the object world, independent of their relationship to the subject. Hood and Bloom (1979) discussed that a child first refers to actions by self and others as aspects of his or her own egocentric world. Later, the child's development continues to extend to both actions and intentions of self and others; it is no longer merely restricted to the egocentric world. Hood and Bloom (1979) also stated that a child's causal reasoning continues to be qualitatively different from the adult's until age 7 or 8 (Piaget, 1926, 1928, 1930; Werner & Kaplan, 1963). In other words, a child's causal reasoning develops until it approaches the adult's concept of causality around 7 or 8 years of age.

It is critical not to assume that because we understand causal relationships, they are equally obvious to the children we teach. Indeed, it is probably the case that most children under age 8, and older children who have cognitive deficits, will not understand them exactly as adults do. Some common examples of statements in voice therapy that may need to be reexamined in relation to this are: "If you yell and scream, you'll get bumps on your vocal cords"; "If you talk too much, you'll hurt your throat"; "If you don't breathe deeply, you'll run out of air"; "If you talk softly, no one will hear you."

Champley (1977) studied the way that preschool children could be helped to process the instructions given during tasks to elicit vocal samples. For children in the preoperational stage of cognitive development, intellectual processing is marked by intuitive assimilation and accommodation. According to Neubauer (1965), "intuitive cognitive functioning refers to an implicit, relatively imprecise and informal type of understanding" (p. 18). In the preschool child, this is marked by the relatively nonverbal character of cognitive functioning and a reliance on overt manipulation of concrete–empirical props when attempting logical operations (Neubauer, 1965). Because of this, it is necessary to provide young children with the means for processing verbal directions at a concrete level.

Imagery research offers some insights concerning the representation of abstract ideas. Reese (1970) suggested that information can be presented to children in two ways to foster acquisition:

1. in a meaningful linguistic content rather than in isolated terms, with some kind of spatial relation or meaningful interaction between objects and
2. with a cue for response that is concrete rather than abstract, pictorial rather than verbal. (pp. 404–414)

Writers in the areas of teaching mathematics and music (Jeffrey, 1958; McMahon, 1961) to young children have provided further pertinent insights concerning specific use of visual cues and relationships to represent abstract ideas. Welsh and Harvin (1976) suggested a developmental hierarchy of visual representations in mathematics proceeding from the most concrete representation to the most abstract:

1. Concrete, manipulable objects
2. Color photographs
3. Black-and-white photographs
4. Colored pictures
5. Line drawings
6. Diagrams
7. Symbolic representations (includes written symbols)

Schiffman (1976) said that discrimination of auditory stimuli is one of the most important psychologic processes involved in learning, and one about which we know very little. It may develop as a Gestalt-like abstraction through experience or through a gradual extraction of differentiated attributes. It is clear, however, that young children's ability to process information and instructions related to vocal behavior depends to a large extent on the type of visual clue used to represent the focal attributes of the signal. The younger the child, the more necessary the visual clue is and the more concrete that clue needs to be. Although the use of the visual-clue method may provide a child with a means for a more overt manipulation of abstract ideas, some degree of verbal mediation is usually still required. The simplest form of verbal mediation is the basic model-response paradigm. The use of modeling is an integral part of speech-language-voice therapy programs. The classic psycholinguistic definition of modeling refers to an imitation of vocalizations "which occur in close temporal proximity" to a given target (Prutting & Connolly, 1976). Elicited imitation, according to Prutting and Connolly, refers to "those imitations which occur when a child responds to an examiner's request to 'say what I say' and repeats a model" (p. 415). Elicited imitation has long been used in language evaluations and allows a great variety of language stimuli to be investigated (Carrow, 1974). The assumption has not been explored fully in relations to voice evaluation techniques. Nonetheless, it seems the only feasible method with very young children because it eliminates the need for verbal and symbolic mediation and emphasizes sensory decoding and encoding of the vocal model. Imitation of vocal patterns is a practice that children engage in from early infancy. Champley (1977) found that the use of a vocal model was especially critical in vocal tasks involving pitch and loudness.

Visual cues are important, especially for younger children, and equipment that provides biofeedback and electroacoustic monitoring can be used most successfully with children. Any noninvasive instrument can be used safely in school settings; however, the portability and cost of such equipment often limits widespread acceptance in schools.

Bales and Sera (1995) studied young children's ability to distinguish between stable characteristics that anchor personal identity and changeable ones that can vary within an individual, using pictures and question tasks. Their findings provide information about how children understand and misunderstand the status of personal attributes. Generally, the preschool subjects had the most trouble with changeable rather than stable characteristics, and they performed relatively well on tasks where questions emphasizing mechanisms of change were used. The questions were designed to focus the child's attention on the possibility of change across a time interval and did not require a same–different judgment. For example, "Can someone go from being happy to being sad?" emphasized a process of change from one state to another. The question "if a person is happy, does he have to stay happy forever and ever?" emphasized the stability of a particular feeling state across time.

The results of this study and others focusing on changeable characteristics suggest that the way children understand voice characteristics could be probed in similar ways.

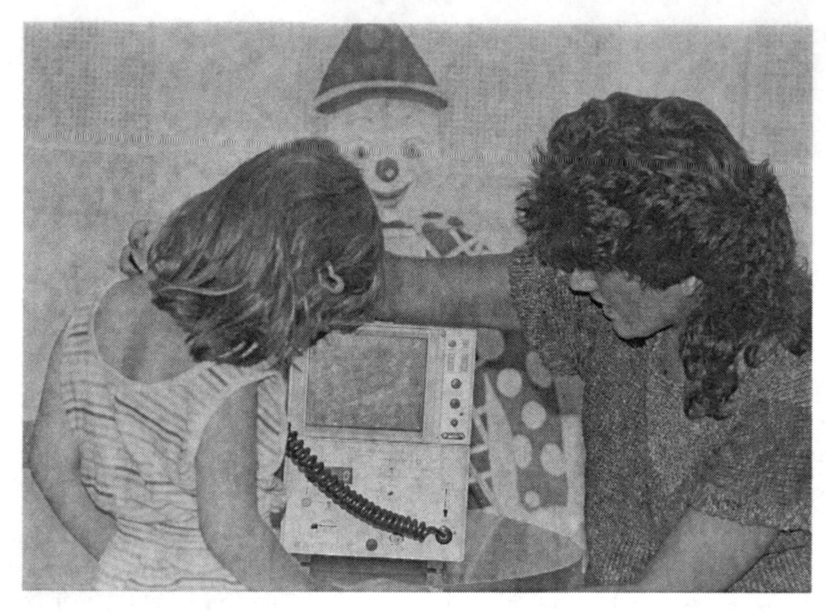

The Visi-Pitch machine allows for a target production in view while the child attempts to match it.

For example, "if a person sounds happy, does he have to sound happy forever?" "Can someone go from sounding happy to sounding sad?" and "can someone go from sounding sad to sounding happy?" Bales and Sera's (1995) subjects were more consistently accurate when the questions were framed in a way that suggested the possibility of change. This has implications for the way we present questions to young children in voice treatment. We might start with an identification game when the child uses happy–sad stickers to identify the feelings in a stimulus voice repeating the same words. Then the clinician could proceed with questions to focus on the possibility of mood change to focus attention on the changeability of the vocal characteristic. Other characteristics inherent in vocal signals such as sleepy–wide awake, loud–soft, rough–smooth, and so on could be attempted. For example, "If John's voice sounds loud, does it always have to sound loud?" "Why not?" Children's justifications and explanations can help determine if they are attending to processes of change and how well they understand the variability of the property. Such information allows us to refrain from proceeding too quickly into production activities before the cognitive scaffold is in place to support learning.

Linguistic Development

Let us consider some of the simplest descriptive terms used in voice therapy. Adjectives or antonyms such as *loud, soft, high,* and *low* name poles on a continuum of perceptual judgments of frequency or intensity. They are called *relational terms* because they describe perceived relationships. Appropriate receptive and expressive use of such terms requires at least a partial understanding of certain complex relationships. The terms also can be used in more than one sense. We do not know the ages at which normal children acquire these terms, but it is likely, for example, that they acquire *high* and *low* initially in the spatial sense and only later apply these words to auditory events. Similarly, the word *soft* is probably learned first in association with tactile stimuli.

Clark (1969b, p. 206) stated that the senses of certain positive adjectives, such as "good" and "long," are stored in the memory in a less complex form than the senses of their opposites. Many writers have noted that a number of antonymous adjectives are not symmetric opposites (Clark, 1969a; Greenberg, 1966; Lyons, 1963; Sapir, 1944; Vendler, 1968). The scale is named in many cases by the unmarked "positive" member of the pair of adjectives when both adjectives describe the same dimension. Also, in many pairs the positive adjective is neutralized at times. For example, "How high is it?" simply asks for information, but "How low is it?" seems to imply that the object is expected to be low. Both the unmarked and the marked adjectives can be used in a contrastive sense such as "Pete's voice is loud" and "Bill's voice is soft." In this way, the terms specify the dimension, contrast with each other, and imply an assumed standard. Sapir said that even when an unqualified relational term is used (for example, "Your voice is loud", it is no less relational than when a standard is given ("Your voice is louder than mine"). Sapir called it the unqualified "ungraded" term when it depends on a comparison with a norm relevant to that particular subject. Therefore, "Motorcycles are loud" implies in relation to other vehicles; "That motorcycle is loud" implies in relation to other motorcycles.

When the terms *loud* and *soft* are compared, it appears that *loud* is unmarked, and *soft*, as it is used to describe a pole on the scale of loudness, is marked. *Loud* can possess neutral qualities for use in a nominative sense, as in "How loud is the TV?" as well as in a contrastive sense, "That TV was loud." *Soft* seems to be used only in a contrastive sense. When using the terms *high* and *low* to describe tonal stimuli, *high* appears to be the unmarked term, whereas *low* is marked. It is apparent that "How high is the man's voice?" is not a neutral question, however. Both high and low can be marked when applied to descriptions of the postpubertal human voice, depending on the gender of the speaker.

When the comparative constructions of the terms are used ("Your voice is louder" or "Which one is highest," for example) the problems of implied standards and complex relationships are compounded. Although it may seem that young children should easily understand the simple descriptive terms used during voice therapy, it may not necessarily be so (Andrews, 1975).

Discussion of the Problem With the Child

It is interesting to observe children's responses to hearing recordings of their voices. Unless they have had a great deal of listening training, they seem to respond not to any specific attribute of the auditory signal, but to the total sound as a symbol of self. Thus, the child is likely to say "That's me, isn't it?" or "That's not me" rather than "That's my voice" or "That's not my voice." Such evidence of the strong association of self with voice reminds us that it is certainly ill advised to use any negative terms such as *wrong, bad,* or *unpleasant* to describe vocal symptoms. It is also apparent that in attempting to describe the possible effects of inappropriate vocal behavior, words such as *hurt, harm,* or *damage,* which suggest bodily injury, should be avoided.

It is probably reasonable to refer to a child's voice as "different" when attempting to make him or her aware of the problem. It is important, however, that the parameter to be focused on is clearly understood. When selecting terms to be used in describing the target vocal parameter, it is probably wise for a clinician to avoid using the same terms for more than one parameter. For example, *low* is sometimes used to refer to both pitch and loudness levels. It is also helpful if the words used to describe the parameter under discussion can be applied readily in changing situations. For example, *inappropriate* is a term that relies heavily on context. A voice that is inappropriately loud in the library may be perfectly appropriate or even necessary outdoors. Even the use of the word *too* before a descriptive adjective (e.g., "too loud") also implies that the child has internalized some kind of standard for both the loudness and the situation. It is helpful if the clinician uses terms that can later mark points on a realistic continuum when finer contrasts are demanded. Clinicians can become trapped by their own terminology if this has not been considered in advance.

Attempts to Make Therapy More Concrete

It seems easiest to find suitable nonauditory representations of the intensity parameter; more variety is found in materials used to illustrate various loudness levels. Visual feedback can be provided by pictures, instruments with needles or lights reflecting changes in intensity (e.g., the sound-level meter and the decibeloscope), and objects of various sizes. Pictures most frequently used generally fall into one of the following categories: size difference, facial expression, or gesture showing speaker effort, or listener reaction (e.g., hands cupped around mouth or finger to lips), effect on an object (e.g., a vibrating drum or slammed door), and varied distances between speaker and listener.

McDonald and Chance (1964), referring to therapy for children with cerebral palsy, advocate the use of role-playing activities in which the child pretends to be whispering a secret, giving an order as a policeman would,

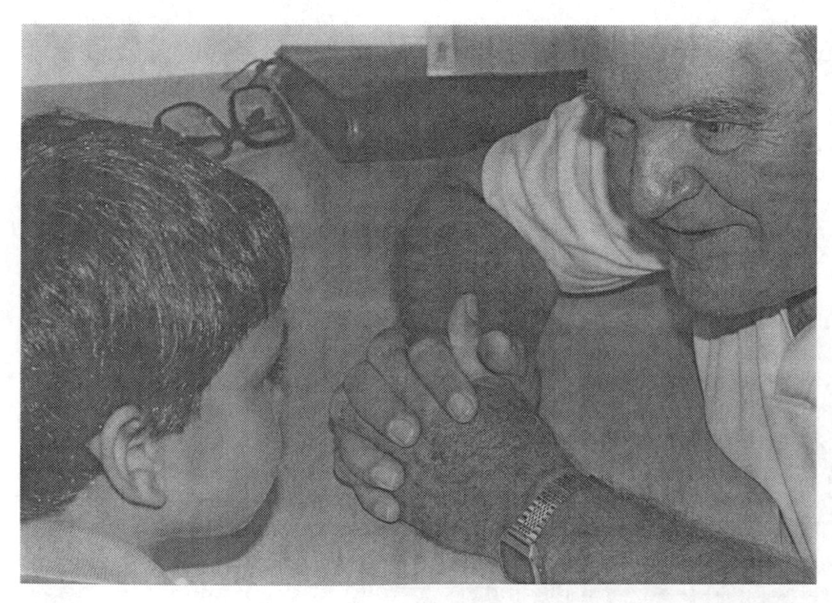

The clincian's nonverbal behavior during discussions with the child adds to the effectiveness of the communication.

and so on. In this way, the context or interaction helps define the loudness level.

When pitch or quality are under consideration in therapy, however, fewer options are available. Pitch differences may be depicted spatially by using pictures of stairs, ladders, or, as Wilson (1972) suggested, children standing on rocks of different heights or using puppets. The sizes of the puppets can be related to differences in pitch levels. Quality differences may be represented pictorially with type of movement, such as pictures of palm trees moving gently or vigorously in the wind (Wilson, 1972) or by using differences in texture, such as grains and materials representing a variety of tactile sensations (Andrews, 1973) and acoustic patterns.

There seems to be no way to make perceptual evaluations tangible and concrete or to make imitation of vocal patterns as clear-cut as the imitation of the placement of articulators can be made. Voice therapy can never be absolutely clear and direct in its approach because of the obviously inaccessible sound source. It nevertheless is reasonable to assume that procedures can be refined and realistic expectations for children developed if the complexities of the concepts and linguistic terms used in voice therapy are considered.

Affective Development

Our voices reflect our feelings, and our ability to understand the feelings of others depends, in part, on our ability to perceive significant cues in their vocal expression. Studies of parent-child interactions have shown that even infants and very young children adapt their vocal behavior in response to the vocal patterning of the adult. In a study reported by Lieberman (1975) infants modified their pitch levels to approximate the adult model. They vocalized at a lower pitch when interacting with the father and used a higher pitch when babbling in response to the mother. This study, and studies of recognition of speaker's voices by infants (see Aslin, Pisoni, & Jusczyk, 1983, p. 657), illustrates the importance of the effect of vocal models on the child's learning of vocal expression.

There is another interesting line of research that has relevance to our understanding of how children learn about the expression of their own and others' feelings. This involves the ways an individual learns to identify his or her own emotional state (Schacter, 1975). Skinner (1971) stated that children initially identify emotion in terms of external cues. This continues until the linguistic community draws their attention to the less salient cues associated with the external circumstances. If we accept the premise that the linguistic community plays an important part in shaping the child's focus on the more subtle cues, we would assume that considerable variation exists in the way children learn to attend to variations in vocal expression. There would also be the potential for some young children to identify cues inaccurately or fail to attend to certain cues.

It seems that young children are usually unaware of the possibility that different feelings and emotions may be felt by different individuals responding to the same external cues. They assume that everyone feels and reacts the same way they do in a given situation. Their descriptions of their feelings are concrete and specific to the external situation or event. For example, when asked to explain "happy" a young child might say, "I feel happy when it's my birthday." It is obvious that the emotion is defined specifically in terms of the situation. The emotion itself is seen as a predictable consistent part of that event. The underlying assumption that everyone feels or reacts the same way is revealed in answers to questions such as, "Does your friend feel happy then, too?" Frequently a young child will reply, "Yes, she knows it's my birthday."

It is only as children grow older that they begin to understand that it is possible for people to hide their true feelings. Ekman and Oster (1979) discussed this aspect of affective development. They said that older children acknowledge that sometimes one is unaware of another's true emotion or might mislead another person regarding an emotion. Lazarus (1968, 1975) states that strategies might be employed not only to manipulate the external signs of the emotion but also to reduce or augment the emotional experience itself.

Some knowledge of emotions and the ways in which they are expressed is probably an important prerequisite to success in modifying certain kinds of vocal behavior. If we do not understand that our own behavior may be affected by our feelings or recognize the feelings of others, it is difficult to focus on vocal behaviors that reflect a part of a general emotional response. Voice clinicians frequently need to help children increase their understanding of feelings generally and then help them learn how feelings are reflected in specific vocal behaviors. Some information about the sequence of development of children's understanding of emotion is therefore relevant to voice therapy programming.

Harris, Olthof, and Terwogt (1981) investigated the existence of marked changes with age in children's knowledge of situational, personal, and strategic factors. Concepts of happiness, anger, and fear were explored. In this study, subjects in three age groups (mean age 6, 11, 15) responded to questions. The responses were analyzed with respect to the use of cues to identify each emotion, the strategies of self-control, and the effects of the emotion on other psychologic processes.

Results indicated that the number of children defining emotion in terms of situational cues declined with age, and the citing of mental cues increased with age. The older children, but not the youngest group, concentrated on the observed rather than the observer. These results confirmed the speculation that many of the younger children had difficulty imagining a situation in which an observer might be unaware of another person's emotion. The two older groups of subjects were also more able to realize that another person's detection of their emotion is contingent on how they behave. There was also evidence to suggest that a child's detection of emotion depends on the nature of the emotion. The revealing of the positive emotion is more likely to occur through actions, whereas negative emotions are more likely to be revealed through answers in which an inner state, distinct from outward expression, is implied. Both the younger and older subjects conceived of the intentional display of emotion through actions, statements, and facial expression. The older children were more sensitive to the possible conflict between inner and outer states; however, the younger children focused on the outer display of emotion only. In addition, the three age groups demonstrated different strategies when asked how they could change their emotion. Although subjects of all ages suggested changing the situation, only the two older groups proposed cognitive strategies, such as redirecting one's thoughts.

Results of this and other studies indicate a progression in the development of the conception of emotion. One pattern predominates among young children, and this pattern changes somewhere between the ages of 6 and 11 years. By 11 years of age, most children have begun to move from the conceptualization that can be described as standard behavioristic (or stimulus-response) described by Skinner (1971) to what Miller Galenter, and Pribram (1960) have described as subjective behaviorism. In other words, the young child focuses on publicly observable components of emotion—the eliciting situation and the overt behavioral reactions. Children age 11 and older consider not only the observable components, but also the hidden mental aspect of emotion.

It may be helpful to summarize children's knowledge of emotion in terms of two distinct developmental stages (adapted from Harris, Olthof, & Terwogt, 1981):

Stage I: Younger Than 6 Years of Age

Emotion = situation + own behavioral reactions

happy	birthday	laughing
sad	pet's funeral	crying
angry	quarrel	yelling

One's own emotion is identified by noting either the situation or one's reactions. *Another's emotion* is identified by noting his or her reactions; correct identification is seen as restricted only by the location of the observer and his or her attentiveness to those reactions. *Control over emotion* is accomplished in either of two ways: (a) may pretend by displaying a reaction different from one normally elicited by the situation (e.g., joking after a quarrel); (b) may alter the emotion itself by changing the situation, giving rise to the emotion in the first place (e.g., making up after a quarrel).

Young children view the *effects of emotion* in simple terms: Positive emotions have positive effects, and negative emotions have negative effects. There is no attempt to explain them.

Stage II: 11 Years and Older

Emotion = situation + own and others' behavioral reactions + inner mental states

One's own emotion is best identified by reference to inner mental states. *Another's emotion* is difficult to identify because visible reactions are seen as an unreliable guide to inner mental states, and an observer may fail to identify another's emotion accurately. *Control over emotion* can be exercised in several ways:

1. The child may pretend by displaying a response different from that normally elicited by the situation; such a pretense is complicated, however, by the resulting conflict between outer display and inner mental state.
2. The child masks the inner state.
3. The child redirects the inner state.
4. The child alters the situation to control the experience of the emotion.

Older children provide more mentalistic explanations of the *effects of emotion.*

As noted earlier, it is possible that some children with voice disorders also may have problems with interpersonal relationships. Sometimes they may not understand how their own emotional responses are perceived by others or the need to consider the effect of their feelings on their vocal behavior. The information in the preceding section may help the clinician to recognize the child's stage of awareness concerning the feelings he or she and others may be experiencing. It may also help the clinician plan therapy strategies to teach children to identify their feelings and describe them as they relate to vocal expression and productive coping strategies.

Social Development

One of the most important skills young children need to learn is that of gaining entry to a group of peers during play. This is a critical social task for children, and it is probable that vocal behavior significantly affects the process of assimilation into groups. The group entry process has been referred to as "assimilation" (Phillips, Shenker, & Revitz, 1951), "access" (Corsaro, 1981), and "initiations" (Vandell & George, 1981). Whatever the process is called, it is evidently a difficult one to learn. Kindergarteners were studied by Corsaro, who found that young children's initial efforts to enter a peer group were rebuffed by their peers approximately 50% of the time. Studies have also shown that there are developmental changes in the strategies children use to enter groups and that as children grow older the strategies become more sophisticated.

Although differences in strategies used by children have been studied in relation to the child's age and stage of development, they also have been studied in other ways. Richard and Dodge (1982a) found that popular children generated more strategies, as well as more competent strategies, than did children who were unpopular with their peers. Putallaz and Gottman (1981a, 1981b) studied second-grade children and found that unpopular children were more likely to use "hovering" behavior and self-referent speech than did popular children. Neither of these strategies resulted in acceptance by peers. Coie, Dodge, and Coppotelli (1982) subdivided unpopular children into two groups. They referred to children who were not liked by peers or who were actively disliked as rejected children. Those who were not liked but were not disliked either were called neglected children. Dodge, Coie, and Brakke (1982) found that rejected and neglected children behave differently from popular children, both in the classroom and on the playground.

Studies of children in laboratory situations and naturalistic settings have resulted in some interesting findings about the strategies employed by children categorized as popular, rejected, and neglected. The group entry behavior of rejected and neglected children seems less likely to involve group-oriented statements and more likely to involve self-oriented statements and behaviors. Peers seem to perceive the rejected children as aggressive and disruptive. This appears to be related to the frequency with which rejected children try to enter a group with active or loud behavior that interrupts the group's activity. They also seem more often to respond negatively to statements initiated by peer hosts or established group members. Neglected children, however, engage in fewer entry attempts than other children. Neglected children appear to employ nonassertive approaches, such as waiting and hovering around a peer group. Hovering was the most frequent strategy used by neglected children, even though it is typically ignored by peers. The different entry strategies used by popular, rejected, and neglected children only partially explains the responses of peers. Researchers have also noted that peers may be favorably biased toward popular children because of other factors, such as physical attractiveness.

Although documentation of social competence is incomplete, studies of entry behaviors have yielded some findings that are of interest to the clinician designing voice therapy intervention programs. Undoubtedly, individual children vary in the degree of social awareness and competence they exhibit. Some children who develop vocal problems related to abuse may also exhibit patterns of social behavior similar to those described by children categorized as rejected. Similarly, children who are handicapped because of vocal disorders may at times exhibit nonassertive approaches to group entry and be ignored by their peers in the same way that children described as neglected are ignored. The part played by vocal behavior in the perception of general physical attractiveness is also not completely understood at this time. More research is needed before we can explain the part the voice plays in the process of peer acceptance. Nonetheless, it is certainly useful for us to review the strategies that psychologists have identified as entry behaviors and consider the way in which voice use may or may not contribute to their success. Then, when we identify children with voice problems who are repeatedly unsuccessful in their attempts to gain access to peer groups, we can teach alternative patterns of vocal use and relate them to meaningful social goals. A coding system explained by Dodge, Schlunt, Delagach, and Schocken (1982) and developed from systems used by others (Dodge, 1981) isolates strategies such as those listed below. Such a list may be used by the voice clinician to observe children's behavior (see Table 5–4). It also provides useful information that can be helpful in enhancing motivation and structuring discussion of reasons for changing behavior during implementation of voice therapy programs.

Table 5–4. Strategies children use to approach peers.

Strategy	***Identifying Behaviors***
Wait and hover	Approaches a group Observes activity for more than 3 seconds Does not speak
Attention getting	Verbal or nonverbal attempts (nonaversive) Tries to attract attention Tries to interrupt play (Example: bounces a ball on the table where other children are playing, clowning, shouting, etc.)
Group-oriented statements	Verbalizations Refers to the children or the play activity (Example: "That looks like a fun game you are playing")
Question	Child directs a question to the group members Requires or expects a response (Examples: "What are you doing?" "What is your name?")
Self-referent statements	Verbal statement referring to self Verbal statement describing self (Examples: "I've got lots of cars like that" "I want a turn")
Disruption	Verbal or nonverbal aversive behavior Interrupts peers' play Disrupts peers' play (Examples: grabs toys knocks over building blocks)
Mimicking	Imitation of the behavior of the group Attempts to integrate by engaging in same behavior as group (Examples: parallel play with toys playing basketball singing)
Other	Any other behavior initiated by entry child

Group-oriented statements and behaviors (e.g., questions and statements about the group or the activity) are the most effective strategies and are used more by older children and by children perceived as popular. Dodge et al. (1982) have suggested that such strategies are related to the Piagetian process of decentration. To make a statement that is group-oriented rather than self-oriented, the child must adopt the frame of reference of the group. This involves orientation to the behavior of others over oneself and is not consistent with egocentric thought. Deviant children are more likely to use strategies (such as disruptions and attention getting) that draw attention to themselves. They are less likely to use group-referenced strategies. Researchers have noted that deviant children frequently move from peer group to peer group, attempting to gain entry but failing to join in. Dodge, Coie, and Brakke (1982) have observed that in the classroom and on the playground, deviant children—particularly neglected children—approach each other infrequently. They suggest that the withdrawal of these children may occur as a result of a series of failures to establish positive peer relationships. Such children therefore may not respond to encouragement to join in. They may need to be specifically taught alternative strategies for initiating peer contacts.

A low-risk strategy, one in which the probability of a decisive outcome (either positive or negative) is small in comparison to the probability of a neutral outcome, is usually tried first, especially by children who are not acquainted. The best example of a low-risk strategy is hovering around a peer group and waiting to be invited to play. The peer-group entry process is one of taking increasing risks as the entry process proceeds. Dodge et al. (1981) have proposed that children employ low-risk strategies during initial stages of the entry process and higher risk strategies during later stages. Some common sequences of children's strategies are:

1. Waiting and hovering ⟶ group-oriented statement
2. Waiting and hovering ⟶ mimicking of peer group
3. Disruption ⟶ disruption
4. Waiting and hovering ⟶ mimicking ⟶ statement regarding peer group (most successful)

Similarly, it seems easier for children to use high-risk strategies with children with whom they are already acquainted. Examples of high-risk strategies include making statements, asking questions, and mimicking the behavior of the group during the approach. Children seem to minimize the risk of rejection by employing such strategies only after they have been successful with lower risk strategies. It is possible that socially incompetent children have not learned the progression from low-risk to high-risk strategies. They may either remain at the stage of employing low-risk strategies or jump too soon into high-risk strategies. The former pattern may be perceived as shyness and the latter as disruptiveness. McFall and Dodge (1982) have observed that correct employment of such a progression involves the ability to observe accurately the responses of other children.

The successful child is the one who manages to avoid drawing attention to himself or herself during entry and focuses on the group. Putallaz and Gottman (1981a, 1981b) stressed that any strategy that drew attention away from the group was most often met with rejection. Continual group reference may involve such cognitive skills as role taking and empathy, skills frequently associated with social competence (Chandler, 1973; Staub, 1975). Activities that include opportunities for children to engage in perspective taking are helpful in facilitating the development of social competence.

Summary

We have reviewed some of the information drawn from various areas of child development that may have relevance to voice therapy. Some generalizations can be made concerning the way our knowledge of developmental stages can affect the way we approach intervention. For example, some interesting changes occur in children's ability to understand certain concepts around age 8. Additional research is needed before we can progress to a more complete understanding of the best approaches to remediation with children of different ages. It is probably wise to assume that children younger than age 8 require a more concrete presentation of therapy tasks and may need help with some of the concepts and language used in voice therapy.

Additionally, assessing the child's social and emotional development and how that child's voice use is helping or hindering him or her in dealing with feelings, in interactions with peers, and in attempts to satisfy basic needs for acceptance and attention can provide important information to the clinician. Observation of the child's behavior not only in the therapy room but also in the classroom and on the playground may yield significant information, for example. This information can be used to enhance motivation for change by ensuring that therapy activities are meaningful and relevant in terms of the child's level of interpersonal skill.

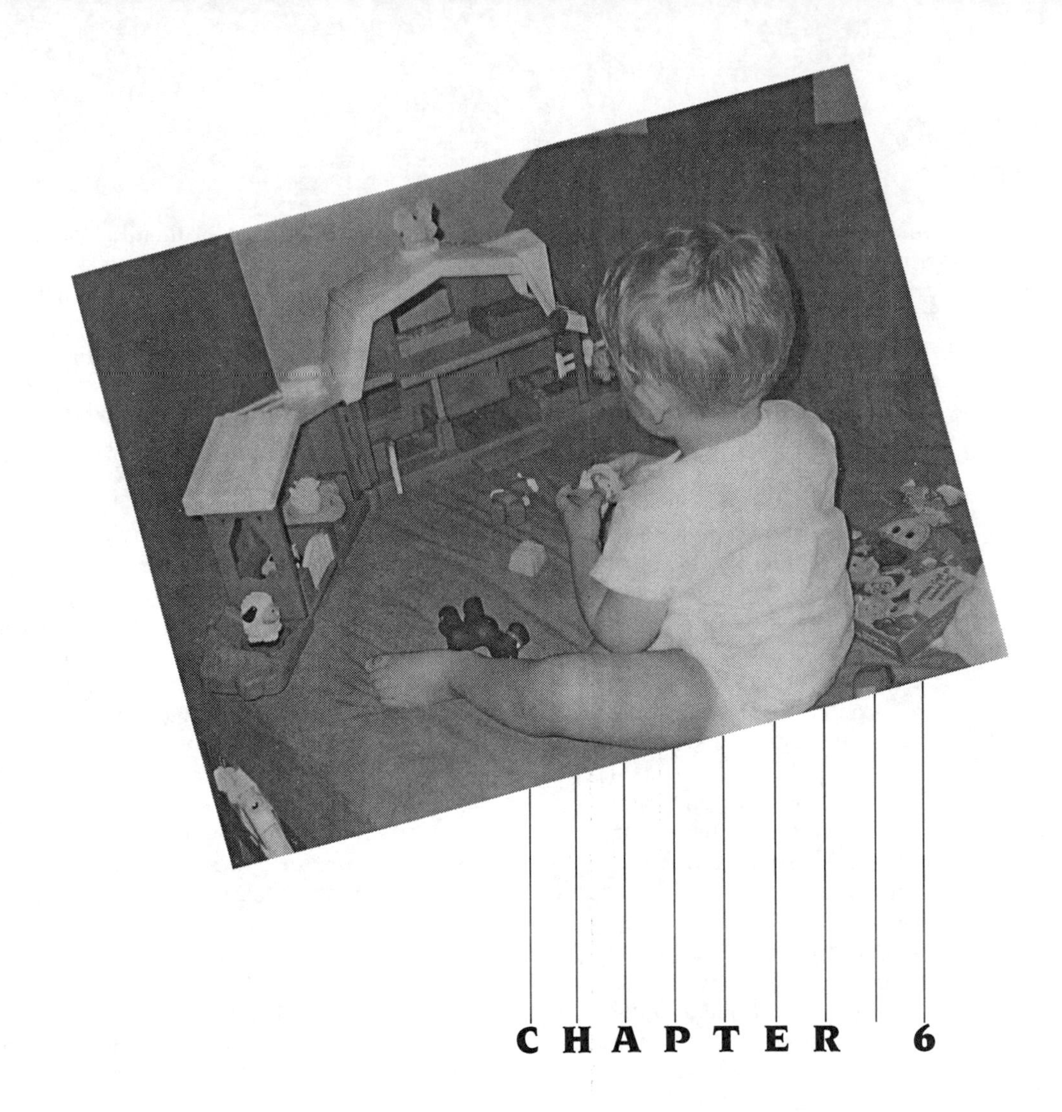

CHAPTER 6

Behaviors Related to Vocal Production

Voice disorders may be categorized in different ways. Pannbacker (1984) provided an excellent review of classification systems. We may decide, for example, to categorize the disorder according to our perception of etiology. Many writers have used the organic–functional dichotomy to group disorders this way. Other writers have noted that disorders usually exist on a continuum and that organic difficulties usually include some emotional components, and functional problems frequently result in tissue change if faulty habits are perpetuated across time.

Another method of categorizing voice disorders is to group them into perceptual categories according to the problem. Wilson (1972) stated that voice problems traditionally have been classified as quality problems, resonance problems, loudness problems, and pitch problems. Deviations in rate may be regarded as a fifth category or classified as a problem of articulation and rhythm. Symptoms also may be described in terms of pattern of muscular activity. Boone (1983) referred to hyperfunctional behavior patterns that occur when there is excessive muscular contraction and force of movement in respiration, phonation, or resonance. He described the ways in which hyperfunctional symptoms are exhibited in relation to varied anatomic sites and physiologic functions. The opposite set of symptoms, hypofunctional behavior patterns, occur when there is too little effort or muscle weakness frequently associated with neurologic impairment.

Another method of categorizing voice disorders is by referring to sets of voice characteristics subsumed under or associated with a primary classification or syndrome. For example, Montague and Hollein (1973) found that children with Down's syndrome typically exhibit more breathiness, roughness, and hypernasality than other children do. Mysak (1971) described the typical voice characteristics of children with cerebral palsy as forced or intermittent voicing, phonation on inhalation, difficulty coordinating the initiation of phonation with breath groups, difficulty in shifting from vegetative to phonatory breathing, difficulty with pitch control and stability, breathiness, and spasms of the vocal cords. Similarly, children with severe hearing losses frequently exhibit a similiar type of voice quality, which results from difficulties in monitoring the vocal behavior of self and others. Thus, children with hearing losses often are described as having distortions of pitch, loudness, and rate, and cul-de-sac resonance. Children with "adenoidal" problems are noisy breathers, exhibit hyponasality, and sometimes have laryngeal symptoms related to postnasal drip or dryness of the vocal tract resulting from mouth breathing. Velopharyngeal insufficiency results in a set of voice symptoms that includes hypernasality, reduction in oral breath pressure affecting articulation, and nasal emission.

In medical journals, particularly in articles written by otolaryngologists, changes in the vocal mechanism that result in changes in vocal behavior usually are categorized according to the type of condition that is manifest. Because these terms may be used frequently in medical reports, it is useful to discuss them here. The first is *congenital,* which refers to any alteration in the structure of the mechanism that was present at birth. Thus, cleft palate, laryngeal web, and laryngomalacia are examples of congenital conditions. The second is *traumatic,* which refers to any condition that results from injury (as in the case of intubation when a child is given oxygen and the folds are damaged) or accident. A larynx may be damaged through trauma in a car accident, or a palate may be injured if a child falls on a sharp stick. The third general category is that of *inflammatory diseases.* Inflammatory and ulcerative changes in the mechanism can be bacterial, viral, or fungal. An example of a fungal disease is histoplasmosis, which is carried by pigeons. *Allergic conditions* affecting the mechanism are considered to be another category, as are *neoplastic* (new growth) conditions. When new tissue is added to the existing mechanism, that tissue may be malignant or benign. Fortunately, malignant tumors are rare in young children. Benign growths, such as nodules, are the additive lesions that occur most frequently in school-age populations. Hemorrhages sometimes occur between the muscle and the squamous lining of the vocal folds. These concentrations of blood in one area, or generalized bruising of an entire fold, also may be described as additive lesions of the folds. An additional category is that of conditions related to the presence of foreign bodies. Examples are physical reactions that occur when a child swallows a safety pin or a fish bone or gets a pea lodged in the nasal cavity. The final category used by physicians is *psychosomatic*, and this encompasses any changes in the state or use of the mechanism that are directly related to an individual's reaction to stress or emotional disturbance.

The Relationship Between Classification of Problems and Their Treatment

The way we view or describe a set of symptoms sometimes affects our approach to treatment. A comprehensive framework that allows us to look at a child's problem with a wide-angle lens may be the most valuable. As speech–language pathologists, frequently we are called on to coordinate the intervention program or at least to discuss the total problem with the child, the family, the teachers, and other professionals. Obviously, we always need to be sure that a child receives appropriate medical referrals because some problems require specific surgical and medical treatments. (Congenital conditions frequently can be helped by surgical procedures or prosthetic devices. Inflammatory conditions, such as bacterial infections, respond to medication, such as a series of antibiotics prescribed by a physician; in some severe cases, steroids are used to reduce inflammatory reactions. Psychosomatic problems frequently require help from a psychiatrist, psychologist, or social worker.) We also must be alert to our role in explaining to the child why it may be necessary for him or her to see various specialists, in preparing the child for procedures that may be frightening if the child is unaware of what is to be expected, and in providing ongoing support and encouragement. In addition, we need to assume responsibility for evaluating the extent of the behavioral compensations adopted or perpetuated by the child. Inappropriate vocal strategies will be maintained by some children even after they have been treated successfully to remove the root cause of their problem. Elimination of a medical problem does not always mean that a child automatically reverts to a pattern of normal vocal behavior. We always need to remember that, as educators, we are concerned with maximizing the child's abilities and coping skills in all aspects of an intervention program.

Thus, it is probably useful for us now to consider the basic areas of behavior that are important in the development and maintenance of appropriate vocal performance. When we evaluate any child with a voice problem, we need to be aware of his or her abilities in the following critical areas: respiration, phonation, resonance, and psychodynamics. We shall discuss each of these areas in turn. Because speech-language pathologists are familiar with basic anatomy and physiology, however, and because other texts are available for a review of this information, we shall not focus on the normal anatomic and physiologic processes of respiration, phonation, and resonance. Rather, we shall highlight some of the important abilities in these areas that affect the way an individual's voice is used and perceived. We shall note the contributions of each area, the way behaviors are coordinated and sequenced, and factors that affect or limit the production of appropriate vocal patterns. In addition, we shall focus attention on some of the abilities related to the area of psychodynamics that can affect vocal expertise. This will provide a backdrop that will be useful later when we discuss specific procedures for diagnosis and management.

Areas of Behavior Related to Voice Production

Respiration

The primary function of the respiratory system is biologic. Through ventilation our blood gases are continually adjusted. The other important function of the respiratory system is to provide controlled and regulated airflow for the production of acoustic signals. Breathing at rest is more frequent (more breaths per minute) and also more rhythmic (more even inspiration and expiration phases) than breathing for speech or singing. Because we phonate during exhalation, the inspiration is usually quicker and the expiration is lengthened during speech breathing. If the vocal signal is to be adequate, the air supply must be carefully controlled and regulated.

Baken (1979) listed several criteria that must be met if the airflow is to be controlled sufficiently to produce adequate voice during speech. First, the quantity of air impounded during inspiration must be matched to the anticipated utterance. Utterances vary with respect to length and phonemic structure. Most people replenish air supply at phrase boundaries; however, there may be differences between individuals and between performance on reading and conversational speech tasks. Second, the air reservoir must be refilled quickly so that disruptions in the flow are minimized. Third, the pressure of the alveolar gas must be appropriate. During vegetative breathing through a relatively open vocal tract, the pressure demands are not great. When voice is produced, however, air is passed through high impedances, and the amplitude of the sound is related to pressure variations. Thus, the fourth criterion is that the pressure not only must be adequate but also must be regulated. Fifth, all these criteria must be met with the least expenditure of energy so that the system operates with maximal efficiency. Finally, all of the above must be accomplished within constraints imposed by the individual's metabolic gas-exchange requirements.

The foregoing discussion reminds us of some of the abilities that children need in the area of respiration for voice. When we observe children's respiratory behavior, we need to consider the movements of the chest wall (rib cage and diaphragm–abdomen) in relation to each other during both inspiratory and expiratory activity. It is also useful to observe how much air a child expires during expiration when we are considering chest-wall movements. If laboratory equipment is not available, an estimate of the child's ability to prolong the expiratory phase can be made by asking the child to prolong phonemes and timing the duration. It is usually useful to compare durations of phonemes where there is both high and low impedance (e.g., voiced vs. unvoiced continuants). We also need to observe the child's respiratory behavior during connected speech. As Baken (1979) observed, a speaker must be able to achieve an acceptable interaction of the vocal tract, rib cage, and abdomen to achieve muscle forces that are both effective and efficient with respect to the amount of energy expended (see also Baken, 1977, 1979b, 1981).

Some children may try to talk on the inspiration of air rather than during the expiration. Others may not have developed respiratory muscle control sufficient to regulate the airstream in response to specific speaking demands. This may be particularly apparent when the child tries to vary the loudness level of utterances or when utterances of varying lengths and phonemic complexity are attempted. Itoh, Horii, Daniloff, and Binnie (1982) found that during trains of repeated syllables individuals with hearing impairment used speech breathing in much the same way normal hearers do but that they expended more volume per syllable. The results of kinematics analyses reported by Forner and Hixon (1977) suggested that speakers with hearing impairment initiate speech at lower lung volumes than do normal hearers, and many utterances are initiated within the tidal volume range.

An important aspect of respiratory behavior to observe is the way in which a child replenishes the air supply during connected speech. As a young child develops language and joins words into sentences, the timing of pauses and the use of those pauses to replenish the supply of available air assumes greater importance. As utterances increase in length, the demands on the respiratory system during speech also increase. If a child inhales before every two or three words, the flow and rhythm of speech are disrupted. If a child inhales at the beginning of an utterance and not again until the tidal or reserve volume is depleted, the voice may be affected by the gradual reduction of available air across time. For example, it may fade or become strained or quavery at the ends of sentences. Most children seem to take in their largest amount of air spontaneously during a deep inspiration when they first begin a sentence and then use phrase pauses to take smaller or replenishing breaths as the meaning allows. These replenishing breaths are sometimes called *catch breaths* and ensure that the available air supply is never markedly reduced until the opportunity for the next deep inspiration occurs. Some children may not acquire this respiratory expertise for sustained connected speech spontaneously. They need to be taught the concept of replenishing breaths if they are to sustain appropriate voicing during continuous speaking or reading.

A useful analogy when explaining replenishing breaths to young children is that of filling a car with gas during a trip. At the beginning of a journey, the driver fills the gas tank. As he travels, he stops to "top off his tank" before it is completely empty. The driver uses this strategy to ensure that he will never run out of gas before he has finished his journey.

The analogy of the car engine fueled with gas and the voice motor driven by the airstream is also useful when explaining to children another important aspect of respiratory behavior related to voice—the coordination of the exhaled airstream with the onset of phonation. The larynx acts as a valve in the respiratory tract, and the timing of the onset of the exhalation of the airstream and the smooth initiation of phonation involves exquisite precision.

In some children with voice disorders the smooth, easy initiation of phonation may be inhibited because of the inappropriate coordination of respiration and phonation. Like an inexperienced car driver who steps too abruptly on the accelerator, some speakers set the vocal folds abruptly into motion with excessive force. An opposite, although also inappropriate, problem is that of attempting to phonate before the airstream reaches the larynx. Thus, in addition to the amount of available air, the coordination of the emitted airstream with initiation of phonation is critical.

Clinical evidence suggests that persons with communication disorders vary in terms of the ways they use their respiratory systems for speech production. Sapienza and Stathopoulos (1994) studied respiratory function in women and children with bilateral vocal nodules. They suggested that individuals with nodules might be compensating by using larger lung volume excursion because of higher than normal glottal airflow during phonation. They hypothesized that if the nodules resolved, appropriate lung volume excursion would occur as a result of better control of laryngeal airflow. More research is needed, but at this point in time, it does not appear as if specific speech breathing abnormalities can be directly tied to specific speech disorders in any consistent way.

Before leaving the topic of respiration, let us consider other general points that are relevant to our discussion. Many children with voice disorders are noisy inhalers or even mouth breathers because of the frequent congestion they experience in the nasal cavities. Some reasons for noisy or labored inhalation or the complete inability to inhale through the nose are chronic allergic or infectious rhinitis or sinusitis and enlarged tonsils and adenoids. Labored inhalation, in addition to being distracting to the listener, may affect the efficiency of the inhalation phase of speech breathing. Children with chronically enlarged adenoids that obstruct the nasopharynx usually present a number of identifiable symptoms. They may exhibit pinched nostrils, sleepiness in school, pallor, circles under the eyes, enlargement of the bridge of the nose, snoring during sleep, and habituated mouth breathing at rest. The mucous membranes of the vocal tract may be dry because of the mouth breathing; this dryness, sometimes in association with an irritating postnasal drip, may also result in hoarse voice quality. (Some of these symptoms also may be noted in children with partial blockages of the upper respiratory tract caused by intermittent allergic or infectious conditions causing swollen tissue.)

An extensive study of the habits, behavior, and breathing patterns of children with adenotonsillar hypertrophy was reported by Baranak, Potsic, Miller-Bauer, and Marsh (1983). Parents of patients completed questionnaires before and after adenotonsillectomy. In addition, sleep sonography was performed to determine nocturnal respiratory patterns. Parents' responses to the questionnaires indicated significant postsurgery improvement in breathing and sleep patterns; children snored less, had fewer episodes of obstructed inspiration, moved less in their sleep, and abandoned unusual sleeping postures (head hanging over side of bed, legs raised, and so on, assumed in attempts to position the body so that inhalation could occur more easily). The conclusions were supported by the sonographic analyses of respiratory patterns tape-recorded during sleep. About 67% of the sample showed clear improvement (i.e., less inspiratory effort and greater periodicity of respiration, and virtual elimination of episodes of obstructive apnea) after surgical removal of tonsils and adenoids. Another study of 100 children with adenotonsillar hypertrophy, reported by Pasquariello, Potsic, Miller, and Corso (1983), indicated that this population frequently demonstrates significant diet and nutrition problems. When enlargement of the tonsils and adenoids persisted for a long period of time, some children experienced difficulties and discomfort when eating. They were reported to be slow eaters and preferred soft foods. When the children's growth records were reviewed, more than 25% were below the 10th percentile for weight, although heights were generally age appropriate. Increased appetite and weight gain were reported following adenotonsillectomy.

The findings of studies such as those noted above remind us that when we suspect that a child may have enlarged tonsils and adenoids, we should question parents concerning the child's respiratory behavior during sleep. When the child is upright, the airway may be less obstructed than when the child is horizontal. Periods of sleep apnea, difficulty when eating, or low weight for age may be considered evidence that medical attention should be sought.

Deep, relaxed breathing is considered by some authorities in allied health fields to be important in achieving general relaxation and reduction of physical and mental tension. The ability to relax and breathe deeply and efficiently at rest may need to be taught to some children with hyperfunctional voice problems. It may be a part of teaching general or specific relaxation techniques. In addition to appropriate breathing patterns at rest, some children with voice disorders may need specific help in developing and maintaining appropriate speech breathing abilities. As noted, these include the manner and depth of the inhalation, the control and length of the exhalation, the use of replenishing breaths, and the coordination of the emission of the exhaled air with the onset of phonation.

Phonation

Changes in the subglottal air pressure (affected by actions of the thoracic and abdominal muscles and recoil forces that change the volume of the lungs) also change the sounds produced by the larynx. An increase in the subglottal pressure increases sound intensity (Isshiki, 1964). Also, the myoelastic-aerodynamic theory of phonation (Broad, 1973) associates increases in subglottal air pressure with increases in fundamental frequency. Nonetheless, Titze (1980), in his review of refinements of theory regarding myoelastic-aerodynamic fundamental frequency control, believed it to be primarily myoelastic because stiffness and mass are controlled by muscular contractions. The ability to produce normal phonatory patterns is related both to respiratory control and regulation and to healthy vocal fold structure and function.

Vocal Fold Pathology

The human vocal fold consists of a muscle (the vocalis) and the mucous membrane that covers the muscle. The mucous membrane, or mucosa, consists of the epithelium and the lamina propria. The lamina propria is divided into three layers: superficial, intermediate, and deep. Hirano (1981) described these layers in the following way: The superficial layer appears loose and pliant, and it is here that edema often develops. The intermediate layer is made up primarily of elastic fibers. The deep layer is dense with mostly collagenous fibers. The entire structure consisting of the intermediate and deep layers of the lamina propria is known as the *vocal ligament.* The epithelium and the superficial layer of the lamina propria is described as the *cover.*

Histologic descriptions such as the one provided by Hirano (1981) help us understand some of the ways in which pathologic states affect the laryngeal sound. Most lesions discussed by Hirano (1981) that occur frequently in children seem to invade the cover and affect mass and stiffness. The vocalis muscle does not move as vigorously as the mucosa during vibration of the folds. Thus, alterations in the mucosal cover seem to affect how the voice is perceived. Hirano (1981) listed the following aspects of pathologic states that may interfere with normal vibratory function: location of the pathology, glottal incompetence, symmetry of the bilateral vocal folds, uniformity within each vocal fold, layer structure, mass and stiffness of each layer, and interference with vibratory movement of the fold on the opposite side. He noted marked interference with vibratory movement of the fold on the opposite side when the following pathologies occur: polyp, polypoid vocal fold, cyst, epithelium hyperplasia, papilloma, and carcinoma. Fortunately, carcinoma is rarely found in children. Histologic manifestations of nodules and polyps vary; intratissue bleeding, hyaline degeneration, edema, fibrosis, and cell infiltration were seen in the adult larynges examined by Hirano. Nodules and polyps did not invade the vocal ligament, however. The mass of the superficial layer of the lamina propria increased, and stiffness changes could be observed. For example, when edema predominated, stiffness decreased, whereas fibrosis, intratissue bleeding, hyaline degeneration, and cell infiltration sometimes increased stiffness. Epithelial hyperplasia (any pathology causing hyperplastic thickening of the epithelium as the chief lesion) also increases mass and stiffness of the cover, as does papilloma, a benign neoplasm originating from the squamous cell epithelium. Papilloma usually enters the superficial layer, and occasionally the intermediate and deep layer, of the lamina propria. Hirano noted that it sometimes also may invade the vocalis muscle itself.

When Hirano (1981) studied acoustic measures and tried to relate the findings of laryngeal mirror examinations of 200 patients to patterns of vocal fold vibration and perceptual impressions, the only direct relationship that emerged was that with fundamental frequency. Increased mass results in a lower fundamental frequency. Hirano stated his impression that if you can detect a pathology using acoutic analysis, you can also hear the differences in voice and see the pathology with the laryngeal mirror. This statement is reassuring for the speech–language pathologist working in school settings where opportunities for laboratory analysis are limited. A trained ear and awareness of the importance of laryngeal examinations by a physician are of utmost importance for the voice diagnostician.

Changes in the physical dimensions and characteristics of the vocal folds influence the sound produced. The fundamental frequency of the voice is controlled by changes in thickness, mass, tension, and length. We have just seen how some pathologic states can change an individual's ability to make laryngeal adjustments. Most of the neoplastic pathologies result in increased stiffness and mass of the folds. Mass and stiffness are also affected by variations in the length of the folds. Longitudinal tension is increased by stretching the vocal folds, and the fundamental frequency of the voice increases as length is increased. Variations in vocal fold length result from contraction of the cricothyroid muscles (Gay, Hirose, Strome, & Sawashima, 1972; Shipp & McGlone, 1971); but there is also an anteroposterior movement by the arytenoids. The movement of the arytenoids is the result of activity by the interarytenoid and posterior cricoarytenoid muscles, which occurs most frequently during the production of higher frequencies in the modal register (Hollien, 1983).

Broad (1973) summarized some of the ways that changes in vocal fold dimensions affect the laryngeal sound. He said that the vocal fold dimensions are determined largely through the motions of the cricoarytenoid and cricothyroid joints. The ability to vary the width of the glottis is determined mostly by the adduction and abduction movements of the arytenoid cartilages. The medial compression of the vocal folds is determined by the adductory squeeze of the arytenoids. Vocal fold length is determined primarily by the rotation in the cricothyroid joint. Vocal fold tension and thickness also are determined largely by the relative rotation between the cricoid and thyroid cartilages. Pathologies or neurogenic or psychogenic conditions that influence children's abilities to make these adjustments in vocal fold dimensions affect the sound of the voice.

Perceptions of Phonatory Behavior

When we listen to a child's voice, we usually make some perceptual judgments about the way it sounds. We compare the individual's voice to the voices that we have heard of other children of similar age and gender.

The average perceived pitch, or the acoustic measurement of the fundamental frequency of a person's voice, is affected by anatomic and physiologic factors. The length and thickness of the folds is influenced by such factors as the individual's age, gender, and physical size. Thus, the most frequently used pitch level, sometimes called the *habitual pitch,* is usually structurally determined. Other factors in addition to the basic structural constraints, need to be considered; however, imitation, faulty learning, and excessive tension in the larynx may affect the way that the structures are habitually used.

In addition to the pitch level used most frequently by a speaker, we may need to be interested in the entire range of pitches available to that speaker. Again, the limits of the range are structurally determined. We need to remember that there are both physiologic and musical limits of the voice. At both ends of the entire pitch range, it is possible to emit sounds that are not musical.

The lowest musical sound that can be produced by a speaker is defined as *basal pitch.* At the upper limits of the musical range, postpubertal males can produce falsetto voice and some trained sopranos can produce what is known as a *laryngeal whistle.* Falsetto is produced with a vibratory pattern that differs significantly from the regular vibratory mode. The vocal folds are stiff, narrowed bands, tightly approximated, and the airstream forces them to vibrate rapidly along the extreme edge of the approximating surfaces. Beyond the top of the musical range, it is possible to produce nonmusical sounds, such as those emitted during emotional states involving a high degree of tension. Shrieks and cries fall into this category.

Herzel and Reuter (1997) reported on high-pitched vocalizations produced by a healthy 9-year-old boy. With forceful expiration, he produced high-pitched phonation with jumps from falsetto to whistle register (1000 to 1700 Hz whistle vocalizations). He phonated at a maximum fundamental frequency of 950 Hz during regular phonation. They found frequency jumps and biphonation (two fundamental frequencies), which they interpreted in a nonlinear dynamic framework and suggested that instabilities occur in the transition region between a whistle register and falsetto. The hypothesis of vortex-induced vibrations was supported by the observation that strong airflow is needed to sustain whistle phonation. Herzel and Reuter, therefore, have demonstrated that a normal prepubertal larynx can produce whistle register with harmonics like falsetto but with different driving mechanisms. Another nonmusical sound that can be produced at the lower end of the pitch range is referred to as *vocal fry.* This sound is difficult to describe and is usually likened to the sound made by a creaky door or by popcorn popping. We can describe vocal fry physiologically as the sound made when the folds are extremely relaxed and loosely approximated. This pattern is different from the vibratory pattern used during regular phonation. It is important to remember that true vocal fry is a completely relaxed sound. Our voices sometimes trail off into vocal fry when we are tired or speaking with minimal effort. It should not be confused with the tense, strained, irregular vibrations produced during hyperfunctional voice use. Children will sometimes use glottal fry when they are playing and making sound effects with their voices. They also, of course, will use strained vocalization patterns that sound somewhat similar when they are imitating engines and trucks. The differentiating feature between true vocal fry and other nonmusical sounds produced is the absence of tension associated with vocal fry.

Many clinicians investigate the extent of the pitch range during voice evaluations. It has been noted that individuals with voice disorders frequently exhibit a restricted pitch range. Conversational pitch range, or the limits of the rise and fall of the voice during conversational speech, is also of interest to the clinician. Some speakers have a restricted conversational range because their entire available range is limited. Other speakers may use a narrow conversational pitch range, or monotone, because of factors unrelated to the availability of other pitches.

Occasionally, pitch breaks will also be observed in children. They are not considered to be a problem if they occur around the time of puberty. Curry (1949) found that they occur when rapid pubertal changes take place. If pitch breaks occur in children who are not pubertal or approaching puberty, they may reflect the use of an inappropriate pitch level. Clinical experience suggests that when the level is too low, the voice breaks upward, and when the level is too high, it breaks downward, hence the clinical dictum that "the voice breaks in the direction it wants to go."

When we listen to children's voices, we are interested in habitual level, available range, variability, and the way pitch changes reflect meaning and feeling.

The loudness level of a child's voice during conversational speech is also of interest to a clinician. We are interested in the level that the child habitually uses and the ways in which the child can vary his or her loudness in response to situational and contextual demands. It is usually important to consider respiratory behavior, pitch, mouth opening, body position, and the amount of effort that the child appears to expend when making judgments concerning children's abilities with respect to loudness levels habitually used, the range of available loudness, and the use of loudness variations.

Mucosal Wave

Quality deviations may be due to the alteration in the mucosal wave during phonation. When the mucosa covering the vocal folds is not loose and pliant, it does not move freely during the vibratory cycle. Laryngeal lesions, as well as scar tissue, may inhibit the mucosal wave. The absence or distortion of the mucosal wave significantly influences voice quality.

Although all human voices, in contrast to synthesized voices, exhibit some slight variations in periodicity, deviations in periodicity are typically greater in adults' pathologic voices than in normal voices. Measures such as jitter or F_0 perturbation, shimmer that is cycle-to-cycle variations in amplitude, and harmonic-to-noise ratio (HNR) have been used to try to differentiate healthy and disordered voices on the basis of these acoustic changes. Information concerning periodicity tells us about the consistency of cycle-to-cycle variations. Pabon (1991) showed that the distribution and amount of perturbation usually varies across the voice range and changes as a function of pitch and loudness.

Karnell, Scherer, and Fischer (1991) demonstrated that methodologic factors, such as sampling frequency, window duration, and method of F_0 extraction affected jitter values. Aperiodicity measures are also affected by the sensitivity and accuracy of the recording equipment used to obtain the voice samples. McAllister, Sederholm, Ternstrom, and Sundberg (1996) examined the relationship between F_0 perturbation and hoarseness in children's voices during continuous speech. The samples were perceptually rated for hyperfunction, breathiness, and roughness, and the subjects demonstrated different degrees of hoarseness. High correlations were found between hoarseness and both hyperfunction and breathiness. Results showed low correlations between perturbation measures and perceived hoarseness. The authors speculated that factors such as the severity of hyperfunction (Klingholz & Martin, 1985), which does not seem to yield high jitter values, and the high F_0 of children's voices may affect the measurements. Whereas Steinsapir, Forner, and Stemple (1986) found that children in their earlier study tended to exhibit higher perturbation measures on sustained vowels than did adults, this was not seen in the samples obtained during running speech by McAllister et al. Both perturbation measures used by these experimenters correlated poorly with perceived hoarseness, hyperfunction, breathiness, and roughness, but the perturbation values for running speech were higher than those for sustained vowels, even with the removal of the effects of pitch variability.

Voice Profiles

Bohme and Stuchlik (1995) obtained voice profiles of the voices of 277 untrained healthy children's voices between the ages of 5 and 14 years and developed a standard childhood voice profile for the untrained voice between the ages of 7 to 10 years. They found that they could not obtain valid responses from children under 7 years of age or over 10 years. Between 7 and 10 years, however, they found that boys phonated louder than girls. Nonetheless, no age-related changes were noted in the maximal and minimal loudness levels across the different frequencies or the upper and lower limits of the frequency range. They estimated the voice range of both boys and girls to be 29 musical semitones. The sound pressure level (SPL) of the maximal and minimal intensity increases, however, when the frequency and dynamic range narrows near the upper and lower limits of the voice range. Voice range profiles, sometimes referred to as VRPs or phonetograms, chart how loudly and how softly the subject can produce a range of pitches. This technique, useful for singing teachers, allows the documentation of subsequent increases in vocal range abilities that may result from training, maturation, or both. These profiles also are useful for voice clinicians, as a reference showing the capability, graphically, of young children's available pitch and loudness ranges (see chapter 9).

Changes in VRPs related to vocal pathology also have been identified. McAllister, Sederholm, Sundberg, and Gramming (1994) found, for example, that there was a reduction from 25 to 19 semitones in the frequencies available to children with nodules. They assume that the VRP contours are related to the structural properties of the vocal fold mucosa and that developmental physiologic factors explain the smaller ranges exhibited by children compared with adults. Only the mutational voices approximated the upper frequencies of adult voices. All premutational children had smaller ranges with higher lower limits and lower higher limits. Vocal nodules, as well as restricting pitch range, also cause an elevated phonation threshold in the VRP. This finding is consistent with perceptual data on children with vocal nodules who have difficulty phonating softly and at high pitches. Differences in normal VRPs were also reported by McAllister et al. (1994) when children with hoarseness in the absence of nodules and children with glottal chinks were examined. Parents were asked for data regarding pubertal status of the 60 ten-year-olds who participated in this study and if the growth spurt for the previous year exceeded 10 cm/year, it was assumed the child had entered puberty. See Taranger, Engstrom, Lichtenstein, and Svennkerg-Redegren (1976) for a discussion of this index. Heylen et al. (1998) found differences between a group of 94 normal children and 136 children with vocal pathology aged 6 to 11 years. These researchers used an indexed approach to differentiate their two groups on the basis of several variables. Results suggested that the gender of the child was not salient but that both age and vocal pathology significantly influenced most of the defined VRP characteristics. The number of semitones available in modal register was significantly decreased in children with nodules, cysts, or edema. Also their highest frequency was significantly less than the high limit of the frequency range in normal children. Thus Heylen et al. concluded that their Voice Range Profile Index for Children (VRPIc) was useful for screening children and to qualitatively assess the efficacy of voice treatment.

In addition to pitch and loudness variations produced by the adjustments of the vocal folds, there is an overall quality of the voice perceived by the listener. This perceived quality, or timbre, of the voice is affected by airflow, the laryngeal structure and function, as well as by the resonance characteristics. The size and mass of the folds, as we know, change across time because of predictable factors related to age and gender. There are also intermittent changes that are less predictable and occur as the result of the way an individual's laryngeal structures react to emotional states, physical conditions, and environmental influences and demands. Thus, an individual's voice quality may vary at different times of a day, week, or year.

The way in which the folds approximate, or come together at the midline, is important in any consideration of quality deviation. Normal, healthy vocal folds approximate evenly along the free margins during vocal fold adduction. We have seen that edema and growths change the margins of the folds and interfere with normal laryngeal adjustments. When the folds approximate to some extent, but vibrate intermittently or irregularly, and the smoothness or evenness of the vibratory pattern is disrupted, we describe the behavior as *dysphonia.* The phonation is present, but it is disturbed. In some cases, an individual's vocal behavior may be predominantly dysphonic with periods of complete aphonia occurring intermittently or occasionally. *Aphonia* is the term used to describe the absence of voice during attempted phonation.

We have probably all experienced short periods in our lives when we have tried to talk with an acutely irritated vocal tract and felt that our voices "cut out" during a sentence. When children are aphonic for relatively short periods of time, this distressing loss of voice is usually the result of acute infections or prolonged or intense use of the voice (e.g., cheering at ballgames). If aphonia occurs for longer periods of time, it may be the result of neurologic or psychogenic difficulties or severe structural deviations.

Fairbanks (1960) used three descriptive terms to describe quality deviations. One is *breathiness.* Spectrographic analyses of breathy voice usually show reduced definition of a periodic soundwave. The listener usually hears an audible escape of air, suggesting that the free margins of the folds are not approximating optimally. There are, of course, degrees of perceived breathiness, ranging from what some children describe as "a very airy voice" to an almost imperceptible degree. Boone (1983) wrote that we frequently hear breathiness at the beginning of an utterance and that the vocal folds may approximate slowly after the initiation of the outgoing airstream has already begun.

Hoarseness is the term used most frequently to describe laryngeal-quality disorders. Moore (1971) said that hoarseness may be related to mucus, additional mass on the folds, or relative flaccidity of one or both folds. Some writers differentiate between hoarseness and *harshness* by suggesting that more tension is present in harshness. Others, such as Darley (1965), say that a hoarse voice quality combines the acoustic characteristics of harshness and breathiness. Harshness is difficult to describe, but it usually creates an unpleasant reaction on the part of the listener. The speaker seems to be using too much effort to speak, may exhibit observable tension in the neck, and may initiate phonation with hard glottal attacks. In Boone's 1983 description of harshness, he also referred to the frequent presence of "metallic aspects of resonance" that are sometimes observed in a harsh voice.

Spectrographic analysis is useful when describing the characteristics of quality deviations because the aperiodicity of laryngeal vibration can be seen.

Visual displays of the acoustic signals are sometimes useful for providing both diagnostic information and feedback to the child during therapy. Changes in periodicity of the signal and differences in types of voice onset can be demonstrated and improvement can be quantified when instrumentation is available. Quantification is especially important because vocal symptoms frequently occur inconsistently and vary in terms of perceived severity. When instrumentation is not available, the speech–language pathologist will need to define symptoms carefully and help children chart the occurrence of specific symptoms using perceptual scales.

Hoarseness is sometimes reduced when the loudness level of the voice increases because the speaker adducts the folds more vigorously. An increased pitch level also can sometimes improve the extent of closure, reduce the aperiodicity in the vibratory pattern and decrease perceived hoarseness.

It is not uncommon for a child who has additive lesions of the vocal folds, such as vocal nodules, to produce a clearer voice quality when talking or singing loudly. The voice also may sound clearer on higher pitches. This is usually most noticeable when the lesions (either unilateral or bilateral) are small or moderately sized. As the lesions increase in size, greater and greater effort is necessary in order for the child to adduct the folds forcefully enough to compensate for the lesions during fold closure. Also, as the size of the lesions increases, their effect on increasing the mass of the vocal folds and consequent lowering of the habitual pitch of the voice may be more obvious.

Thus, when children are dysphonic because of vocal nodules, there is always the danger that they will compensate for their hoarseness by learning to overadduct the folds and talk more and more loudly. In such cases, the problem is exacerbated by excessive effort and strain. When such behavior is habituated, the place where the folds first make contact at the point of their maximum excursion (i.e., the junction of the anterior one third and posterior two thirds of the folds) is repeatedly irritated. Therefore, although this effortful production may make the voice sound clearer in the short term, the long-term effect will be that the nodules may increase in size, and the vocal quality will deteriorate.

Other compensations that are sometimes adopted by dysphonic children are the frequent use of glottal stops. When a glottal stop is produced, the arytenoid cartilages are completely adducted to close the glottis. The sudden release of the blocked air results in a characteristic burst, which is perceived as a pop or click. This sound may be heard as a substitution for a plosive (as in the word "bo*tt*le") and is similar to the abrupt phonatory onset heard when children initiate stressed vowels at the beginning of words with a hard glottal attack. This abrupt, almost grunting sound differs significantly from a normal easy onset of phonation. It also differs from a breathy attack, which occurs when the airstream begins to pass through the laryngeal valve before the folds approximate. Because the breathy attack is diametrically opposed to the hard glottal attack, it is usually taught as a substitute technique during the beginning stages of therapy to eliminate hard attacks. Both kinds of voice onset, however, may be described as the result of deviations in the exact timing and coordination of the airstream with the beginning of the vibratory cycle.

Phonation breaks are sometimes noted in association with quality deviations. This term is used to describe short periods of aphonia that occur on syllables, words, or phrases. It is usually associated with hyperfunction and may appear most frequently on unstressed syllables when the speaker reduces his or her effort level. It also may be related to difficulty maintaining appropriate air pressure (e.g., on the final syllable of a breath group). Sometimes it signals vocal fatigue if the speaker has been attempting to increase effort (e.g., by raising the pitch, trying harder to talk) during a prolonged period of talking. Sometimes the speaker will try throat clearing, coughing, or swallowing to remedy the problem.

Throughout our discussion of phonation, I have referred to the effect of size, mass, and tension changes in the folds and the extent of vocal fold closure on perceptions of pitch, loudness, and quality. It has been noted that the laryngeal structures react to environmental and physical changes. The laryngeal surfaces are composed of mucous membrane and are frequently subject to irritation by airborne substances and viral and bacterial infections. Reactions of the laryngeal structures can range from extreme dryness of the membranes to excessive secretion. Both dryness and wetness can lead to irritation of the structures, inflammation, and swelling. When such conditions are present, an individual is particularly at risk if abusive vocal behaviors occur repeatedly. It is important to remember that abusive vocal behaviors include the use of excessive amounts of effortful talking or singing, hard glottal attacks, inappropriate use of loudness or pitch levels, and excessive throat clearing and coughing. Compensatory behaviors adopted by an individual trying to talk with an irritated or altered laryngeal mechanism sometimes lead to habituated hyperfunctional vocal behavior that exacerbates the original problem. Children's abilities in the area of phonation should always be considered in relation to available medical information concerning conditions (e.g., allergies and infections) that may increase their susceptibility to adopt abusive compensatory practices. Although the majority of voice problems in children are related to vocal abuse, it should be emphasized that children will also present with organic problems unrelated to abuse. Other structural deviations, such as papilloma, laryngeal webs, and paralyzed vocal folds, may be seen. In these cases, as in other less frequently seen organic pathologies, the medical report will be the critical factor in evaluating and treating the problem. In some cases, emotional problems and faulty learning will result in abnormal use of the vocal mechanism. Whatever the etiology of a disorder involving abnormal use of the laryngeal structures, the vocal symptoms themselves need to be described specifically. This includes a description of the onset, the extent of vocal fold adduction, and the smoothness and evenness of the perceived vibratory pattern.

Resonance

The complex laryngeal tone is modified still further by the supralaryngeal structures. The voice is affected by the size, configuration, and coupling of the supraglottal cavities. Adjustments of the shape and acoustic properties of the vocal tract are known as *articulation.* The vibrating airstream may be changed by variations in tension size and shape of vocal tract structures. Direct emission may be through the nose or the mouth, depending on the position of the velopharyngeal closure mechanism, and the vibrating column of air may be converted to a series of speech sounds. As we know, when the lips, tongue, or palate block the airstream, plosive sounds are generated; when the airstream is constricted and turbulence occurs, fricative sounds are produced.

Because many of the same structures influence both articulation of speech sounds and resonance, it is sometimes difficult to discuss resonance independently. This is why many writers say that resonance problems are actually articulation problems. One distinction that can be made is that between speech intelligibility and vocal acceptability. These two aspects are obviously related, and yet there are some advantages in considering them separately. Intelligibility of speech sounds is a function of the distribution of energy within the speech sounds. This is accomplished by precise predictable movements of vocal tract structures (such as the lips, tongue, and palate) that are capable of generating recognizable phonemes. The distinctive features of speech sounds are well known and are similar for all speakers of a language. Problems with speech intelligibility can result from inadequate velopharyngeal closure during the production of oral sounds. In such instances, vowels may be produced nasally, and consonants requiring oral breath pressure are frequently distorted. The acceptability of the voice quality is also affected and perceived as hypernasal. When voice is perceived as hyponasal, substitutions such as b–m, d–n, and g–ŋ are frequently noted and attributed to obstruction of the nasal cavities. Thus, when speech intelligibility is affected, the misarticulations are generally also accompanied by a perceived change in the acceptability of the voice quality. An acceptable voice during speech involves an appropriate balance of both oral and nasal resonance. In addition to specific articulatory adjustments necessary for intelligible production of speech sounds, however, there are changes in the configuration of the vocal tract itself that contribute to the production of acceptable voice.

Let us consider the way that resonance characteristics are altered during voice production. The musculo-membranous tube above the larynx is made up of the laryngopharynx, the oropharynx, and the nasopharynx. This pharyngeal cavity is lined throughout with mucous membrane and communicates with the tympanic, oral, laryngeal, and nasal cavities, as well as with the esophagus. Because of the softness of the tissues lining the pharynx, reinforcement of overtones is not a major contribution of this cavity during voice production. Because of the presence of the pharyngeal constrictor muscles, however, this cavity can be differentially tensed or relaxed. There are individual structural differences in the length, size, and shape of the pharynx, and individual differences in the muscular tension of the walls of the pharynx during voice production. The fauces, the oral cavity itself, and the buccal cavity also are lined with mucous membrane and are highly variable in shape and dimensions. Individual differences occur with respect to basic structure of these cavities and range of variability during voice production.

It is obvious that the mouth is certainly the most movable and adjustable of the cavities of the vocal tract. The degree of mouth opening and movement during communication significantly affects oral resonance, affects facial expression, and provides important visual cues that supplement vocal communication. The mouth's most important biologic function is, of course, to provide a port between the external world and the respiratory and digestive tracts. It initiates the digestive process through the production of saliva. On occasion we encounter a child in voice therapy who has problems with excess saliva production or inappropirate swallowing of saliva. Excessive moisture in the corners of the mouth or obvious drooling may be observed. When such symptoms are noted, it may be necessary to observe such relevant behaviors as head position (because gravity may be a factor), mouth closure at rest, and frequency of swallowing (children should swallow at least once every 40 seconds). At the Hospital for Sick Children in Toronto, Canada, important work has been done on the treatment of drooling problems in children, and this work reminds us of the importance of considering the biologic as well as nonbiologic functions of the oral cavity.

The nasal cavities are paired and separated by the nasal septum. They communicate with the exterior by way of the nares, with the nasopharynx through the velopharyngeal port, and with the paranasal sinuses. The surface of the nasal cavities filters, moistens, and warms the air as it is inhaled. Nasal passages may become dried out, irritated, or both under certain conditions, or they may produce excess secretions that diminish or block nasal resonance.

During normal voice production, there is a shifting balance of oral resonance and direct and indirect nasal resonance. Let us consider some of the terms used to describe resonance patterns.

Vowel sounds and all consonants in English with the exception of /m/, /n/, and /ŋ/ are produced with a preponderance of oral resonance; in other words, the direct emission of the vibrating air column through the mouth. Because the velopharyngeal port is closed during the production of oral sounds, there is minimal direct air emission through the nasal cavities, so we can say there is no direct nasal resonance. Nevertheless, some indirect nasal resonance may occur during the production of oral sounds. Vibrations may sometimes be felt on the bones of the face and nasal cavities during projected speaking or singing of oral sounds. These vibrations reverberate through the craniofacial bone structures and add richness and color to the tone. In order to maximize indirect nasal resonance, some teachers and singing coaches use images such as "place the sound in the mask" or "use forward projection of the voice" or "think that the sound is vibrating the bones of the head." It is usually suggested that "forward tone focus" or concentrating the resonating energy in the front of the face helps a student to maximize both oral resonance and indirect nasal resonance.

During the production of /m/, /n, and /ŋ/, when the velopharyngeal port is open and the vibrating column of air is emitted directly through the nose, there is a preponderance of direct nasal resonance in the voice. If the nasal cavities are obstructed because of structural constraints (e.g., enlarged adenoidal tissue) or the presence of foreign bodies or excess secretions, the voice is described as denasal, hyponasal, or "blocked." This is the sound we hear when someone sounds as if he or she has "a cold in the nose."

In a study by Rastatter and Hyman (1984) perceptual judgments of denasality were found to be dependent on speaking task. The results suggest that the listeners were able to categorize nasal resonance problems accurately when they were caused by rhinologic disorders such as edematous adenoids and allergic rhinitis. Both VCV syllables using the nasals /m/, /n/, and /ŋ/ and loaded sentences proved the best tasks for listeners to detect hyponasality because when denasal children prolonged isolated vowels, the listeners judged them to be exhibiting nasal resonance characteristics close to normal. Another interesting finding was reported by Rastatter and Hyman on six children ranging in age from 8 to 14 years who each had an anteriorally deviated septum of traumatic origin. Listeners judged these children to have essentially normal resonance. The researchers point out that these results should not be overgeneralized, because deviated septums vary with respect to severity and origin and may accompany other pathologic nasal conditions.

Whereas hyponasality describes too little direct nasal resonance on /m/, /n/, /ŋ/, hypernasality refers to an excessive amount of direct nasal resonance on sounds other than /m/, /n/, and /ŋ/. Hypernasality is always the result of inefficient valving of the velophyaryngeal sphincter mechanism. This may be the result of structural or neurologic deficits or may be functional in origin. The degree of the velopharyngeal insufficiency and the nature of the compensations adopted will influence whether speech sound generation also is impaired.

Assimilated nasality is the term used to describe a resonance pattern that results from imprecise timing of the movements of the velopharyngeal valving system during running speech. Assimilated nasality is usually a behavior learned through imitation (as in the case of speakers representing certain regional speech patterns) and is usually not considered to be a resonance disorder unless a speaker aspires to a career in professional voice use. It is sometimes observed in speakers who have mild velopharyngeal inadequacy or faulty learning where speech-sound intelligibility is not impaired but resonance characteristics are. Essentially, assimilated nasality results from the influence nasal consonants exert on adjacent or neighboring oral sounds. For example, if a vowel is preceded or followed by a nasal sound and the velopharyngeal port is not opened or closed quickly or precisely enough, some hypernasality may occur during production of the vowel itself. Similarly, if an oral consonant is embedded in a cluster of nasal consonants, such as in the word "ven*t*nor," nasal emission or plosion may occur on the /t/.

The perception of appropriate oral–nasal resonance balance in speech depends on the interplay of a number of related factors. Rapid connected speech involves a series of precise articulatory and resonatory adjustments. When we observe a child's behavior in the area of resonance, we consider his or her ability to generate both oral and nasal phonemes appropriately and to adjust the size, shape, tension, and configuration of the oral and nasal cavities. It is important to remember that only excessive nasal (hypernasality) or oral (hyponasality) resonance is of clinical concern.

The most important prerequisite for appropriate resonance is an intact and operational velopharyngeal closure mechanism. If any doubt exists concerning the efficiency of this mechanism, velopharyngeal assessment should be obtained (e.g., X-ray study, cinefluorography, nasopharyngoscopy).

Psychodynamics

Communication takes place when a message is transmitted by a speaker to a listener. This interaction between speaker and listener is basic in the true communication of information and feelings. When communication attempts involve little regard for the listener, the act may provide satisfactory self-expression or even catharsis for the speaker, but satisfying communication rarely occurs. A self-absorbed speaker does not capitalize on the responses of the listeners, and the communicative interaction is therefore inhibited.

Vocal communication involves the transmission of meaning on a number of levels. The sounds and words produced carry semantic content, and their arrangement in phrases and sentences, or the syntactic pattern, adds further information. In addition to the phonological, semantic, and syntactic factors, however, information is provided by the paralinguistic aspects of the utterance. Such features as rate, timing, stress, and prosodic patterns add immeasurably to the transmission of meaning and feeling. It is interesting to note that the larynx is acutely sensitive to the emotional state of the speaker. We all know from experience that the intensity and degree of feeling affect our ability to control the sound of our voice voluntarily. When we are just a little anxious or nervous, for example, we can usually manage to prevent our anxiety from affecting our vocal communication. If, on the other hand, we are absolutely terrified, our control diminishes. At such times it is unlikely that we even think about how our voice sounds to a listener, and if we do attempt to conceal our emotional state voluntarily, our attempts do not succeed.

Speaker Characteristics

Researchers such as Davitz (1964) and Fonagy (1981) have summarized some of the predictable phonatory patterns associated with intense emotional states. Studies have focused on the acoustic analysis of intensely emotional speech patterns in real-life situations, as well as in lines spoken by actors and actresses. Many different languages have also been studied, and the generalizations reported here are consistent across languages. Some writers have suggested that the biologic function of the larynx, described by Darwin (1872) in his discussion of the "flight or fight" phenomenon, may account for the consistent laryngeal patterns observed. Fonagy stressed the dynamic nature of distinctive features occurring during emotive speech and said that if the symptoms of emotive behavior are vestiges of a once purposive activity, vocal and prosodic features may be interpreted in terms of symbolic bodily movements.

We shall summarize some of the behaviors that Fonagy (1981) associated with specific emotional states beginning with his description of anger. Forceful expirations and very intense activity of the expiratory muscles are observed. There is imperfect phonation, such as breathy voice. The speaking rate is faster than normal. Fonagy also noted that the vocal strategy is entirely different for aggressive versus tender emotive speech. Tender voice is characterized by a complete but smooth contact of the vocal folds, and the false folds and laryngeal ventricles are widely separated. In contrast, in hatred the laryngeal ventricles are compressed, probably because of the spasmodic contraction of the adductor muscles. Thus, in anger, it is likely that the false folds are approximated and may disturb the vibrations of the true folds. Because of the extent of the muscle contractions, and despite the high subglottal pressure caused by the effort of the expiratory muscles, the intensity of the sound produced may be less than a sound produced with much less effort during tender speech. Slower rate and slower gradual pitch changes are observed in affectionate tender speaking. During a prolonged state of fear or anguish, the use of an extremely narrow pitch range is observed consistently.

Fonagy's research findings support some of the vocal stereotypes commonly held in our society. There is no doubt that certain stereotypes or sets of vocal characteristics associated with certain personality types exist. These are learned as part of the acculturation process, and there are some similarities and differences between cultures. For example, many American female speakers are perceived as speaking too loudly by members of Asian cultures. Within the American culture, particular vocal patterns have become associated with certain personality stereotypes. These have not been exposed to extensive empirical scrutiny but seem to have achieved some measure of general acceptance. For example, the effeminate male voice is generally characterized by high pitch level, exaggerated pitch inflections, prolongation of vowels, and light vocal timbre. The *macho* male voice is described as having a low pitch level, less vocal variety, shorter and less elaborate sentence structures, and a larger proportion of falling inflections (denoting decisiveness) at the ends of sentences. The sensuous female voice is characterized by a breathy quality, higher pitch level, reduced loudness, slower rate, and increased frequency of pauses. Aggressiveness in women is characterized by greater loudness, lower pitch level, fewer questioning or tentative inflectional patterns, faster rate, and precise articulation. In general, slow rate, increased frequency of pauses, and restricted variability of both pitch and loudness tend to suggest lower cognitive function in speakers of both genders.

The importance of the media in establishing and reinforcing vocal stereotypes cannot be estimated precisely, but it is undoubtedly significant. Anyone who has listened to the Saturday morning cartoons on television can identify the "good guy" and the "bad guy" voices, even when not watching the picture on the screen. Children undoubtedly are influenced by all the voice models to which they are exposed and probably internalize and identify them with certain vocal patterns. Thus, as we consider a child's vocal behavior, we need to be aware of the influences that contribute to his or her cultural conditioning. We also need to be aware of the close relationship that exists between children's emotional state and level of general physical tension and its relationship to voicing patterns. Although it is expected that vocal behavior will fluctuate across time in response to varying feeling states, the presence of consistently excessive emotional and physical tension reflected in vocal behavior may be diagnostically significant.

Listening Responses

As mentioned, true communication involves an interaction between a speaker and a listener. In other words, a message has to be received and processed as well as transmitted. A good communicator, therefore, is an effective listener as well as an effective speaker. An effective listener is usually an active listener; that is, messages are received, processed, and acknowledged. Clinical experience suggests that listening responses, those verbal and nonverbal responses that indicate a message has been processed, may be developed late in the sequence of language acquisition. Very young children seem to demonstrate few listening responses that are not purely egocentric. If one observes preschool children, and even children in the early elementary school grades, one may notice that they rarely verbally acknowledge that they have processed what has been said to them. Older children and adults usually provide evidence of active listening by facial expressions, gestures, interjections, questions, and confirmations such as "I see." This may be because as one's communicative competence grows, one's awareness of the need to provide more explicit feedback to the listener develops. For example, an adult who is working on a project in the backyard will usually respond when someone calls from the house to say lunch is ready. The need to assure the speaker that the message has been received is acknowledged, either by a wave or other nonverbal signal or by a sentence such as, "I'll be there in a minute." A young child playing in the backyard when called for lunch may give no indication that the message has been received. This may be why a parent sometimes feels compelled to call, "Did you hear me?"

This example provides a vivid reminder to many of us of the frustration we feel when someone to whom we are speaking is unaware of the need to provide us with feedback through listening responses. One could speculate that listening responses are the highest and, therefore, the last aspect of communicative behavior to be mastered. Some individuals may never fully master this communicative skill, even as adults. Lecturers are often grateful for members of an audience who demonstrate a high frequency of nonverbal listening responses. Those are the audience members who nod, smile, laugh, and otherwise indicate active processing of the information they are receiving. Because such active listening is reinforcing and reassuring to a speaker, a lecturer may tend to look at, or focus attention on, listeners who actively respond. If we think about people with whom we enjoy talking in one-to-one or small-group conversational settings, we also realize that the reassurance that our thoughts and feelings are being received and processed is always important. We gain most satisfaction from talking when we feel we have the active attention of our listeners. We know listeners are attending to us when they acknowledge us and to our messages through their listening responses. Eye contact is probably the most critical listener response. In our culture, we expect the listener to look at us when we are talking and to demonstrate continued interest by maintaining eye contact. We react to a listener's wandering gaze by thinking that he is losing interest. If a listener's eyes wander and there are other signs (such as rising from a chair, shifting the feet, or moving away from the speaker), we usually assume that the conversation is being terminated. Naturally, depending on the level of awareness of the speaker, these signs may be interpreted and

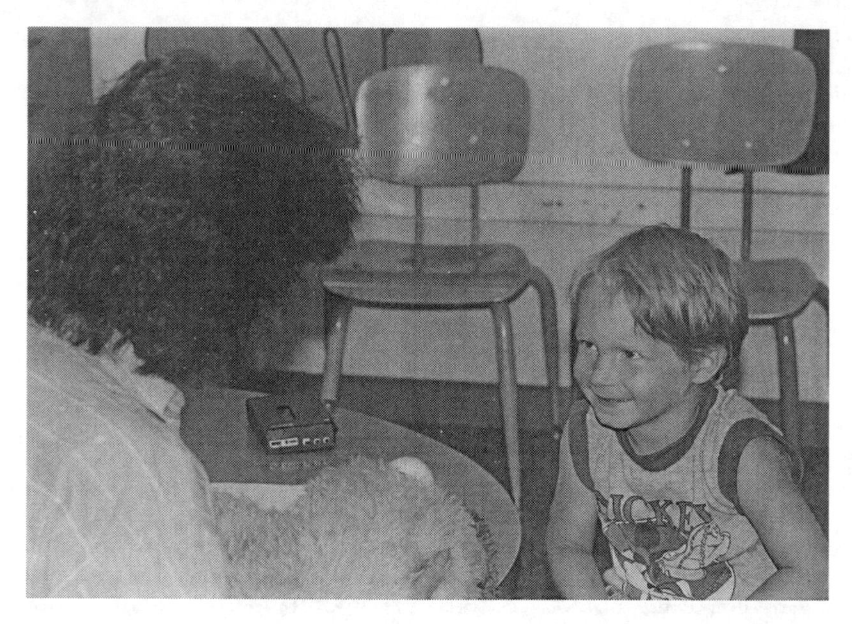

Figure 6-1. Eye contact is probably the most critical listener response.

acted on or not. Some speakers will immediately interpret such nonverbal signals as meaning that the conversation is terminated. Others may try to compensate for the wandering attention of the listener by talking more quickly, more loudly, or more dramatically. Some speakers, and we have all encountered them, seem completely unaware of the reactions of the listener and continue talking ad infinitum, choosing to ignore all but the most blatant verbal evidence of communication breakdown.

When children talk incessantly and ignore listening responses, it is important to consider the reasons that might be causing such behavior. If they are very young, it is possible that they may not yet have developed expertise in attending to and interpreting nonverbal signals. Children 8 years old and younger may not yet have learned either to transmit or to interpret a variety of explicit listening responses. Children who are older may also at times demonstrate a lack of awareness and skill in this area of communicative competence. In such cases, the behaviors may need to be taught to them by explicit demonstration, analysis, and discussion.

There may be some elementary school children who seem to have developed the communicative competence to encode and decode listening responses, and who understand both the semantic meaning and the emotional tone of messages and yet they frequently ignore listening responses. Of course, all children do this occasionally when they are extremely uptight or upset. The emotionality of the moment may obscure everything else. An example of this occurs when a child bursts into a classroom and interrupts a teacher who obviously does not want to be interrupted. If the child is extremely excited or anxious, the need to tell the teacher what has just occurred on the playground is so intense that the teacher's initial negative reaction is disregarded completely. When this behavior occurs frequently, however, it may be assumed that a particular child's anxiety level or need for attention is unusually strong. Frequent interruptions, incessant bids to seek and hold attention, very loud or very fast talking, and repeated disregard of listener responses may indicate not only immature communicative skills but also unresolved emotional conflicts or inadequate satisfaction of basic human needs.

The most satisfying communicators vary their listening responses according to the needs of the speaker. They observe and respond appropriately to the verbal, nonverbal, and paralinguistic features of a speaker's messages. For example, when a speaker is very upset or agitated, a sensitive listener is aware of that speaker's need to express his or her feelings or tell his or her story in an uninterrupted manner. Thus, such a listener, sensing that the goal of the interaction is primarily catharsis, provides understanding by murmuring supportive responses and sympathetic interjections that reflect acceptance of the speaker's feelings. A less sensitive or less skillful listener, in a similar situation, by attempting to interrogate or give advice might antagonize a speaker who has a primary need to ventilate his or her feelings and to be understood. Thus, listening responses are usually geared to the interaction that is occurring: At times, they are reflections of understanding a speaker's situation; at other times, they may be more direct attempts to clearify or analyze or debate issues.

It is important for clinicians to consider the range of communicative behaviors used by the children they teach. Some children with voice disorders may not demonstrate a well-developed range of listening responses. Such children may be so intensely involved with their own anxieties or needs that they are unable to focus on the demands of varied communication settings or on the needs of others. For example, the frequent use of talking primarily for self-expression may sometimes be seen in children referred to the clinician because of vocal abuse. Incessantly loud talking or other abusive vocal behaviors sometimes may be related to immature listening skills or may be a symptom of unsatisfied personal needs. Such one-sided attempts at communication rarely result in satisfying interpersonal interactions.

Question-Asking Skills

As we have seen, many questions are primarily listening responses. There are many types of questioning behaviors, however, and these need to be considered. The informational question appears very early during language development, and the *Why*? question is frequently heard in young children's speech patterns. We know from our study of language acquisition that tag questions ("That's mine, isn't it?") appear earlier than interrogative reversals ("Isn't it mine?"). Children ask questions to find out information, to gain attention, to seek comfort and reassurance, to elicit repetitions of pleasing verbal patterns and make verbal connections with others. Questioning is a strategy for coding personal experience. We check our own perceptions and understanding of feelings and events in this way. Bloom's 1956 taxonomy provides us with a model of the different levels of questioning that teachers may use. Questions can be designed to elicit information ("What is today's date?") or can involve interpretation ("What is important about today?"). Questions can also elicit analysis and synthesis of information. For example, a skillful analytical question can encourage the listener to break down information in different ways, and synthesis questions can encourage reorganization of ideas in a variety of formats. An example of an analytical question is, "What times during the day do you talk a lot?" An example of a synthesis question is, "If you talk most during recess, how much recess talking-time do you have each week?" Evaluation questions that involve some judgment are the most complex question forms to answer. To evaluate and form opinions, children must first organize their thoughts and consider pertinent information. Therefore, a question such as, "Why are some people better listeners than others?" might prompt a child who has been discussing specific listener behaviors to form opinions about specific behaviors that seem especially important. The child might respond, "Some people are better at showing you they are listening to you. They look at you, nod when they agree, and ask questions about what you are saying."

The Amount of Talking

The amount of time that a child spends talking each day varies according to situations and opportunity. The classroom organization and the amount of discussion and oral activity encouraged by the teacher are, of course, significant factors during school hours. The peer group and play activities engaged in during free time also exert an influence, as does the kind of family interaction. In addition, each child has a unique personality, and some children are naturally more verbal than others. The amount of self-generated talking varies from individual to individual. We can break down the amount of self-initiated talking further by considering the purposes of the talking. Some children will spend the greater percentage of their talking time in self-expression. Others will spend less time telling about themselves, and their talking may involve fewer purely egocentric statements and a greater number of oral attempts to manipulate the listener. The range of purposes exhibited and the variety of topics covered allows us to gain further insight about the child's needs and his or her strategies for need satisfaction through vocal behavior.

We therefore can describe the child's vocal behavior by considering how much he or she talks and how often he or she initiates conversation. We can further analyze it by observing how much of the talking is self-expression, how many questions are asked, the type and purpose of the declarative and interrogative forms used, and the type and frequency of what seem to be satisfying communicative exchanges.

Specific Components of the Four General Areas

Vocal Production

We have already discussed the four general areas of behavior that provide the support framework for vocal communication. For vocal production to occur optimally, all parts of the mechanism must be structurally intact and exhibit a maturity and level of function commensurate with the chronological age of the child. The importance of the anatomic and physiologic state of the mechanism is especially important in the areas of respiration, phonation, and resonance. Although we have discussed these three systems separately, it is obvious that during voice production, the child must be able to coordinate the contributions from each area of behavior. Implicit in the notion of adequate function is the ability to sequence a series of behaviors efficiently, smoothly, and with appropriate timing. The mechanics of optimal voice production depend on the presence of intact functional structures capable of supporting coordinated sequences of respiratory, phonatory, and resonatory activity. This aspect of production, the generation of signals or messages, is referred to in communication theory as *encoding*. Some of the components that contribute to optimal vocal encoding are listed below.

A. *Respiration*
   1. Intact respiratory structures
   2. Adequate breathing patterns for speech
      a. Depth of inhalation
      b. Type of inhalation
      c. Length of exhalation
      d. Control of airflow (stopping–starting/decreasing–increasing)
   3. Appropriate timing
B. *Phonation*
   1. Intact laryngeal mechanism
   2. Ability to make precise adjustments
      a. Vocal fold excursion/closure
      b. Vocal fold mass/stiffness
      c. Vibratory onset/termination
      d. Smooth continuity of vibratory pattern
   3. Appropriate timing—durational aspects
   4. Adequate sensory feedback
   5. Coordination of respiration and phonation
      a. Adjustment of airflow
         i. Loudness
         ii. Pitch
         iii. Duration
      b. Appropriate pausing for air intake
         i. Deep inhalations
         ii. Replenishing breaths
      c. Synchronized muscle activity
C. *Resonance*
   1. Intact supraglottal tract structures
   2. Adequate coupling of oral and nasal cavities
   3. Precise adjustments of velopharyngeal sphincter during oral–nasal, nasal–oral transitions
   4. Adequate oral breath pressure for production of speech sounds
   5. Adequate sensory feedback

We have listed some of the optimal components subsumed under the respiratory, phonatory, and resonatory systems. These three systems could be described as providing the technology of voice production. To produce an appropriate voice, the "machinery" must be structurally and functionally viable. In addition to possessing the appropriate technological potential for encoding and monitoring voice signals, however, an individual must operate in a psychologic domain. It is this psychologic domain that we discuss next. Technicians can build machines, such as voice synthesizers, to generate a variety of voice signals, but dynamic vocal behavior seen in its interpersonal context is uniquely human.

Psychodynamics

The fourth area of behavior, that of interpersonal factors affecting voice, relates to the decoding aspects of vocal behavior. Vocal performance, or the encoding of signals, does not occur in a vacuum. There is always an effect on self, on others, or both. Depending on the level of competence we have achieved, we are able to monitor, understand, modify, and evaluate our vocal products and respond appropriately to the feedback provided by others. Our competence or our knowledge of the rules of vocal and nonvocal behavior is developed by observing others, from explicit instruction, and by trial and error. A child's level of competence will be affected by such factors as age and cognitive and affective development. Some examples of rules concerning vocal behavior that are internalized as competence develops are (a) when to talk and when not to, (b) how loudly to talk in a given situation or context, (c) the ways in which emotion is expressed in voice, and (d) the rules for expressing emotions appropriately. Vocal competence, as an aspect of total communicative competence, is reflected in the way the child adapts vocal behavior in response to personal needs, the reactions of others, and the constraints of his or her world.

Some important interpersonal factors that contribute to the development of effective vocal behavior are listed below. The list is certainly not exhaustive.

Interpersonal Factors

1. Appropriate emotional adjustment/self-esteem
2. Awareness of feedback from others
   a. Listens to others' words, meanings
   b. Observation of nonverbal aspects
      - eye contact
      - facial expression
      - gestures, postures
      - use of space
      - loudness
      - pitch
      - intonation
      - silence, pauses
3. Providing feedback to others
4. Seeking feedback from others
   a. Asks questions
   b. Checks to see if meaning is understood
   c. Pauses to allow others to respond
   d. Talks slowly enough so that others can process information
5. Shares talking time
   a. Takes turns
   b. Does not interrupt
6. Awareness of differences between people
   a. Adapts to status of listener
   b. Adapts to needs of listener
   c. Adjusts production if listener does not understand or respond
7. Awareness of differences in situations
   a. Adapts to physical constraints
   b. Adapts to formal–informal aspects
   c. Shares or controls feelings appropriately
8. Awareness of needs and interests of others
   a. Shows interest in what others are doing or feeling
   b. Respects others' property, ideas, feelings
   c. Allows others to finish what they are saying
   d. Does not talk only about self
9. Understanding of the relationship between vocal output and own feelings and needs
10. Understanding of the relationship between vocal output and effect on others

Summary

We have described the four general areas of behavior that are important for appropriate vocal production. We have emphasized certain abilities that contribute to efficient function in each area.

Chapter 7 provides a more detailed format for analysis of children's behavior, and Chapter 8 describes in-depth assessment techniques.

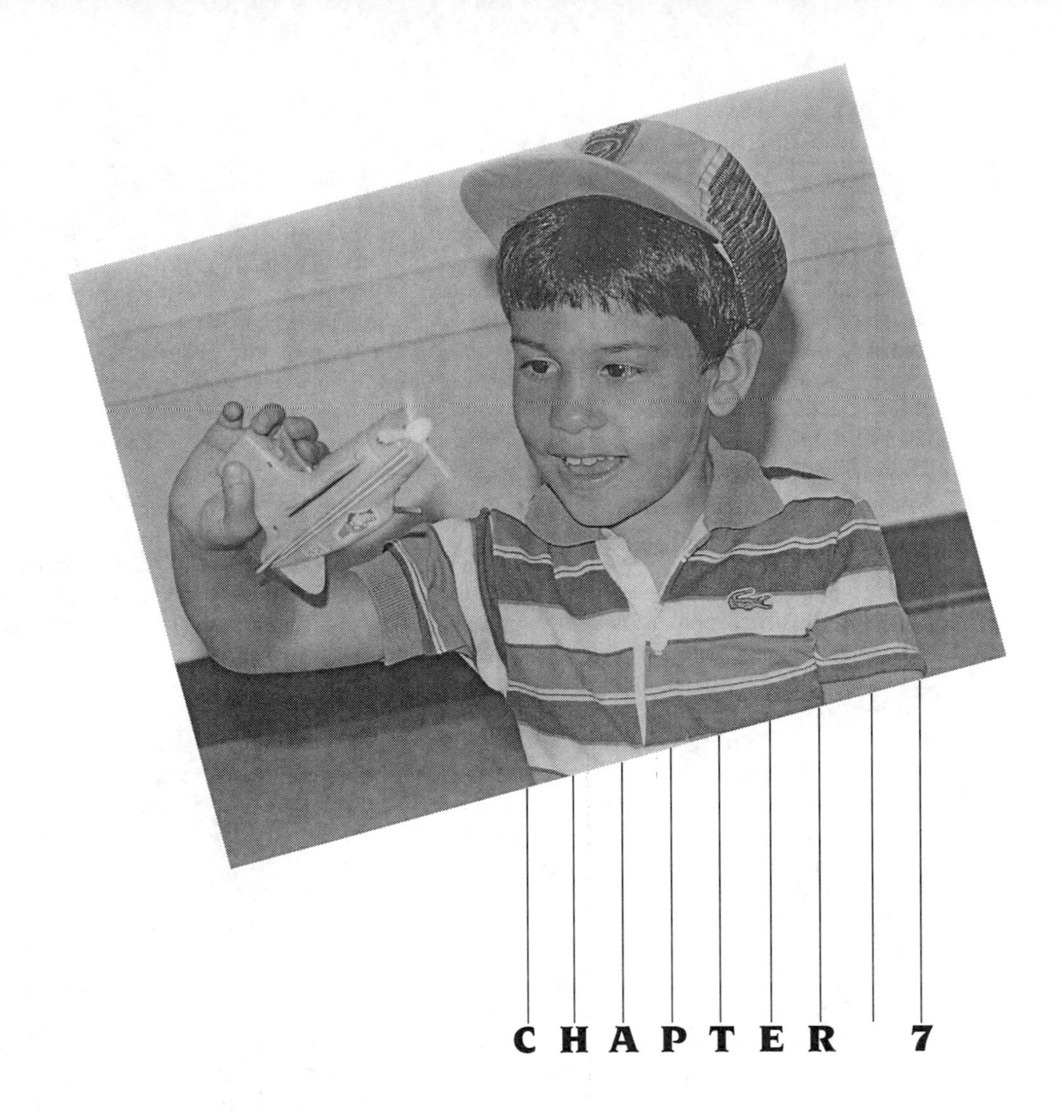

CHAPTER 7

Theoretical Bases for Decision Making

When we start out on a car journey, we usually have some idea of our final destination and a map to guide us in finding our way. If we have been there before, we may have a cognitive map rather than one drawn on paper. Similarly, as we consider the assessment of children, it is helpful to have some kind of map or framework to guide us. Basically, assessment is a data-gathering process, and we gather two general kinds of data: We observe behavior, and we consider relevant information. We can observe the child's behavior either in naturalistic settings (e.g., playground, lunchroom, classroom) or in a structured way in the therapy room as we elicit samples, ask questions, and present specific tasks. As a result of what we see and hear, we first identify certain symptoms or signs. Symptoms or atypical signs are like red flags that alert us. We then begin to look at the supporting behaviors that may be generating or perpetuating these symptoms. We develop hypotheses concerning the way the mechanism is being used, the appropriateness of individual pieces of behavior, and the sequencing of the behaviors during voice production. We look at the coordination of various areas of activity and make inferences about the ways one part of the mechanism may be compensating for another. We consider the effectiveness of the general communication strategies used and how these strategies are helping or hindering the satisfaction of personal needs. The medical report and case history and the results of instrumental tests (see chapter 9) also provide important information that help us interpret the behavior we observe.

Therefore, the first step in the decision-making process is direct observation. As clinicians, we are trained to focus on the observable aspects of children's behavior. We watch and listen and make an initial judgment concerning the appropriateness or inappropriateness of what we see and hear. If we decide that there is something inappropriate about the child's voice, we move to the next stage of the process of assessment, that is, we make inferences concerning the underlying behaviors that may be generating or maintaining the observable symptoms. Our inferences are educated guesses or hypotheses that we develop concerning the possible reasons for the symptoms we observe. Inferences usually arise from our direct observations of behavior and then are checked against additional information we glean from such sources as case histories, instrumental analyses, and reports from other professionals. As we sift through the salient clues obtained from direct observation of the child and the pertinent background information, we are looking for patterns. Our past experience and training help us do this. Our knowledge of anatomy and physiology and the four areas of behavior important in voice production help us to zero in on any negative aspects of critical behaviors that may be demonstrated. We then look at the interrelationships between critical behaviors and speculate about the possibility that some negative aspects may be compensatory devices. We also consider the way behaviors are sequenced and coordinated. Finally, we develop some additional inferences concerning the relationship between the child's vocal production and his or her overall communicative effectiveness.

When we have developed a set of inferences based on direct observation and checked those inferences against relevant background information, we arrive at the next stage of the decision-making process: the formulation of our clinical impressions concerning the nature and scope of the problem. Clinical impressions are generalizations that can be supported by our available data. We formulate our generalizations against a backdrop of our previous direct experience and our knowledge of the literature. It is important that evidence support our generalizations. In our assessment reports, we always need to summarize the data we have collected to substantiate the generalizations we make. This organization of the data also helps us to think about each individual child's pattern in relation to the overall available body of knowledge concerning children with voice disorders. For example, what does this pattern suggest in relation to etiology? What referrals should be considered? What approaches to remediation have been described in the literature as especially helpful for patterns of this type? Our data-referenced generalizations help shape our approach to management. Some children's patterns will not resemble any others that we have seen or read about. These cases are the ones that prompt us to search for additional information, new sources, and second opinions. A schematic representation of the assessment process can be seen in Figure 7–1.

Generalizations Concerning the Voice Mechanism

It is important to look for patterns in children's behavior during the assessment process. Some symptoms cluster together, and we can sometimes identify commonalities in behavioral patterns.

Although each child is unique and each voice is different, it is convenient to group negative aspects of behavior frequently observed in children with voice disorders. This is useful for review purposes because it focuses attention on some predictable patterns and accommodations. An example of symptoms that typically occur in combination is the hypernasality of voice quality and the distortion of consonants requiring oral breath pressure that occur in the presence of velopharyngeal inadequacy. Similarly, certain predictable compensations or accommodations correlate with some specific deficits. To compensate for velopharyngeal inadequacy, many children attempt to valve the airstream by using laryngeal movement (i.e., glottal stops), pharyngeal movement (i.e., pharyngeal fricatives), and alae constriction (i.e., nasal grimaces). See Kummer and Lee (1996).

In the last chapter, we discussed the four general areas of behavior that are important to voice. We also listed some optimal behaviors under each of the four areas. We noted that although it is not always necessary for each child to exhibit all of the optimal behaviors to have an adequate voice, a knowledge of some of the optimal behaviors is useful for the clinician in planning remediation programs. Similarly, it is useful to know some frequently occurring patterns involving negative aspects of behavior that are observed under the four general areas. This enables us to be alert for them when we are assessing an individual child's pattern.

Patterns of Muscular Activity

One way to characterize behaviors is to describe the level of muscular activity inherent in the mechanism during vocal production. There is an optimal state of muscle tension and amount of effort used during appropriate voice production. It is also possible to demonstrate an inappropriate degree of tension and effort. Boone (1983) has referred to hyperfunctional voice problems as those characterized by too much force and contraction of muscles concerned with respiration, phonation, and resonance. A child who is using too much effort may be working hard at the task of producing voice and yet failing to produce a result that is pleasing. The harsh sound that is heard (symptom) results from an excessive level of muscular activity in the mechanism that may be localized in one site or may be pervasive. If a *hyper*functional pattern of behavior is habituated, the muscle

Figure 7–1. Stages in the assessment process.

A. *The child's behavior*

Behavior	Clinician's role
Observable symptoms audible visible	Clinician's observations of what is seen and heard.
Negative aspects of critical behaviors respiration phonation resonance	Clinician's inferences concerning maladaptive uses of the mechanism.
Patterns of behavior sequencing coordination compensations	Clinician's inferences concerning the interrelationship between behaviors.
Communicative effect personal adjustment interpersonal factors	Clinician's inferences concerning relationship between vocal behavior and satisfaction of needs.

B. *Information about the child from pertinent medical and case history information*

Information	Clinician's role
Case history information family models family history of voice problems environmental factors educational factors psychosocial factors	Clinician's generalizations concerning the nature and severity of the participating and maintaining factors.
Medical information anatomical constraints medical conditions medication	

Clinician's decisions re:
1. referrals
2. consultations
3. programming

state will "feel" normal to the child. The opposite state is that of *hypo*function where the degree of tension during muscle contraction or effort is insufficient to produce appropriate voice. This state occurs less frequently and is usually associated with neurologic or emotional disturbance. We shall summarize some important considerations to bear in mind in relation to both hyperfunctional and hypofunctional patterns of behavior.

Hyperfunctional Patterns

Listed below are some generalizations that can be made concerning hyperfunctional patterns of behavior.

1. May be desirable or undesirable accommodations to structural deviations (e.g., malformation, laryngeal web, papilloma, paralysis, tracheostomy, velopharyngeal inadequacy)
2. May be temporary or habituated responses to acute or chronic medical conditions of the upper respiratory tract (e.g., allergies, infections, effects of medications)
3. May or may not result in tissue change (e.g., swelling, hemorrhage, hyperkeratosis, polyps, nodules)
4. May involve use of false (ventricular) folds
5. May be related to deviant sensory system (e.g., hearing loss, neurologic impairment)
6. May be related to social or emotional adjustment (e.g., aggression, anxiety, inappropriate self-concept, faulty learning)
7. May be related to cognitive function (e.g., developmental delay)
8. May be a component of cerebral dysfunction (e.g., spasticity in children with cerebral palsy)

The following negative behaviors may occur in association with hyperfunctional patterns:

A. *Respiration*
   1. Quick, shallow inhalation
   2. Inspiratory voicing
   3. Inefficient control of exhalation
      a. Talks on residual air
      b. Does not take replenishing breaths
      c. Runs out of air at ends of sentences
      d. Air escapes in a rush at beginning of utterances

B. *Phonation*
   1. Abrupt initiation of phonation (hard glottal attacks)
   2. Folds approximated too tightly; voice sounds strained or pressed
   3. Adduction of false folds
   4. Limited use of rate and pause variation
   5. Observable tension in neck muscles
   6. Loudness level inappropriate for situation
   7. Loudness variation limited to increases
   8. Pitch level inappropriate
   9. Phonation breaks
   10. Pitch variation limited to getting higher
   11. Uses laryngeal valve (not respiratory muscles) to control exhaled air
   12. Sounds hoarse, harsh, diplophonic, ventricular

C. *Resonance*
   1. Tension in supraglottal resonators
   2. Sounds strident, muffled
   3. Lack of reverberation of sound on bones of face
   4. Minimal mouth opening, tight jaw
   5. Insufficient balance of oral-nasal resonance
   6. Tense or posterior carriage of tongue, or both.

D. *Interpersonal communication*
   1. Talks too much; does not take turns
   2. Tries to get and hold attention by talking loudly
   3. Limited awareness of effect of own tense behavior on others
   4. Does not ask questions or asks them constantly
   5. Few "other"-referenced statements
   6. Does not adjust vocal behavior to feedback

It is important to remember that any one child with a hyperfunctional pattern will not exhibit all the negative behaviors listed and that there will, of course, be differences in the severity. In some cases, excessive tension can be observed in only one area. In other cases, more than one area may be involved, but a pattern of generalized tension can be observed in only one area. In still other cases more than one area may be involved, and a pattern of generalized tension can be seen across areas.

Hypofunctional Patterns

Listed below are some generalizations that can be made concerning hypofunctional patterns of behavior.

1. May be secondary to structural deviation or damage (e.g., bowing of folds, neurologic impairment, atrophy of folds, postintubation changes, surgery)
2. May be related to accommodations to acute or chronic upper respiratory tract conditions (e.g., soreness)
3. May be indicative of social or emotional adjustment (e.g., reticence, hysteria)
4. If severe, may necessitate use of substitute communication system (e.g., ventricular phonation, artificial larynx, sign language)
5. May occur in combination with altered sensory feedback (e.g., dysarthria, dyspraxia, impaired hearing)
6. May be a component of cerebral dysfunction (e.g., weakness or flaccidity in children with cerebral palsy)
7. May occur subsequent to prolonged hyperfunctional use

Wilson (1979) described hypofunction as resulting from overly lax muscular tonus. This may be specific to one area or generalized across areas. For example, children who are severely hypotonic may have difficulty maintaining an erect head, neck, and thorax, as is sometimes observed in children with cerebral palsy. The following negative aspects of behaviors can sometimes occur in association with hypofunctional patterns:

A. *Respiration*
   1. Inhalation insufficient in depth and timing
   2. Exhalation weak
   3. Exhalation of short duration
   4. Inadequate control of exhaled air
   5. Weak muscle tone and movement
   6. Inadequate use of replenishing breaths

B. *Phonation*
   1. Breathy initiation of phonation
   2. Inadequate laryngeal valving
   3. Excessive air escape during phonation
   4. Voice sounds breathy, aphonic
   5. Weak laryngeal tone
   6. Low pitch levels
   7. Minimal vocal variety
   8. Low vocal intensity
   9. Voice fades at ends of phrases

C. *Resonance*
   1. Inadequate amount of oral resonance
   2. Inadequate amount of nasal resonance
   3. Minimal movement of lips and tongue to shape oral cavity
   4. Vibrating column of air not projected forward
   5. Voice sounds thin, weak
   6. Lack of resonance may affect intelligibility of speech sounds
   7. Inadequate movement of velopharyngeal sphincter mechanism

D. *Interpersonal communication*
   1. Initiates spontaneous speech infrequently
   2. Minimal facial movement or expression
   3. Does not adjust loudness level to situation or listeners' needs
   4. Withdrawn, reticent
   5. Responds minimally to questions
   6. Does not volunteer for participatory activity
   7. Does not share feelings

Factors Related to Daily Use

A number of factors can be identified that, individually or in combination, may negatively affect the state of the vocal mechanism. Appropriate vocal hygiene involves avoidance of excessive demands on the mechanism, particularly at times when it is especially vulnerable. The mechanism seems to be especially at risk when there are changes in the mucosa—redness, swelling, dryness, or the presence of excessive mucus—as a result of physical, emotional, environmental, and chemical factors. If a child engages in demanding or prolonged vocal activity during times when an atypical condition already exists in the larynx or upper respiratory tract or in both, the effect of the vocal activity will be more pronounced than when the tissues are healthy. Thus, the condition of the mechanism during the time that it is in use influences the possible effect of that use. Punt (1967) discussed the importance of adequate lubrication of the vocal tract. Too much mucus may lead to frequent coughing and throat clearing; too little may cause dryness and heighten susceptibility for irritation of vocal structures if folds are adducted vigorously or with excessive tension. Persistent mouth breathing (e.g., when a child is congested or has enlarged adenoids), medication (such as antihistamine and decongestant), a dusty dry environment, or restricted fluid intake may all contribute to dryness of the vocal tract. The effect of vocal abuses can be magnified if structures are already dry or irritated, and increased hydration should be recommended.

Characteristic patterns of vocal abuse in relation to the demands made on the mechanism have been noted by clinical writers. Wilson (1979) distinguished between vocal abuse (sudden straining of the voice or continuous use of harmful practices) and vocal misuse, which involves incorrect pitch and loudness. Use may be influenced by a child's interests and lifestyle (e.g., athletic activities, choir, drama group, cheerleading), permanent or temporary alterations in the mechanism (e.g., compensations), medical conditions (e.g., infections), emotional and social adjustments (e.g., vocalization style and frequency of vocalization), and vocal models (e.g., learned behaviors). The term "phonotrauma" is sometimes used to describe the effect on the mechanism of inappropriate voice use.

With respect to assessment of factors influencing susceptibility, the clinician should be alert for any indications of temporary or permanent conditions affecting the vocal mechanism and try to discover if there is a repetitive pattern in the child's amount or kind of voice use. The identification of situations and interactions with the potential for negative vocal practices should be attempted during interviews with parents and teachers. Open-ended questions that elicit descriptions of children's preference for, and participation in, various activities seem to yield the most useful information.

The lists below show negative behaviors that can be ascertained from informants and observed by clinicians.

A. Negative behaviors to be ascertained from informants
   1. Protracted talking above noise
      a. in cars with windows open
      b. over TV or music
      c. competing for attention in groups
   2. Excessive talking and singing
      a. amount of talking time
      b. activities involving vocalization
      c. time spent in quiet activities
   3. Habituated responses
      a. repeated vomiting (e.g., bulimia)
      b. sound effects and imitations
      c. scaring others (shrieks and screams)
      d. emotional outbursts (tantrums, prolonged crying)
      e. expressions of anger, excitement, etc.
      f. coughing, throat clearing, wheezing
      g. yodeling
      h. smoking
B. Negative behaviors to be observed by clinician
   1. Excessive amount of talking
   2. Very loud talking
   3. Hard glottal attacks
   4. Fillers (ahs, ums produced with strain)

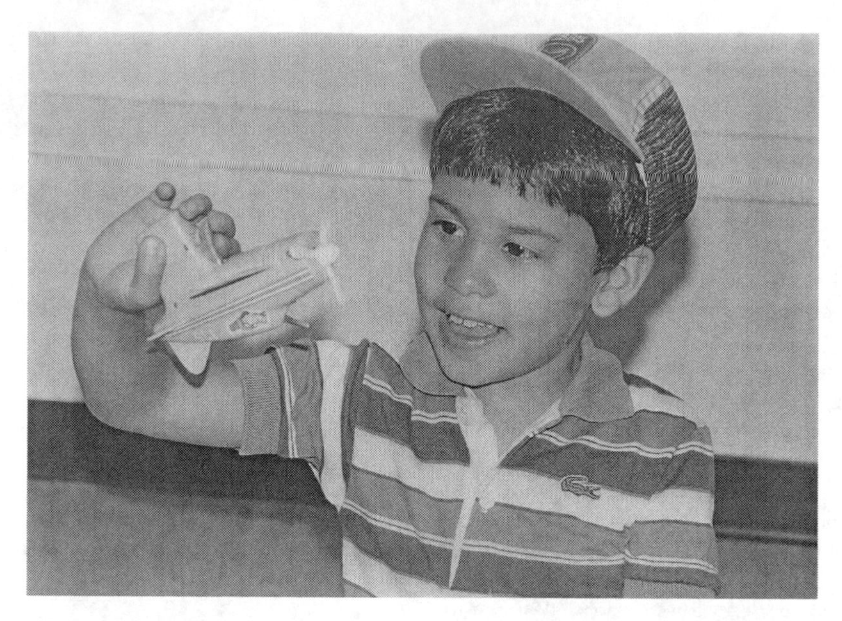

Figure 7-2. Some sound imitations can be produced without abuse to the vocal mechanism.

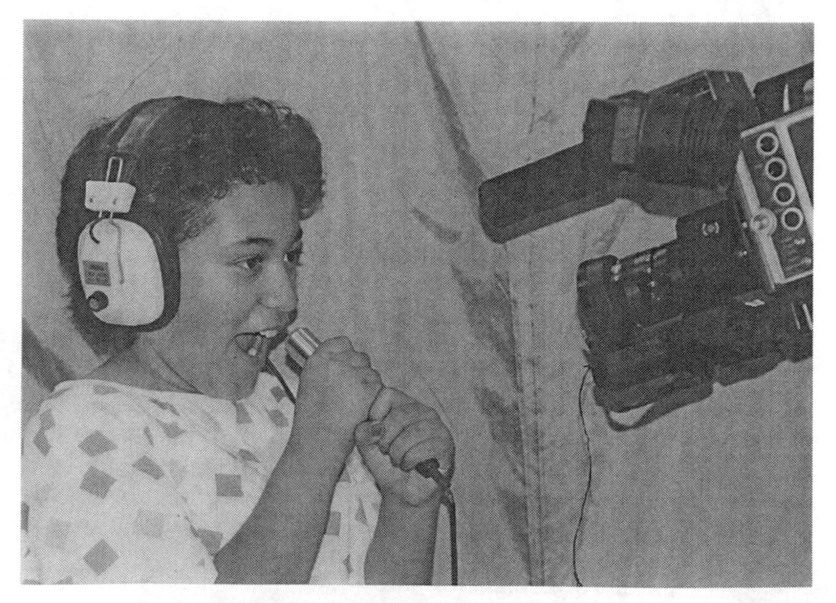

Figure 7-3. Prolonged or strained loud singing accompanying records or cassettes is a frequent form of vocal abuse.

5. Strained vocalizations
6. Sudden shrieks
7. Forced laughter, overloud laughter
8. Shouting, screaming, cheering
9. "Funny" voices used to get attention
10. Throat clearing, coughing, wheezing
11. Imitation of nonspeech sounds
12. Strained singing, very loud singing

Atypical Sound Production (A Substitute Sound Source—Dysphonia Plicae Ventricularis)

A maladaptive behavior sometimes observed is the effortful compensatory strategy of phonating with the false vocal cords. This compensation is seen in children who do not have true vocal folds or who have congenital malformations of the folds. Brodnitz (1971) said it may be adopted also by children who have had surgery to remove benign tumors of the true folds or children who have suffered from laryngitis. Parisier and Henneford (1969) reported that dysphonia plicae ventricularis occurred in a patient who had surgery for removal of juvenile laryngeal papillomas. These wartlike growths on the laryngeal structures are thought to be caused by a virus and may be potentially life threatening if they impede the airway. Papillomas are not related to vocal abuse or misuse, although hoarseness may be a symptom of their presence. Parisier and Henneford's 1969 patient with papillomas subsequently had surgery also to remove a laryngeal web. Later, a laryngologist observed his use of the false folds for phonation. Children sometimes use the false folds for phonation to draw attention to themselves or because of other psychogenic problems. Sometimes phonation of both the true and the false folds occurs simultaneously, and the listener perceives a "double voice." The predominant characteristics of ventricular phonation are extreme tension, hoarseness and aperiodicity, and restricted pitch range. When the child is seen under laryngoscopy, the false folds approximate during phonatory activity but do not approximate during quiet breathing or vegetative activity such as throat clearing, coughing, laughing, or crying. Ventricular phonation may be viewed as an extreme phonatory compensation, often associated with a general pattern of hyperfunctional activity. Tension in the shoulders, neck, and jaw may be observed, and the respiratory pattern sometimes is found to be shallow, tense, and inefficient.

Consistency of Symptoms

Another characteristic of patterns of behavior that is diagnostically significant is the consistency. When a child exhibits the symptom of hoarseness, for example, we are interested in the frequency of occurrence and the situations in which it occurs. Intermittent hoarseness may be the result of accumulation of secretions on the folds if it occurs in an allergic child at certain times or seasons of the year. If the voice is hoarse only in the morning and clears as the day wears on, drainage from the nasal cavities may occur during sleep. If the voice is clear in the morning and becomes hoarse at the end of the school day or after participation in or attendance at athletic activities, the symptom may be related to abusive or excessive voice use. If the onset of symptoms occurs in close association with a psychologically traumatizing event in the child's life or is observed only when a child is in a particular context or speaking to particular listeners, emotional factors may be diagnostically significant. Intermittent symptoms also may suggest that permanent tissue changes have not occurred.

Intermittent symptoms that occur in association with fatigue may suggest that there is a neurologic component to the problem (e.g., a child who begins to read a passage quite clearly but who becomes increasingly hypernasal as the reading progresses and the control lessens).

The Influence of Fatigue on Vocal Behavior

Children who do not enjoy restful sleep are handicapped in terms of their attentiveness in school during the day. Fatigue also may affect their vocal behavior. Additionally, if they are mouth breathers at night, they may experience dryness of the vocal tract and therefore be more susceptible to vocal fold irritation and/or abuse if the vocal folds are used vigorously. A number of conditions may contribute to sleep interruptions, and clinicians usually question parents about possible symptoms of these behaviors during parent interviews and history-taking sessions if a child has voice-quality problems. Sleep disorders can haunt children during their waking hours, and any possibility that such a disorder may exist should be carefully investigated so that treatment can be obtained if warranted.

Sleep Apnea

Sleep apnea is the most common form of apnea (or absence of breathing) in children. It affects 1 in 50 children. There are cessations in rhythmic breathing caused by obstruction in the upper airway. Enlarged tonsils and adenoids are the usual causes of such obstruction. Surgical removal of the tonsils and adenoids is effective 85 to 90% of the time. Parents may report that children thrash around during sleep, sleep in positions such as sitting up or with their heads hanging off the bed to breathe better, snore loudly, eat slowly, experience daytime fatigue, have circles under their eyes, are pallid, are below average in height and weight, or display a combination of these behaviors.

Sleep Terrors

Sleep terrors are another form of episodic interruptions of children's sleep during the night. A child emitting a piercing scream characterizes this condition. The child appears to be terrified when the parent enters the bedroom and exhibits signs of disorientation and unresponsiveness.

Unlike a child who has had a nightmare, a child with night terrors will have no recollection of the event in the morning. Reassurance that everything is all right is the only thing a parent can do at the time the event occurs. Sleep deprivation may be a significant factor in triggering night terrors, so parents are advised to put the child to bed earlier or to try to allow the child to sleep longer in the morning to compensate. Children usually outgrow the problem.

Sleepwalking

Sleepwalking is a condition where a child is floating between consciousness and unconsciousness. Parents should ensure that the environment is safe if a child is a sleepwalker by locking windows and removing sharp objects. During the episode, a parent should not try to interact with the child. Trying to calm a child down may make the child more upset or confrontational. In severe situations, where the child may harm himself or others, the physician can prescribe medication. By puberty, most children seem to have ceased sleepwalking.

Insomnia

Insomnia is sometimes seen in children who do not seem to be able to relax enough to drift off to sleep. Young children may have this condition because they are worried or stressed by a problem, real or imagined. Physicians usually do not prescribe medications for children with insomnia but suggest behavioral and environmental modifications. Parents can establish routines before and at bedtime, remove televisions from bedrooms, provide high protein snacks, reduce stimulation by reading quietly to children before they sleep, and adapt good attitudes and models regarding sleeping practices.

Bedwetting

Bedwetting (enuresis) may not be classified as a sleep disorder, but it occurs during sleep and often interrupts rest. It is a very common problem. Even 5-year-old children have a 20% incidence of frequent bedwetting. Physicians are usually reluctant to treat the problem before 7 or 8, however, when it can become a source of embarrassment. It is important for parents not to make children feel they are doing something wrong because this increases anxiety and exacerbates the problem. Withholding fluids and waking the child to go to the bathroom usually does not help. Behavioral modification strategies such as using moisture-sensitive pads that sound an alarm have been used successfully with some children. Some physicians may prescribe medications, such as antidepressants and an antidiuretic hormone that reduces urine outputs at night.

Changes in the Mechanism Related to Abuse

Organic changes that can be linked to effortful vocal practices include thickening of the folds, vocal nodules, polyps, and hyperkeratosis. Wilson (1979) discussed these pathologies in detail and noted that vocal nodules are the most frequently observed pathology in children. A child's susceptibility for developing additive lesions of the folds may be affected by constitutional factors (Arnold, 1963; Kelly & Craik, 1952; Luchsinger & Arnold, 1965). There seems to be evidence that additive lesions occur more frequently in some families than in others. It is unclear whether this is because of a constitutional predisposition or a pattern of learned behavior; however, Table 7–1 illustrates the incidence of vocal-fold pathology by type and gender. The total number of children examined was 612.

It can be seen from the Baynes' data that structural changes in the mechanism occur with a higher frequency in boys than in girls. Senturia and Wilson (1968) reported that voice deviations occur twice as often in boys as in girls and that laryngeal nodules and localized hyperplasia are the most common benign lesions in children. The same researchers also noted that secretion is present in the nasal fossae, and the arytenoids are reddened, edematous, or both in a high percentage of children with deviant voices. It is unclear why some children seem to be particularly at risk, whereas others who engage in frequent strenuous vocal activity remain unaffected (Anderson & Newby, 1973). Wilson (1979) concluded that nodules are probably the result of a combination of factors. It may be that a number (or certainly more than one) of the high-risk factors noted below may contribute to a pattern of heightened susceptibility for the development of these additive lesions of the folds. Attention to the possibility of gastroesophageal reflux as a significant risk factor is warranted especially if the arytenoids and other posterior laryngeal structures are red.

High-Risk Factors Relating to the Development of Vocal Nodules

Clinical writers have noted that some of the following factors may predispose an individual to develop vocal nodules:

Table 7–1. Incidence of vocal fold pathology.

Type	*Boys*	*Girls*	*Total*
Nodules	126	36	162
Thickening	122	26	148
Polyps	15	6	21
Other	15	7	22
Total	278	75	353

Note: Baynes, R. A. (1967). *Voice therapy with children—A global approach.* Paper presented at the American Speech and Hearing Association convention.

1. Constitutional tendency (Arnold, 1963; Kelly & Craik, 1952)
2. Chronic upper respiratory problems (Withers, 1961)
3. Psychological living environment (e.g., size of family; Wilson, 1979)
4. Physical living environment (e.g., air pollution; Wilson, 1979)
5. Personality and adjustment (Arnold, 1963; Sederholm et al., 1995)
6. Endocrine imbalance, especially thyroid (Withers, 1961)
7. Vocal abuse: sudden straining of the voice (Wilson, 1979); continuous use of abusive practices (Glaze, 1996)
8. Vocal misuse: incorrect pitch and loudness (Wilson, 1979)
9. Gastroesophageal reflux (Gumpert et al., 1998)

Nodules appear on the edge of the free margin of the fold at the junction of the anterior and middle thirds. There is a progression of development from a slight swelling and reddening in the initial stages, then gradual thickening, and finally fully developed growths consisting of fibrotic tissue (DeWeese & Saunders, 1973). Grey (1973) and Withers (1961) have provided additional information about the maturation sequence of nodules. Although nodules are never painful, they result in size–mass changes that affect evenness of adduction and the vibratory pattern of the folds. As the nodules increase in size, vocal symptoms such as hoarseness become more apparent. Moore (1971a) noted the relationship between the size of the mass and the amount of air leakage, or breathiness, but said that the hardness of the nodule is also a factor. A noncompressible nodule may result in audible symptoms even if it is quite small in size. To compensate for the nodules, children often use more effort in adduction, thus pressing the folds more tightly together to minimize the irregularity in the margin of the folds. By talking more loudly or at a higher pitch level, some children compensate for the alteration in size and mass. These strategies tend to exacerbate the condition of the mechanism, however. Eventually, if the nodules become larger, the child may exhibit periods of aphonia.

Negative Behaviors Associated With Vocal Nodules

1. *Phonation*
   a. Hoarse or breathy phonation, or both
   b. Pitch level may appear low for age and gender (increased mass)
   c. Aphonia on unstressed syllables
   d. Hard glottal attacks on words beginning with vowels

e. Voice clearest when phonating loudly; poorest when phonating softly
f. Voice clears somewhat in upper part of pitch range
g. Reduced phonation time on prolonged /a/
h. Difference in duration time of unvoiced versus voiced continuants
i. Restricted pitch range
j. Hyperextension of head and neck
k. Repeated nonproductive throat clearing
l. Vocal variety limited to increases in loudness
m. Intermittent diplophonia (two-toned sound caused by uneven distribution of weight on folds)

2. *Respiration*
a. Shallow inhalation
b. Inefficient use of exhalation

3. *Interpersonal*
a. Aggressive style of vocal interaction
b. Incessant talking

Because vocal nodules are the most frequently occurring vocal pathology in school-age children (Baynes, 1967; Senturia & Wilson, 1968; Wilson, 1971; Wilson, 1979), it is useful to discuss some of the behaviors such children frequently exhibit. Figure 7–4 summarizes assessment information obtained following an evaluation of an 8-year-old boy who was referred by his classroom teacher.

Brett was a typical vocal abuser who personified many of the characteristics noted in the literature. His demands on his vocal mechanism were excessive, and he exhibited few of the optimal behaviors necessary to support loud vocalization combined with strenuous activity. An allergic condition increased his susceptibility for irritation of the mechanism. He compensated for his poor respiratory support for sustained speaking by increasing the effort he was using in the laryngeal area. Supraglottal resonance was not well developed, and lip and tongue movements were minimal. His attempts to improve intelligibility were limited to using more laryngeal effort and increasing the tension in his whole body. Brett needed to learn to use more productive vocal strategies, since the compensatory behaviors he was using were not effective. Telling Brett he should never talk loudly was not a feasible solution, given his lifestyle.

Brett's profile is a typical one, frequently seen in active, talkative boys of his age. We have noted some negative behaviors under the "interpersonal" category of Brett's profile. We do not mean to imply that there is necessarily a causative relationship between these behaviors and the development of vocal nodules, although there is some evidence (Green 1989) in the literature to indicate the possibility. Nonetheless, clinical experience suggests that some children with vocal nodules need to develop improved interpersonal skills to facilitate vocal improvement. It is also possible that a child such as Brett may need even better interpersonal skills than other children to protect and improve his voice.

Constraints That Reduce Volitional Control

Affective Constraints

Because the voice is a bridge between an individual and his or her world, disturbances in voice and the withholding of voice have been noted in the literature as symptoms of affective disorders. Voice reflects emotional states and reactions to life stress. Goldfarb (1961) studied children with schizophrenia and described a variety of vocal characteristics. In a later study (Goldfarb, Braunstein, & Lorge, 1976), also with children with schizophrenia, no specific set of symptoms was observed, but there was a basic loss of control and regulation of speech.

The terms *elective* and *selective mutism* have been used in the psychologic literature

Figure 7–4. A profile of Brett—age 8 years.

A. Behavior
- 1. Audible and visible symptoms
  - i. Hoarseness (lessens as loudness increases)
  - ii. Hard glottal attacks
  - iii. Excessive loudness level during conversation
  - iv. Observable tension in neck and jaw
  - v. Observable tension in shoulders
- 2. Negative behaviors
  - a. Respiration
    - i. Clavicular inhalation
    - ii. Short exhalation phase
    - iii. Inefficient control of exhaled airstream
  - b. Phonation
    - i. Leakage of air during phonation
    - ii. Aperiodic vibratory pattern
    - iii. Inappropriate initiation of phonation
    - iv. Variety limited to getting louder
  - c. Resonance
    - i. Reduced oral resonance on sustained continuants (z, ʒ, ð)
    - ii. Reduced nasal resonance on sustained continuants (m, n, ŋ)
    - iii. Reduced mouth opening
    - iv. Inappropriate tone focus
    - v. Tension of supraglottal structures

  Pattern = hyperfunctional

  Excessive effort and muscular tension observed in all three areas
- 3. Compensations
  - i. Uses laryngeal valving to compensate for lack of respiratory muscle control during exhalation
  - ii. Uses excessive laryngeal effort to compensate for reduced resonance and articulatory precision
  - iii. Uses increased loudness as only means of "clearing" tone and varying voice

  Hearing sensitivity within normal limits bilaterally
- 4. Interpersonal behaviors
  - i. Does not listen well
  - ii. Uses few "other-referenced" statements
  - iii. Uses many "self-referenced" statements
  - iv. Does not adapt to feedback or situational constraints
  - v. Does not share talking time
  - vi. Uses loud talking to get and hold attention

B. Information
- 1. Medical report
  - i. Matural bilateral nodules
  - ii. Allergic to mold; cat and dog dander
- 2. Family history
  - i. Youngest of five children
  - ii. One older sister (a cheerleader) had vocal problems
- 3. Environmental
  - i. Has a dog that sleeps in his room
- 4. Vocal demands
  - i. Active in neighborhood peer group; sporting activities; church choir
- 5. Other
  - i. Teacher reports that he is a very active, noisy child in class

(Kolvin & Fundudis, 1981) to describe the withholding of voice and speech by young children. Psychiatrists suggest that such children have severe psychologic disturbances, frequently come from conflicted families, and may use withdrawal behaviors to manipulate their environment. In most instances of mutism of this type, the children have previously developed speech and language and may continue to use voice in certain situations or with certain people but withhold oral communication consistently for long periods of time. Cline and Baldwin (1994) believe the best incidence estimate is 0.9 per 1000 children if a 6-month persistence criterion is used. They also believe that there are probably many hidden cases and that the ratio is higher among immigrant or ethnic minority families and in rural areas where families are isolated. Girls also appear to become mute more often than boys do (Lebrun, 1990; Wright, Miller, Cook, & Littman, 1985). Hayden (1980) reported that boys, however, were referred for treatment earlier because clinging, passive, and shy behavior may be seen as more appropriate in girls than in boys. Selectively mute children have a higher incidence of speech problems than other children, and it is always possible that fear or embarrassment may keep children from exposing their speech to peers. Although it is usually difficult to test these children, a receptive language test is often administered, and parents can be questioned concerning speech intelligibility; as much information as possible about language and speech skills should be obtained. Cline and Baldwin (1994) provided a review of the communication patterns and relationships in families of selectively mute children.

This lack of voice or disordered voicing may be viewed as a manifestation of psychologic disequilibrium. Extreme anxiety, depression, conversion reaction, or personality disorder can interfere with normal volitional control over phonation (Aronson, 1980). Wilson (1979) said that hysterical aphonia is not common in children, although dysphonia is relatively common. In some children, a normal voice returns quickly, whereas other children require help from a clinical psychologist or counselor. Wilson (1979) also noted that some children may have bowed vocal folds as a result of a hysterical condition. In older children, mutational falsetto is thought to be related to a conflicted response to sexual maturity (Van Riper, 1972) or problems in a relationship with the parent of the same gender. For example, a postpubertal boy may maintain a high-pitched voice because of a reluctance to identify with his father.

In very young children, when voice use is withheld completely or restricted because of psychological factors, the problem may at first seem to be merely shyness. An example of this kind of problem can be seen in the following case history:

Rosie, a 5-year-old kindergartener, was referred to the speech–language pathologist by her classroom teacher because she did not talk at all during the school day. She smiled when people spoke to her, hung her head, or used gestures. Great effort was expended by school personnel to coax Rosie to talk. She was given extra privileges and treats and special attention, which she seemed to enjoy, but she could never be encouraged to vocalize. She was neat and careful in her written tasks and assignments and seemed extremely cooperative and well behaved. The speech–language pathologist interviewed the parents and described to them some of the problems that Rosie's "excessive shyness" was causing her. The parents' response was surprising. They smiled and said, "So she's making fools out of you all at school here. We don't have any problem at all at home. She talks to us all of the time. It's just at school and on the bus that she won't do it. You're the experts, and it's your problem obviously." The parents' reaction indicated that a psychologic consulation was needed, and the family was eventually persuaded to seek family therapy. The psychiatric report to the speech–language clinician indicated that it seemed likely that the parents were hostile to authority figures and were subtly encouraging Rosie's responses. It was recommended that school personnel (including the bus driver, lunchroom supervisor, etc.) refrain from becoming caught up in the "game" of coaxing Rosie to talk because such attempts were seen as rewarding to her and were in fact reinforcing the undesirable behavior. Instead, it was suggested that Rosie be rewarded for any nonverbal attempts to relate positively to others and that significant adults at school should try to establish warm, accepting relationships with her. It was two years before Rosie used appropriate vocal behavior in the school environment.

In Rosie's case, the child's withholding of vocal behavior was related to a severe psychologic disturbance that involved a conflicted pattern of family interaction. The example emphasizes the need for team assessment of such problems and the fact that the reactions of all school personnel are important in determining the way the symptoms are maintained. Rosie's "aphonia" was a response to entering a different (i.e., school) environment. In other cases, the appearance of such behavior can occur suddenly after many years of vocalizing appropriately in a particular environment. Such was the case of Misty, who exhibited a sudden onset in response to traumatizing occurrences in her home life.

Misty, age 11 years, was in a special education classroom for mildly developmentally delayed children. She had been enrolled in language therapy for some years and exhibited normal patterns of phonatory behavior and articulation, but depressed receptive and expressive language skills. She had been seen by the speech–language pathologist for her regular session on a Friday and participated normally in the session. When Misty came to school on Monday, she seemed withdrawn, offered no voluntary communication, and responded in a whisper when she was asked questions by her teacher. When Misty's occasional whispering continued to be her only attempt at communication, a case conference was scheduled. The mother reported that Misty could not be encouraged to vocalize at all at home. She attributed Misty's withdrawal to the father's sudden departure from the family. Psychiatric counseling further revealed that Misty had recently begun to menstruate and had been frightened and apprehensive. Her depressed language skills made it more difficult for her to understand and cope with the physical and emotional changes that occurred. After 6 months of counseling in combination with speech–language therapy, Misty's appropriate vocal behavior was reestablished.

As can be seen in the preceding examples, the way a voice is not used, or withheld, can be indicative of an individual's psychologic adjustment. It may be important to consider the child's relationships with significant adults in the home and school environment because such relationships are critical in helping a child cope with adjustments to painful events and situations.

Neurologic Constraints

The volitional control of voice may be diminished by impaired neurologic functioning resulting from disease or congenital problems. Kereiakes (1996) provides a review of how an extensive history and physical examination is necessary to diagnose the problem correctly. Also see Colton and Casper (1990), Dobres, Lee, Stemple, Kummer, and Kretschmer (1990), Harvey (1996), and Rosin, Handler, Potsic, Wetmore, and Tom (1990). Occasionally, young children will be seen with myasthenia gravis (Wilson, 1979). Poor control of the musculature results in hypernasality, dysphonia, and reduction of loudness levels. Symptoms increase as the system fatigues. More commonly, the effect of impaired neurologic function is seen in children with cerebral palsy. Mysak (1980) has described the variety of voice problems occurring in this population. The symptoms depend on the type

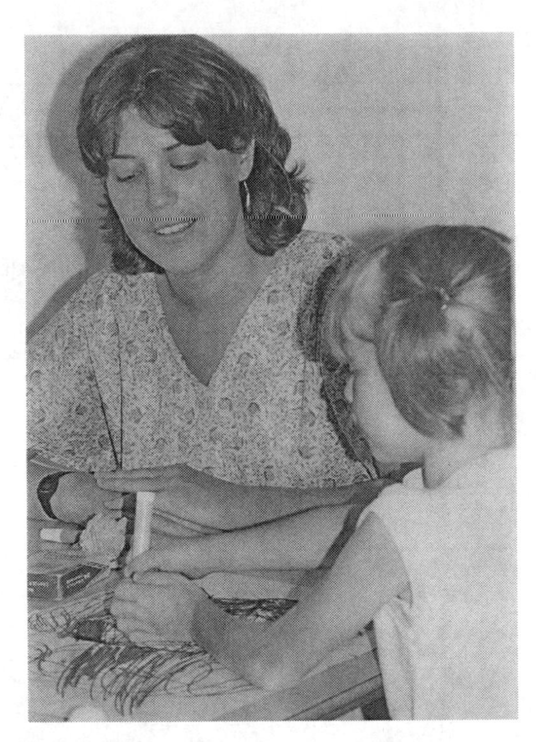

Figure 7-5. Children who withhold vocal communication may be encouraged to express their feelings through nonverbal tasks. A warm, trusting relationship with the clinician can then develop gradually.

and severity of the condition. Westlake and Rutherford (1961) provide some helpful guidelines for assessing the voluntary control necessary for sustained voicing. Table 7–2 is adapted from their ideas. Phonation may be observed during periods of involuntary activity (such as laughing, crying, sighing, coughing) and in voluntary tasks. See Table 7–3.

Cognitive Constraints

The incidence of voice problems in developmentally delayed children is higher than in the general population. Voice symptoms associated with Down syndrome have been studied by Montague and Hollein (1973), Novak (1972), and Weinberg and Zlatin (1970). Although developmental delay is not the primary cause of voice disorders in children with Down syndrome (Novak), some evidence suggests that modal frequency levels may deviate from normal levels; hearing loss occurs with greater frequency; and breathiness, roughness, and hypernasality often are observed. In Novak's 1972 study, laryngeal examination found only slight thickness of the vocal fold mucosa but signs of atrophy and dryness in the pharyngeal mucosa.

Metabolic disorders are sometimes seen in connection with developmental delay. The

Table 7–2. Respiration.

Prerequisite Behaviors	*Inadequate Behaviors*
1. Voluntary control of inhalation	Panting: fewer than three quick breaths in 5 seconds. Reverse breathing (upper chest depressed during inhalation).
2. Voluntary control of exhalation	Involuntary movements during exhalation.
3. Sufficient air to sustain phonation	Fewer than 4–5 seconds exhalation.
4. Breathing rate that allows for continuous phonation	A rate of 30 breaths per minute or higher in children over 2 years.

Table 7–3. Phonation.

Prerequisite Behaviors	*Inadequate Behaviors*
1. Ability to initiate phonation rapidly	Less than once per second (repeated /ha/).
2. Sustain phonation for phrases of more than 2 or 3 words	Fewer than 5 seconds. Normal children can sustain for 10 seconds or longer.
3. Voluntary control of laryngeal movements	Erratic involuntary spasms and movements of laryngeal muscles (heard in fluctuations and breaks in sound).
4. Appropriate muscle tonus in head, neck, torso	Unable to lift head easily when shoulders are held down (weak neck flexors). Hyper- or hypotonicity of musculature. Inappropriate posture.
5. Differentiation of muscle activity	Vocal-fold adduction associated with extensor patterns (e.g., hypotonic child may extend trunk and neck to assist adduction; hypertonic child may hyperextend jaw).

thyroid, an endocrine gland, produces thyroxin, which regulates the body's metabolic rate. Individuals who suffer from hypothyroidism have a lowered metabolic rate. Their voices may be excessively low in pitch because of edema of the folds (Aronson, 1980). Brodnitz (1971) stated that some vocal symptoms of extreme thyroid deficiency are roughness and hoarseness. Cognitive deficits also may affect children's ability to understand the language used during assessment and therapy and to process feedback and adjust behavior.

Sensory Constraints

Voice problems frequently result from difficulties in monitoring one's own voice and the voices of others. Auditory, visual, and kinesthetic awareness can be disturbed in a variety of ways. Some disturbances are transitory; others are permanent. Children with structural abnormalities of the vocal mechanism, supraglottal tract, or both receive distorted sensory feedback during the speech-learning period. An example of this is the child with a cleft palate. Tactile, kinesthetic, and auditory feedback is affected even during prespeech vocalization. In most instances, specialists try to alleviate this by the early fitting of speech appliances and early initiation of surgical procedures. Because multiple procedures frequently are needed, these children are constantly adapting to changes in the structures and consequent changes in feedback over a period of years. Another example is that of a child with enlarged tonsils and adenoids who undergoes a tonsillectomy and adenoidectomy. It is commonly believed that some children with a normal velopharyngeal mechanism can take up to 6 weeks to adjust their behavior and exhibit normal resonance following surgery. Before surgery, they may have made closure against the enlarged adenoidal pad. After surgery, they sound hypernasal until they adopt more vigorous velopharyngeal movement. During the adjustment period, they are adapting to altered auditory and proprioceptive feedback. Children who have laryngeal surgery also need time to make adjustments in their motor behavior as they learn to adapt to new sensory information. This is why we need to be alert, for example, to possible problems in children who have multiple surgeries to remove papilloma.

The most dramatic examples of voice deviations resulting from altered feedback are seen in children with hearing loss. Fuller (1970) noted that voice quality is disturbed when children have flat audiograms with threshold levels greater than 50 dB. It is also disturbed if losses are 40 dB or greater in the low frequencies accompanied by a greater loss in the high frequencies. Some factors that affect the extent of the voice problem include the severity and type of loss, the use of amplification, the training received in use of residual hearing (Calvert & Silverman, 1975) and the emphasis given to voice in speech–language therapy. Ling (1975) stated that it is important to focus on the control of breathing and vocalization early in the remediation program. Frequently, if too much emphasis is put on language stimulation and articulation skill, and respiration, phonation, and resonance patterns are ignored, inappropriate voicing patterns become habituated. Audiologists frequently consider inappropriate loudness levels to be clues that are of interest diagnostically. A child with a conductive loss may speak too softly because he or she is able to monitor through bone conduction, and a child with a sensorineural loss may need to speak very loudly, even in quiet environments, to monitor the voice auditorally.

Vocal Symptoms Associated With Hearing Loss

Some vocal symptoms identified as occurring in persons who have impaired hearing are listed below. The degree of loss affects type and severity of symptoms.

A. Faulty resonance
  1. Hypernasality
  2. Hyponasality
  3. Cul-de-sac resonance
  4. Posterior tongue carriage
  5. Insufficient velopharyngeal closure
  6. Oral–nasal imbalance
  7. Difficulty habituating appropriate patterns
B. Inappropriate loudness
  1. Level
  2. Variation
C. Inappropriate pitch
  1. Modal pitch
  2. Variation
D. Inappropriate rate
  1. Breath groups
  2. Prolonged duration and diphthongizations
E. Inappropriate initiation of phonation
  1. Not matched with expiratory cycle
  2. Hard attack
F. Tendency to develop nodules
G. Inappropriate prosodic patterns

Constraints Resulting From Specific Structural Deviations

Velopharyngeal Inadequacy

Because the velopharyngeal closure mechanism is responsible for separating the oral and nasal cavities, an inadequate mechanism results in hypernasality of vowels and nonnasal consonants and distortion of consonants. Consonants that require intraoral breath pressure are particularly affected. When the velopharyngeal mechanism is structurally intact but functionally impaired, as in the case of paralysis, the problem is usually referred to as *velopharyngeal incompetence.* When the term *velopharyngeal insufficiency* is used, it suggests structural deficiency. Structural defects include unrepaired clefts of the palate (overt, submucous, or occult), short palates (congenitally short or the result of surgical repair of a cleft), lesions due to trauma, abnormally large or inactive pharynges, and inappropriate relationships between structures (sometimes seen in craniofacial anomalies associated with a variety of genetic syndromes; see Kummer & Lee, 1996).

A team approach to assessment is usually the procedure of choice. Velopharyngeal adequacy is best evaluated in a medical center where information from videofluoroscopic, endoscopic, or radiographic analyses is available. There are also a number of noninvasive instruments, such as accelometric devices, that can provide information concerning the adequacy of velopharyngeal closure. These instruments are sometimes available in speech science laboratories in universities and medical centers. The plastic surgeon, orthodontist, and prosothodontist play important roles in the assessment and habilitation process. Surgical procedures and the various kinds of speech appliances and obturators have been described in the cleft-palate literature. A secondary surgical procedure that is sometimes used with good results is the construction of a pharyngeal flap. In this procedure, a piece of mucosal tissue from the pharynx is permanently attached to the velum to form a bridge. When air is emitted through the nose (as in breathing or the emission of nasal consonants), it passes on either side of the flap. To accomplish closure of the port, pharyngeal wall activity is necessary so that the sides of the pharynx close around the bridge of tissue. Bzoch (1972) reported that hypernasality and problems with nasal emission were reduced in patients who had undergone this surgery. We mention this secondary procedure not because it is necessarily the method of choice for all patients but because it is a fairly common example of a permanent alteration in structures that requires accommodation and relearning.

Negative Behaviors Associated With the Velopharyngeal Inadequacy

Negative behaviors frequently associated with velopharyngeal inadequacy and problems that cause difficulty for children who have undergone procedures to improve insufficiency are listed below. In some cases, symptoms persist even after structural adequacy is achieved. In other cases, procedures do not always produce the desired result. We must emphasize that although certain behaviors occur frequently in such a population, each child must be evaluated carefully and individually. Following surgical or prosthetic intervention, periodic reevaluation is encouraged. In some instances, revisions may be necessary. See Lewis et al. (1993) for a discussion of the vocal characteristics of children with velopharyngeal incompetence.

A. *Phonation and resonance*
   1. Breathiness
   2. Hoarseness

3. Hyperfunctional use of phonatory mechanism
4. Laryngeal attempts to compensate for inadequate velopharyngeal valving (e.g., glottal stops)
5. Nodules
6. Hypernasality of vowels (especially apparent on high vowels /i/ and /u/
7. Hypernasality of oral consonants
8. Hyponasality of nasal consonants (sometimes apparent subsequent to pharyngeal flap surgery); if accommodation does not occur as a result of therapy, revision may be necessary
9. Nasal emission of airstream

B. *Articulation*
1. Distortions of consonants dependent on intraoral breath pressure, particularly fricatives and affricatives
2. Substitutions most frequent on plosives (e.g., glottal or pharyngeal stop)
3. Voiceless consonants more difficult than voiced
4. Consonantal blends misarticulated frequently
5. Nasal snort—posterior nasal fricative
6. Nasal grimace—constriction of nares; /s/ may be lateralized, palatalized, or produced with pharyngeal friction
7. Omissions of pressure consonants
8. Substitution of nasals for pressure consonants
9. Connected speech may be unintelligible

Vocal Fold Paralysis

Paralysis of the vocal folds is relatively common in children (Holinger & Brown, 1967) and may be congenital or acquired. It represents about 10% of all congenital anomalies of the larynx and may be bilateral or unilateral. Laupus and Pastore (1967) noted that the abductor muscles are most usually affected. If one or both folds are fixed in an abducted position, breathing is not restricted, but voice use may be impaired. Symptoms will depend on the degree of involvement and the compensations that are possible with respect to closure. For example, if only one fold is affected and the other is able to approximate it, the leakage of air during phonation will be minimized. Some degree of breathiness will be present if one or both folds are fixed in the paramedian position. If one fold is fixed at the midline, voicing will not be impaired because the other fold will move to the midline appropriately during phonation. Some difficulty in breathing, especially during physical activity, will be noted, however, because the airway is reduced. If both folds are fixed at the midline, and the airway is blocked, the child will need to breathe through a tracheostomy tube. Such a child may need help dealing with the disturbance in respiratory and phonatory activity and in personal and interpersonal adjustment.

Vocal cord paralysis is a common cause of stridor and hoarseness in infants and children. Rosin et al. (1990) presented data on 51 cases and noted that they found that pediatric vocal fold paralyses were different in etiology from those seen in adults. In children, the etiologies most commonly seen were central nervous system abnormalities (especially Arnold-Chiari deformities with associated meningomyelocele and hydrocephalus), congenital cardiovascular disease, and idiopathic and local trauma. Neurologic difficulties usually led to bilateral paralysis. Unilateral paralysis occurred most often from trauma or cardiac abnormalities. Rosin et al. also noted that postinfancy cases of vocal fold paralysis might result from blunt or neurologic trauma including near drowning. Of the 51 children they studied, 29 were diagnosed with bilateral paralysis, and on follow-up, 16 had normal voice quality, 2 remained hoarse, 1 child had a soft voice, 1 had no communication, 2 used esophageal voice, and 2 used sign language. Unilateral paralysis patients' follow-up revealed that 50% had normal voice, 14% were hoarse, and 9% were softer than normal; no nonverbal methods of communication were reported, although not all of this group could be contacted. The left vocal fold was more often involved than the right, which is explained by the longer course of the left recurrent laryngeal nerve that makes it more susceptible to injury, especially when a child has congenital cardiovascular anomalies. Intubation trauma is also implicated in some cases of laryngeal paralysis in chronically sick children. Cavo (1985) demonstrated that the recurrent laryngeal nerve was vulnerable to pressure injury between the endotracheal tube and the superior portion of the thyroid cartilage. The physician must palpate the arytenoids to differentiate between vocal fold paralysis caused by intubation and cricoarytenoid fixation or posterior glottic stenosis because both of these conditions also may result from intubation.

Symptoms Associated With Vocal Fold Paralysis

Respiratory difficulties; stridor, cyanosis, apnea
Breathiness; hoarseness, aphonia
Reduced loudness levels
Reduced vocal variety
Hyperfunctional compensations
Personal adjustment difficulties
Impaired interpersonal skills
Ventricular phonation
Feeding problems
Stoma noise (if tracheostomy necessary)
Nonverbal (substitute) communication

Laryngeal Trauma

It is difficult to generalize about the patterns of symptoms displayed by children who have undergone traumatic experiences affecting the larynx because the insults vary considerably with respect to the type of damage. Prolonged intubation is a common cause of trauma in children. Clinicians should be alert to the need to question parents concerning episodes of respiratory distress in a child's medical history or surgeries that may have involved intubation. Endotracheal tubes and nasotracheal tubes can result in temporary or permanent damage, as can aspiration of foreign objects, direct trauma to the neck, or inhaling toxic substances.

Bent and Porubshy (1998) reported on 10 cases of pediatric laryngeal trauma with a mean age of 9 to 7 years. Eight cases suffered blunt trauma, whereas two suffered penetrating trauma. Traumas included motor vehicle accidents, strangulation, gunshot, clothesline, go-cart, and falling injuries. These authors believe that the anatomic characteristics of the immature larynx, along with social factors (e.g., car seats), reduce the incidence and severity of injury. Recovery of voice, although 80% good in their series, is related to the severity of the injury.

Summary

We have discussed some typical symptom patterns that are sometimes seen in association with specific etiologies. We also have listed a wide range of symptoms that can occur in conjunction with some of the most common problems. We emphasized the importance of always considering each child as a unique individual. It is certainly unwise to assume that one can ever be sure that a child with a specific problem will automatically exhibit a predictable set of symptoms. Nevertheless, it sometimes helps us organize our thoughts and our planning strategies if we are cognizant of the way some symptoms cluster together. In Chapter 8, we describe specific assessment strategies.

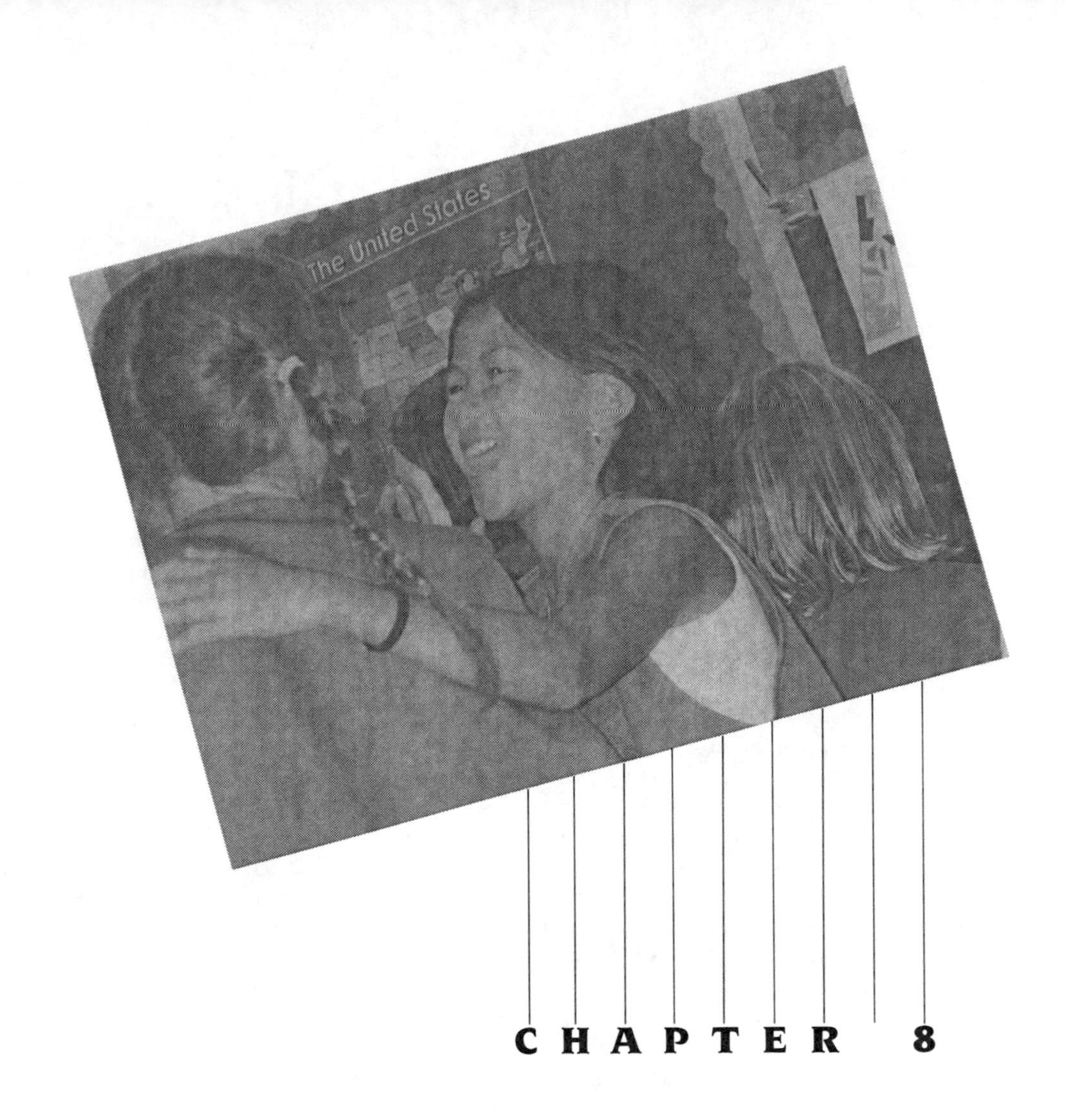

CHAPTER 8

Techniques for Evaluating Vocal Behavior

The first step in the evaluation process is usually screening. In many school districts, screening of all children is conducted by the speech-language pathologist at regular intervals. At such times, the voice screening is a part of a process that also involves hearing, articulation, and language. The clinician, for example, listens to the child's voice during brief conversation, reading, or both, or asks the child to count. Many screening forms have been developed by clinicians as aids to sharpening their focus on specific aspects of behavior. Most forms include the opportunity to note any deviations in pitch, loudness, quality, and resonance. Many clinicians include prolongation of vowels in the screening to check duration time and any deviations, such as breaks in the continuity of voicing. The *s–z* ratio (Eckel & Boone, 1981) is also popular as a screening technique and is used if quality deviations are suspected. If, during the screening, the clinician is unsure that a problem is permanent or transitory (as in the case of a child with an upper respiratory tract infection), then a follow-up screening is usually scheduled.

In school districts where periodic screening of all children is not standard procedure, the speech–language pathologist must rely on referrals. These referrals are made primarily by teachers; but sometimes parents, school nurses, and physicians ask that a child be seen for voice evaluation. When clinicians depend on referrals alone, they need to ensure that information concerning voice disorders is disseminated. Regular in-service programs for teachers and other school personnel need to be organized so that symptoms of vocal disorders can be identified. Programs on voice hygiene for music teachers, physical education teachers, nurses, bus drivers, lunchroom supervisors, parents, and others can be provided. Posters and notices can be used effectively to raise awareness. For example, one innovative clinician placed small, colorful signs on each table in the teachers' lounges in one school district. On each stand-up sign was written: *If any children you know have voices that sound unusual (e.g., hoarse, raspy, nasal), please send them to the speech teacher to be checked.* Informal discussions with individual teachers can also stimulate interest and help focus attention on vocal behavior.

It is usually helpful to initiate and maintain cordial professional relationships with otolaryngologists in the community. When new physicians move into the clinician's district, a friendly call or letter describing the services available for children with voice problems may be mutually advantageous. Some established physicians who rarely refer for voice therapy may nevertheless respond positively to invitations to lecture to speech–language pathologists. Question–answer periods following such lectures can help generate interest in improving communication between physicians and teachers. Clinicians may find it rewarding to ask physicians to participate in team presentations with speech–language pathologists on such subjects as ear, nose, and throat problems for PTO or PTA groups. Improved communication between physicians and speech–language pathologists usually heightens the physicians' awareness of the speech–language pathologists' areas of expertise and consequently may increase the number of children referred for voice therapy. When physicians do make referrals for voice therapy, they usually respond favorably to short follow-up reports. Some clinicians routinely write to thank physicians for referrals. They use the opportunity to note that they enjoy working with children with voice problems and would appreciate future referrals.

Most clinicians want to be sure that they have obtained adequate information on the child's abilities before they make a medical referral. This enables them to send a description of their findings with the child when he or she visits the otolaryngologist. A referral form is helpful because a form that asks the physician to provide specific written feedback to the clinician concerning his or her findings streamlines the communication between professionals. Most school districts have their own medical referral forms, and frequently the best forms are short and simple so that a busy physician can complete them in a few seconds. It is also important, however, to try to provide as much information as possible concerning the speech–language pathologist's findings. This can help focus the physician's attention on pertinent information that the clinician thinks may be relevant to the medical diagnosis. The physician's evaluation report shown in Figure 8–1 allows information of this type to be transmitted to the physician.

Evaluation Procedures: Trained Perceptions

Unfortunately, no standardized tests are available for clinicians to use during voice diagnosis. Much work remains to be done in this important area of evaluation. We have to rely on our trained perceptual evaluations of the child's behavior. These are different from the perceptual judgments made by others who observe the child because of our training in the normative aspects of communication behavior, our familiarity with the research literature, and our skills developed in the practice of speech–language pathology. In the next chapter, we will see how technological advances have allowed us to supplement our perceptual evaluations with additional information obtained by using instrumentation. For example, our ear may tell us a child's pitch in inappropriate for his or her age and gender. We can then analyze the voice patterns acoustically and compare the frequency characteristics the child exhibits with those documented in the literature for age and gender. In this example, the clinician's ear identifies the nature of the problem and the acoustic measure corroborates it. Here we will begin by describing how the clinician begins the evaluation using trained judgments.

We shall note some of the relevant behaviors subsumed under our four general areas and explain some ways in which these may be elicited. Remember as you read the suggestions that the tasks provided are designed to help the clinician formulate subjective impressions about children's behavior. In the absence of normative data for each task, we have no objective method of comparing an individual's responses with other children of similar age, gender, or socioeconomic level. Similarly, our impression of a child's poor performance on any one task is not in itself evidence that a pathology exists. Patterns of difficulty on a number of tasks, however, may help us to formulate hypotheses concerning the nature of the problem and the possible etiology. These hypotheses help us to decide (a) whether the child has a problem that requires further assessment or warrants intervention; (b) whether additional information or help is needed, and, if so, what referrals should be made; and (c) which specific behaviors should be translated into possible goals for therapy.

We find it convenient to use the form shown in Figure 8–2 to record the results of our evaluation. This form is divided into sections pertaining to respiration, phonation, resonance, and high-risk factors. At the beginning of each section of the recording sheet, the clinician decides whether detailed information needs to be recorded before proceeding to the next section. The cover sheet of the form is completed last. The check marks on this page indicate areas of concern and help us focus on information that is important to us when we formulte our treatment plan. Following the Andrews Voice Evaluation Form are examples of methods that we have found useful for eliciting samples of relevant behaviors.

Figure 8–1. Physician's evaluation report (voice).

Child ______________________________ Age ________

School ______________________________ Grade ________

This child has been evaluated by the speech pathologist. Because of voice symptoms that could be related to physiologic or neurologic conditions affecting communication, a physician's statement concerning pertinent medical information is requested.

Speech–Language Pathologist's Findings: ______________________________

____

____

Date of Evaluation: ______________________________

Description of Voice: ______________________________

____

____

I. Physical conditions that may be pertinent (circled)

allergies	frequent upper respiratory infections	craniofacial anomalies
surgeries	excessive mucus	broken nose
medications	thyroid condition	hearing loss
deviated septum	enlarged tonsils and adenoids	dryness of tract
previous intubation		GERD
mouth breathing		

other: ______________________________

II. Abusive practices (circled)

throat clearing crying, screaming excessive talking loud talking
sound imitations impersonations coughing smoking yodeling

other: ______________________________

III. Demands inherent in lifestyle–environment (circled):

voice models noisy environment cheerleading sporting activities
choir solo singing dramatics stress
other: ______________________________

Please complete the following information and return the entire form as soon as possible. Thank you.

____

Speech–Language Pathologist

Results of physician's evaluation (e.g., condition of larynx, tonsils, adenoids):

____

____

Does the child need medical care related to the communication disorder (e.g., surgery, prosthesis, medication)? Yes _____ No _____ If yes, please explain:

____

____

Please describe any health or medical problems that could affect the communication training: ________

____

Comments: ____

____

____

Date: __________ Signature of Physician: ____________________________________

Please return to: Stamped Name:

(Clinician's name and address)

____

Suggestions for Eliciting Samples of Respiratory Behavior

1. Length of inhalation may be assessed by having a child inhale through a straw while keeping a piece of tissue attached to the end of it.
2. When checking a child's depth of inhalation, provide a model and cues. For example, demonstrate lower chest expansion with the clinician placing his or her hands on the child's chest. A few practice trials may be needed.
3. Depth of inhalation, as well as length of exhalation, can be observed by using the activity of blowing through a straw into a glass of water. The clinician should model an exhalation of at least 10 seconds, stressing the relationship between depth of air intake and length of time the bubbles can be blown in the water.
4. When the clinician is observing the length of a child's exhalation, it is important that the child understands the concept of continuity. Give instructions such as "Keep going as long as you can" or "Keep making the sound until my finger reaches the end of the table." For young children, it is helpful to use an object moving toward a destination to elicit the prolongation (e.g., "Say the /s/ until the snake gets to his cave" or "Say the /z/ until the bee gets to the hive"). Silly Putty can also be stretched to suggest prolongation.
5. When the clinician presents tasks involving control or segmentation of exhaled airflow, a model and clear explanations of the purpose of the activity are necessary for all children. For younger children, a picture of a little pig huffing and puffing a house down (e.g., "He takes in a lot of air—then he lets out one huff like this

Figure 8–2. Andrews voice evaluation form.

Child's name ______________________ Date(s) examined: ______________________

Birthdate: ______ Age: ________ Time of day: ______________________

School: ________ Grade: ________ Examiner: ______________________

Siblings' names and ages: ____________ Room/teacher: ______________________

______________________ Hearing testing results: ______________________

____

Cold or allergic reaction at time of testing? Yes _____ No _____

____

Synopsis of Diagnostic Results
(check areas of concern)

Respiration
Type and depth of inhalation _____
Length of exhalation _____
Control of airflow _____
Use of replenishing breaths _____

Phonation
Vocal fold abduction–adduction _____
Vocal fold mass/tension adjustments _____
pitch _____
loudness _____
Onset of phonation _____
Evenness of vibratory pattern (quality) _____

Resonance
Oral resonance _____
Nasal resonance _____ Transitions between orality and nasality _____
Tone focus _____
mouth opening _____
tongue movement _____
lip movement _____

Interpersonal Factors
Motivation _____
Environmental factor _____
Psychodynamic factors _____
Referral needed: Medical _____ Psychological _____
Enroll in therapy? _____ Yes _____ No

Rate
Phrasing _____
Length of pauses _____
Too rapid _____
Too slow _____

High-Risk Factors
Relevant _____
Irrelevant _____

Respiration
Respiration for speech appears:
appropriate _____ inappropriate _____ (if inappropriate, complete section that follows)

Figure 8–2. (continued)

Characteristics of Breathing Patterns:

1. Coordination of inhalation and exhalation in spontaneous speech:
   rhythmical _____ jerky _____ noisy _____ other _____
2. Chest wall movements: appropriate _____ inappropriate _____
3. Tension sites: none _____ chest _____ neck _____
4. Length of exhalation (average of three trials)
   a. Can count on one breath to _____
   b. Sustains s-s-s _____ sec
   c. Sustains z-z-z _____ sec
   d. Sustains /a/_____ sec
   e. Sustains /i/_____ sec
5. Control of exhalation (stopping and starting airflow per breath)
   a. Number of /p/ productions per exhalation _____
   b. Number of /t/ productions per exhalation _____
   c. Number of /g/ productions per exhalation _____
   d. Number of /tʃ/ productions per exhalation _____
   e. Number of /h/ productions per exhalation _____
6. Use of replenishing breaths
   a. Number of breaths taken while counting to 50 _____
   b. Number of breaths taken while reading (50 words at child's reading level) _____
   (Child's reading rate appears: appropriate _____ fast _____ slow _____)

Phonation

Phonatory behavior for speech in the following areas appears:

	quality	onset	loudness	pitch	rate
Appropriate	_____	_____	_____	_____	_____
Inappropriate	_____	_____	_____	_____	_____

(if inappropriate, complete section below)

1. Quality in spontaneous speech sample

	Mild	Moderate	Severe
a. Normal _____			
b. Breathy _____	_____	_____	_____
c. Harsh _____	_____	_____	_____
d. Hoarse _____	_____	_____	_____

   e. Related observations: pitch breaks _____ phonation breaks _____
   aphonia _____ glottal fry _____ diplophonia _____ tremor _____
   other: _____________________________________
   f. Hard attacks noted in spontaneous speech: _____ yes _____ no

2. Onset of phonation

Single Words	*Appropriate*	*Breathy*	*Hard Attack*
a. arm /a/	_____	_____	_____
b. eggs /e/	_____	_____	_____
c. umpire /ʌ/	_____	_____	_____
d. out /au/	_____	_____	_____
e. ooze /u/	_____	_____	_____
f. eight /eɪ/	_____	_____	_____
g. apple /æ/	_____	_____	_____

Figure 8–2. (continued)

Sentences	*Appropriate*	*Breathy*	*Hard Attack*
a. Uncle Eddy eats eggs.	_____	_____	_____
b. Is everyone angry?	_____	_____	_____
c. Amy Anderson always understands.	_____	_____	_____
d. Aunt Ellie ate out.	_____	_____	_____

3. Loudness
   - *a.* Prolonged vowel /a/ loudly: _____ seconds
   - *b.* Prolonged vowel /a/ softly: _____ seconds
   - *c.* Can say the days of the week softly: yes _____ no _____
     Can say the days of the week loudly: yes _____ no _____
   - *d.* Sustained vowels gradually increasing and decreasing loudness (e.g., police car siren coming closer and fading)
     Ability to control loudness: yes _____ no _____
     Limited loudness range: yes _____ no _____
     Tension present: yes _____ no _____
   - *e.* Counting from soft to loud; loud to soft
     Ability to control phonation: yes _____ no _____
     Limited range: yes _____ no _____
     Tension present: yes _____ no _____
   - *f.* Sustained level during reading passage:
     overstrong _____ weak _____
     fading _____ lacking in variety _____
     inappropriate to meaning _____ appropriate _____
   - *g.* General conversational level: appropriate _____ inappropriate _____
     Describe if inappropriate:
     Comments:

4. Pitch
   - *a.* Reading and conversation: habitual level:
     Appropriate to age and sex _____ too low _____ too high _____
     Voice breaks to higher pitch _____ Voice breaks to lower pitch _____
     Variability: appropriate _____ limited _____ monotone _____
   - *b.* Ability to imitate extremes of pitch range (isolated vowels):
     good _____ fair _____ poor _____
   - *c.* Ability to discriminate pitch differences (pitch pipe; noise makers):
     good _____ fair _____ poor _____
   - *d.* Ability to imitate a given pitch (isolated vowels):
     good _____ fair _____ poor _____
   - *e.* Ability to imitate a sequential pitch pattern (isolated vowels: e.g., low/high/low):
     good _____ fair _____ poor _____
   - *f.* Ability to imitate pitch inflections (phrases):
     e.g., It's mine? It is? She's eaten it?
     It's mine! It is! She's eaten it!
     good _____ fair _____ poor _____
   - *g.* Consistency of appropriate pitch level, range and variability in conversational speech:
     always _____ sometimes _____ never _____
   - *h.* Does the child's age and physical development indicate the possibility of pubertal voice changes?
     Yes _____ No _____

Figure 8–2. (continued)

Resonance

Overall resonance in reading and conversation appears:
appropriate _____ inappropriate _____ (if inappropriate, complete section below)

1. Ability to sustain a hum: nasal resonance present _____ weak _____ absent _____

2. Word pairs (vowels in nonnasal vs. nasal contexts)

	appropriate	*hypernasal*	*hyponasal*	*assimilated nasality on vowels only*
hat/ham	_____	_____	_____	_____
pat/mat	_____	_____	_____	_____
bat/man	_____	_____	_____	_____
towel/town	_____	_____	_____	_____
cow/now	_____	_____	_____	_____
pout/noun	_____	_____	_____	_____

3. Oral sentences (to check for hypernasality)

She eats cheese chips.	(nares open)	same _____ different _____
" " " "	(nares occluded)	
Charley has a fat cat.	(nares open)	same _____ different _____
" " " " "	(nares occluded)	

4. Nasal sentences (to check for hyponasality)

My mommy makes me mad.	(nares open)	same _____ different _____
" " " " "	(nares occluded)	
Ned knows Nancy's not nice.	(nares open)	same _____ different _____
" " " " "	(nares occluded)	

5. Circle observed characteristics of possible velopharyngeal inadequacy:
   snorts/grimaces   nares constriction   nasal emission
   bifed uvula   palatal deviations   distortion of pressure consonants
   Comments:

6. Circle observed characteristics of possible nasal obstruction:
   dark circles under eyes   noisy breathing   mouth breathing
   blocked nostril   swelling of nasal bridge   discharge   congestion
   enlarged tonsils   slow eater
   Comments:

7. Oral-nasal balance:
   appropriate _____ hypernasal _____ hyponasal _____ mixed _____

8. Circle observed characteristics of neurological dysfunction:
   absent gag   weak cough   asymmetrical palatal movement
   Comments:

Figure 8–2. (continued)

9. Tone focus (when counting)

	seated near clinician		*projecting voice across room*	
	adequate	inadequate	adequate	inadequate
mouth opening	_____	_____	_____	_____
lip movement	_____	_____	_____	_____
tongue movement (retracted?)	_____	_____	_____	_____
supraglottal tension	_____	_____	_____	_____

High-Risk Factors

High-risk factors appear:
present _____ absent _____ (if present, complete section below)

1. Physical conditions that may be pertinent (circle):

allergies	frequent upper respiratory infections	postnasal drip	paralysis, paresis
surgeries	GERD	dryness of tract	spasms, tremors
medications	excessive mucus	hearing loss	deviated septum
bifed uvula	thyroid condition	mouth breathing	broken nose
cleft palate	craniofacial anomalies	enlarged tonsils and adenoids	

uncoordination of muscles of face or mouth
other: ____________________________________

Comments:

2. Abusive practices (circle);

throat clearing	crying, screaming	excessive talking
loud talking	sound imitations	impersonations
coughing	smoking	yodeling

other:____

Comments:

3. Demands inherent in lifestyle–environment (circle):

voice models	noisy environment	cheerleading	sporting activities
choir	solo singing	dramatics	stress

other:____

Comments:

4. Psychodynamic factors (circle):

talking too much	ignoring feedback	not seeking feedback
ignoring differences between people	ignoring differences in situations	family problems
ignoring needs and interests of others	poor self-esteem	
aggressive behavior	reticence	

other: ____

Comments:

____

/huh/ and stops—then lets out some more") or similar visual aids are helpful.

6. When the clinician wants to see the number of syllables, words, or numbers emitted in one exhalation, ask children to count or say the alphabet as far as they can in one breath. For younger children, ask them to name colors of beads threaded on a string. See if they can manage to name more beads (as clinician moves them) in successive trials.
7. To help older children understand the concept of replenishing breaths, the clinician may need to use a reading passage and mark pauses in different places to illustrate how the meaning is enhanced or changed depending on where we pause to breathe.

   The use of visual aids (e.g., cars stopping at gas stations, trains stopping at stations, elevators stopping at various floors to let more people in) can help younger children understand the concept of periodically refilling or refueling the air supply.
8. To see whether children are stimulable and can produce changes in their behavior when they have an understanding of the concept of replenishing breaths, try the following: Ask older children to read a passage and note their use of replenishing breaths. Then ask them to mark places in the passage where it makes sense to pause and take in air. After they have marked the pauses, ask them to reread the passage and note if their behavior has changed since the first reading (count pauses for breaths in each instance; also note appropriateness of pauses in terms of meaning of passage). For younger children who cannot read well, use objects or colored blocks or beads arranged in a continuous array. When they "read" them (e.g., "a red bead, a blue bead, a yellow bead"), demonstrate how they can be arranged in groups so that there is time to stop and breathe. See if they can arrange them in manageable breath groups. Then ask them to say them again.
9. In children exhibiting disturbed respiratory patterns (e.g., neurologic impairment) it may be valuable to assess the child's vegetative breathing pattern. This can be accomplished by making the following observations:

   a. Number of breaths per minute at rest—
   bpm's
   (count number during 20 seconds and multiply by 3)

   b. Rhythmic deep breathing (with cues)
   slows rate to ______ bpm's
   appropriate movement of chest wall
   ______ yes ______ no
   extends exhalation phase during rhythmic breathing when cued
   ______ yes ______ no

   c. Physical observations
   posture
   appropriate ______ inappropriate ______
   hyperextension of neck
   ______ yes ______ no
   concave chest ______ yes ______ no
   extraneous movements
   ______ yes ______ no
   noisy ______ yes ______ no
   ______ other

   d. Ability to understand
   concepts ______ yes ______ no
   instructions ______ yes ______ no

Suggestions for Eliciting Samples of Phonatory Behavior

If a structural anomaly is present or if tissue change has occurred as a result of irritation, abusive habits, or both (i.e., nodules, polyps, thickening of the folds), the child may have difficulty approximating the folds evenly. He or she may therefore be unable to produce a clear tone unless using considerable effort. If so, the voice will sound *best* when loud and poorest when soft. In such cases, aphonia on unstressed syllables may occur during soft talking.

1. Ask the child to count from 1 to 40. Ask him or her to do it softly, then loudly. (If the tone is clearest when the child counts loudly, it is possible that there is some pathology present.)
2. Ask the child to sustain the vowel /a/ for as long as he or she can. (Most young children can do this for 10 seconds. If the child lasts less than 7 seconds on repeated trials, sounds clear *only* when loud, has voice breaks or diplophonia, it may be a sign of pathology.) Younger children will need help to ensure that they understand the concept of prolongation. The clinician may say, "Keep going until my pencil stops moving across the paper," and so forth. Another technique would be to use visual aids and say, "Here is the big brown bear." (Present bear.) "He says /a/ for as long as he can. You be the big brown bear and say /a/ for as long as you can. Like this. . . ." (Examiner models 10-second production of /a/.)
3. Ask the child to produce the /s/ sound for *as long as he or she can.* Then ask the child to produce the /z/ sound continuously. If, on repeated trials, the child always sustains the unvoiced /s/ for *longer* than the voiced /z/, it may be a sign of pathology (Eckel & Boone, 1981). Because the child has the same amount of available air for both phonemes, it is significant if the phoneme /z/, requiring approximation of the folds, is the more difficult.

   Examples of techniques that may be useful for young children include:

   a. "Sammy Snake goes /s/." (Present snake and place house 3 feet from snake.) "Keep going until Sammy Snake gets into his house." (Examiner models 10-second production of /s/ while moving snake into house.)
   b. "The car goes /z/." (Present car and place garage 3 feet from car.) "Keep going until it gets to the garage." (Examiner models 10-second production of /z/ while moving car into garage.)
4. Onset of phonation may be affected by the loudness level that the child is using. Therefore, in addition to asking a child to produce individual words, it is helpful to ask the child to say the sentence "Uncle Eddie eats eggs" softly and then loudly. Listen to see if he or she begins each word with a hard glottal attack.
5. If a child appears to be using excessive effort during phonation, note any observable signs of tension in the jaw, neck muscles, and so forth. Then, place your fingers under the child's chin above the larynx. Ask the child to swallow. Then ask him or her to sustain a vowel. If you feel the same muscles being used in phonation as are used in swallowing, it may indicate that the child is using excessive muscular effort.
6. A child who uses excessive effort when phonating because of edema or additive lesions that make adduction difficult may phonate best when talking loudly or producing the stressed syllables in a word. To check for this, ask the child to repeat multisyllabic words (e.g., Mississippi, Alabama, Mrs. MacIntyre, Mr. Johnson). Note if the child is aphonic on the unstressed syllables.
7. To determine the effect of a more relaxed production on the quality of the sound, ask the child to yawn while producing a vowel sound. For a young child, the following technique may

help the child understand the concept: "Look at Baby." (Present baby doll.) "She is yawning. She is tired. Let's pretend you are tired. Take a big breath. Yawn and say /a/." (Examiner models behavior.)

8. Children who are intermittently aphonic may have difficulty with adduction or simply may be running out of air. More air is lost during soft phonation than during loud phonation when the folds are closed for a longer portion of the vibratory cycle. To check to see if there is a pattern in the aphonic production, ask the child to read a passage or tell you about a picture. If, during connected speech, the vocal quality is poorest at the ends of sentences, it may indicate that the child needs help in improving breath support. Make sure you get samples of both soft and loud speech.
9. If aphonia or hoarseness is related to vocal abuse, the folds may be more swollen after prolonged use. On one occasion, test the child late in the day to assess the effects of use and fatigue on the voice.
10. Ask the child to vary loudness, for example, starting loudly and becoming softer (diminuendo) or starting softly and becoming louder (crescendo). Younger children may need the analogy of a siren coming closer or getting fainter as it moves away (e.g., a police car goes "Whoo . . ."). For younger children, the following technique may be used to assess loudness variations: "Look, the garage is on fire!" (Present garage.) "Here is a fire engine." (Present fire engine.) "It goes 'Whoo.' It is coming. It is getting louder. The fire engine is going home. It is getting softer." (Examiner models production of "Whoo" at a soft intensity level, followed by an increase in loudness and then decrease. Phonation is accompanied by corresponding movement of the fire engine.) "You pretend you're the fire engine. Start at home, put the fire out and go back home. Remember, it goes 'Whoo.'"
11. To determine if a child understands the concepts of loud and soft, it is sometimes useful to pair a loud sound with a large puppet and a soft sound with a small one. (Present large Mr. Bert puppet. Play the following tape recording.) "His voice sounds loud: /u/." (Present small Mr. Bert puppet. Play the following tape recording.) "His voice sounds soft: /u/. Show me who said this." (Examiner plays tape recording of loud /u/. Repeat for soft /u/. Randomize trials.)
12. Ask the child to hum on a variety of different pitches after being given a model. If the higher pitched hums are clearer, it may mean that the child can approximate the folds best when there is greater stiffness. This may indicate some tissue change affecting the adjustments of the folds.
13. Ask the child to sing a simple song (e.g., "Happy Birthday"). Note whether the child can vary the pitch of his or her voice appropriately. Restricted pitch variability is sometimes a sign of vocal pathology. Be cautious—this child may just have a "tin ear"!
14. If a child is young or seems to have difficulty with the concepts of high and low pitch levels, it may be advantageous to use visual aids and techniques similar to the ones below:
    a. (Place Mrs. Chicken on top of steps. Play the following prerecorded tape.) "This Mrs. Chicken talks in a high voice /i/." (Place Mr. Bert on bottom of steps. Play the following

prerecorded tape.) "This Mr. Bert talks in a low voice /i/. Show me who said this." (Examiner plays tape recording of high /i/. Repeat for low /i/. Randomize trials.)

b. (Present sheep and steps.) "Mr. Sheep says /a/. He goes up the steps." (Examiner moves sheep up steps, producing /a/ one tone higher on each step.) "Make Mr. Sheep go up the steps. Mr. Sheep says /a/. He goes down the steps." (Examiner moves sheep down steps, producing /a/ one tone lower on each step.) "Make Mr. Sheep go down the steps."

For additional discusson of eliciting voice samples from preschool children, see Andrews and Champley (1993) and Andrews and Summers (1993).

Suggestions for Eliciting Samples of Resonance Behavior

1. When the clinician is testing for the presence of hypernasality, the following techniques may prove useful:
   a. Ask the child to say [a-ŋ] vigorously. Does the velum move up for [a] and down for [ŋ]? Does the velum move symmetrically?
   b. Ask the child to sustain nonnasal sounds (e.g., vowels and fricatives). Listen to see if there is any difference when nostrils are occluded and unoccluded. (Place thumb under child's nostril to occlude.) There should be no perceived difference on nonnasal sounds if there is adequate velopharyngeal closure.
   c. Ask the child to say sentences with no nasal sound, for example:

      "She keeps cheese chips."
      "Charley has a fat cat."
      "Lisa teases Chris."

      Does the resonance sound appropriate? Is there any difference when the nostrils are occluded and unoccluded? (If a child is hypernasal, there will be a difference in the sound when the nostrils are occluded. If a difference is heard, it is an indication of velopharyngeal incompetence during connected speech.)
   d. Do an articulation analysis of the sounds requiring oral breath pressure (e.g., plosives, fricatives, and affricatives). Children with velopharyngeal problems often have the most trouble with these sounds. (The Iowa Pressure Test is useful.) Additional sentences with pressure sounds and including high vowels are these:

      "Chip bits of ice." "Louise has skis."
      "Kitty has fleas." "Fix the scissors."
      "She eats three cookies." "Squeeze the chopsticks."
      "Freeze the peas." "See Chris kiss."
      "Cross the t's." "She sells six geese."
2. When the clinician is testing for the presence of hyponasality, the following techniques may prove useful:
   a. Observe whether the child is a mouth breather. This may indicate nasal obstruction. Are there signs of tonsilar or adenoidal enlargement? (Does the child snore loudly at night? have circles under eyes? have pinched nostrils? have enlarged bridge of nose? appear listless? have frequent upper respiratory tract infections?) Does the child have allergies that cause nasal congestion? Can air be emitted through both nostrils, one nostril only, or not at all?

b. Can the child produce nasals (e.g., /m/ and /n/) with appropriate nasal resonance and vibration in nasal area? (Place hands on nasal area to feel vibrations.)

c. Ask the child to say a sentence loaded with nasals (e.g., "My mommy makes me mad"). Does the resonance sound appropriate? Is it the same whether or not nostrils are occluded? If it sounds the same, the child must not be emitting the nasal sounds through the nose. Additional sentences are these:

"Mr. Norris never knew."	"Coming home is fun."
"My neighbors moved."	"Ring in the new year."
"Don't knock Juan's knees."	"My nose never runs."
"Sing and hum in tune."	"Notice Kevin's nostrils."
"Time my running."	"Hammer nine nails."

d. Ask the child to prolong a humming sound. (For young children, move a toy car toward a garage.) Inability to hum may indicate nasal obstruction.

3. When the clinician is testing for the presence of assimilated nasality, it is important to listen to the production of vowel sounds adjacent to nasal consonants and those adjacent to oral consonants. Observe how the nasal consonants influence the production of the oral sounds. The following suggestions may be helpful:

a. Does the resonance sound appropriate when the child says a sentence (e.g., "Charley has a black hat") in which there are no nasals present? Children with assimilated nasality will do this appropriately.

b. Ask the child to say word pairs and observe the quality of the vowel sounds when they are adjacent to nasals. Compare the production of the same vowels in oral contexts. For example:

at	am	dough	know
cat	mat	pat	pam
rig	ring	see	knee
bake	make	beat	meat

c. To observe the child's production at the single word level without a model, have the child supply the missing word. For example:
Mother is a woman, Daddy is a _______.
I hit the baseball with a _______.
It doesn't belong to you, it belongs to _______.
With my ears I hear, with my eyes I _______.

d. Ask the child to say sentences such as "Go downtown now, Mrs. Brown." Observe whether the perception of the oral-nasal balance changes during connected speech.

Eliciting Samples of Interpersonal Behavior

1. Engage the child in conversation with one or more other children in the speech room. Try to introduce topics in which the child will become emotionally involved, for example, "Some people think school should continue all summer." "Should the whole class miss recess when one or two children misbehave? Why not?" (Observe amount of talking, turn taking, interruptions, etc.)

2. Notice feedback. Ask children to tell the true meaning of sentences spoken different ways. (Observe their ability to respond to cues.)

a. I like school.
(frown; flat intonation)
(puzzled look; questioning inflection)

b. He's a good person.
(negative facial expression; hesitant rate)
("He's" prolonged; questioning intonation)

c. Girls giggle a lot.
(tight mouth; duration of "girls" prolonged)
(happy face; questioning inflection)

3. Ask questions. Ask children individually to ask you any five questions that they would like you to answer (or use this technique with a small group of children questioning each other). (Observe the child's ability to formulate questions, take turns, and engage with others.)
4. Adapt to different situations. Show the child pictures of different situations, for example, a library (looking at book); a movie theater; a playground (fight); an art gallery. Ask the child to use the same words but say them in a manner that would be right for the different places; for example, "I'm going to tell my mother all about this." (Observe the appropriateness of the child's response.)
5. Show the child pictures of different people and ask him or her to choose the person the clinician is talking to when saying, "I need to talk to you" (e.g., point to the picture; older children may be asked to say why they chose a specific picture)—for example, elderly person, young child, doctor or nurse, police officer, school principal, bus driver, mother. (Observe the child's ability to interpret the vocal behavior used by the clinician. The clinician may also question the child about why certain choices were made.)
6. Tell the child a sample story and ask him or her to tell you why things worked out the way they did. Ask the child to retell the story with a different ending. (Observe the child's analysis of the needs and interests of others.)

a. Jim was playing with his train set. His young brother Billy kept asking him if he could play, too. Jim ignored him. Finally, Billy grabbed the caboose and threw it on the floor. Jim yelled at him, "You dummy—you've broken my caboose—I'll get you for that."

b. Greg and Tom were playing ball. Greg hit the ball over the fence into a neighbor's yard. The neighbor was annoyed because the ball broke a tomato plant in his garden. When he looked over the fence, Greg yelled, "It's not my fault—it's Tom's ball."

c. Juanita and Maria were giggling on the subway and forgot to get off at their stop. When they were late getting home, their mother was angry. They were scared, so they told her their teacher kept them, and they missed the train home. Their mother said she would go to the school and complain to the principal the next day. Maria yelled at her mother, "The principal will just think you're crazy!"

Additional Suggestions for Eliciting Samples of Voice During Conversational Speech

1. Describe your best friend.
2. Tell me four things you did in school today.
3. Describe the plan of your house. Start at the front door.
4. How will it be different when you are in grade ________?
5. What will it be like to be a teenager?
6. Who are the important people in your life? Tell me about them.
7. How would I recognize your family if I met them on the street?
8. Tell me about a movie you saw recently.
9. What would you like to do on your birthday?

10. What are the best and the worst things about this school?

Additional Topics to Elicit Discussion of the Child's Feelings

1. What do people misunderstand about you most?
2. What is something that really bugs you?
3. What do you think about when you can't fall asleep?
4. Say something you like about yourself.
5. What feelings do you have the most trouble sharing?
6. What is something someone did for you today that you especially liked?
7. Who are the people you most like to talk to? What is it about them that is special?
8. What have you done recently that you are proud of?
9. What are you looking forward to this week?
10. What would you most like to change about yourself? your family? your friends? your teacher?

Summary

Naturally, the information we obtain in the voice diagnostic evaluation is considered together with the results of the oral peripheral examination, the hearing testing, the medical report, and the case history. As we put all the pieces together, we obtain a pattern of the child's abilities, current level of functioning, the context in which he or she is operating, and the most pressing needs and priorities for the remediation program.

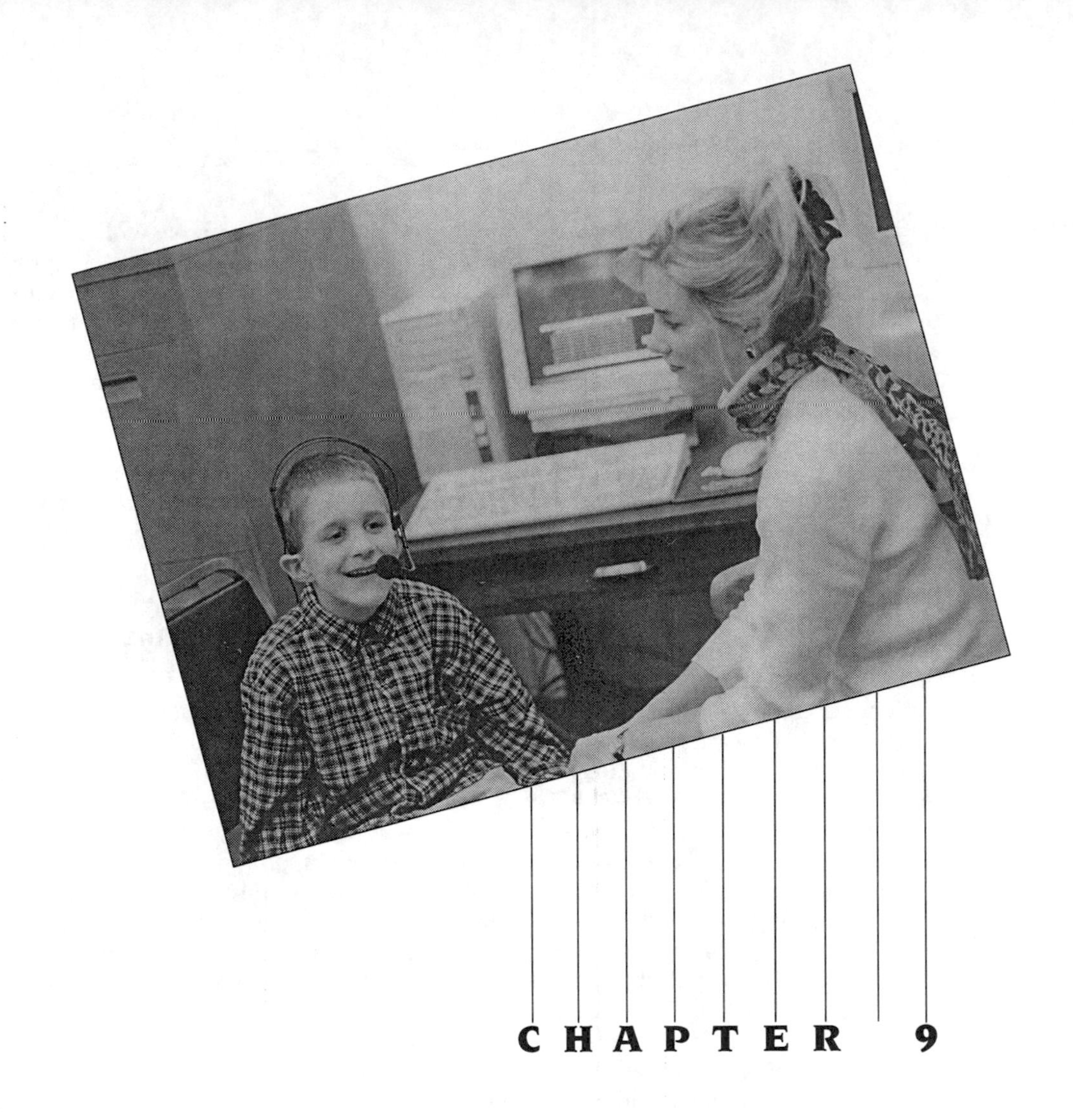

CHAPTER 9

The Analysis of Voice Using Instrumentation

Rahul Shrivastav, M.Sc., CCC-SLP

In the previous chapter, we described noninstrumental techniques for the evaluation of children's vocal behavior. Improvements in digital technology and the subsequent availability of personal computers in recent years have led to an increase in the application of technology to the study of voice. Quantifiable measures relevant to the evaluation of voice have become a routine part of many voice assessments. These measures are frequently referred to as "objective" measures because the data is obtained through the use of instruments. However, because the instruments are operated by human beings and because the results obtained are subject to human interpretation, some degree of subjectivity is always involved. Nevertheless, objective data provide us with opportunities to discover salient information to supplement and document clinicians' observations.

Instrumental analysis of voice can help clinicians study vocal behavior in a more comprehensive and detailed way than is possible just by observing a child. It allows clinicians to gather information and make quantitative measurements related to the functioning of various subsystems involved in voice production. This helps them amass more information pertaining to the cause of the voice problem and to strengthen documentation of the changes occurring during the treatment period. Because children often are unable to describe the nature of their disorder as accurately as adults, instrumental analysis of voice often provides critical additional information during the diagnosis and management of voice disorders in the pediatric population. Many instruments allow noninvasive monitoring of vocal behavior, making testing painless, easy, and relatively inexpensive. Further, Zajac, Farkas, Dindzans, and Stool (1993) noted that children today are more exposed to computers and other electronic devices, making them less "technophobic" and more willing to allow clinicians to use instrumental devices for voice analyses. In this chapter, we will review the theoretical bases underlying the development and refinement of measures that are used to quantify aspects of voice and voice-related behaviors. Specifically, we will review perceptual, aerodynamic, physiologic, and acoustic approaches and the tools that have been used in clinical settings. The advantages and limitations of various instruments also will be addressed. Additionally, precautions to assist clinicians in obtaining reliable results will be reviewed.

Perceptual Voice Analysis

Clinical evaluation may be divided into two categories: Perceptual evaluation, which involves trained auditory judgments made by clinicians, and instrumental analysis. Perceptual analysis of voice involves the clinician listening to the client's voice and assigning it a value on a given scale. Various scales are used for individual parameters, such as pitch, loudness, and quality. More comprehensive scales, such as the GRBAS scale proposed by the Japan Society of Logopaedics and Phoniatrics (Hirano, 1981) and the Wilson-Rice Voice Profile (Connelly, Wilson, & Leeper, 1970; Wilson & Rice, 1977) have also been proposed. These scales have multiple dimensions that are rated by the clinician to provide overall evaluation of the subject's voice. Recent studies by Kreimann and Gerratt (1998) have demonstrated that most scales used for perceptual ratings of voice quality have very poor reliability, especially in their midranges. In other words, although the reliability of these scales is fairly high when severely disordered voice samples are rated, the reliability tends to fall off for mild to moderately disordered voice samples. The authors also pointed out that the validity of such rating scales has never been empirically tested. Although such shortcomings underscore the need for more research, this should not lead us to believe that perceptual ratings are not important. When used by trained clinicians, perceptual ratings are always an important part of the process of classifying and describing disordered voices.

Instrumental Voice Analysis

Instrumental analysis of voice involves the use of various instruments to make objective measures of acoustic or physiologic signals to provide information about vocal behavior. Such analyses typically give results in the form of some numbers (e.g., fundamental frequency in Hertz or intensity in decibels), waveforms, or both. It is advantageous for clinicians to have results that are easily quantifiable, but numbers or waveforms produced by computers are always dependent on the clinician's interpretation. In this sense, these measures still have some amount of "subjectivity." To minimize subjectivity, the clinician needs to have a thorough knowledge about the instruments and procedures used to obtain specific measures and an understanding of how to interpret them accurately. Additionally, the accuracy of the measures depends critically on the way the signals are obtained and the quality of the recording equipment and procedures.

Most clinicians would agree that instrumental and perceptual analyses of voice, when used together, provide the most comprehensive picture of vocal behavior. An ideal voice evaluation should thus include both of these types of analyses. Supporting this notion, Hillman, Montgomery, and Zeitels (1997) stated:

> It has been our experience that, when used appropriately in conjunction with a team approach, objective measures of vocal function can result in more accurate and thorough diagnoses; better quantification of the impact of a disorder on vocal function; objective documentation that can assist in subsequent evaluation of treatment effectiveness; development of more comprehensive and better coordinated treatment plans; enhancement of ongoing efforts to design and improve treatment procedures; and efficient support for clinical research. (p. 175)

The advantages offered by instrumental evaluation of voice disorders have led to its increased use in clinics. Nonetheless, although there is a high incidence of voice disorders in children and successful use of instrumental measures in the pediatric population has been established, there is a lack of normative data for children (Geralyn, 1997).

For appropriate use of voice measurements, the clinician using these measures needs to be aware of the nature of the measures, the kind of information provided by the measures, and the shortcomings of each technique being used. We will review some of the commonly used techniques and equipment used for instrumental analyses of voice, the rationale underlying their use, the nature of the information provided by these measures, as well as some precautions for clinicians to avoid making errors in interpreting the results.

The human voice is a product of several subsystems. The respiratory system provides the power for voice production. The inspiratory and expiratory muscles act together to maintain a constant expiratory air pressure below the glottis, which provides the driving force for vibration of the vocal folds. This vibration of the vocal folds leads to the generation of an acoustic signal. Any pathology constraining the laryngeal system can affect how the expiratory air stream is modified to produce the glottal acoustic signal. Constraints on the system include commonly seen laryngeal changes, such as additive lesions and vocal fold swelling. The acoustic signal produced by the larynx is further modified by the supralaryngeal cavities to produce what a listener finally hears as the human voice. Disordered voice may thus be characterized by inadequate or inappropriate functioning of one or more of the subsystems, by a lack of coordination between various subsystems, or both. An ideal voice evaluation, therefore, should review the adequacy of function of each subsystem involved in voice production, as well as the coordination between the individual subsystems.

Measures of Air Volumes

Volume is a measure of the *quantity* of a fluid. The quantity of air managed by the respiratory system may be defined in terms of "lung volumes" and "lung capacities." These can be subdivided and described as tidal volume, vital capacity, inspiratory capacity, expiratory capacity, and residual capacity. The importance of making measures of these respiratory volumes for assessing speech and voice disorders has been questioned by Colton and Casper (1990), who pointed out that, although comprehensive detailed measures are important for the respiratory physiologist, these measures do not provide much information for the diagnosis or management of voice disorders, as long as the patient has the capability to create sufficient volume for speech. Rather, it is more important to determine how the volume of air is used during voice production (Boone & McFarlane, 1994).

When the volume of air used during phonation is measured along with the duration of phonation, it can be used to estimate the mean airflow rate (MAF; see Measures of Airflow later in this chapter for a description of this measure). By dividing the volume of air exhaled by the duration of phonation, a voice scientist can obtain the mean airflow per unit time.

$$\text{Rate of Airflow} = \frac{\text{Volume of air exhaled}}{\text{Duration of phonation}} \quad (1)$$

Instrumentation for Measuring Volume

A variety of instruments can be used for measuring volume. The *spirometer* is one of the oldest and simplest of such instruments. Different kinds of spirometers are available and are broadly classified as "wet" and "dry." The principle behind the use of a wet spirometer is simple. The subject exhales into a hollow cylinder that is placed in water and balanced for its weight by attaching a counter weight. As the subject exhales, the cylinder fills with air and rises. By determining how much the cylinder rises, the voice scientist can determine the volume of air exhaled by the subject. Dry spirometers (called "dry" because they do not use any water) are of different kinds but the principle underlying the way they work is similar to that of the wet spirometer. The volume of air exhaled moves some mechanical device, and the amount of movement reflects the volume of air being exhaled. Rau and Bekett (1984) compared measurements from a wet spirometer with those from some portable dry spirometers and found the results to be comparable.

Spirometers are inexpensive and easy to use. They are commercially available from several companies and are routinely used for tests of respiratory function. Modern spirometers have been integrated with digital technology and enable the user to obtain several measures and printable figures with the touch of a button. Spirometry is of limited use in voice measurement due to some of its shortcomings.

Shortcomings and Precautions

The most serious shortcoming of spirometers is their low sensitivity and poor temporal resolution. In other words, these instruments cannot measure small changes in volume and changes that occur over a brief period of time. Measurements for voice usually involve very rapid and relatively small changes in flow and volume. Clinicians cannot, for example, determine the changes in the airflow that occur within each individual glottal cycle. Thus, a spirometer is only useful for measuring relatively large changes in volume, occurring over relatively longer periods of time. Spirometry requires the subject to exhale or phonate into a face mask that collects the airflow and delivers it to the spirometer. It is essential for clinicians to ensure that the mask fits well around the patient's face and that there is no leakage of air from the edges because such leakage leads to an error in measurement of the volume. Clinicians must take care to use appropriately sized face masks and to present the mask in a way that does not cause anxiety for the child. Some of these measures, such as the measurement of vital capacity, require the subject to perform *maximal* inspiration and exhalation. Often, instead of maximum inspiration or expiration, young children tend to perform the maneuver only to a comfortable degree. Therefore, clinicians need to be extra cautious while making these measures, focusing on making the child understand the task correctly and observing the child during the procedure to ascertain if maximal inspiration and expiration were indeed achieved.

Measures of Airflow

Measuring the rate of flow of air through the glottis can help determine how the exhaled air is being utilized by the laryngeal system to produce voice. Flow refers to the movement of a volume of air per unit time; in this case, the movement of air that needs to be measured is that across the glottis. It can be seen from equation (1) that the volume of air exhaled is directly related to the rate of the airflow and the duration of the airflow. By a simple algebraic rearrangement of the terms in equation (1), the voice scientist also can determine the volume by measuring the airflow.

$$\text{Volume} = \text{Rate of Airflow} \times \text{Duration of Phonation} \quad (2)$$

Most modern, commercially available devices for the measurement of airflow have high sensitivity and excellent temporal resolution, thus allowing measurement of small and rapid changes in airflow and volume. These instruments are sturdy and relatively easy to use and are fast replacing the spirometers in clinics. The success of aerodynamic assessment in the pediatric population has been addressed by Lotz, D'Antonio, Chait, and Netsell (1993), who reviewed the results of more than a thousand aerodynamic evaluations in the pediatric population and found the success rate to be as high as 84% for 2-year-olds, with an increase to 100% in the 6- to 9-year-old age group.

Measurement of airflow can be used to obtain several different measures. The MAF is the average airflow across several glottal cycles. This measure represents the total airflow for voice production over a relatively long period of time. Studies such as that by Hirano, Koike, and Von Leden (1967) have shown that high MAF is an indication of poor glottal closure. However, MAF has been found to vary significantly across subjects and to be affected by factors such as the fundamental frequency and intensity of phonation. It is therefore necessary to follow a standardized protocol for measuring MAF (Baken & Orlikoff, 2000). Koike and Hirano (1967) reported that the MAF differed significantly between adult men and women and suggested that this was due to differences in the vital capacity between the two genders. To minimize this variability, Koike and Hirano proposed a measure called the *Vocal Velocity Index* (VVI), which they defined as the ratio of MAF to vital capacity. They suggested that by normalizing the MAF by vital capacity, the gender differences in MAF can be minimized. VVI is not a commonly used measure, however, and little data are available on it (Baken & Orlikoff, 2000). VVI findings in children have not been reported, and its usefulness in this population is questionable because studies such as that by Beckett, Thoelke, and Cowan (1971) have not found any significant differences in mean airflow in children of either gender. In children, therefore, measure of MAF may be sufficient to document the use of expiratory air by the laryngeal system.

Several measures can also be determined by studying the cyclic variations in glottal airflow. To do this, a specialized transducer with high frequency and temporal resolution is used. Glottal airflow is obtained by *inverse filtering* of the airflow measured at the oral cavity to remove the influence of the supralaryngeal tract from the measured signal. Because the airflow is measured in front of the lips, the signal obtained is a sum of the glottal airflow, as well as that of the effects of the oral cavity. By applying the inverse filter, the effects of the supralaryngeal cavities are minimized, and we can obtain an estimate of the airflow through the glottis. More details of this procedure are subsequently discussed under Correlates of Vocal Fold Motion.

Koike, Hirano, and Von Leden (1967) used measures of airflow to determine the volume of air consumed during three modes of voice onset—"breathy," "soft," and "hard"—and found that the airflow consumption at voice onset was significantly different for the three conditions. The air consumption during voice onset therefore may be useful in monitoring the type of glottal attack.

Instrumentation for Measuring Airflow

Two instruments commonly used for measuring airflow are the *pneumotachograph* and the *warm wire anemometer*. The most common device used to measure the airflow is the *pneumotachograph*. It is based on the fact that when an air stream flows through a resistance, it leads to a fall in pressure across the resistance. Simply stated, when the air stream flows across a barrier that offers resistance to the airflow (such as a wire mesh), the pressure due to the airflow is greater before the mesh and less on the other side. This drop in pressure depends on the resistance offered by the barrier, as well as the amount of airflow. Because in a pneumotachograph the resistance to the airflow is kept constant, the pressure drop is proportional to the flow of air. By measuring the pressure drop across a resistance, the pneumotachograph can determine the flow of air through it. *Warm wire anemometers* work in a different manner. These instruments have a heated wire that lies in the path of the air stream. As the air flows over the heated wire, it changes its temperature and thus its electrical resistance. The flow of air can be determined by measuring the change in the resistance because greater flows cause larger changes in electrical resistance.

Shortcomings and Precautions

Like spirometry, measurement of airflow requires the subject to phonate into a face mask. The face masks used for obtaining these measures should be large enough to allow easy jaw movement for speech but should also fit well enough to prevent any leakage of air. These face masks are available in different sizes, and care must be taken to choose the appropriate size for children. To minimize anxiety, the procedure must be carefully explained to the children. It is often helpful for the clinician to demonstrate to the child how the mask will be used by wearing it herself or by fitting it on another person before attempting to test the child. For all measures of flow and volume, it is important for the clinician to ascertain that there is no leakage of air from the edges of the mask. When the clinician is using a pneumotachograph to measure the airflow, care must also be taken to ascertain that the resistance offered to the airflow remains constant. The water vapor in the exhaled air can condense on the wire mesh barrier, which leads to an increase in resistance to airflow. To avoid this, many pneumotachographs have an electrical circuit to heat the wire mesh and prevent water condensation. Baken and Orlikoff (2000) described the shortcomings of a warm wire anemometer to include (a) lack of linearity (i.e., the relation between the flow and the change in electrical resistance is not constant), (b) a poorer frequency response than the pneumotachograph, (c) different sensitivity to ingressive and egressive airflows, and (d) the possibility of obtaining erroneous results as the flow becomes turbulent in nature. Advances in engineering have minimized many of the aforementioned shortcomings of warm wire anemometers, but nevertheless the pneumotachograph remains the instrument of choice for measuring airflow in most clinics at this time.

Measuring Air Pressure

Pressure is defined as the force per unit area. During vocalization, the vocal folds are held closed while the respiratory muscles contract to exhale the air from the lungs. Adequate subglottal pressure is essential for normal voice production and is especially important for intensity variation. The most reliable estimates of subglottal pressure can be obtained by direct measurement such as those obtained through a tracheal puncture. For routine clinical use, however, techniques for measuring subglottal pressure need to be quick, painless, and noninvasive. Two such techniques are commonly used in clinics.

1. The most popular approach to estimate the subglottal pressure is to measure the oral air pressure during the production of a voiceless plosive. During the production of a voiceless plosive, the vocal folds are wide open, but the oral cavity is completely closed. Thus, the pressure in the oral cavity is the same as the subglottal pressure. Measuring the peak oral pressure during a voiceless plosive (typically /p/) provides an estimate of the subglottal pressure (Rothenberg, 1973; Smitheran & Hixon, 1981). The subject is instructed to repeat a train of CV syllables with a voiceless plosive (e.g., /pi/-/pi/-/pi/-/pi/-pi/) and a pressure transducer that is connected to the oral cavity through an appropriately positioned tube measures the oral pressure. The pressure in the oral cavity during the plosive is approximately the same as the subglottal pressure during phonation of the vowel.
2. Another technique for measuring the subglottal pressure is to suddenly interrupt the airflow externally (Sawasimha, Kiritani et al., 1983). The subject phonates into a face mask attached to an external device that has an arrangement to stop the airflow momentarily. When properly controlled, the pressure measured when the airflow is interrupted reflects the subglottal pressure.

Instrumentation

A variety of pressure transducers are commercially available. These differ in their construction and their capabilities with respect to their sensitivity and frequency response. Except for some specially designed pressure transducers, these devices are placed outside the body and are coupled to the measurement site by a probe or a tube (Baken & Orlikoff, 2000). Tubing commonly used for coupling the pressure transducers to the oral cavity is flexible and has a small diameter and can be placed in the oral cavities of even very young children without much discomfort.

Shortcomings and Precautions

The most critical issue in the measurement of air pressure using the plosive production task is the placement of the pressure sensing tube. Care must be taken to place the tube perpendicular to the direction of airflow; otherwise the pressure measure tends to interact with the airflow and this leads to an error in measurement. The direction of this error (positive or negative) depends on the direction of the sensing tube in relation to the direction of airflow. Maintaining the appropriate placement of the tube is not easy because movements of the tongue and lips tend to displace the sensing tube during speech tasks. To minimize the displacement of the tube, it is positioned in the posterior oral cavity. The recommended approach to placing the sensing tube in the posterior part of the oral cavity is to pass it lateral to the lower gums and around the last molar. Although the sensing tube does not interfere much with the movement of the articulators, the presence of a foreign body in the oral cavity may cause some discomfort in children. Sometimes younger children tend to displace the tubing with their tongues, thereby affecting the measures. Explaining the procedure to the child and encouraging them to avoid moving the tube can help minimize the errors due to inappropriate placement of the tube. Clinicians should also be aware of the possibility of saliva blocking the sensing tube, which might give erroneous results.

Visualizing the Larynx

Visualization of the larynx has become an important aspect of the diagnoses and management of voice disorders. Visualization allows the clinician to look for lesions on the vocal folds and for aberrant vibratory behavior. Historically, laryngologists have observed the larynx using a laryngeal mirror; however, such examination does not allow for the observation of the vibratory characteristics of the vocal folds because vocal fold vibration is simply too fast to be observed by the naked eye. The use of stroboscopic light to observe vocal fold movement and the development of the fiber-optic endoscope has revolutionized examinations of the larynx during voice production. Recent advances in ultra-high-speed photography and the development of videokymography have also been promising developments and may overcome some of the shortcomings of stroboscopy. All of these techniques enable clinicians to observe the vocal folds for the presence of any mass lesions, the nature of the vocal fold margins (whether they are smooth or rough), the symmetry and regularity of vocal fold movement, patterns of glottal closure, the amplitude of vibration, as well as the presence or absence of the mucosal wave. Such observation of the vocal folds during voice production was not possible previously with the laryngeal mirror examination or with endoscopy using a constant light.

Two kinds of endoscopes are commonly used. One is a "rigid" endoscope that is inserted into the oral cavity, and the other is a "flexible" endoscope that is inserted through the nasal passages. Both the rigid and flexible endoscopes offer some advantages, and the use of one over the other often is based on the purpose of the evaluation. Many clinicians use both of these endoscopes for clinical evaluations, unless certain circumstances prevent the use of one. For example, the rigid endoscope, which is placed in the oral cavity, may touch the pharyngeal wall or the base of the tongue and elicit a gag reflex, making it difficult to visualize the larynx. However, the rigid endoscope has a larger diameter and generally provides a larger and clearer picture of the larynx than the flexible endoscope. Also, during examination of the vocal folds, the rigid endoscope tends to lie closer to the larynx, thereby providing a better image. The rigid endoscope limits the movement of the tongue and jaw, however, and restricts the speech tasks that can be performed during the evaluation. Unlike the rigid endoscope, the flexible endoscope has the advantage of allowing the patient to freely move the tongue and jaw, thus enabling the examiner to observe laryngeal behavior during connected speech. Flexible endoscopy frequently is used when the gag reflex prevents the use of rigid endoscopy or when vocal fold behavior during continuous speech needs to be observed. Nasoendoscopy may not always be possible in young children due to the small size of the nasal passages, however. Nasoendoscopy using a flexible endoscope may also cause greater anxiety, particularly in children. Successful use of the flexible endoscope, however, has been documented in several studies such as that by Shprintzen and Golding-Kushner (1989), who reported that young children can tolerate a thin, flexible endoscope when it is used with mild topical anesthesia. Lotz, D'Antonio, Chait, and Netsell (1993) reported successful nasoendoscopic exams in children as young as 2 years old. Nonetheless, the success of such examination is influenced greatly by the training and the experience of the examiner.

Instrumentation

Videostroboscopy

Videostroboscopy has become the gold standard for the diagnoses of laryngeal pathology in most clinics, and it allows the clinician to observe laryngeal movement during vocalization. Videostroboscopy involves the use of a fiber-optic endoscope to view the larynx. Instead of viewing the larynx under steady light, this procedure uses rapid flashes of light to view the vocal folds. These light flashes are coordinated with the glottal cycle, so that the successive light flashes occur at a frequency that is slightly lower or slightly higher than the frequency of phonation. The result, therefore, is that the vocal folds appear to move in slow motion. It is important to remember, however, that the observed movement is not truly seen in slow motion but is the sequencing of a series of "snapshots" taken from different glottal cycles. The vocal folds only appear to move in slow motion as the eye visualizes the chain of selected images as a continuous pattern. The equipment used for videostroboscopy has two basic components, a light source to emit light flashes and a camera unit attached to a video recorder or computer for recording the obtained images. Because the strobe light needs to be coordinated with the glottal cycles, a contact microphone or an electroglottography (EGG) unit is used to determine the fundamental frequency of phonation. The microphone (or EGG electrodes) is attached to the subject's neck with an elastic band to make contact with the larynx. When the subject phonates, the fundamental frequency of phonation is determined, and the strobe light is pulsed at approximately the same frequency. The camera is attached to a fiber-optic endoscope that is used to view the vocal folds. Figure 9–1 shows a fiberoptic cable cut out to reveal the glass fibers inside. These fibers transmit light, while allowing some flexibiity to the cable. A complete videostroboscopy unit is shown in Figure 9–2.

Ultra-High-Speed Photography

Ultra-high-speed photography involves photographing the vocal fold movement at rates as high as 3000 to 5000 frames per second. When films are viewed at a regular frame rate, the vocal fold motion can be seen in slow motion. Unlike stroboscopy, this technique shows the vocal fold movement in true slow motion; it does not need stroboscopic illumination and consequently eliminates the need to determine the fundamental frequency of phonation. Although researchers have used ultra-high-speed photography for many

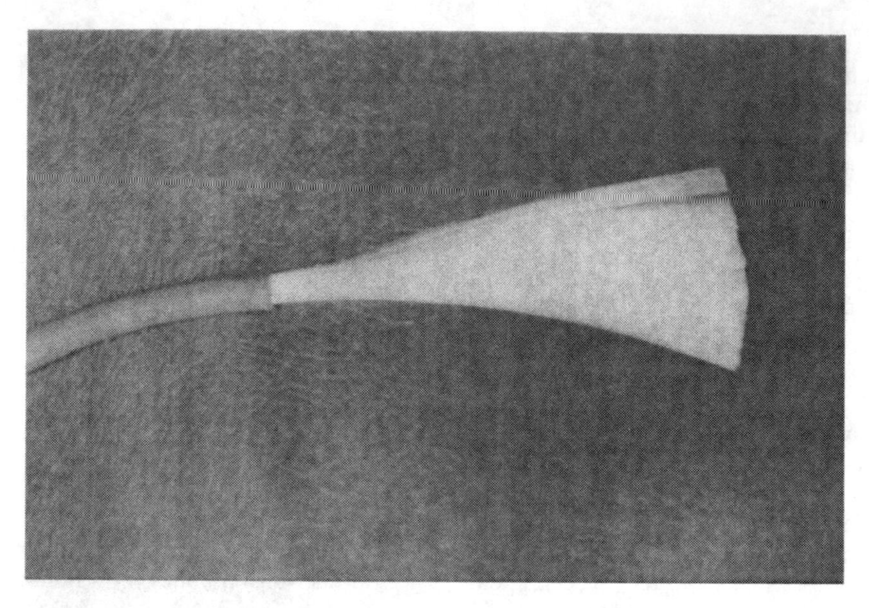

Figure 9–1. The fiberoptic cable of the endoscope cut out to show the individual glass fibers inside. Each of these fibers is capable of transmitting light.

years, it is rarely used clinically. This is mainly because of the extremely high cost, large size, and complexity of the equipment. Recent developments have made the equipment smaller, less expensive, and much easier to use. It is possible that the use of ultra-high-speed photography for routine clinical evaluation of the larynx will increase in the near future.

Videokymography

A recent development in techniques of the visualization of the larynx is that of videokymography (Schutte, Švec, & Šram, 1998; Švec & Schutte, 1996). This technique trades off spatial resolution to improve time resolution when imaging laryngeal movement. Thus, instead of obtaining a relatively large image of the larynx at 50 or 60 frames per second, this technique images a single line at frame rates of approximately 8000 frames per second. Because of the high-speed imaging, this technique also does not require stroboscopic illumination for viewing vocal fold movement. Videokymography can provide information about the movement of the upper margin of the vocal folds, the mucosal wave, and asymmetry between the left and the right vocal folds. Videokymography also shows promise of becoming more useful in clinical evaluations in the future.

Shortcomings and Precautions

All three methods of visualizing laryngeal movement involve relatively expensive equipment. Videostroboscopy is the most commonly used method for visualization of the larynx and presently the easiest to obtain commercially. The most serious shortcoming of this method is the fact that the images obtained are not truly slow motion. Because

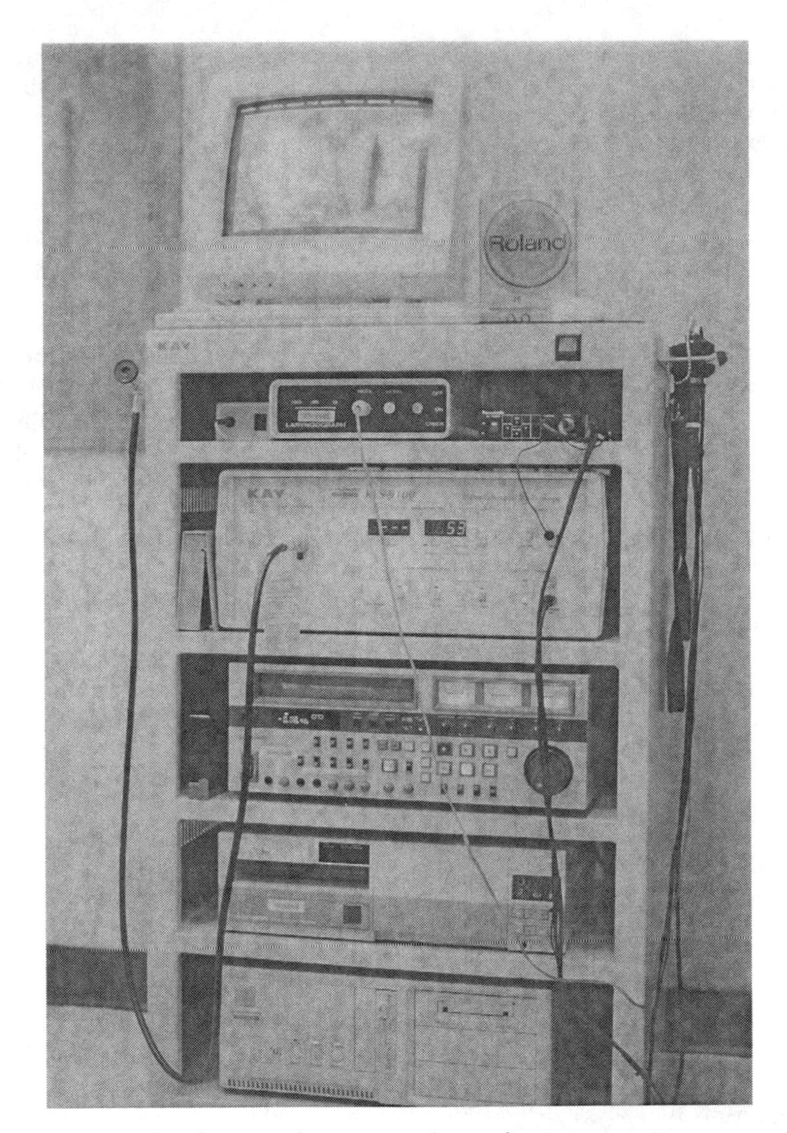

Figure 9–2. The Kay Elemetrics videostroboscopy system.

stroboscopy involves coordinating the light flashes with the fundamental frequency of phonation, such assessment works only for periodic vibration of vocal folds. In patients with voice disorders, the glottal cycles are often too irregular to coordinate the light flashes and the glottal cycles, and videostroboscopy fails to "slow down" the visualized movement of the vocal folds. Ultra-high-speed photography, on the other hand, does not require fundamental frequency extraction and can be successfully used for all patients with voice disorders, regardless of the severity and nature of their pathology. At the present time, the complexity and high cost of the equipment prevents its wider clinical application. Recent advances in engineering and digital technology have made it possible to miniaturize the hardware and reduce the cost of the equipment for ultra-high-speed photography of the vocal folds, and wider application may thus result. Videokymography is a low-cost alternative to ultra-high-speed photography and offers many of the same advantages over stroboscopy. There is no need for extraction of the fundamental frequency of phonation, and hence it can be successfully used with all patients with voice disorders. Videokymography only provides information about a single line on the vocal folds, however, and Baken and Orlikoff (2000) pointed out that movement of the endoscope or of the larynx can change the line that is under observation.

Correlates of Vocal Fold Motion

Direct observation of the larynx is not always possible because it always involves some degree of invasiveness. Furthermore, quantification of the images that are observed is difficult. The cost of equipment required for direct observation of the larynx is still relatively high, and it requires expert clinicians who usually work in a team that includes laryngologists. Another way to obtain information about vocal fold movement without direct observation of the vocal folds is to measure changes in some parameters that are directly related to the vocal fold movement. Because all of these techniques use some measure that covaries with the vocal fold movement, Baken (1987) categorized these techniques as "correlates of vocal fold motion." Such techniques include *electroglottography* (EGG) and *inverse filtering* of the oral airflow or of the acoustic signal. *Photoglottography* (PGG) is another such technique, but it is not widely used in clinics. The result obtained by using these techniques is usually a waveform corresponding to some measure of the laryngeal system such as the glottal contact area or the glottal area function. Although a study of normal voice using any of these techniques typically shows a periodic, quasitriangular pattern, depending on what exactly is being measured, these waveforms can give very different information. The overall pattern of these waveforms can contribute significant information about the vibratory behavior of the vocal folds. Characteristics of the waveforms can also be quantified in terms of various phases or quotients. Some commonly used instruments of this type are described in the following sections.

Instrumentation

Electroglottography

Electroglottography is based on the application of Ohm's law to monitor vocal fold motion. Ohm's law states that the current flowing through a resistor is directly proportional to the voltage applied across it and is inversely proportional to the resistance offered by it. A pair of electrodes is placed externally on either side of the subject's thyroid cartilage. One of these electrodes emits a small current into the tissue. The opposite electrode collects the current being emitted. Because the body tissues can conduct electricity, the current flows through the vocal folds from one electrode to the other. As the subject phonates, the vocal folds open and close repeatedly. When the vocal folds are open, the area of contact between the two vocal folds is small, and there is air in between the vocal folds. Because air is a poor conductor of electricity, less current flows through. On the other hand, as the vocal folds close, they come in greater contact with each other, and more current can flow through the tissues. Thus, the amount of current reaching the collecting electrode varies with the movement of vocal folds. The electrical current emitted by the EGG unit is very small in magnitude, does not cause any unusual sensation or pain, and is not harmful to the body. Because the EGG waveform is based on the current flowing through the vocal folds when they come in contact, it is a measure of the relative *glottal contact area*. An EGG unit is shown in Figure 9–3, and the EGG waveform obtained from a normal speaker is shown in Figure 9–4.

Childers, Hicks, Moore, Eskenazi, and Lalwani (1990) have shown that the EGG waveform reflects vocal fold vibratory behavior. The waveforms obtained using EGG can be interpreted based on changes to its overall shape, which are related to the underlying vocal fold behavior. Studies have been done to relate the changes in the vocal fold behavior to the shape of the EGG waveform for normal as well as for disordered voices (Childers, Hicks, Moore, & Alsaka, 1986; Titze, 1984). Additionally, the EGG waveform can be quantified in terms of various phases or quotients. Although measures such as the open quotients and open phase have been applied to the EGG waveform, these may not be appropriate because the EGG signal does not give information about the open phase (Baken & Orlikoff, 2000). This is because the EGG signal is a measure of glottal contact, and the open phase may not involve any contact between the vocal folds. Instead, alternative measures such as the relative contact duration and contact quotient have been proposed to describe the information obtained from the EGG signal (Titze, 1984). A thorough understanding of vocal fold physiology and the principles underlying the EGG can help the voice scientist

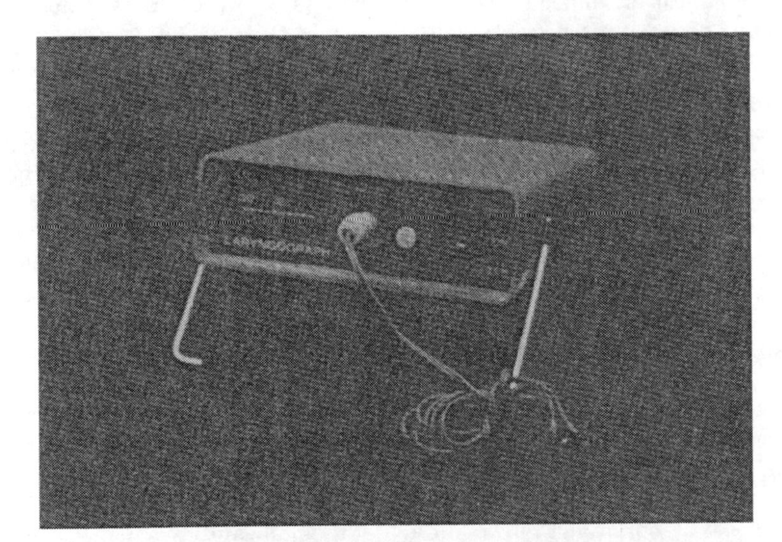

Figure 9–3. The "Laryngograph" from Kay Elemetrics. (From *Manual of Voice Treatment: Pediatrics Through Geriatrics*, 2nd ed. [p. 32], by Moya L. Andrews, 1999, San Diego: Singular Publishing Group. Copyright 1999 by Singular Publishing Group. Reprinted with permission.)

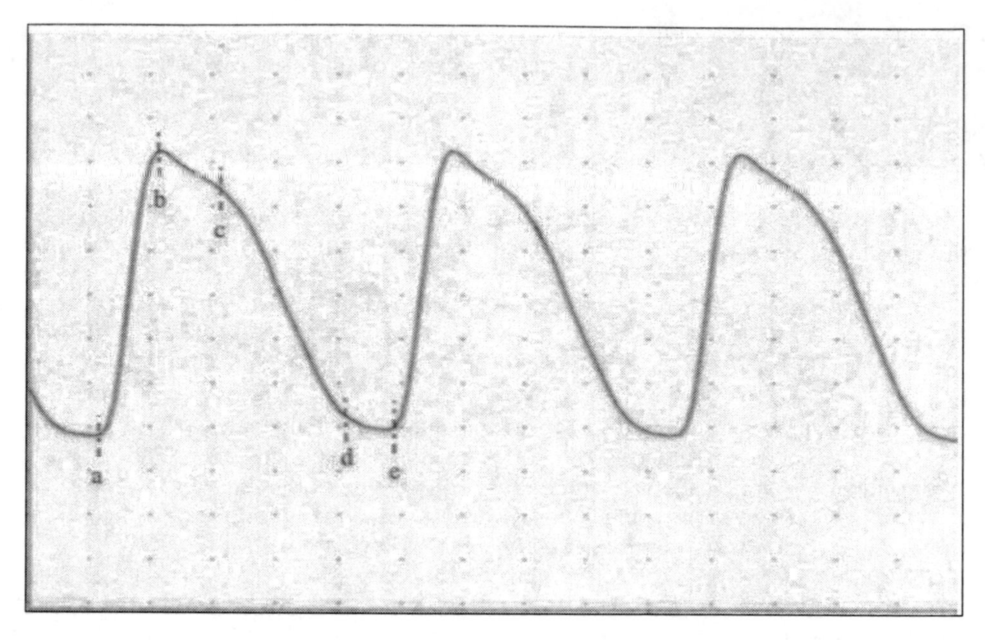

Figure 9–4. The electroglottographic waveform obtained for the vowel /æ/. The first cycle has been marked to show various phases in the glottal cycle: (*a-b*) vocal folds adduct, (*b-c*) maximal contact between the two folds, (*c-d*) vocal folds abduct, (*d-e*) minimal contact between the two vocal folds.

interpret various "features" of an EGG waveform in terms of the vocal fold behavior. The EGG is an excellent method for objective assessment of vocal function in the pediatric population because of its noninvasiveness, low cost, and ease of use. Additionally, it proves to be a good tool to use in clinics and perhaps also in schools because it is not affected by environmental noise and is portable (Cheyne, Nuss, & Hillman, 1999).

Inverse Filtering

Another method of obtaining information about the laryngeal behavior is through the use of *inverse filtering.* This technique can be used with the airflow signal or the acoustic signal measured at the level of the lips. The purpose in making these measures is to obtain information about the events occurring at the level of the glottis. As the airflow (or the acoustic signal) passes through the oral cavity, it acts as a filter allowing some frequencies to pass through, while attenuating others. Changes occur in the acoustic or airflow signal as it passes through the oral cavity because of the resonance associated with these cavities. By using certain computations, it is possible for the examiner to determine the filter characteristics of the oral cavity at a given time. Once this is done, a new filter with characteristics that are the *inverse* of the oral cavity resonance is created. When this *inverse filter* is applied to the original signal, it negates the contributions of the oral cavity and a waveform reflecting the changes occurring to the airflow at the glottis is obtained. Thus, inverse filtering of the airflow, or the acoustic signal, can provide information about the behavior of the vocal folds during voice production.

Inverse filtering of the flow signal requires a modification of the pneumotachograph that was developed by Rothenberg (1977). This requires a circumferentially vented mask (also known as the "Rothenberg mask"), shown in Figure 9–5 along with the transducers. Examples of the oral airflow and inverse filtered waveforms are shown in Figure 9–6. Measures obtained from such inverse-filtered airflow include the DC flow (minimum flow), peak flow, AC/DC ratio, and various phases (e.g., open phase, closed phase) and quotients (e.g., open quotient, closed quotient, speed quotient) of the glottal cycle. *DC flow* is the amount of airflow measured when the vocal folds are completely closed. *Peak flow* is the maximum flow in a glottal cycle. The *AC/DC ratio* (Isshiki, 1981) is a measure of the glottal efficiency. As with the EGG waveform, the various glottal phases and quotients reflect laryngeal vibratory characteristics during vocalization. Inverse filtering of the acoustic waveform has proven difficult, because it tends to introduce several distortions in the glottal wave. Therefore, it is not commonly used clinically.

Photoglottography

An additional technique that has been used for indirectly determining vocal fold movement is *photoglottography.* Photoglottography uses light sensors to monitor the amount of light passing through the glottis. As the vocal folds open and close, the amount of light passing through the glottis varies. Measurement of the changes in the amount of light gives information about the vocal fold

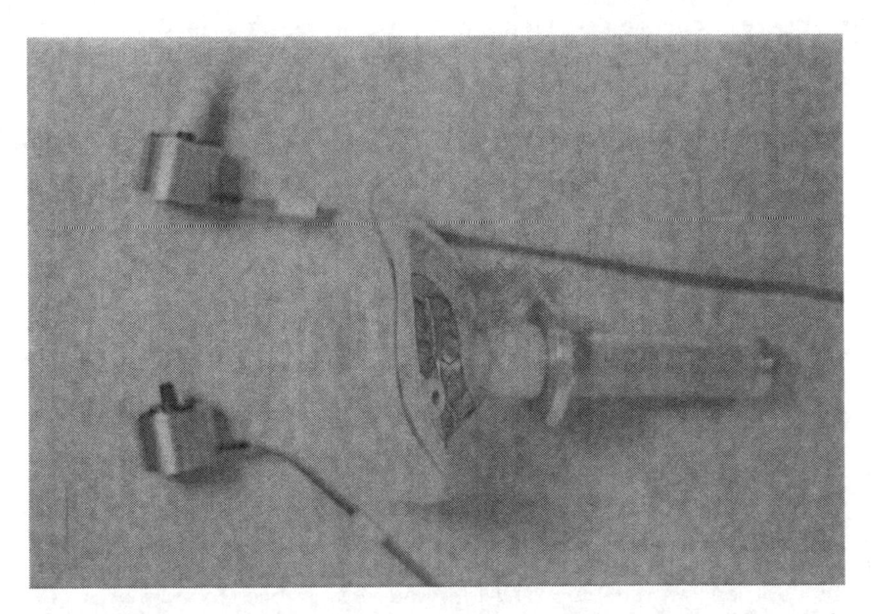

Figure 9–5. The circumferentially vented "Rothenberg mask" shown with the transducers used for measuring oral airflow. This mask allows high-frequency resolution during measurement of oral airflow.

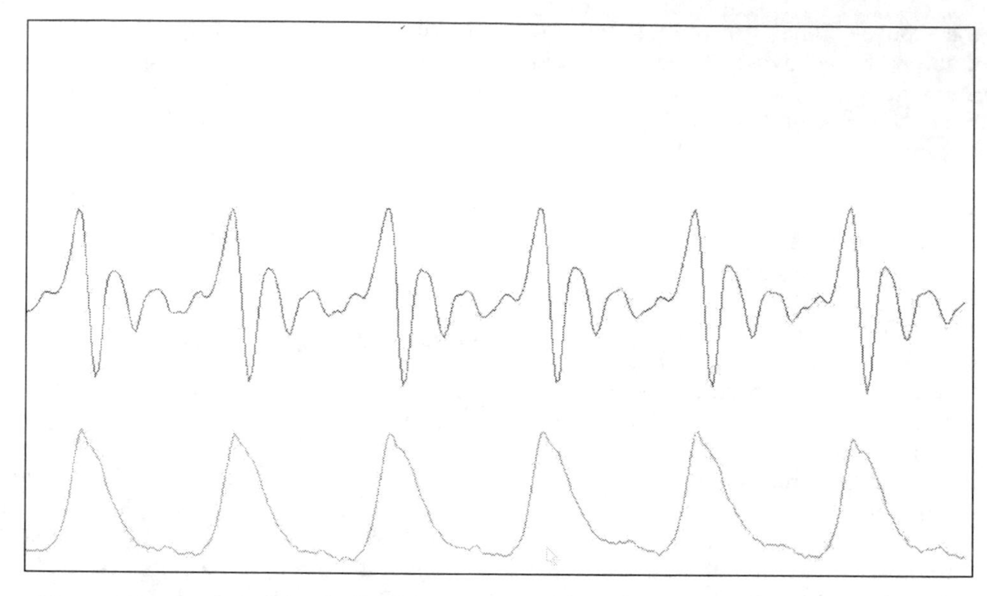

Figure 9–6. The oral airflow waveform for the vowel /æ/ and its inverse filtered waveform.

movement. Its use in clinics is very limited at this time, however.

Shortcomings and Precautions

Electroglottography is a popular technique in many voice clinics. It is noninvasive and relatively inexpensive. Precautions that should be taken by an examiner when obtaining an EGG signal include appropriate placement of the EGG electrodes and avoiding head movement during signal acquisition. Careful and appropriate placement of the electrodes improves the accuracy of the signal obtained. The thyroid lamina is easily located in most adults; however, in children visual inspection alone may not be sufficient to locate the thyroid cartilage. In such instances, the clinician can manually feel for the laryngeal structures by placing his or her hand on the subject's neck. Additionally, the movement of the thyroid cartilage during swallowing can help locate the thyroid cartilage more easily. Appropriate electrode positioning can also be achieved by moving the electrodes and monitoring the signal until the signal with maximum amplitude is obtained (Baken & Orlikoff, 2000). Unnecessary movement of the head can introduce extraneous noise in the EGG signal and must be avoided. This can be accomplished by having the subject use a headrest for support. Nevertheless, EGG is not free of problems, and questions have been raised about the interpretation of electroglottographic results. Although the EGG signal can be used to determine the fundamental frequency (and frequency perturbation measures), the validity of numerical measures such as the open quotient has been questioned, and their use has been discouraged (Baken, 1992). Furthermore, it has been found that EGG waveforms are relatively more difficult to obtain in female subjects and in younger children. This may be because of the wider, shorter larynges in women (Colton & Conture, 1990) and the relatively greater amount of fat tissue in children. Fatty tissue is a poor conductor of electricity and thus interferes with the flow of electrical current that is essential for obtaining precise EGG signals.

Perhaps the most significant shortcoming of inverse filtering is the difficulty in determining the vocal tract filter characteristics. Unless this is determined correctly, the resulting glottal flow or acoustic wave will not be accurate. Several computer algorithms for determining the vocal tract filter have been used, but further work to improve their reliability needs to be done. Additionally, inverse filtering provides more accurate results for steady phonation when the vocal tract and laryngeal behavior is relatively steady. Automatic inverse filtering has not been found to be useful with running speech, but efforts to improve results continue (Strik & Boves, 1992).

Measuring the Final Product: Acoustic Assessment

Acoustic analysis of the vocal signal is probably one of the most commonly used objective measures. The equipment required for this is more readily available in clinics and laboratories, and it is relatively inexpensive. Furthermore, advances in computer hardware and software have increased its use significantly because most personal computers come equipped with "sound cards," microphones, and speakers. Such equipment also can be purchased in the electronic or computer department of many stores. Programs that can carry out a variety of analyses can also be purchased for a relatively small price. Although improvement in technology and its widespread use is commendable, the use of acoustic measures by a clinician without a proper understanding about the theory behind the measures and the factors that affect the measures can unfortunately lead to erroneous results. Fortunately, most universities now include an in-depth study of acoustic analyses of voice and speech and their clinical applications for students in current training programs. Measures made from the acoustic signal can be classified as measures of (a) frequency and frequency perturbation, (b) intensity and intensity perturbation, and (c) spectral measures.

Measures of frequency and frequency perturbation include mean fundamental frequency during phonation and speech, frequency range during phonation, and jitter. *Mean fundamental frequency* of phonation is the average frequency of the glottal cycles and corresponds to the perceived pitch. The unit of measurement for fundamental frequency is hertz (Hz). It may be measured from steady vowels or during speech or reading tasks. The mean fundamental frequency shows age-related changes; during childhood, it falls gradually at first and then shows a sharp fall at puberty, especially in boys. The *frequency range* is the difference between the highest and the lowest pitch that a subject can produce and is an indicator of the pitch capabilities of a larynx. Conversational frequency range is measured during running speech, and the total range is usually measured during phonation of vowels at the limits of the range. *Jitter* is defined as the cycle-to-cycle variability in the fundamental frequency and is therefore a measure of frequency perturbation. Frequency perturbation measures focus on the variability in the voice that is not under voluntary control. Because running speech has inherent variability that can be attributed to stylistic and intentional changes in fundamental frequency, jitter is measured only from steady vowel samples. Many different methods of calculating frequency perturbation have been suggested, but there is no clear consensus regarding the method that should be used. Absolute jitter has been shown to be frequency dependent, and therefore most voice researchers and clinicians tend to use measures such as the *jitter percent* or the *jitter factor*, which are relatively independent of the fundamental frequency of phonation. Because of the many different methods available to calculate frequency perturbation, clinicians must be careful when comparing these measures and should be specific about the methods used when reporting the findings.

Measures of intensity and intensity perturbation include the mean intensity of phonation, the range of intensity, and shimmer. The *mean intensity* of phonation is measured in decibels (dB) and corresponds to the perceived loudness. It can be obtained for steady vowels and for speech or reading. The *intensity range* is the difference between the softest and the loudest note that a person can phonate, and as with the frequency range, it is a measure of the limits of the laryngeal system. Intensity perturbation is measured as *shimmer*, which is defined as the cycle-to-cycle variability in intensity.

The frequency and intensity range can also be calculated in a step-by-step manner. The subject is asked to phonate at specific frequencies, and the minimum and maximum intensity that can be produced at each of these frequencies is determined. This gives a complete profile of the vocal capabilities of the individual and is known as the *voice range profile* (VRP). The VRP is an excellent method to measure and record the capabilities of a subjects' larynx and has been used in clinics and also for research. For example, Hacki and Heitmüller (1999) obtained the VRP of 180 children between 4 and 12 years of age to study the development of their voices across time. VRP has the advantage of showing not only the frequency and intensity ranges that an individual can produce, but also the interaction between the two. Böhme and Stuchlik (1995) obtained normative data for VRP for 7- to 10-year-old boys and girls, which are presented in Figures 9–7 and 9–8. McAllister, Sederholm, Sundberg, and Gramming (1994) observed that 10-year-old children with disordered voices presented with VRP that differed from that of control subjects, thus demonstrating that VRP may be a suitable tool to characterize disordered voice in the pediatric population.

The VRP procedure, however, tends to be time consuming because it requires the subject to phonate at a number of different frequencies and intensities. Thus, the VRP has been used infrequently in voice clinics because the time available for testing is relatively limited. Furthermore, the nature of the tasks required to obtain VRP is relatively difficult and its use with children is constrained by the child's compliance level and cognitive development. Children often find the repetitive nature of the task monotonous, may not understand the task, and have short attention spans.

Besides measures of frequency and intensity, several spectral measures also can be determined. These are widely believed to reflect voice quality. The simplest spectral representation is the *spectrogram*. A spectrogram is a three-dimensional representation of speech, with time and frequency on the abscissa and the ordinate, respectively, and intensity marked as the darkness or color of the markings. Spectrograms can either be broadband or narrowband. Broadband spectrograms filter speech with larger bandwidths and are useful for resolving the vowel formants. Narrowband spectrograms filter speech into narrower frequency bands and therefore are useful for resolving individual harmonics. Examples of broadband and narrowband spectrograms are shown in Figure 9–9. Changes in voice quality such as hoarseness lead to increased noise in the spectrogram (Yanagihara, 1967). Although spectrograms are excellent tools to observe a visual pattern of the nature of speech, it is difficult to quantify these observations di-

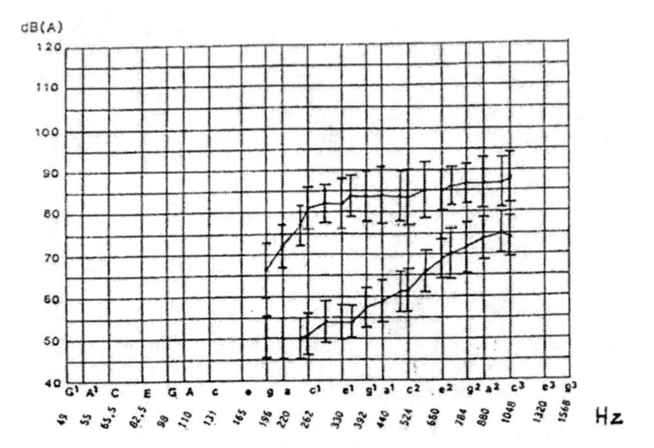

Figure 9–7. Voice range profile in 7- to 10-year-old boys. (From "Voice Profiles and Standard Voice Profile of Untrained Children," by G. Böhme and G. Stuchlik, 1995, *Journal of Voice*, 9, 304–307. Reprinted with permission from Böhme and Stuchlik.)

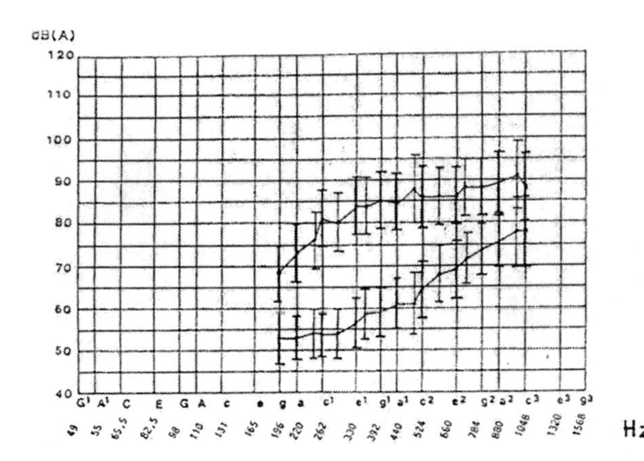

Figure 9–8. Voice range profile in 7- to 10-year-old girls. (From "Voice Profiles and Standard Voice Profile of Untrained Children," by G. Böhme and G. Stuchlik, 1995, *Journal of Voice*, 9, 304–307. Reprinted with permission from Böhme and Stuchlik.)

rectly. In certain other measures, such as the *harmonic-to-noise ratio* (HNR), such characteristics are more easily quantified. HNR and other similar measures (e.g., glottal noise energy [GNE], normalized noise energy [NNE]) have been developed to measure the amount of noise in the voice. As with the frequency perturbation measures, several algorithms

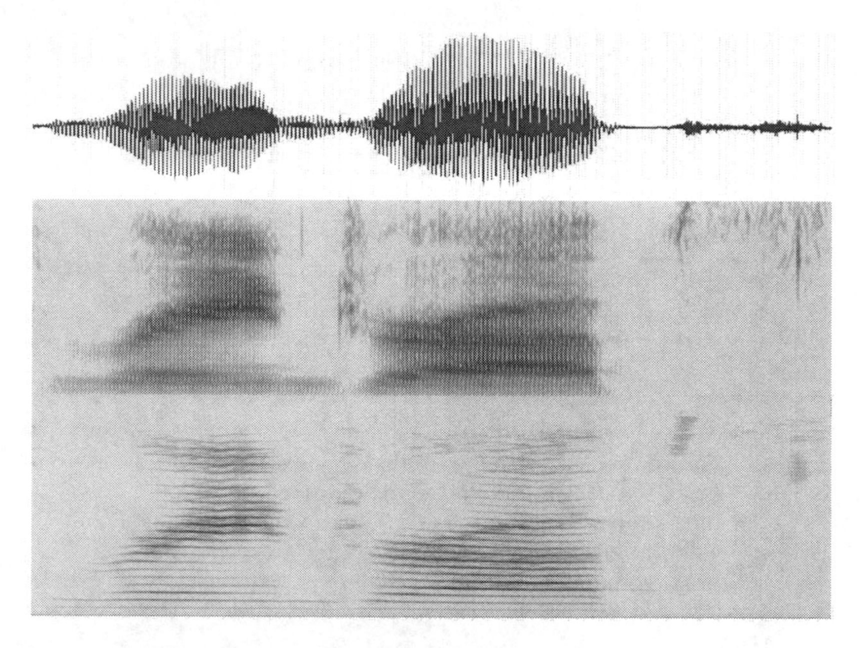

Figure 9–9. The acoustic waveform (*top panel*), the wideband (bandwidth = 300 Hz) spectrogram (*middle panel*), and the narrowband (bandwidth = 50 Hz) spectrogram (*lower panel*) of the word "raindrops." Notice that the narrow band spectrogram resolves individual harmonics in speech, whereas the wide band spectrogram displays formants more clearly.

have been proposed for this calculation, but there is, as yet, no consensus regarding which measure to use. Many of these measures to determine the amount of noise in the voice acoustic signal have been found to covary with the frequency and intensity perturbation measures, suggesting that the perturbation measures affect the calculated HNR. Some algorithms reported more recently, such as the GNE (Michaelis, Fröhlich, & Strube, 1997), have been found to be relatively independent of the perturbation measures and may be a useful measure of the amount of noise in the signal. Hanson (1998) and Hanson and Chuang (1999) have shown that certain other spectral measures correspond to the pattern of glottal closure and may be associated with voice quality changes. These include the *H1-H2 ratio* (difference between the level of the first and the second harmonic), the *H1-A1 ratio* (the difference between the level of the first harmonic and the intensity of the first formant), and the *H1-A3 ratio* (the difference between the level of the first harmonic and the intensity of the third formant). Hanson (1997) and Hanson and Chuang (1999) reported that the H1-H2 ratio is related to the open quotient, H1-A3 corresponds to the presence of a posterior glottal chink, and the H1-A3 ratio reflects the spectral tilt. These measures have only been studied in adults, however, and their validity in children still needs to be established.

Hard glottal attacks are associated with many voice disorders (Heuer, Towne, Hockstein, Andrade, & Sataloff, 2000), so reliable documentation of their occurrences in children's voice use is advantageous for clinical documentation of treatment outcomes. Peters, Boves, and van Dielen (1986) demonstrated that the intensity rise time (defined as the time taken for the vowel intensity to rise from 10% to 90% of the maximum intensity) correlated highly with the listener's perception of the degree of glottal attack and suggested the measurement of intensity rise time as a simple method to identify hard glottal attacks. Shrivastav (1999) found that the correlation between listener's ratings of the strength of glottal attack and acoustic characteristics of voice improved when intensity rise times as well as frequency fall time were considered simultaneously. Although the exact method for simultaneous use of both intensity rise time and frequency fall time for clinical use is not yet clear, it may be possible to use a combination of these measures to monitor the presence or absence of hard glottal attacks. However, both these studies report data obtained from adults, and findings for children's voices need to be studied.

Instrumentation

The instrumentation used for recording and analyzing acoustic signals includes a microphone to collect the signal, a medium to record the signal, and appropriate software to complete the necessary analyses (see Figure 9–10). The results obtained from any analysis depend on the quality and maintenance of the equipment used to make the measurements. It is important to remember that the final result will always be limited by

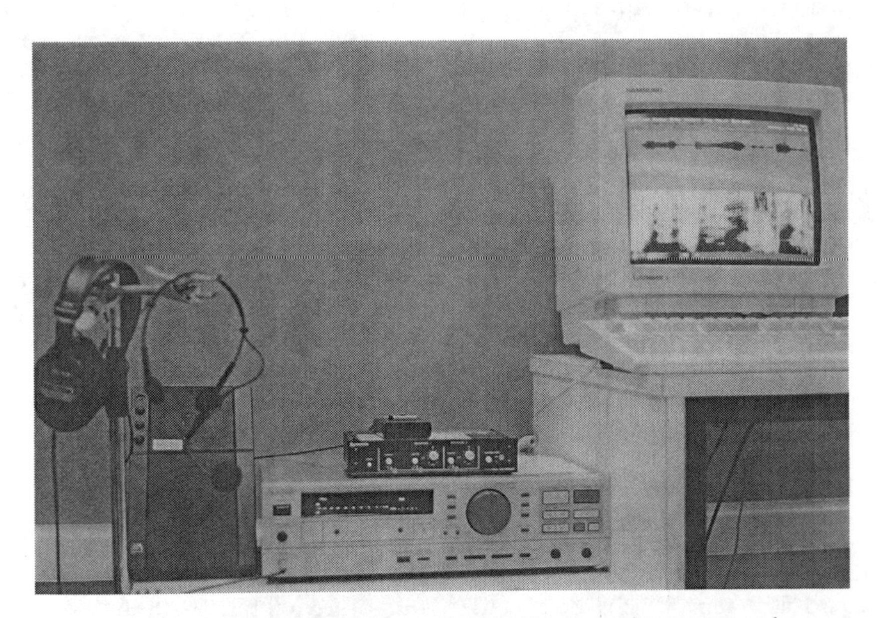

Figure 9–10. Setup for acoustic analyses of voice. This picture shows a head-mounted microphone, a preamplifier, a digital audiotape recorder used for data collection and storage, and a computer with appropriate software for analyses of the recorded signals.

the accuracy of the weakest component in the system. One cannot obtain valid measures, for example, by using a perfectly good analysis device if the sound signal was initially recorded using a poor-quality microphone. One must always be aware of the limitations of the system used for analyses. For example, some commercially available "sound cards" may not meet the criteria to obtain valid measures, and acoustic recordings and analyses performed using faulty hardware may not be accurate. Many mistakes can be avoided if the clinician carefully follows the guidelines provided by the manufacturer of the analysis package. Most analysis programs either come with their own specially designed hardware, or have specific recommendations regarding the hardware that should be used. It is also helpful to review available research findings concerning the reliability of various types of equipment and to consult with experts in the field of voice analyses.

The first component of a recording system is the microphone. Many different kinds of microphones (varying in their construction, sensitivity, and frequency response) are commercially available. Most commercial suppliers of recording and analysis systems recommend specific microphones for use. If no specific microphone is mentioned, however, a few points need to be kept in mind before obtaining one. A good frequency response, low distortion, and low noise are important features of a good microphone, and it is wise to choose the best available. Clinicians also should inquire about the "impedance rating" of the microphone and select a microphone that matches their recording system. Titze and Winholtz (1993) found that the distance and the angle of the microphone from the mouth could also significantly affect some acoustic measures. Thus, a constant lips-to-microphone distance and angle should be maintained to minimize such variability. Use of a head-mounted microphone may be helpful in this regard because it allows the subject to move the head freely while still maintaining a constant distance and angle from the microphone. Finally, it is usually sensible to be cautious about "special features" built into some microphones such as those built to work with automatic speech recognition software. Many of these microphones have noise reduction circuitry that may affect the voice signal, and therefore they may not be suitable for subsequent acoustic analyses of the voice samples.

Traditionally, audio cassettes have been the most commonly used medium for the recording and storing of voice samples. Although the quality of audiotapes has improved over the years, tapes may not be the best option. Doherty and Shipp (1988) found minimal distortion while extracting average fundamental frequency and average intensity using audio cassette players, but the perturbation measures (jitter and shimmer) were adversely affected. Most experts now suggest that a better alternative is to record and store voice samples digitally. Digital audiotapes are specially designed for recording and replaying signals in the audible frequency range while minimizing distortion and providing a satisfactory signal-to-noise ratio. Portable and larger models of digital audiotape (DAT) recorders are readily available commercially. A more recent development is that of the minidisc (MD). Minidisc players are being marketed as an alternative to the "Walkman" and the portable compact-disc players. The technology used in MD is similar to that used for compact discs and provides high-fidelity reproduction of sounds. However, unlike the compact disc, MD allows the user to erase and rewrite the data on the disc. Winholtz and Titze (1998) compared output from a DAT with that of an MD and found the two to be equally good for perturbation measures, but the signal-to-noise ratio was poorer by 10 dB for the MD output. With computer memory becoming increasingly compact and inexpensive, it is even possible to record and store data directly on a computer hard drive. Recording directly on to a computer hard drive provides high-quality recordings and makes it easy to access and analyze data when needed by the clinician.

Once the signal has been recorded, it can be analyzed to obtain a variety of measures. Several of these measures depend on the extraction of the fundamental period of the signal. Unfortunately, extraction of the fundamental period of phonation has proven to be a remarkably difficult task, especially for pathological voice samples. Hence, many acoustic measures cannot be correctly determined when the clinician attempts analyses of voice samples where the fundamental period cannot be estimated accurately. Based on the application of nonlinear dynamics to vocal fold vibration (Titze, Baken, & Herzel, 1993), Titze (1995) suggested classification of acoustic recordings of vocal signals into three categories: (a) periodic with small random perturbations (Type 1), (b) periodic with subharmonic structures and modulation (Type 2), and, (c) nonperiodic or "chaotic" signals (Type 3). Baken and Orlikoff (2000) suggested further classification of each of these three categories into two or three subtypes. Classification of signals into these three types can be done by observation of the acoustic or EGG waveforms or a narrow band spectrogram (Herzel, Berry, Titze, & Saleh, 1994). Both of these methods can show the presence of *bifurcations* and *chaos*, which are the basis of classifying the signal into the three types mentioned previously. Bifurcation and chaos are concepts described by the theory of nonlinear dynamics, which promises to have a significant influence on our understanding of vocal fold behavior (Baken & Orlikoff, 2000). It has been recommended that perturbation levels should only be measured when the acoustic signals can be classified in the first category. Signals that fall under the second category can be subjected to spectrographic analyses, whereas the chaotic signals are best judged perceptually (Karnell, 2000). The criteria for dividing the signals into these three categories are not clearly defined, however, and this classification of signals is as yet not widely practiced. Thus, at this point, it is strongly recommended that clinicians consider the type of sample and make a decision regarding its periodicity before subjecting it to further analyses.

Shortcomings and Precautions

Although recording and analyzing the acoustic signal is inexpensive and easy to perform, it is important to remember that it gives limited information about vocal fold physiology per se. Nonetheless, some measures such as the H1-H2 ratio may be more closely related to known physiological findings than others. Additionally, the relationship between the acoustic findings and the perceptual ratings of voice quality is not well understood. Various studies that were aimed at identifying a specific acoustic-to-perceptual relationship have yielded widely varying results. Thus, it is prudent for clinicians to ensure that the signal they obtain is of sufficient quality to inspire confidence in the results of acoustic analyses. Adherence to guidelines such as recording in a quiet environment and the use of appropriate devices (microphone, recording medium, etc.) is important. Maintenance of correct recording levels must also be monitored. If the signal is recorded at a very high intensity, for example, a part of the signal is lost. This is referred to as "clipping." Signal clipping restricts the measures that can be obtained from that sample. Appropriate recording levels can be maintained by using the "VU meter" that is available in most professional recording systems. A "VU meter" displays when the intensity level of the signal is within the appropriate range for adequate recording. Some knowledge about digital signal processing also can help the examiner understand how to use various measures and to interpret them appropriately.

Measuring Nasality (Assessment of Velopharyngeal Function)

Evaluation of velopharyngeal function and nasality has proven to be a complicated task. Although many techniques have been proposed for clinical evaluation of nasality, the relationship between the perceived nasality and velopharyngeal function is not straightforward and makes it difficult to relate the findings of these techniques to the final percept. Methods that have been proposed for evaluating velopharyngeal function vary from endoscopic evaluation to observe the velar movement, to the measurement of nasal airflow, acoustic, or accelerometer signals.

Endoscopic evaluation of velopharyngeal function can be accomplished using the flexible endoscope. Appropriate positioning of the flexible endoscope in the nasal cavity allows a view of the soft palate from above. The movement of the soft palate during various speech and nonspeech tasks can then be observed. Nonetheless, such evaluation is subjective and requires experienced clinicians. Furthermore, because of its invasive nature, young children may not tolerate flexible endoscopy. Several noninvasive measures to quantify nasality in speech also have been proposed. Measures such as the *Horii oral nasal coupling* (HONC; Horii, 1980) and *the oral nasal acoustic ratio* (TONAR; Fletcher, 1970) measure the ratio of the nasal to oral accelerometric and the acoustic signals, respectively, and provide some indication about the velopharyngeal function. Nasal airflow, or the ratio of nasal to oral airflow during production of different sounds, also has been measured as an indicator of velopharyngeal functioning. Spectrographic analyses of voice can also provide several cues that suggest nasalization. These include the presence of "antiformants," decreased overall energy, and an increase in formant bandwidths (Kent & Read, 1992). Spectrograms of a nasalized and non-nasal vowel are shown in Figure 9–11.

Instrumentation

The instrumentation for measuring velopharyngeal function is based on the same principles as that described under previous sections. The flexible endoscope used for the assessment of velopharyngeal function is similar to that used for observing the larynx. Acoustic measures such as the TONAR capture the acoustic energy being radiated from the mouth and the nose and is recorded using two appropriately placed microphones, one for the nose and the other for the mouth. Measures like the HONC require the use of an accelerometer, which detects tissue vibrations caused by sound. Flow measures used for quantifying nasal emissions can be detected using a pneumotachograph. The critical issue in all these measures is the separation of the nasal and the oral signals. This can be done by using a special partition between the two transducers, for example, the use of a baffle between two microphones. Similarly, flow-collecting face masks can have a partition for separating the nasal from the oral airflow.

Shortcomings and Precautions

Perceived nasality is a result of many different factors and the relationship between the perceived nasality and the various objective measures is not linear. Measurement of nasality requires the use of instruments and principles that are used for measuring certain other functions such as the airflow or the acoustic signal. Thus, the shortcomings and the precautions that clinicians need to be aware of are similar to that of those instruments. The spectrographic cues for nasalization tend to

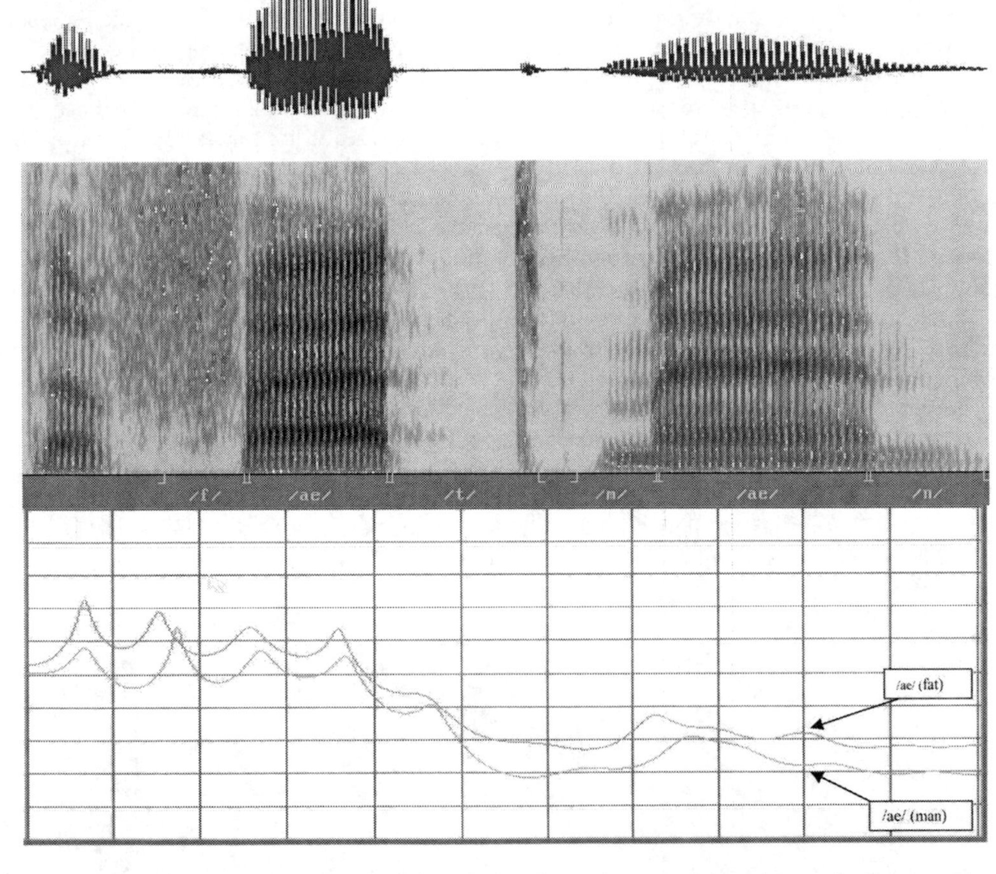

Figure 9–11. Spectrogram (*top*) and LPC waveform (*bottom*) of the phrase *the fat man*. Observe the difference in formant intensity for the vowel /æ/ in the words "fat" and "man" due to coarticulatory effects of the nasal consonants. Also note the presence of the low frequency "nasal formant" in the word "man."

be highly variable from subject to subject and can be difficult to quantify.

Use of Instrumental Measures in Therapy

Instrumental measures are useful not only to understand the nature or characteristics of normal and disordered voice, but also to provide feedback during voice treatment. Additionally, they can be used to compare pre- and posttreatment patterns to document treatment outcomes. The use of biofeedback in voice therapy involves providing tangible feedback to help the patient focus on and control specific incorrect behaviors. The feedback is then gradually eliminated while the patient learns to maintain appropriate behavior without the help of any external support. With the capability to use high-quality graphics, computer technology has enabled many objective measures to be incorporated into programs to emulate video games that are popular with children. Programs demonstrating changes in vocal parameters, such as fundamental frequency and intensity, or the presence or absence of voicing and nasality, have been developed. The display of one such program is shown in Figure 9–12. Other measures such as videoendoscopic images, electroglottographic wave- forms, electromyographic (EMG) signals, chest and abdominal wall movement, and galvanic skin response or blood pressure (to estimate levels of anxiety) have been used more directly without any special interface and therefore are often more applicable with middle or high school students. Many of the aforementioned measures have been converted to the visual mode so that the subject can see the graphic representation on a computer screen or a cathode ray tube in real time. Some measures such as the galvanic skin response have also been converted to the auditory mode. For example, the patient's galvanic skin response can be converted into a series of clicks, with the rate of clicks being directly related to the magnitude of the signal. The Facilitator (see Figure 9–13) is another instrument that allows auditory feedback. Developed by Kay Elemetrics in association with Dr. D. R. Boone, the Facilitator is capable of five different kinds of auditory feedback, including amplification, delayed auditory feedback, metronome pacing, masking, and loop feedback. Further research on the clinical efficacy of specific cues and types of feedback that supports behavioral changes is still needed.

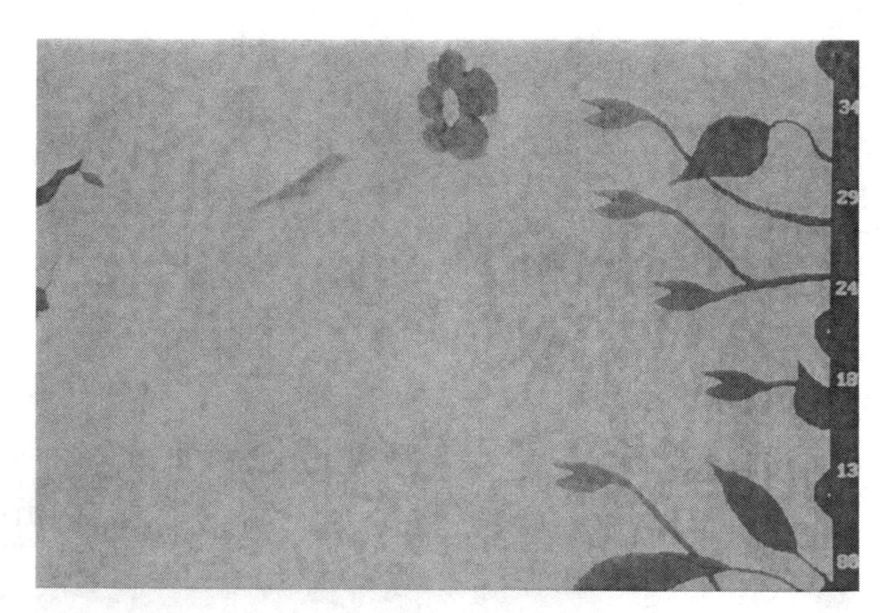

Figure 9–12. Screenshot of the Visi-Pitch III developed by Kay Elemetrics. This instrument provides visual feedback regarding certain acoustic parameters with gamelike graphics and can be used for voice therapy with children.

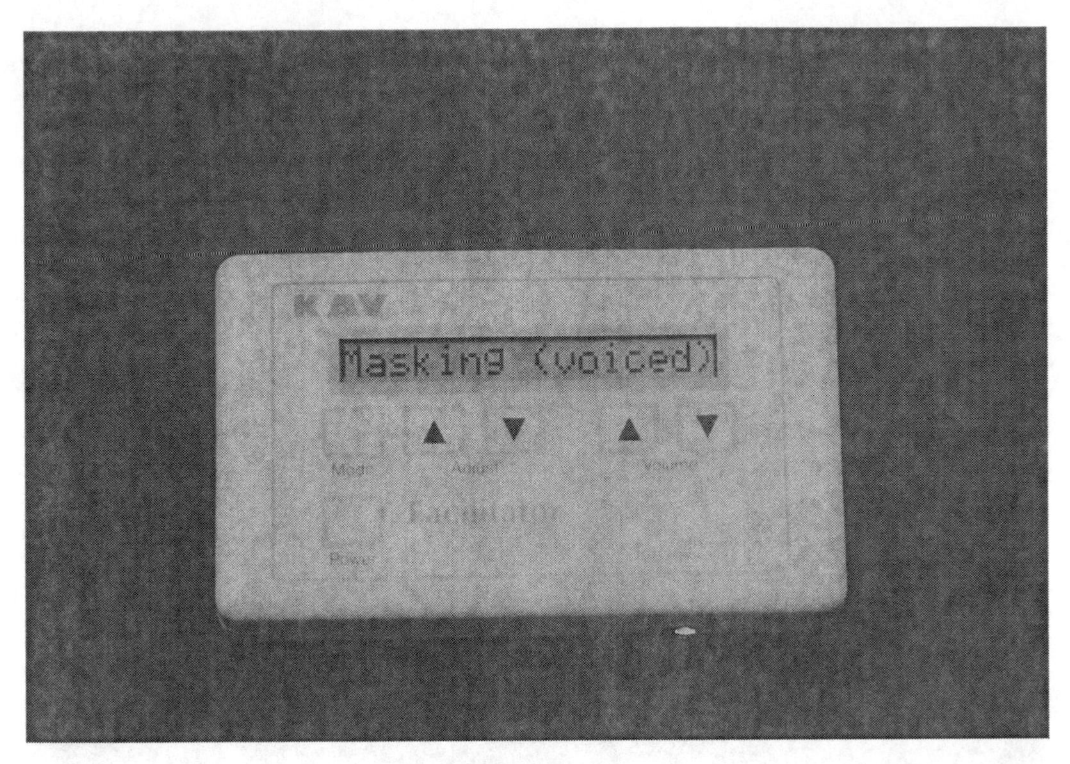

Figure 9–13. The Facilitator, developed by Kay Elemetrics in association with Dr. D. R. Boone, can provide five kinds of auditory feedback. (From *Manual of Voice Treatment: Pediatrics Through Geriatics*, 2nd ed. [p. 143], by Moya L. Andrews, 1999, San Diego: Singular Publishing Group. Copyright 1999 by Singular Publishing Group. Reprinted with permission.)

Summary

In the last two decades, a variety of instrumental measures to assist clinicians in the diagnoses and management of voice disorders have been developed. These measures make it possible for clinicians to test the adequacy of function of specific subsystems involved in voice production. These measures also help clinicians by providing alternative sources of information to supplement trained clinical observations during the decision-making process. Thus, assessment and documentation regarding the cause of the voice problems and their nature and severity are enhanced. Objective measures also provide quantifiable evidence of changes in voice patterns over time. There is continuing research aimed at refining instrumental measures, and rapid advancements in technology have made them easier to perform, less expensive, and more reliable.

In this chapter, we have reviewed perceptual, physiological, aerodynamic, and acoustic approaches to vocal assessment and treatment, and we have described the theoretical bases underlying the development and application of specific types of instrumentation. We also have discussed the shortcomings of certain procedures, and the precautions that clinicians need to take to maximize accuracy and reliability of the measures obtained through the use of various types of instrumentation. We have emphasized the need for carefully controlled conditions during the collection and recording of voice samples, and for informed interpretation of the results of instrumental analyses. History taking, trained judgments of observable behaviors, traditional approaches to stimulability, and voice assessment tasks are necessary components of a voice evaluation. This comprehensive approach allows a clinician to develop clinical impressions and hypotheses about etiology, severity, voice status, and prognosis. The addition of instrumental measures of voice and voice-related functions provides another important dimension to corroborate and document diagnosis and management of children presenting with voice disorders.

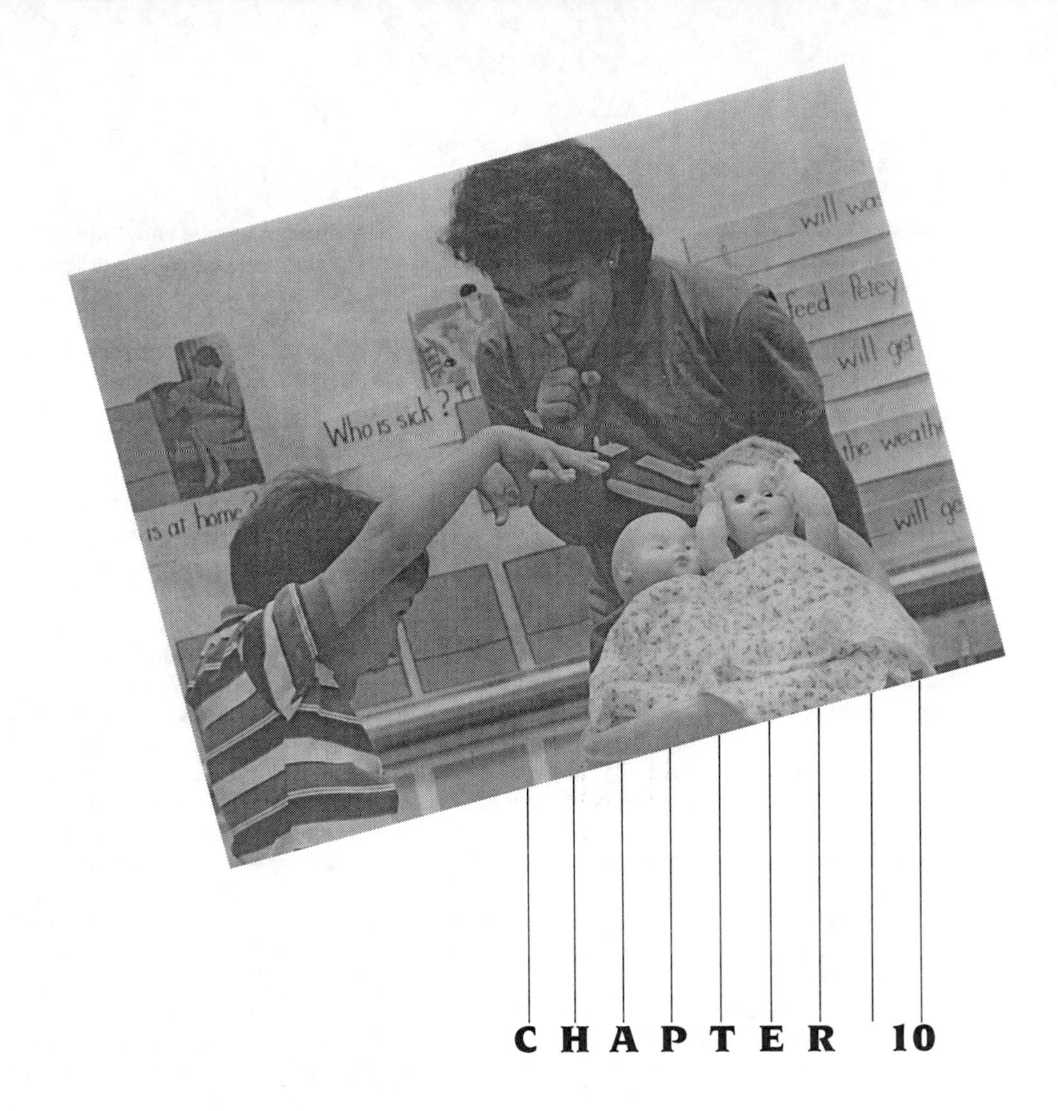

CHAPTER 10

Program Planning and Approaches

We looked at some of the components of the four general areas of behavior relating to voice. We constructed checklists of some aspects of vocal production and vocal competence that contribute to optimal patterns of vocal behavior. The checklists are helpful for noting the presence or absence of components when we observe children's behavior. They can also be used to record descriptions of inappropriate or atypical characteristics and to note if an absent, immature, or distorted behavior could be elicited in its appropriate form. In Chapter 8, we discussed in-depth assessment procedures. At this point, however, we need only concern ourselves with a possible repertoire of behaviors that may or may not be observed. The reason we want to call attention to these behaviors is that as prized components of vocal behavior, they may, on occasion, be behaviors that handicapped children need to acquire. An inventory of various components of each of the general areas related to voice is helpful as we consider objectives for therapy. In voice therapy, our aim may be to teach behaviors that are absent, substitute appropriate behaviors for inappropriate ones, strengthen behaviors that are weak or inconsistent, and shape and refine behaviors until prized characteristics are habituated. If, as a result of a sequence of treatment (usually referred to as a *program*), we believe a child could acquire particular behaviors, we may state those desired terminal behaviors as our *program objectives*. When we select our objectives, we need to be cognizant of (a) the constraints imposed by any structural or medical conditions; (b) limiting factors such as development stage, ability, motivation, parental support, available time; (c) the repertoire of optimal behaviors from which to choose; and (d) the developmental progression of normal acquisition.

One more point should be made before we turn to the specifics of program planning, and that is the importance of always considering the vocal demands inherent in the child's lifestyle. We shall illustrate this by some examples. Consider the need for optimal performance in the area of respiratory control. Many children will not need to demonstrate optimal respiratory support to produce adequate voice production. If a 7-year-old girl uses her voice mainly in conversational situations and has few demands for projected sustained speaking, it may not be necessary to select objectives from among the optimal behaviors in the area of respiration. Minimal skill may suffice. On the other hand, should a child be active in strenuous athletic pursuits and frequently engage in loud sustained talking in conjunction with physical activity, the demands on the respiratory system may be such that optimal support may indeed be required. Similarly, the child who is the star in the school operetta and makes great demands on the vocal mechanism during singing and speaking may need to develop optimal respiratory behavior to avoid the deleterious effects of strenuous unsupported laryngeal activity. Optimal levels of function may indeed be realistic targets for such a child because interests and needs may enhance motivation for improvement.

Because we have included a listing of optimal behaviors, we do not want to imply that every child we teach must, should, or can achieve all of them. Expectations for each child are always tempered by what is realistic and sensible for the individual. Program objectives must always be individualized. Optimal target behaviors should not be considered as a set of behaviors that all children must acquire. They could be considered as landmarks that define potentials for growth and change.

Program Objectives

Depending on the nature of a child's problem, objectives are usually drawn from one or more areas. If the child exhibits deficits in all areas, the decision to work on objectives from each area simultaneously or sequentially will be made based on the child's level of functioning and the priorities established by the clinician. Some children can handle work on all areas at once and benefit from an approach that emphasizes interrelationships; others may be confused by such an approach. The selection of the objectives is based on what seems to be realistic for a child to achieve in a given period of time. The objectives are the long-term goals, or the behaviors the child will have achieved by the end of a therapy program. They are always stated in terms of the child's behavior, and action verbs are used because the behaviors must be specific and observable. Standards and criterion levels are also needed. It is usual and helpful to develop a task that can be used as a pretest and a posttest for each objective. This test then enables the clinician to measure the progress made as a result of the therapy program.

Once the terminal objective has been stated and the pre- or posttest has been specified, a behavioral hierarchy is established. We look at the overall behavior that we hope the child will finally learn and break it up into an orderly sequence of smaller pieces of behavior. These pieces of behavior are arranged in a sequence proceeding from the simplest or easiest to learn to the hardest or most complex. Our knowledge of the normal acquisition of the behaviors helps us develop this sequence. We know, for example, that children use vegetative breathing before they develop speech breathing; we also know that vocalizing isolated vowel sounds is easier than vocalizing words, phrases, or sentences. Each individual behavior that we select and arrange in a cumulative series of difficulty becomes a short-term or intermediate goal. These short-term goals are the building blocks of the program plan. They specify the prerequisite behaviors, or the foundation, necessary to achieve the objectives of the overall program. The following example illustrates what we do first, that is, specify the overall objective and pretest–posttest:

General Area: Laryngeal behavior.

Specific Symptom: Limited vocal variety.

Terminal Objective: Child will produce "word pictures" on verbs, adjectives, and adverbs with 90% accuracy; one per sentence.

Pretest–Posttest: Fifteen simple sentences read and tape recorded. Count sentence correct if underlined word is emphasized in any of the following ways (pitch, loudness, or rate changes).

Once the terminal objective is stated, we then state the short-term goals and arrange them in a meaningful sequence.

The following list illustrates a behavioral hierarchy that might constitute short-term goals of the first part of the therapy plan. You will notice that this is an "awareness" not a "production" hierarchy.

1. Identification of "picture words" and "nonpicture" words (verbs, adjectives, adverbs versus articles, prepositions, pronouns)
2. Identification of voice strategies to make picture words (e.g., loudness, pitch, rate changes)
3. Matching picture words with a strategy (e.g., noisy = loud voice; velvety = soft voice; crawled = slow voice; galloped = fast voice; dropping = voice goes down; climbing = voice goes up)
4. Choosing picture words to underline in simple sentences

5. Describing strategies another person demonstrates
6. Judging the appropriateness of another person's word pictures
7. Describing better strategies for another person to use (e.g., "You could make the word longer")

Short-Term Goals and Examples of Strategies

In addition to stating what behaviors the child will learn and the order in which they will be acquired, we need to plan how the steps will be mastered. Each behavior needs to be taught, and so a teaching strategy must be developed for each goal. A strategy operationalizes a goal. The common strategies we use in voice therapy are the same as those used in other forms of therapy. We explain and describe and model the target behaviors. We also provide stimulation and cues (visual, auditory, tactile, and kinesthetic) to facilitate learning. We always need to know what we are planning to say and do (the stimulus) and what we expect the child to say and do (the response). We need to know in advance whether we will accept an approximation of the target response or whether we expect perfect accuracy. We need to plan the number of trials, the kind of trials, and the method of scoring and evaluation. The strategy we use is really our lesson plan. It is a script we follow as we work with the child. There are many lesson-plan formats, but most of them require that the stimulus and the response and the criteria are stated explicitly. The materials we use and the reinforcement provided are also stated on many lesson-plan forms. An example of a short-term goal with a matching strategy is as follows.

Short-Term Goal

The child will hum with appropriate tone focus and resonance for 10 seconds, given a model and visual and tactile cues (100% accuracy, five trials)

Strategy

1. The clinician will model the sound while holding the child's hand against the clinician's face and lips. The clinician will explain how her lips "tickle" as the sound vibrates. The clinician will ask the child to produce the sound, pressing the child's lips against the clinician's hand and against her own hand.
2. The child will hum (while the clinician watches the secondhand of the clock) for 10 seconds. The child will press her lips against her own hand to feel the vibrations.
3. The clinician will time five trials. Verbal descriptive statements will be used as reinforcement, for example, "I can feel the tickling on my hand as you hum. I can feel the vibrations on your face. Your humming sounds rich and full. I can hear how the sound is tickling your lips."

It will be helpful now to discuss some specific behavioral goals and describe a variety of strategies that may be used to achieve them. We shall select goals from only one general area, that of respiration. Our terminal objective might be for the child to demonstrate appropriate speech breathing by the end of the therapy program.

Terminal objective: The child will use appropriate breathing patterns (100% correct on 15 trials) when speaking spontaneous sentences.

Pretest–posttest: Fifteen sentences spoken by the child; clinician rates (a) type of inhalation; (b) efficient use of exhalation. Sentences elicited by use of 15 picture cards[1] and the instruction "Tell me what is wrong in this picture."

Short-Term Goals and Strategies to Achieve Them

1. To increase the depth of the inhalation
2. To increase the length of the exhalation
3. To increase control of the exhaled airstream

Strategies or techniques to achieve these goals can be described according to their effectiveness in highlighting specific aspects of the targeted behaviors. For example, techniques that emphasize the sensory and kinesthetic awareness of the desired behavior usually involve postural change that facilitates appropriate movement and provides heightened awareness of a particular part of the body. We shall explain only a few of the basic strategies used to modify respiratory behavior in order to develop efficient patterns of speech breathing and will describe why some techniques are helpful in achieving goals.

Strategies to Achieve Increased Depth of Inhalation (Goal 1)

The most common mistake that children make during deep inhalation is moving the shoulders and upper chest instead of increasing the depth and width of the lower chest cavity where the lungs inflate most efficiently. Therefore, any posture that decreases the likelihood of movement in the shoulders and upper chest can be used to help achieve this goal. Exercises that involve postural change to decrease the likelihood of excessive movement or tension of the shoulders and upper chest frequently position the upper part of the body so that gravity assists. For example, an exercise undertaken by a subject lying flat on the floor facilitates a lowered, relaxed carriage of the shoulders and decreases the likelihood of movement in the upper chest during inhalation. Postural positioning also is used to increase kinesthetic awareness of movements of the abdominal and lower thoracic muscles. Contact of the abdomen and lower chest with hard surfaces or other body parts provides a form of biofeedback that helps an individual monitor the presence and extent of required movements. For example, an inhalation achieved as the individual rests the upper part of the body against the thighs ensures that the chest movement is felt on the thighs and upper legs. Such an exercise begins with the candidate seated in a chair. The upper part of the body is then moved forward until the torso rests on the upper legs. Deep inhalation is then repeated so that the movement of the lower chest is felt against the upper legs. Variations of this exercise that use pressure against hard surfaces include sitting the subject in a chair in front of a desk or table so that forward movement of the thoracic wall results in pressure against the table or desk edge. When an individual lies in a prone position on the floor and inhales, the pressure of the movement of the abdominal and thoracic muscles is felt against the floor. This effect can also be achieved to illustrate movement of the back of the chest cavity by having the subject stand against a wall or lie with the back flat on the floor. Movement of the sides of the thoracic cavity can also be monitored by placing the hands on the sides of the lower chest above the waist so that the upward and outward movement of the rib cage is felt. Resistance in the form of a loose elastic band

[1]"What's Wrong Here?" Level 1, Catalogue #85–230 (Hingham, MA: Teaching Resources, n.d.).

tied around the rib cage so that the elastic stretches during inhalation can also heighten kinesthetic awareness during inhalation. Naturally, it is important that a child engaging in this kind of exercise not wear restrictive or tight clothing. Belts and tight waistbands that cramp the movements can detract from the efficacy of the technique.

Another approach to monitoring the desired movements of the respiratory muscles during deep inhalation is through the placement of an object on the lower chest. If this object moves as the direct result of thoracic expansion, a child can see, as well as feel, the effects of the desired movement patterns. Young children seem to enjoy lying on the floor on their backs and watching an object (e.g., a stuffed animal) moving up and down as they breathe in and out. A book is often used in a similar way with older children.

Some children experience difficulty with deep volitional inhalation. This difficulty sometimes is seen in children who are neurologically impaired or extremely tense. Children who are developmentally delayed also may need more specific cues related to the onset of the inhalation task. We know that forceful explusion of air from the lungs is a means of capitalizing on the internal versus external air pressure differential. We also know that there is elastic recoil of the lungs that encourages air intake subsequent to air expulsion. We use this information when we apply techniques such as pressing down on the lower chest and abdominal cavity just before instructing a child to inhale. Another similar facilitating technique is to ask a child forcefully to "snort out" all the air in his or her lungs before inhalation. "Snorting out air" involves expelling the air through the nose with the mouth closed. The respiratory muscles help force the air out as the chest walls collapse and the abdominal wall moves in. Reverse movements occur as the child inhales and the abdominal wall moves out and the thoracic walls expand. Five or so rapid "snorts" alternated with deep air intakes can be used to demonstrate the contrasting physiologic states. Sometimes two or three "snorts out" are suggested prior to deep inhalation to create an intense need for a deep inhalation to follow. (Caution needs to be exercised to ensure that children do not hyperventilate.)

Coordination of Inhalation and Exhalation

The tying together of the contrasting patterns of exhalation and inhalation and repeated practice of the rhythms of slow, deep breathing is a beneficial transition from goal 1 to goal 2, which is to increase the length of exhalation. In the initial stages of teaching speech breathing, it is usually beneficial to slow down the rate of vegetative breathing (i.e., decrease the number of breaths per minute). As the rate of breathing slows, the depth of breathing increases. With the length of the inhalation equaling the length of the exhalation during slow rhythmic breathing the child can be asked to concentrate on how the body feels. The teacher then verbalizes descriptions of what is happening in the body during the "in" and "out" phase. Repeated quiet descriptions of this kind can help a child understand the concepts and associate each idea with a specific sensory awareness. Such an activity has the added benefit of relaxing the child and developing in the child a feeling of the naturalness and ease of the behavior. A child who may be predisposed to try too hard "to do the exercises" and becomes tense as a result can thus experience the naturalness of act. A teacher can assist in this by quietly repeating such statements as "Your body *knows* how to breathe—relax and feel how easily your muscles move. The muscles help your chest grow big as the lungs fill with air, then grad-

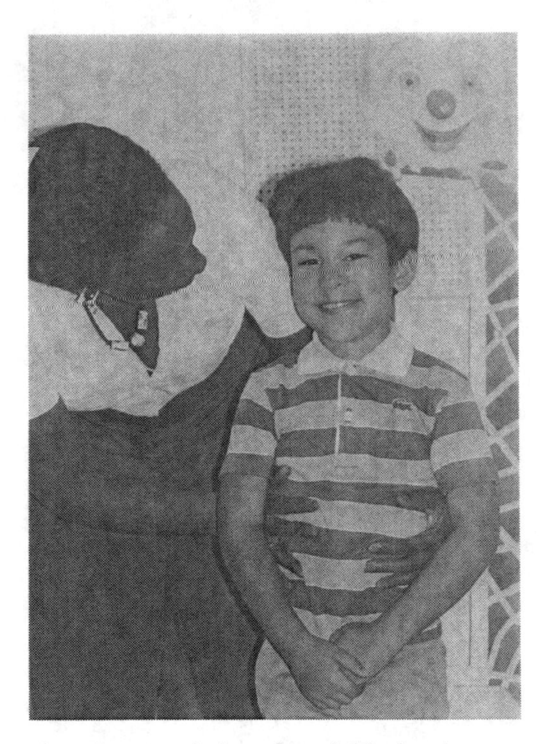

The clinician helps the child develop an awareness of the movement of the lower chest during deep relaxed breathing.

ually the air is going out again—in—out—in—out—one, two, three in—one, two, three out."

Images also can be used for vividness of understanding. For example, "Your lungs are like two balloons slowly growing bigger and bigger. Now they are growing smaller and smaller." Once an awareness of the even rhythm of vegetative, quiet breathing has been learned, the next step in the sequence is to shift gradually from the "equal in–equal out" phases of nonspeech breathing to the "quick, deep in—long, controlled out" phases of speech breathing. This can be accomplished by changing the counting rhythm. For example, "This time we will take longer to breathe out. Breathe in, one, two, three and out, one, two, three, four, five."

Strategies to Achieve Goals 2 and 3

A common mistake that children make when they do not use the exhaled airstream efficiently for speech is to allow too much air to rush out during the first few words, leaving them with insufficient available air to finish the sentence. Thus, some children need to learn to conserve the air that they have inhaled and to ration it out across an entire utterance. The concept of a steady stream of air exhaled gradually can be learned by practicing exercises that focus on the gradual

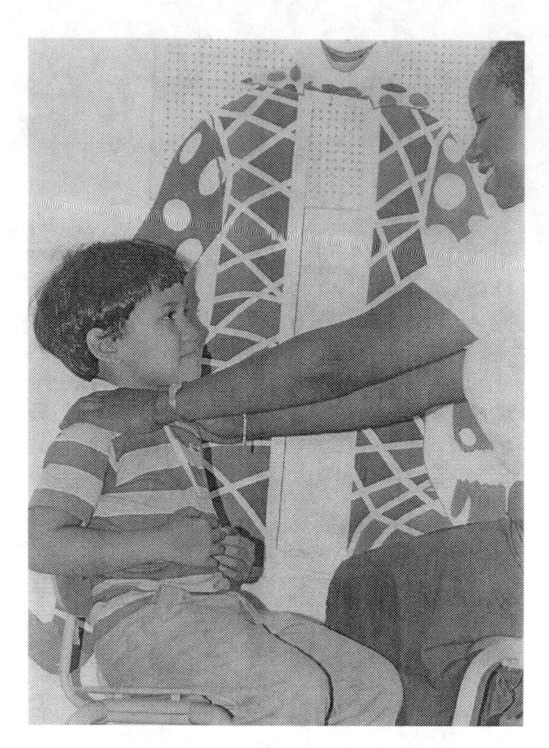

Upward movement of the shoulders is discouraged during deep inhalation.

emission of air for increasing durations of time. Another mistake some children make is to attempt to control the emission of the airstream by blocking the flow with excessive tension in the larynx. When this occurs, the valving action of the larynx is used to compensate for ineffective respiratory muscle action.

Exercises to achieve both increase in the length of the exhalation (goal 2) and control of the exhaled airstream (goal 3) therefore can be described in terms of their helpfulness in avoiding the likelihood of such errors. Any exercise that emphasizes the gradual elongated emission of air and simultaneously prevents the control of the airstream by closure of the vocal folds is optimal. Examples of such exercises are prolongations of unvoiced continuant fricative consonants. Prolongation of /s/ for increasing lengths of time (measured in seconds) is an excellent strategy to use to help achieve goal 2. The advantages of this strategy include the open glottis because /s/ is unvoiced, the opportunities for monitoring the evenness and continuity of the air emission by tactile (feeling the airstream), visual (watching the effect of the airstream moving a feather, etc.), and auditory feedback. Other consonants that can be used are /0/ and /θ/. These breathed continuants, because of their place and manner of articulation, share the advantage of focusing the child's attention on the forward projection of the airstream, which helps to distract attention from the laryngeal area. This side benefit is especially helpful if the child is inclined to use excessive laryngeal tension. The use of such fricative sounds has the added advantage of allowing for a smooth transition to the next goal in the therapy process. After the child has achieved competence in emitting a lengthened controlled flow of air, the addition of voicing is easily achieved by requiring the child to produce the voiced cognates of the unvoiced phonemes. Thus, a child can be instructed to add voice to /s/ and prolong /z/ instead. Similarly /θ/ can become /ð/ and /ʃ/ can change to /ʒ/. The adding of voicing midway through the emission of the airstream, initially, can be especially helpful in creating the appropriate preparatory set with respect to respiratory control, before the addition of laryngeal activity.

Another set of exercises sometimes used to help achieve goal 3 involves activities related to the segmenting of the exhaled airstream. Skill in "chunking" the airstream is required because speaking involves a series of modifications of the exhaled airstream. Thus, exercises such as producing as many short /p/ productions as possible during an exhalation phase are useful. Because /p/ is an unvoiced bilabial, its production is helpful in focusing the attention on the lip movement rather than laryngeal valving. Again, the subsequent addition of voicing results in the production of the cognate /b/, and the alternation of /p/ and /b/ allows for practice of seriated unvoiced and voiced productions during a single exhalation. It is possible to count the number of products achieved during one exhalation and thereby to work toward increasing both length and control of the exhalation phase. Other techniques sometimes used to establish improved control of the air available for exhalation include emission of the air in two, three, or four segments. In other words, a child might be instructed to divide his or her available air into equal halves, thirds, or quarters. If the child uses an unvoiced phoneme, such as /h/, to emit the "air chunks," he or she is forced to rely on respiratory muscle control alone because no valving of the airstream occurs at the laryngeal or articulatory levels.

Unique Aspects of Voice Therapy Programming

We have reviewed some of the basic terms used in programming. Although it is apparent that voice programming is similar to other kinds of programming, some important differences need to be mentioned. In articulation therapy, when a child misarticulates a phoneme, the target phoneme is already known to the clinician. When a child exhibits a voice disorder, the identification of the target vocal behavior is sometimes more complex. The standard used to judge the child's best voice is less clearly defined. Vocal behavior varies depending on age, gender, and anatomical and psychological constraints. Sometimes there are anatomical constraints that are permanent and irreversible. Examples of such constraints are severe structural malformations or neurological impairments. In such instances, a child's best voice may never be a perfectly "normal" voice but a voice that is the result of the best possible compensations. The task of eliciting a target voice may frequently involve the manipulation of a number of different behaviors. Thus, the clinician and the child together must embark on a trial-and-error search for the most efficient vocal production. Compounding the problem is the fact that the clinician's most easily available model is that of an adult voice. Although an adult's production of any specific phoneme is not markedly different from a child's target phoneme, an adult voice is usually different from a child's voice. Thus, at times the use of tape recordings of samples of children's voices may be an important part of a voice therapy strategy.

General Approaches to Developing Task Sequences

There are a number of different approaches to vocal remediation, and one could argue that no single approach is necessarily better than another. Nevertheless, certain approaches will be better suited to some individuals' needs and some patterns of symptoms than others. Much depends on the number of inappropriate symptoms exhibited by the individual child, the severity of the symptoms, and the interrelationship of symptoms. In previous discussions, we have focused on the different areas of behavior, on selecting objectives and goals, and on choosing strategies to achieve those goals. We have also mentioned the need for behavioral hierarchies. We now review some different approaches that affect the way we order our therapy tasks.

One approach to planning task sequences in voice therapy probably grew out of traditional voice improvement programs. This is a holistic approach to remediation based on the assumption that if all of the component parts of voice production are overhauled sequentially, the end result will be an appropriate composite voice. Thus, one begins at the beginning of the physiological process (i.e., with respiration) and proceeds in an orderly fashion to link respiration with the onset of phonation, with sustained phonation, then with resonance and articulation. With this approach, the kind of symptoms exhibited by the child does not alter the progression of the tasks. The order is predicated on the sequence of events occurring during normal vocalization. Thus, because respiration always begins the speech act, respiration training is always attacked first. This is so even if it does not appear that the respiratory behavior is explicitly contributing to the vocal symptoms. Implicit in this approach is the assumption that an understanding of the interrelationship of the system and a strengthening of the control of the behaviors at each level of the entire process will result in an optimal voice. This approach is obviously more time consuming than others and requires a high level of sustained motivation on the part of the student. It probably works best with older children, highly motivated children, or children who exhibit severe symptom patterns that involve the entire mechanism (e.g., children with cerebral palsy).

To illustrate this approach and the other approaches yet to be discussed in this chapter, we shall demonstrate how a task sequence might be developed for a child who demonstrates the symptom of hard glottal attacks. We shall proceed through a typical sequence of tasks that might be used to remediate this symptom. Remember that the task sequence is somewhat abbreviated and will not progress through all the steps. We shall not attempt to continue the sequence to the termination of therapy but shall proceed far enough to illustrate the differences between basic approaches. First, let us consider the holistic approach. (See the box on the next page.)

Another approach to remediation is to zero in on the particular symptoms exhibited by the child and isolate the behaviors to be changed. Thus, for example, if hard initiation of phonation is noted, the phonatory system (or the laryngeal mechanism) would be considered as the primary target system. The behavior to be modified is focused on without reference to its relationship to other aspects of the entire process. This highlighting approach usually involves explicit description of the audible or visible characteristics of the undesirable behavior and contrasts them with the characteristics of the desirable behavior that is to be substituted. This approach is more symptom specific than is the previous approach. It tends to emphasize the behaviors by extracting them from their behavioral context. Verbal descriptions of the

Task Sequence I	**Child's Behavioral Goals**
Respiration	**1.** I can inhale using appropriate lower-chest movement.
Respiration	**2.** I can exhale evenly on /s/ for approximately 20 seconds (airstream smooth and even; length increases during repeated exhalations).
Coordination of respiration and phonation	**3.** I can move smoothly and easily from s-z; h-m during exhalation phase (no breaks or bumps in the flow).
Phonation	**4.** I can prolong *h* + vowel (CVs).
	5. I can stop and start *h* + vowel (CVs) (e.g., hey, he, hi, hoe, who)
Resonance	**6.** I can chant words feeling facial vibrations (e.g., hi/my, he/me, ho/mo, who/moo).
Articulation	**7.** I can prolong voiced sounds while chanting words (e.g., his‿is; she's‿ill; been‿away; gave‿in; beige‿egg; bill‿Emmy).
	8. I can separate word pairs while remembering to begin vowel sound easily (e.g., his/is; she's/ill; been/away; gave/in/; beige/egg; bill/Emmy). (*Cue:* "Think of the sound on the front of the mouth, not in the throat.")
	9. I can say sentences using easy attacks on vowels (e.g., My age is eight; Mom is angry, Amy; May always eats every apple). (*Cue:* "Feel the vibrations on the lips for the /m/ and keep the feeling of the sound there during the vowels.")

behaviors are explicit and concrete and frequently modeled by the clinician and repeated by the child. This approach is often used with young children or with children who are working in groups. (See the box on the next page.)

A third approach that can be employed in voice therapy is that of using specific behaviors from an allied system to cue more appropriate behaviors in another (Shrivastav, Yamaguch, & Andrews, 2000). Thus, we synthesize or link up behavioral patterns to produce a desired vocal effect. This is essentially another way to describe "stimulability" as it applies to vocal production. We are all familiar with the use of facilitating contexts to elicit target phonemes during articulation therapy. Often in voice therapy, we do the same type of thing. We employ associated behaviors, images, or contexts to shape the vocal production. If we think about our example of the child with the hard glottal attacks, we can see that her symptom can be remediated by linking the phonatory behavior to resonance, articulation, or both. We can emphasize easy onset of voicing by focusing attention on "the front of the face" (facial bones) or on the characteristics of voiced continuant consonants. By redirecting the child's attention to another part of the speech mechanism, we accrue an additional benefit of distracting attention from the laryngeal mechanism. Because the articulatory system is less likely to be adversely affected by excessive effort than is the laryngeal system, a child who is using too much effort may be helped by such an approach. It should be noted that this is a frequently used approach

Task Sequence II	Child's Behavioral Goals
Phonation (awareness level)	**1.** I can tell when the voice starts with a hard sound (isolated vowels). "I hear a grunt or click." "The neck is tight."
	2. I can tell when the voice starts with an easy sound (isolated vowels). "I do not hear a grunt or click." "The neck is relaxed."
	3. I can count the hard and easy attacks when other people say words starting with vowels (interpersonal level). any, every, angel, uncle, eggs, insect
Phonation (production level)	**4.** I can feel and describe the difference when I make a hard sound on /a/ and an easy sound on /ha/. *Hard* — *Easy* grunt to start — air comes out first neck tight — neck not tight sounds bumpy — sounds smooth
	5. I can make an easy start on any vowel when I say /h/ before it. I/hi; Ed/head; ill/hill
	6. I can make an easy start on any vowel when I think the /h/ sound and then just say the vowel. (h)ill; (h)is; (h)at
	7. I can make an easy start on words in sentences. (*Cues:* think the /h/ on all of the words. Pause before the vowels.) "Hi, I'm Amy"; "Who are idiots?"; "Hit it anywhere."
	8. I can tell when I've made a hard sound and say it again with an easy sound.
	9. I can tell when I am about to make a hard sound because I know the vowels that trick me most. (*Cue:* Mark the hard words before reading the sentence so that you'll be ready for them.)

that works with many different symptoms. Boone (1977, p. 109) listed 24 "facilitating behaviors" that are useful in voice therapy. We shall illustrate the use of facilitating associated behaviors in the following task sequence designed to eliminate hard glottal attacks. (See the box on the next page.)

A fourth approach to therapy needs yet to be considered. This approach differs from the three already discussed in that it does not focus primary attention on the vocal symptoms. The therapy is aimed at the understanding of the interpersonal dynamics precipitating or maintaining the vocal symptoms. This approach may be used when the clinician feels that the vocal symptoms arise from or reflect problems in personal or interpersonal adjustment. The term *psychogenic* refers to disorders that result from emotional factors, lack of self-esteem, or disturbed

Task Sequence III	Child's Behavioral Goals
Resonance	1. I can prolong a humming sound, /m/, feeling the tickling on my lips and the vibrations on my face.
	2. I can describe the difference between feeling the sound on the front of my lips and face versus all the sound in my throat. (*Cue*: hands on face and lips.)
Articulation	3. I can prolong the /z/ sound, feeling the vibrations on my teeth.
	4. I can prolong the /ð/ and /v/ sounds, feeling the vibrations on my tongue and lip.
	5. I can prolong the voiced continuant consonants + vowels (e.g., za, ði, vo, mu).
	6. I can repeat the five CVs (voiced continuant plus vowel), keeping the vibrations on the front of my face.
	7. I can contrast the forward versus laryngeal tone focus on alternate CV syllables.
	8. I can chant CV + V + V + V, maintaining the forward tone focus even on the vowels that aren't started with the voiced continuant consonant, for example, ma, a, a, a zi, i, i, i
	9. I can chant a sentence, keeping the forward tone focus (e.g., "My mom is mailing money"). (*Cue:* Practice sentence cumulatively, for example, My ____ ____ ____ ____ My mom ____ ____ ____ ____ My mom is ____ ____ ____ My mom is mailing ____ ____.
	10. I can say the sentence maintaining forward tone focus. (*Cue*: Hum "m" before beginning.)
	11. I can say phrases where the first word ends in voiced continuant consonant. (This helps glide into easy start to word beginning with vowel, e.g., I'm eager; I'm anxious; I'm earnest; is Edgar; is Ellie; is Emma; an orange; an apple; an alligator).
	12. I can say phrases pausing before vowel yet maintaining easy, smooth onset. (*Cue:* Think of the vowel sound vibrating in the front of your mouth.)
	13. I can say sentences full of words starting with vowel sounds. (*Cue:* Keep the sound at the front of your mouth.)
	14. I can tell when the vowel sounds at the beginning of words are easy and forward versus hard and in the throat.
	15. I can predict when I am likely to make the vowel sounds hard and with too much effort in my throat.

Task Sequence III (*continued* on next page)

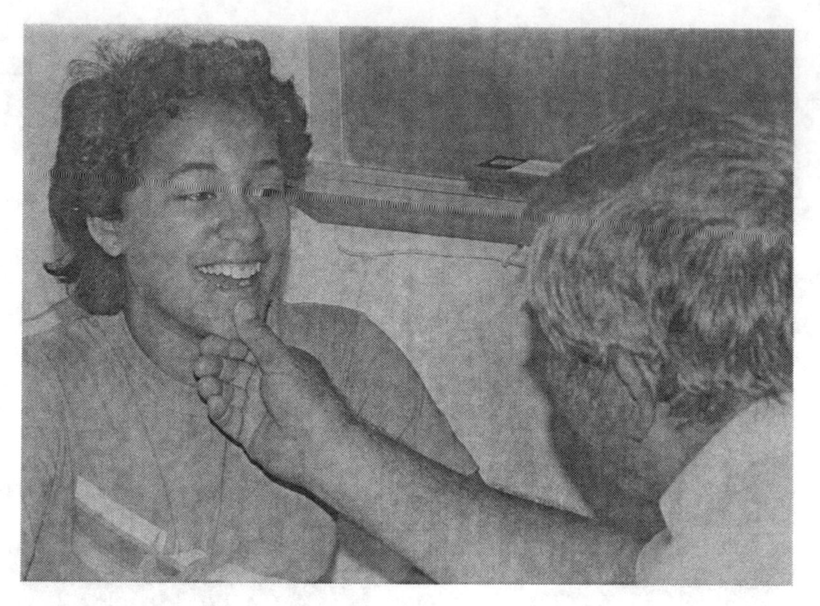

Tactile cues can help to remind the child to keep the voice on the front of the mouth.

Task Sequence III	Child's Behavioral Goals
	16. I can describe what I do to avoid hard attacks on words beginning with vowels, for example: a. Keep the voice on the front of my mouth. b. Prolong voiced continuant (sound carrying) consonants. c. "Think" about linking preceding final consonants to the vowel in the next word. d. "Hum" in my head to place the sound before saying the vowel.

interpersonal relationships. Aronson's (1973) excellent series of tapes illustrating his approach to diagnosis and intervention with adult patients provides insight into the ways in which maladaptive vocal behavior may stem from psychosocial problems. Obviously, severe problems of this kind are best treated by a team approach. Psychological counseling either alone or coordinated with symptomatic voice therapy is frequently the method of treatment used when a complex or severe problem is identified. Some children who exhibit less severe difficulties, however, may benefit from a voice therapy approach that emphasizes analysis of the interpersonal factors influencing vocal behavior. Such an approach focuses on awareness of the way our feelings influence our own vocal behavior and the way our behavior is perceived by others. It involves the effects of physiological and emotional states on vocal strategies. To illustrate this general approach, we will again consider a task sequence designed for a child exhibiting the vocal symptom of hard glottal attacks. In this instance, however, the approach will not focus so much on the vocal symptom but on understanding the underlying basis of that behavior. (See the box below.)

A fifth approach, one that is similar to the preceding approach in that it does not focus attention on inappropriate vocal patterns or on symptom elimination, has been referred to as "cognitive cueing." This approach is particularly useful with children who use limited vocal variation when they speak and has been used successfully with children who speak in a monotone voice, for example, children with hearing impairment (Shrivastav, 1997) and children who have reduced affect due to

Task Sequence IV | **Child's Behavioral Goals**

Interpersonal level

1. I can listen to tape recordings of voices and describe how I feel as I listen to the individual's voices (e.g., tense/relaxed/anxious/annoyed).
2. I can describe specific feeling states associated with certain vocal characteristics, for example,
   angry = loud, tense sound, fast rate
   friendly = pitch variety, relaxed sound, even rate
   scared = soft, quavery sound, pauses, endings fade
   confident = moderate loudness, clear sound, even rate).
3. I can describe the characteristics of voices and behavior of people I like to talk to (e.g., relaxed body, facial expression, and voice; make good eye contact; don't talk all of the time; don't butt in when I'm talking; ask me questions sometimes; seem to really listen to me; voice is easy to listen to; don't talk about themselves all of the time; don't try to be the center of attention always).

Intrapersonal level

4. I can express different feelings while talking (with facial expression and gesture, for example:
   Oh yeah! (angry/happy)
   Answer, anyone! (ordering/coaxing)
   Everyone is out (sneering/questioning)
5. I can explain how it feels and sounds when I talk different ways, for example
   angry "Oh yeah"—neck and jaw tense
   hard attack on "Oh"—voice loud and strained
6. I can describe how listeners respond differently to different ways of saying the same words (e.g., they feel irritated, blamed, put down).

Task Sequence IV (*continued* on next page)

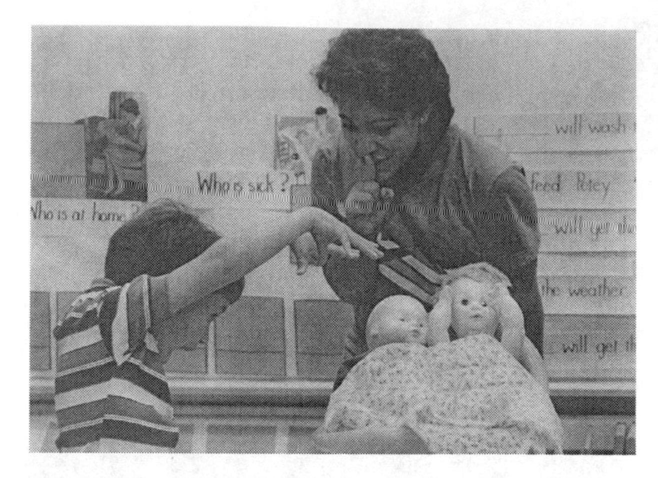

Role playing allows the child to try out a variety of different vocal behaviors.

Task Sequence IV — **Child's Behavioral Goals**

7. I can role play the same dialogue using different feelings in my voice (e.g., friendly/defiant).
   a. I want to talk to you, Al.
   b. I aim to act.
8. I can demonstrate different tricks I can use to make my voice sound: friendly/defiant, relaxed/tense, for example:
   relaxed face and body (versus tense)
   easy attacks (versus hard)
   loud (versus moderate)
   fast (versus slow)
   pauses (versus no pauses)
   pitch rises at end (versus pitch falls)
9. I can role play various situations (switching parts) and analyze the effects I create by using my voice different ways (Tape Record—Play Back—Discuss—Redo).
10. I can match vocal behaviors with specific situations and expected effects (e.g., situation = talking to the principal).
    How do I want to sound?
    What vocal behaviors will be helpful?
    What vocal behaviors will be harmful?
11. I can analyze situations by using the following questions:
    What do I want to gain?
    What risks are there?
    What vocal behavior should I use?
    How will the listener react?

psychosocial difficulties. It has been described by Andrews et al. (2000) as using mental imagery that is specifically suggested or evoked, may be implicit in the semantic content of an utterance, or made explicit by oral instructions. It is the one approach where modeling and imitation of any kind are never used. Thus, this method is useful when the clinician's voice may not be appropriate, for example, if the clinician is an older person or of a different gender. (See the box below.)

In the task sequence below, the child's imagination is used to effect the changes in his vocal behavior. He or she is asked to think about the color of the submarine, whether it hits the bottom with a jolt or settles gently, and so on, rather than thinking about his or her voice characteristics. The lowering of the pitch has the added benefit of relaxing the laryngeal mechanism. The changes in the voice flow from the changes and expansions in thinking about the words or text, just as an actor or singer interprets the literature to be spoken or sung. Thus, when using this approach, the clinician must probe in a way that allows the child's own thought patterns to expand his or her imagery. In this way, individual and natural vocal changes are stimulated that are appropriate for the speaker and that therefore help the child to feel comfortable with his or her productions when they are recorded and played back for discussion and revision. This approach usually works best with older school-age children who can read sentences fluently, although it can be used with younger children if "word pictures" are used on isolated words or short phrases in spontaneous speech.

Task Sequence V	**Child's Behavioral Goals**
Vocal variation with easy voice onset (pitch changes at the sentence level assist easy onset of vowel-initial words)	**1.** I can read the sentence silently and identify the picture words and underline them. I can circle the words that start with vowel sounds. They are tricky to start gently.
"The submarine under water sinks down to the ocean floor."	**2.** I can talk about the images I see when I think about the words I underline.
	3. I can describe how my voice moves downward like the submarine. I can imagine the boat is dark gray and how it settles onto the ocean floor.
	4. I can read the sentence so my voice reflects the sinking of the submarine and shows how still and quiet it is underwater.
	5. I can prolong the vowel sound at the beginning of "under water" and "ocean" so the gentle movement of the submarine is reflected in the way I say the words.

Summary

We have noted that there are many ways to develop task sequences and have illustrated a few different approaches. Obviously, no one approach works with all children, and it is a mistake to think that any specific task sequence will be successful with every child. Even children with the same symptoms respond differently to different techniques. Treatment approaches must be designed, and tasks selected and organized, in response to each child's unique patterns of liabilities and strengths.

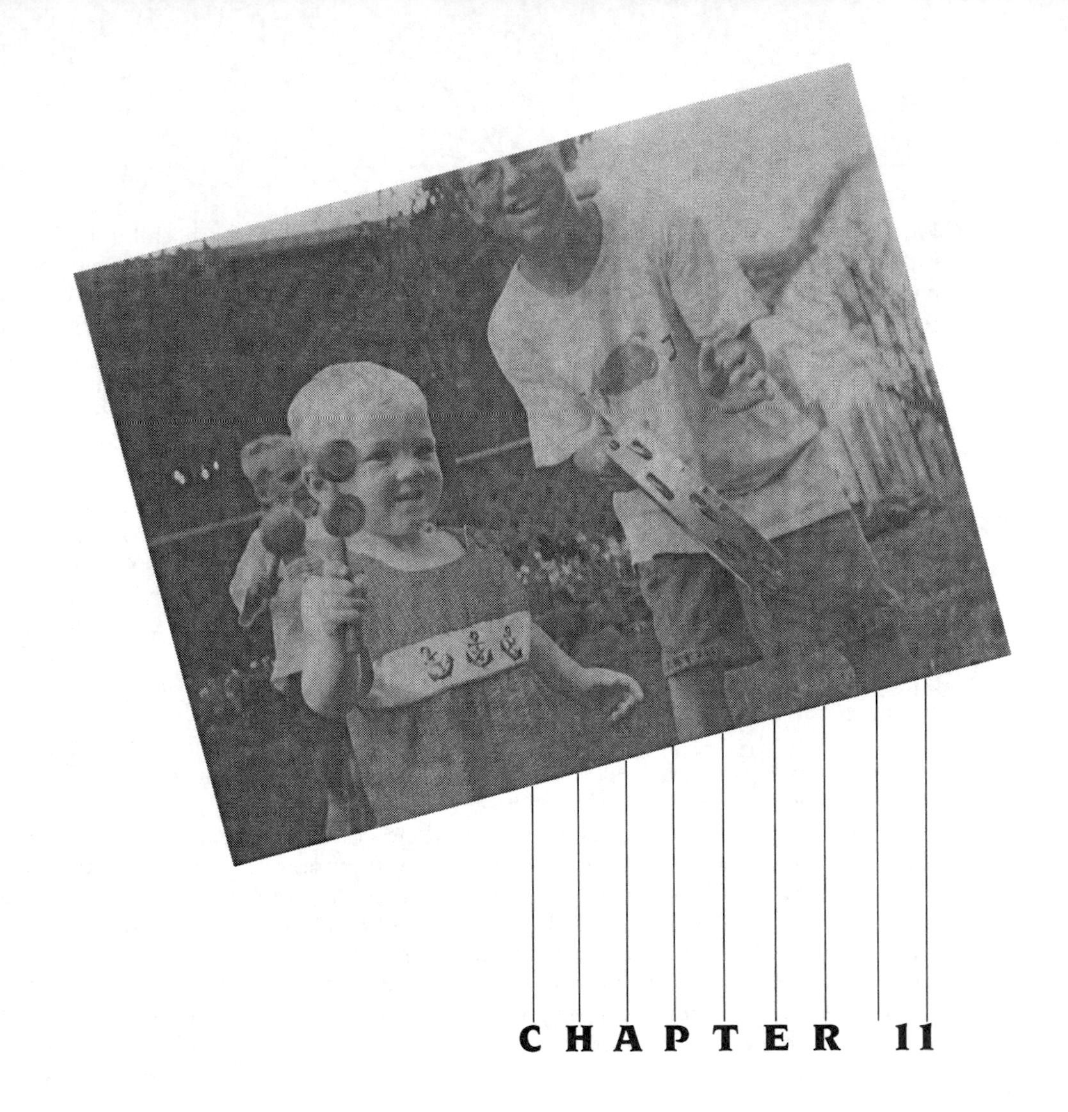

CHAPTER 11

Phases of Therapy Programs

We have just reviewed some different approaches to organizing individual therapy tasks into meaningful sequences. The approach we adopt influences which short-term goals we select, the priority given to certain goals, and the strategies we design to teach the child to acquire the behaviors stated in the goals. Of course, it takes a large number of short-term goals and task sequences to build an entire therapy program. When we take an overview of a complete, well-organized therapy program designed to achieve long-range terminal objectives, we notice that there is usually a discernible pattern. The program is subdivided into sections made up of similar short-term goals and task sequences. These sections are called *phases.*

The amount of time required to implement an entire voice therapy program will vary depending on a variety of factors. Individual phases of the program will be completed along the way, however, and the success of the entire program will depend to a large extent on how these phases mesh in promoting cumulative learning. In the section that follows, we describe and illustrate four distinct phases that are important in voice therapy programming for children. These are (a) general awareness, (b) specific awareness, (c) production, and (d) carryover. Every phase may not always be necessary in every therapy program. Some phases will be more applicable with some children than with others. Nevertheless, it is probably safe to say that there is merit in capitalizing on possibilities inherent in all the phases, not only during the initial stages of program planning but also when problems occur in implementation and program revision seems necessary.

An awareness phase of voice therapy usually involves more complicated planning than does a similar phase in articulation therapy. When a child with an articulation difficulty is taught to focus on distinctive features, the parameters are fairly well defined and are similar for all children. The voice student, however, may present the clinician with a variety of distorted vocal patterns, and some may be rather unusual. In deciding how to describe and define the characteristics of vocal patterns, the clinician is often in uncharted territory. Individual differences in adaptive behavior seem to present more challenges in voice therapy than in articulation therapy. Of primary importance during any awareness phase is the reduction of all behaviors to their simplest form. This enables children to attend to the significant characteristics. Children are taught first to identify characteristics of specific behaviors in others and later to identify what they themselves are doing.

When the clinician first teaches awareness of behaviors produced by others, children are usually better equipped to identify and describe those behaviors in themselves later in the program. An added advantage is the avoidance of feelings of embarrassment and self-consciousness that often result if children are required to focus on their own patterns before they have been trained to observe and describe those behaviors demonstrated by others. One way to approach this kind of observation is to contrast behaviors. When the clinician presents a pairing of basic behaviors, children are given a clear-cut choice, and differences can be made more dramatic. Table 11–1 lists examples of some goals and strategies involving simple behavioral contrasts subsumed under the four different areas of concern in voice therapy. Simple terms are selected and used to describe what is seen and heard, and practice is given in identifying and describing each aspect of the patterns.

We have just illustrated some simple goals and strategies useful for helping children zero in on significant aspects of contrasting behaviors. By pairing the contrasting behaviors, we tried to emphasize the significant differences in characteristics. This technique

Table 11–1. Goals for Awareness Activities.

General Area	Respiratory Behavior	Laryngeal Behavior	Resonance	Interpersonal Skills
Goal 1: Label correctly two contrasted behaviors with 100% accuracy				
(Identification)				
Behavior I	*Upper chest breathing*	*Tense neck*	*Nose voice [m]*	*Angry voice*
Behavior II	*Lower chest breathing*	*Relaxed neck*	*Mouth voice [a]*	*Friendly voice*
Goal 2: Describe the visible signs of the two behaviors in others				
(Description)				
Characteristics I	*Shoulders raised. Lower chest still.*	*Neck muscles move. Jaw thrust out.*	*Mouth closed. Air blows feather near nose.*	*Face frowns.*
Characteristics II	*Shoulders down. Lower chest moves.*	*No movement in neck. Jaw loose.*	*Mouth open. Air blows feather near mouth.*	*Face smiles.*
Goal 3: Describe to others how to change Behavior I to Behavior II				
(Instruction)				
Verbalizations	*1. Keep shoulders down.* *2. Breathe deeper.* *3. Put hands on lower chest and push out.* *4. Move chest walls out at sides.*	*1. Roll head around.* *2. Loosen neck.* *3. Unclench jaw.* *4. Shrug shoulders.* *5. Drop jaw down.*	*1. Open mouth more.* *2. Blow air to move feather.*	*1. Don't frown.* *2. Smile.* *3. Loosen face.* *4. Think friendly thoughts!*

The arrangement of the goals involves a progression from identification to description to instruction.

Strategies that could be used to teach the behaviors stated in the preceding goals might include the following activities:

Goal 1
- A. *Model plus explanation of behaviors.*
- B. *Tell me what one I am doing.*
- C. *You be the teacher and tell me what to do.*

Goal 2
- A. *Tell me how you know which one I am doing.*
- B. *Put a mark beside the label on the chalkboard and tell me why you chose that one.*
- C. *Choose the card with the description that matches what I did. Read it to me.*

Goal 3
- A. *Simon says.*
- B. *Draw a picture of each and explain what you drew and why.*
- C. *You be the teacher and tell me my mistakes and how to correct them.*
- D. *Make up some rules and write them on the chalkboard.*

is frequently helpful in teaching specific awareness of target behaviors. Nonetheless, some children may not be motivated or ready to proceed directly into the specific awareness phase of therapy. Sometimes when we begin to work with a child in voice therapy, a more general orientation to the area to be worked on is necessary first. It is unlikely that all children automatically "know" what they are supposed to be thinking about in voice therapy or why it is important or relevant. Until they develop some basic concepts about the area of concern, they may not be equipped to proceed.

General Awareness Phase

A voice therapy program frequently begins with a *general awareness* phase in which the child is introduced to an area and oriented to significant concepts. If, for example, the area to be considered is respiration, the clinician may begin with a general discussion of breathing: how it is necessary to sustain life, to make sound, and so on. This can by followed by a discussion of how people breathe when they talk or sing; how the amount of air affects the length of the sound; how there are even, smooth sounds or jerky sounds produced when the airstream is emitted in different ways; how air can be taken in and stored by efficient and inefficient methods. If a child is an athlete, the discussion can be linked to the way efficient air use affects athletic performance. If the child plays a musical instrument, the discussion can refer to the relationship between airflow and the musical effect, and so on. What is important is that the child is acquainted with and understands the relevance of the broad area of interest. During the general awareness phase of therapy, we teach the background information that the child needs to understand before beginning work on specific symptoms.

Teacher's Goals

1. To orient the child to the area to be addressed in therapy
2. To develop concepts that are basic to learning in the area
3. To introduce linguistic terms used to describe characteristics and relationships

Child's Objectives

1. The child can identify the area to be worked on.
2. The child can describe why this area is important to all people.
3. The child can describe how this area is important to me in my daily life.
4. The child can explain the basic concepts relevant to this area.
5. The child can define the linguistic terms used in this area.

Steps in the Therapy Sequence

1. The child can identify voice as the area on which I need to work.
   a. Animals, birds, and people all have unique voices.
2. The child can describe why voice is important to people.
   a. we recognize people by their voices
   b. voices tell us important information
      i. age
      ii. gender
      iii. health
      iv. wakefulness/fatigue
      v. emotional state
      vi. intent
   c. people react differently to different voices
      i. familiar/unfamiliar
      ii. pleasant/unpleasant
      iii. natural/artificial
      iv. neutral/emotional

3. The child can describe how voice is important to me in my daily life.
   a. it is the "me" others hear
   b. it can help me feel confident/anxious
   c. it can draw others to me/turn others from me
   d. it can help me/hinder me from getting what I want
4. The child can explain basic concepts relevant to voice (e.g., parameters of voice).
   a. high/low
   b. loud/soft
   c. tense/relaxed
   d. smooth/rough
   e. even/jerky
   f. easy/squeezed
5. The child can define the linguistic terms used in voice (e.g., characteristics of voice behavior).
   a. abrupt/easy onset
   b. slides up/slides down
   c. keeps going/stops
   d. gets softer/louder
   e. too loud/too soft
   f. grunts/clicks/flows/breaks
   g. not enough air/too much air
   h. tight muscles in neck/relaxed neck

Specific Awareness Phase

Once the child has participated in a discussion of the general area and has acquired some understanding of it and its importance, the work on *specific awareness* of individual behaviors can begin. The symptom pattern dictates the selection of the specific behaviors that the child needs to be able to isolate from the behavioral gestalt. During this phase, the clinician models specific behaviors and uses consistent terms to identify and describe relevant behavioral characteristics. The child then practices using this descriptive language. An example of a therapy sequence for specific awareness that is applicable to any behavior and appropriate for any area of voice therapy follows.

During the specific awareness phase of therapy, we teach the child to focus on the part of behavioral patterns that are most relevant to his or her symptoms.

Teacher's Goals

1. To isolate behaviors relevant to the production phase of therapy
2. To discriminate between appropriate and inappropriate behaviors
3. To isolate symptoms to be modified during therapy
4. To describe the auditory, visual, and kinesthetic characteristics of target symptoms
5. To provide pertinent information concerning anatomy and physiology (if applicable)
6. To identify reasons for symptoms
7. To target negative behaviors to avoid or change
8. To describe alternative strategies

Child's Objectives

1. The child will identify behaviors exhibited by others (negative and positive).
2. The child will describe the characteristics of those behaviors.
3. The child will discriminate between the appropriate and inappropriate behaviors.
4. The child will suggest ways others can avoid or change inappropriate behaviors.
5. The child will identify his or her own behaviors.
6. The child will explain the characteristics of the behaviors he or she uses now (auditory, visual, kinesthetic characteristics).
7. The child will explain the correct-incorrect physiology associated with the symptoms.
8. The child will identify symptoms and negative behaviors to change.

9. The child will explain how/why/when he or she uses inappropriate behaviors.
10. The child will describe some ways inappropriate behaviors can be avoided or changed.

When the child has been taught to focus on the characteristics of behaviors that need to be modified and understands the perceptual framework and terminology, he or she is in an advantageous position to experience success on production tasks.

Production Phase

During the production phase of therapy, we teach the child to produce and monitor target behaviors in a highly structured and controlled situation. Initially, cues and monitoring are provided by the clinician. As the production phase progresses, however, the responsibility for cueing and monitoring is assumed more and more by the client.

Teacher's Goals

1. To elicit the target behaviors
   a. in isolation
   b. in simple linguistic contexts
   c. in complex linguistic contexts
2. To describe the child's responses in terms meaningful to the child
   a. how
   b. why
   c. when
3. To provide techniques to shape consistency and accuracy of responses
   a. imitation
   b. extensive cueing
   c. minimal cueing
4. To encourage child's self-monitoring of responses
5. To structure increasingly difficult contexts in which the child can practice target behaviors
6. To reinforce the child's correct responses and attempts at extinguishing undesirable behaviors

Child's Objectives

1. The child will produce a target behavior correctly (in isolation)
   a. with instructions, cues, and model
   b. with instructions and cues
   c. with instructions
   d. spontaneously
2. The child will prolong–repeat the target behavior.
3. The child will stop and start the target behavior at will.
4. The child will demonstrate both the appropriate and inappropriate forms of the behavior (negative practice).
5. The child will produce the target behavior, varying length of utterance
   a. isolated sounds,
   b. syllables,
   c. words,
   d. phrases, and
   e. sentences.
6. The child will produce the target behavior varying complexity of processing:
   a. imitation,
   b. automatic responses,
   c. limited repertoire of responses,
   d. simple self-generated responses, and
   e. complex self-generated responses.
7. The child will produce the target behavior varying the timing of the response:
   a. predictable response time and
   b. unpredictable response time.
8. The child will describe the characteristics of his or her production in terms of
   a. preparatory set,
   b. strategies used,
   c. reactions of self, and
   d. reactions of others.
9. The child will monitor his or her own production
   a. when cued verbally,

b. when cued nonverbally,
c. after practicing aloud,
d. after thinking about it first, and
e. spontaneously.

In voice therapy, the target is usually less well defined than it is in articulation therapy. Thus, the clinician must present opportunities for the child to verbalize descriptions of what he or she is doing to produce the target behavior, and to specify how the behavior sounds, feels, and looks. Monitoring and self-evaluating are achieved most effectively when the processes involved in production are scored and analyzed as well as practiced.

As can be seen in item 4 of the task sequence above, negative practice (Wilson, 1972) may be incorporated into the learning sequence. It is also traditional for the mean length of the response to be gradually increased as a new vocal behavior is learned. During item 5, the traditional progression from isolated sounds (usually vowels or voiced continuants) through gradual combinations of sounds is illustrated. In item 6, we see the graduations that involve cognitive processing. For example, a child who is learning to produce a "new" vocalization pattern usually needs to concentrate full attention initially on the mechanics of production rather than on the ideas expressed. Thus, we require minimal cognitive processing initially and gradually increase the complexity of the processing as skill develops.

When a child first learns to produce a new behavior and that behavior is not yet stabilized, it helps if we give him or her plenty of time to produce the target behavior, or a predictable latency between the stimulus (instructions and/or cues) and the expected response. As skill develops, it is advantageous to begin to vary these demands during practice so that elapsed time between stimulus and response more closely approximates the variability of actual speech interactions. That is why in item 7 of the sample task sequence we include variations in timing. It seems helpful at times to vary timing even when the child is still at the single-sound level. For example, we may wish to employ a strategy such as asking a child to be ready to respond to questions of various lengths with a simple "Oh" or "Ah-hah!" Such an activity, although making simple demands in terms of the length of the target utterance, can be useful in terms of requiring the child to be ready to respond whenever the questioner stops talking. An example of such an activity is given below.

1. Area: Laryngeal behavior
2. Goal: Child will produce an easy vocal tone on single vowels in response to oral questions or statements of various lengths (9/10).
3. Strategy:
   a. Clinician tells the child to be ready to produce an easy voice on [ou] and [ʌ] [a] whenever the clinician stops talking (questions or a narrative may be presented).
   b. Child responds immediately when the clinician pauses. The vowel may be varied in terms of pitch inflections to reflect meaning.
   c. Verbal reinforcement is given. Stimulus materials are as follows:
      i. "I like ice cream, but my sister doesn't. Can you believe that?" [ʌ] (with head shake)
      ii. "The news was exciting today. A bank robber dressed in a ski mask held up the downtown bank and escaped with $100,000!!" [ou]
      iii. "No one was hurt!" [a] (with relief)

The preceding example illustrates the interrelationship that may exist between length of utterance, timing of response, and complexity of processing during voice therapy activities. Although in the sample task sequence presented earlier items 5, 6, and 7 are listed sequentially, the variables of length, timing, and complexity are often difficult to consider in isolation from each other. Because we are always trying to shape behavior so that it will eventually support spontaneous communicative exchange, consideration of conversational timing and interaction between speakers early in the task sequence is often beneficial.

Choosing Materials to Facilitate Responses

We have discussed how we systematically shape the child's responses during the production phase of therapy; however, there is yet another aspect to be considered as we plan therapy during the production phase. We need to choose practice items geared to facilitate correct responses.

The correct choice of appropriate materials to cue responses and to be spoken during practice sessions is an important part of successful planning. It is self-evident, of course, that the level of all materials used should be appropriate to the child's academic achievement level. The child who cannot read fluently needs materials such as rebus stories (pictures interspersed with printed words in sentences). The child who can read needs sentences and passages commensurate with his or her reading proficiency level. Additionally, the content is chosen so as to correlate with the individual child's interests, ethnic and family background, and socioeconomic level. Common sense suggests that the more the child can identify with the characters and the circumstances in stories that he or she is listening to, discussing, or reading, the more involved he or she becomes in the task. Children from single-parent families, for example, may not always feel comfortable reading about or discussing narratives that describe intact family groups. Similarly, children from poor areas may not relate well to pictures from glossy magazines depicting luxurious home interiors. Although most of us are aware of the pitfalls inherent in the examples just cited, we also should be careful to include in stimulus materials pictures of children who match the ethnic characteristics of the children we are teaching.

Choice of Phonemes

Another consideration when we select practice materials is the extent to which the phonemes selected enhance the child's chances of achieving his or her voice production goals. This consideration is a familiar one because we are aware of the importance of using facilitating phonetic contexts when we work with children during articulation therapy. Nonetheless, the effect of specific phonemes and phonemic sequences in facilitating vocal production is somewhat more subtle though equally important. Let us consider some examples of phonemes that are helpful in relation to some examples of specific skills worked on under the various areas that are important in voice therapy.

Respiration

We have talked about the importance of the exhalation phase of respiration. We know that children must be able to prolong and control the airflow during expiration. When we choose sounds for children to practice to increase the duration of the exhalation phase, we need to remember that voiced continuants will be easiest at first. This is because the vocal folds are closed during voiced sounds, thus restricting to some extent the emission of the airstream. We improve the child's chances of success if we ask him or her to prolong sounds such as /z/, /m/, and /v/ because continuant sounds can be prolonged for as long as the air lasts, and the air lasts somewhat longer when the continuant is also voiced. When success has been achieved in increasing the duration of individual voiced continuants, the next step is to proceed to teach the child to prolong unvoiced continuants. We might begin with /s/ /θ/, for example, because the production of these sounds provides the possibility of capitalizing on a kinesthetic awareness of the air passing through the constriction of articulators in the front of the mouth during production of these sounds. The evenness of the airflow can also be demonstrated by the use of visible cues, such as the movement of a feather or paper held in front of the mouth. All of the unvoiced fricative continuants will usually be easier than the glottal continuant /h/, in which the airflow is unimpeded at both the laryngeal and oral levels. Thus, the production of /h/ may best be reserved to practice until last in such a series.

When children have achieved proficiency in prolonging and controlling the airflow during the production of individual continuant sounds, a clinician may wish to introduce tasks that help develop skill in segmenting the exhalation. Because during running speech the exhalation phase is segmented as voiced and unvoiced sounds are sequenced across time, segmentation (or stopping and starting) exercises are frequently valuable. Examples of these exercises may include stopping and starting the voiced continuants practiced previously, as many times as possible during one exhalation. When this exercise has resulted in improvement in performance, production of a repeated plosive during one exhalation may be attempted. Again, the search for the easiest phonemes to practice first should involve a consideration of the features of voicing and the place and manner of articulation. Clinical experience suggests that the most difficult task for children who are working on improving the control of the exhalation may be successive repetitions of the voiceless affricative /tʃ/. Because the oral cavity is relatively open and the vocal folds are apart, the child is required to place more attention on the role of the respiratory muscles. It may frequently be easiest for a child to practice sounds arranged in the following order of difficulty: voiced plosives, voiced affricative, voiceless plosives, and voiceless affricative. Bilabials [p] and [b] that are highly visible provide excellent feedback because a child can look in the mirror and see how the lips are "helping" the respiratory muscles stop and start the airstream. The phonemes produced with a more open oral cavity (e.g., [t], [d], and [k], and [g] and finally [tʃ] and [d_3]) may therefore not be as easy as the bilabials are for some children. Clinicians may find it useful to experiment to see how the features of voicing and the place and manner of articulation affect each individual child's performance on tasks involving repetitions of individual phonemes. In this way, the most facilitating phonemes can be selected for the initial training of segmentation of exhalation.

Phonation

In the area of phonation, certain behaviors may also be facilitated by the selection of appropriate vowel and consonant combinations. One behavior focused on frequently in voice therapy is the onset of phonation. If, for example, a clinician is training a child to use a breathy initiation of phonation, the use of voiceless consonants may be extremely helpful in facilitating appropriate responses. We are familiar with the technique of teaching children to practice CV combinations involving [h] + vowel. Another technique (previously noted) involves the child's practice of smooth transitions from unvoiced to voiced continuants during a single exhalation. This allows the child to begin the flow of air during the voiceless phoneme and then to add voicing gradually. We have found the following combinations useful for teaching smooth transitions into voicing:

s‿z (feel the sound on your teeth)

f‿v (feel the sound on your lower lip)

θ‿ð (feel the sound on your tongue)

h‿m (feel the sound on both of your lips)

The choice of vowel sounds to be used to practice easy initiation of phonation at the syllable and word levels may also be an important consideration. Clinical experience suggests that the /e/, /i/, and /I/ monophthongs (as in "every," "easy," and "ink") seem particularly susceptible to hard attacks when they occur in the initial position of a stressed syllable in words. Because of this, it is often advantageous to begin practicing easy attacks, at the word level, on vowels such as /u/ (as in "ooze"). In general, it sometimes may be observed that the back vowels are more facilitating than the more forward vowels and the lax vowels easier than the tense vowels. With this in mind, the clinician may at times find it helpful to sequence practice materials in an order of difficulty similar to the sequence below:

1. u (ooze)
2. β (Austin)
3. ɜ (Ernest)
4. æ (aspirin)
5. e (any)
6. i (eel)
7. ɪ (it)

Sometimes it may be observed that diphthongs are easiest for a child who is practicing easy attacks on vowels, using the technique of "easing into the vowel" and "lingering" on it. At such times, the diphthong [oʊ] seems more facilitating, for example, than [eɪ]. A facilitating sequence of diphthongs might be similar to that below:

1. oʊ (old)
2. oɪ (oil)
3. aʊ (out)
4. eɪ (ate)

An arrangement of word pairs might then be presented in the following order:

hoe	oh
hoy	oy
how	ow
hay	eh

Selection of vowel sounds that are facilitating is not, of course, a consideration limited only to practice materials associated with the onset of phonation.

When strategies are designed to achieve goals related to quality, pitch, and loudness, the clinician may also need to consider how certain vowel sounds can be helpful in eliciting appropriate target products. For example, the high [i] frequently is used to elicit a high-pitched utterance. In addition to the acoustic characteristics of the vowel itself, words containing [i] vowels frequently evoke helpful associations. Consider words such as "cheep" and "shriek," for example. Similarly, the [ʌ] vowel, as in the word "bump," may facilitate the production of a low pitch. When loudness variations are being taught, a clinician may wish to contrast certain vowel and consonant sequences, such as those in "shush" and "bang," to capitalize on the onomatopoeic effect. The voiceless fricatives will be easier for the child to say softly, and the voiced consonants will lend themselves well to louder, more vigorous production.

If the focus of an activity is the smoothness of the vocal quality, practice materials should be chosen so that open, relaxed vowels are combined with continuant consonants. The liquid [l] is especially facilitating in this regard, as is the semivowel [w]. On the other hand, unvoiced plosives that require interruption in the continuation of the voicing may need to be avoided during early practice trials. Again, the manner and place of articulation need to be considered. Alveolar consonants (so that the movement of the tongue tip can be the focus of the child's attention) may be especially helpful for a child who is practicing avoidance of excessive laryngeal effort. The following word and sentence lists contain some combinations of sounds that facilitate smooth vocal production:

loom	vein	anvil
ruin	honey	mule
oily	oozing	winning
move	mowing	wailing

1. Lily loves lamb and veal every meal.
2. Oh, no, Julie, the oil is oozing away.
3. Now William loves mowing lawns.
4. Honey is flowing smoothly along.
5. Will Mervyn win more money?
6. Whale oil will ruin Merle's loom.
7. Row, row, smoothly over the wave.
8. Ewes, rams, and silken lambs.
9. Millie and Neville wave to Mommy.
10. Lovely smooth raven wings.

Resonance

It is traditional in voice therapy to segregate oral and nasal sounds in syllables, words, and sentences used to test and train children to use appropriate resonance patterns. For example, children who are hyponasal will practice materials loaded with nasal sounds.

1. No, no, not now—never!
2. *Never Say Never Again* may be a mystery movie.
3. My mouth moves more than Mary's mouth.
4. Moaning and groaning, mewing and meowing.
5. My mascot is Mickey Mouse.

Children who are hypernasal may need practice materials involving all oral sounds (and particularly vowels *other* than /i/ and /u/ on which nasality is most frequently perceived) in the initial stages of their therapy program.

1. Go, girl go, row, row, row!
2. Kick the ball over the wall.
3. Pick the apple, pick the pear.
4. The ditch is wide, adjust your stride.
5. Twitch, hop, plop, the rabbit has stopped.

The use of stimulus items involving alveolar consonants and forward vowel sounds emphasizes forward movement of the tongue when tongue retraction is a problem. Materials used to correct this problem might include sentences such as the following:

1. Pit-a-pat, what is that?
2. Eight fat cats sat by the rat.
3. "Itty Bitty," he's Bill's kitty.
4. "Tittle tattle," Betty chatters.
5. Therese baked pies with peas.

In cases of cul-de-sac resonance (or inappropriate tone focus) combinations of sounds that facilitate mouth opening and lip movement can be most helpful; for example, open vowels, rounded vowels, and bilabial and labiodental consonants.

1. Oh, no, Joe, don't go below.
2. One blue bottle plopped off the wall.
3. Two for you and two for Stu.
4. Ah, lady, show off the Barbie doll.
5. "Ahoy," shouted the ship's captain.

When resonance is weak, and a voice lacks sufficient richness and carrying power, chanting is frequently effective in creating a kinesthetic and auditory awareness of increased reverberation in the oral and nasal cavities. Chanting involves the prolongation of vowels and voiced continuant consonants. To maximize the awareness of the "sound carrying" consonants and to emphasize mouth opening and lip movement, practice materials should include a high frequency of continuant sounds that facilitate oral movement.

1. Maisie is marrying Vivian Withers.
2. Rosie revs the engine of the Mercedes-Benz.
3. Lions lying languidly in the zoo.
4. Come now, one and all, come!
5. "Amen" sing the boys as the organ plays.
6. Eve was living in the Garden of Eden.
7. Beams zoom towards the moon.
8. The treasure is golden coins, rubies, emeralds.
9. Hey Ho, Hey Ho, they all are dwarfs you know.
10. Vandals even live in the Virgin Islands.

In cases when children are mildly hypernasal and oral resonance needs to be increased to improve the oral–nasal balance, practice materials should highlight open vowels and voiced continuant consonants that facilitate oral movement, but nasal consonants may need to be avoided in early stages of training.

1. Buzz, buzz, buzz goes the busy fly.
2. Tra la, tra la, a gray and white galah (an Australian bird).
3. Zippidy doo dah, zippidy eh.
4. It is, of course, a lovely day.
5. Hey ho, hey ho, it's off to work we go.
6. "Toto, Toto," called Dorothy, "Where are you?"

The examples cited under the area of respiration, phonation, and resonance illustrate only a few of the ways that clinicians can use their knowledge of the articulation of speech sounds to enhance children's vocal behavior.

Improvement in vocal behavior usually occurs if the movement of specific articulators aids in (a) an awareness of the interrelationship of behaviors, (b) directing attention away from a part of the mechanism being used incorrectly, (c) opening or shaping the oral cavity, and (d) increasing forward tone focus and projection of voice.

Analysis, Self-Monitoring, and Evaluation of Progress

In voice therapy, we usually teach a child a perceptual framework and the descriptive language necessary for monitoring and evaluating behavior during the awareness phases of the program. As we enter the production phase, the child is then equipped with the self-regulating speech patterns (Pellegrini, 1982) that are helpful in mediating behavior. Freeman and Garstecki (1973) discussed the importance of children playing an active part in voice therapy. They demonstrated that children can participate successfully in the process of setting their own goals. When specific behaviors are clearly defined and children actively participate in describing the characteristics of behaviors from the outset, evaluation and self-monitoring are integral parts of the therapy throughout the production phase. Children's own descriptions of behaviors can be used to chart the evaluation sequence. As children progress through a series of self-evaluation activities, they can be encouraged to move from retrospective "after the fact" evaluation of their productions to simultaneous evaluation. Finally, they can arrive at an awareness of how the preparatory set for correct and incorrect products can be identified. This process can be helped by visual aids and charts that allow the progress across time to be concretely documented. In this way, children can be helped to understand where they are going and the intermediate steps along the way.

An example of how self-monitoring skills can be initiated early in the production phase is the way in which cues are explicitly stated during activities to elicit the target behavior. We know that we can stimulate a child to produce a target voice by evoking images that result in modifications of the vocal tract. We can also use many other cues and techniques as well as facilitating articulatory contexts. Whatever technique is most beneficial in eliciting a required response, the child will be helped if a concrete description of it is provided. This description then becomes part of his or her self-cuing and evaluation during subsequent practice.

1. Getting ready: It helps me if
   a. I take in plenty of air.
   b. I relax my neck and chin.
   c. I don't tense my shoulders.
   d. I open my mouth wide.
   e. I think of how it should sound.
   f. my teacher does it first.
2. Starting: It helps me if
   a. my teacher does it with me.
   b. my throat feels open.
   c. I think of honey flowing.
   d. I use an /h/ as the first sound.
   e. I lengthen the vowel.

In questioning a child concerning the characteristics of a response, it is important that the child is asked explicit questions. Vague questions such as "How was that?" and "Do you think that was okay?" are not likely to result in specific answers. It is preferable for the clinician to teach the child to evaluate performance in as concrete a way as is possible. Thus, the techniques used to cue the behavior can be used as a checklist to evaluate that behavior.

1. *Before* you started were you ready?
   Did you have plenty of air?
   Did you relax your neck and chin?
   Did you drop your shoulders?
   Did you think how you wanted to sound?
2. *When* you started what happened?
   Did you feel your throat open?
   Did you think of honey?
   Did you use an /h/?
   Did you lengthen the vowel?
3. What else could you have done to help?

The previous example illustrates the first step in the evaluation process: the identification and description of relevant aspects affecting production. The presence or absence of facilitating aspects are noted. The next step in the process frequently involves the child in a comparative task such as "Was that one better or worse than the last try? Why?" Repeated trials can also involve an element of evaluation. For example, "This time keep doing it until you are sure it is as good as you can make it." The use of audio- and videotape recordings is especially helpful for post hoc analysis of this kind. If videotape equipment is not available, peers in group therapy or mirrors can be used to provide feedback concerning the visual characteristics of the behaviors. The clinician should try not to be the sole evaluator of the behaviors. Independent written scoring of responses with subsequent comparison of the clinician and students' evaluations is a technique that is especially useful in encouraging children to assume responsibility for judging their own productions. When judgments differ, the tape recordings can be replayed and discussed and reasons for discrepancies identified. Evaluation is an active process in which the child is a full and responsible participant, throughout the phases of therapy. But it is during the carryover phase of therapy that the effect of an earlier emphasis on analysis and self-evaluation is most striking. Children who are already comfortable and experienced in analyzing and judging their own behavior seem more likely to demonstrate rapid improvement during the carryover phase of therapy.

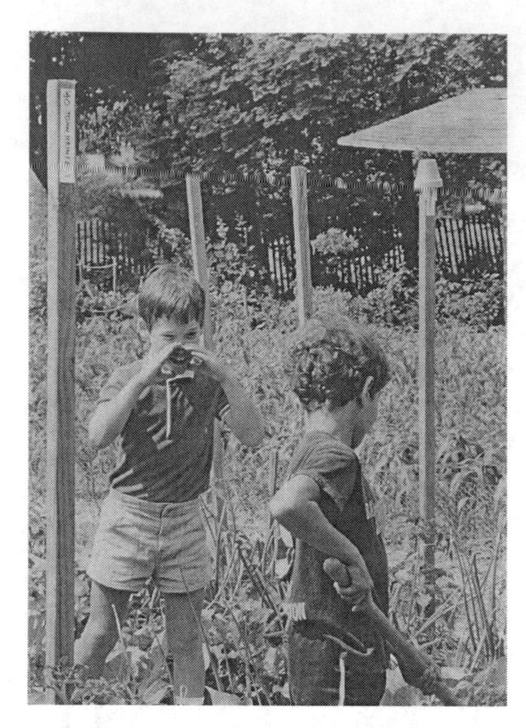

Carryover activities include examples of situations relevant to the child's own lifestyle and interests.

Carryover Phase

During the carryover phase, we teach the child to habituate the target behaviors for increasing lengths of time in increasingly complex interactions.

Teacher's Goals

1. To design a repertoire of rehearsal and practice activities analogous to those encountered in the child's everyday life (e.g., home, school, recreation)
2. To provide a framework for the child to practice analysis and evaluation of voice use in relation to specific situational and interpersonal demands
3. To teach the child to accept responsibility for self-monitoring and evaluation
4. To develop a hierarchy of practice assignments (to be completed outside of therapy) that is meaningful to the child and allows for documentation of progress
5. To provide feedback and reinforcement of the child's vocal behaviors and insights

Child's Objectives

1. I can describe the times in my everyday life when it is hardest/easiest for me to use/maintain my target behaviors:
   a. emotional state
   b. size of group
   c. specific people I know
   d. type of activity
   e. time of day
   f. location of the talking
   g. background noise
   h. physical state
2. I can role play correct vocal behavior (in the therapy room) simulating situations I identify as difficult:
   a. for short interactions
   b. for longer interactions
   c. with the clinician (one-to-one)
   d. with others present (small group)
3. I can analyze my vocal behavior during role playing:
   a. anticipating problems in advance
   b. evaluating behavior after the event
   c. self-correcting during the role playing
4. I can help design easy practice experiences to be completed outside the therapy room:
   a. short duration (e.g., automatic response, asking directions)
   b. neutral emotional contexts
   c. with strangers
   d. with supportive listeners
5. I can keep data concerning my easy experiences and analyze factors affecting my vocal behavior:

a. anecdotal records
b. checklists
c. logs
d. charts

6. I can help design difficult practice experiences to be completed outside the therapy room:
   a. longer duration
   b. competing background noise
   c. larger groups
   d. more demanding listeners
   e. more challenging locations
   f. stressful contexts
   g. when I'm not feeling good
7. I can organize and interpret data concerning difficult interactions and analyze factors affecting my vocal behavior:
   a. generalizations drawn from experiences
   b. coping strategies for specific problems and situations
   c. reinforcement for self (strengths and liabilities) (e.g., "Give yourself a pat on the back")
8. I can accept the help of supportive individuals in monitoring my spontaneous vocal behavior:
   a. my classroom teacher
   b. peers
   c. family members
9. I can adjust my own behavior based on the evaluations of supportive listeners.
10. I can monitor and adjust my behavior without external support.

Teaching Self-Reliance

Throughout voice therapy, it is important to be specific in noting the characteristics of correct responses when reinforcing the child's efforts. When the clinician follows a good evaluation, with a brief explanation of why the behavior was correct, it helps the child focus on the pertinent aspects. For example, "Good, none of the air came out of your nose that time," or, "That's right, you opened your mouth really wide." Sometimes the clinician will describe his or her reactions to the response. An example of this is, "I really like that easy, smooth voice. I feel calm when you use that voice."

It is important also to note feelings and personality characteristics when evaluating children's work in therapy. When we comment on our own feelings of enjoyment or satisfaction arising from our interaction with the child, we enhance his or her self-esteem; for example, "I always enjoy working with you because you don't let problems get you down," or, "You listen so well to my instructions, no wonder you got all of the sentences correct today," or, "One thing I really admire about you is the way you keep trying no matter how hard the task is." Our expressions of confidence in children and in their strengths can help them internalize positive feelings about their part in the therapy process. By our verbal descriptions of the child's predications, insights, and attitudes, we can help significantly in the development of confidence and reinforce feelings of self-worth.

As we progress through the carryover phase of therapy, it is often helpful to state our expectations, not only in terms of the child's achievement of target behaviors but also in terms of his or her feelings and self-evaluations. Our aim in doing this is to encourage the child to rely less and less on others' evaluations. For example, we might say, "Give yourself a pat on the back because you remembered to use your new voice. Isn't it a good feeling to know you remembered all by yourself?" or, "I'm proud of the way you don't need me to remind you to take replenishing breaths now," or, "Although it's always nice when someone else notices how well you're doing, that's not really the main thing. When you know it's right and feel good about it yourself—that's what really counts, isn't it?"

In setting assignments for children to complete outside the therapy room it is often helpful if we include in our instructions some statement concerning our expectations, for example, "Now you might get discouraged if the first time you try this, it doesn't work out. But knowing you, I bet you'll not let that stop you from trying it again." In addition, a positive attitude on the part of the clinician can help children learn to describe their mistakes and failures as opportunities rather than setbacks. For example, "It's a good thing you tried out your new voice in that situation. Now we know the kinds of situations we need to practice today. You'll be ready for it next time." Although we need to code children's experiences in terms that stress the positive aspects, that is not to say that we should avoid discussing the negative aspects at all. We strive to create a climate in therapy in which children can be open and realistic. We need to accept and not discount their feelings of frustration and anxiety in relation to performance on certain assignments. Telling a child, "Don't worry about it," or, "It doesn't matter," may cause the child to feel "put down." It is usually advisable to acknowledge the feelings first, so that the child feels understood, before rushing in with suggestions or advice. A useful strategy is to ask questions to help the child arrive at solutions that are his or her own. For example, "I can imagine how embarrassing that was when your pitch sounded so high in front of the whole class" (acknowledgment of the feeling). "What do you think you could have done differently?" (question focused on child's ability to solve problems). "Is there any other assignment you'd feel more comfortable trying?" (question focused on child's part in planning).

The carryover phase of therapy presents many opportunities for the clinician to teach children to acknowledge and enjoy the rewards of "being one's own person," learning from mistakes and savoring the satisfaction of knowing they can, by themselves, use their own voice the way they want to.

Summary

We have discussed some general principles underlying the preparation of programs for voice therapy. It can be seen that in many respects, planning a voice therapy program is much like planning any other therapy program (see Worksheet 11–1). There are some important differences, however. One is the need to orient the child to the area on which he or she will work and to prepare him or her to deal with the prerequisite concepts and terminology needed during the production phase. We have seen how this can be accomplished during the general awareness phase. Another involves the need to specify the relevant behaviors and their characteristics as concretely as possible. We have reviewed some ways in which this can be dealt with during the specific awareness phase.

It may well be that the ultimate success of an entire voice therapy program for a young child depends significantly on the success achieved in the awareness phases. This is because the understanding and motivation developed during the awareness phases can accelerate progress through subsequent phases. In our discussion of the production phase, examples to illustrate how facilitating materials can be selected to enhance correct responses are provided. We also noted the integral part played by the child's own analysis, self-monitoring, and evaluation of performance. In our sequence outlining the carryover phase, ideas are provided for the gradual removal of external support as the new behaviors are habituated.

Worksheet 11–1. Progress in Self-Evaluation

Child's name __________ **School** __________

Target behavior __________ **Semester and year** __________

I am a careful judge	**Date**
I know when it is right	________
—some of the time	
—most of the time	
—all of the time	
I am able to explain why it is right	________
—some of the time	
—most of the time	
—all of the time	
I know what goes wrong	________
—when my teacher explains why	
—as soon as I've done it	
—while I am doing it	
—as I'm getting ready to start	
—most of the time	
—all of the time	
I can list when I have difficulty	________
—situations	
—types of listeners	
—feelings	
—time of day	
—physical state	
I feel good about my efforts	________
—when my teacher praises me	
—as soon as I've done it	
—while I am doing it	
—as I'm getting ready to start	
—most of the time	
—all of the time	

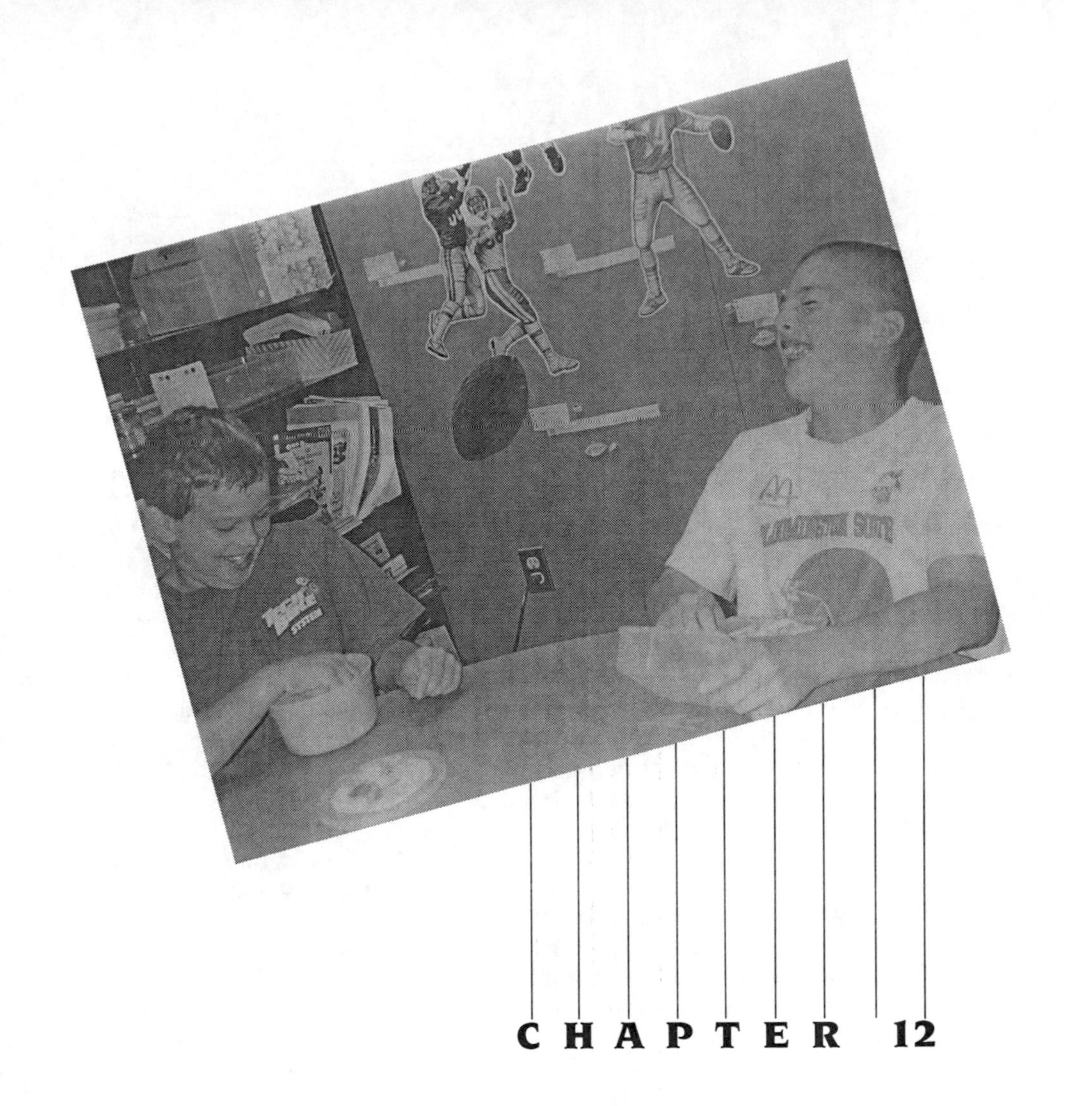

CHAPTER 12

Sequential and Gestalt Approaches to Treatment

In this chapter, we move to a consideration of treatment approaches for children that address a variety of voice problems. Although each child's problem is unique and must be assessed individually, some negative vocal behaviors cluster together. Some are the result of an imperfect mechanism. Others stem from a child's attempts to adjust to short-term or chronic medical conditions or from congenital or acquired structural deviations. Still others may be learned behaviors or manifestations of psychological states.

The approaches presented fall into two categories: Sequential (approaches 1–6) and Gestalt (approaches 7–9). Each approach includes a brief history of the child or children involved, a detailing of the therapeutic goals, and illustrative sample strategies for treatment procedures. These sample strategies are not complete in their presentations; rather, they highlight different aspects of the therapeutic process in each of the plans. They are designed to provide a practical perspective to clinicians engaged in designing individualized programs for children.

At the end of the book, Appendix B contains worksheets we have found useful when working with children.

Treatment Approach 1: Increasing Available Vocal Options

There are many different causes of voice disorders; however, some clusters of symptoms are frequently observed. One such cluster is reduced vocal variety. Cognitive, neurological, and affective constraints can limit a child's learning of appropriate suprasegmental features. Children who have sensory deficits, such as hearing impairment, frequently use limited variation in their voices because their auditory monitoring contributes to imperfect learning. Even children with normal mechanisms sometimes need to be taught how to vary their voices more appropriately. When children habituate only one strategy (such as getting louder) or maladaptive behaviors to get and hold attention, they need help in acquiring a more suitable repertoire of techniques. Thus, we can see that learning about the options that are available to vary the voice can be an important aspect of remediation for children exhibiting problems stemming from many different etiologies.

In the case history that follows, we describe three children who were treated together because they exhibited similar negative behaviors. The causative factors, however, were not similar. The group approach proved to be useful because the children enjoyed the interaction and the stimulation, modeling, and evaluation opportunities implicit in the group activities.

Kurt, Hans, and Brendan: Reduced Vocal Variety

The group consisted of three young boys, all approximately 9 years old. Kurt, a vocal abuser, used an excessively loud habitual level, and his attempts to vary his voice consisted of loudness increases. Hans was diagnosed as "speaking in a monotone," a problem that seemed to be a learned behavior because both of his parents were profoundly deaf. Although Hans himself had normal hearing, he seemed to have habituated some of the characteristics of his parents' speech patterns. Brendan exhibited a mild-to-moderate, high-frequency, bilateral hearing loss.

All three boys were stimulable during their initial assessment period. They were intrigued by the visual feedback provided by the Kay Elemetrics Visi-Pitch, which enabled them to see a representation of their voices on the oscilloscope screen. It was decided to use a therapy approach that relied heavily on associating visual patterns with auditory and proprioceptive feedback. In addition, all associations were coded verbally in simple, concrete language. The boys responded well to the idea that they were going to learn how to "make pictures with their voices." They continued as a group for 1 year, and all made excellent progress on this part of their remediation program. At the end of that time, Hans was dismissed from therapy, and Kurt and Brendan continued to work in individual therapy on additional aspects of their vocal behavior.

Goals

The clinician noted from diagnostic information that the three boys exhibited similar negative vocal behaviors. These included

1. Limited use of pitch variation
2. Limited use of loudness variation
3. Limited use of durational changes
4. Limited ability to describe vocal strategies to express meanings and feelings.

She accordingly decided to address the boys' awareness and use of pitch, loudness, and durational changes in their voices to reflect meanings and feelings. Her three basic goals were to help the boys identify "picture words" in phrases and sentences (nouns, verbs, adjectives, adverbs); to describe vocal techniques to "make pictures" with their voices; and to use vocal techniques to vary pitch, loudness, and duration.

Sample Strategies

Pitch Changes. We know that we can make pictures with our hands. Watch while I draw a bow and arrow. I'll draw the arrow shooting up into the sky. Now I'll draw the arrow falling down to the ground. But did you know that we can also make pictures with our voices? Watch the Visi-Pitch screen while I say the word "arrow." I'll make it go up.

Now I'll make it go down.

Rate Changes. Words can be stretched out. Watch while I write "pull." Now I'll say it, and you can see how long the word looks on the Visi-Pitch screen. Now I'll say "push"—that was a long push. You put your hands on the edge of the table and give a long, hard push, as if you were pushing a car that wouldn't go, while I say the word. Sometimes a "push" and a "pull" can be quick and short. You give a quick push on the table edge, and I'll say the word quickly.

A group of words can also be said quickly or slowly to help the listener get a picture in their mind. Listen to these:

horses gallop   cars race

worms crawl   the tortoise is slow

We can also stop before or after a word to make it important.

Darth Vader . . . arrives!

Ladies and Gentlemen . . . the President of the . . . United States

Loudness Changes. We know about making our voices loud. That is fairly easy to do, for example, "a loud *bang*!" But some people think that getting louder is the only thing you can do to make interesting voice pictures. Some of the best voice pictures are made when we make our voices soft. Listen to these words. I'll say them loudly and softly.

soft and squishy

stroke the kitten's fur

Now let's talk about how they sound best. Why?

Voice Pictures. Let's choose some words that make great voice pictures. The best words are those that make us see the picture in our minds. I'll say some words in special ways, and you tell me what you saw in your mind as I said each one. Close your eyes.

fly (upward inflection)	zoom (downward inflection)
creaky (long duration)	purr (softly)
trot (short duration)	out (loudly, as when calling at a ballgame)
twitch (short duration)	

Look at this ladder. I'll draw a boy on top—he's high up—and one on the bottom—he's down low. When I say the word "boy," you point to the one I am thinking of. I'll say "boy" in a high voice and in a low voice.

Now look at these pictures of a giant and a dwarf. They are both called Fred. The giant is big and has a low voice. The dwarf is little and has a high voice. When I say "Fred," you point to the one I am thinking of. My voice picture will let you know which one it is. I could also show you who I am thinking of by making my voice loud for the giant and soft for the dwarf. Listen while I use this different kind of voice picture. Point to the one I am thinking of as I say "Fred" loudly or softly.

Voice pictures can be made lots of different ways. Voice pictures make the words we say more interesting. We can say words high or low, loudly or softly, slowly (stretching them out) or quickly. We can also stop before a word to make the listener know it is important. Here are some cards with pictures of high-low and loud-soft, long-short and a stop sign. Pick the card that matches the word picture I use (loud and soft can be depicted by a large and small drum being struck or by a listener reacting by cupping an ear or holding both hands over ears; long and short can be shown by lines of contrasting lengths):

giant	quickly	lightning	grab
dwarf	rushing	stretch	reach
fat	lazy	scrunch	twinkle
huge	drop	crash	chirp
little	hole	splash	hiss
sharp	jump	shiver	dark
thick	plop	dive	light
slowly	dungeon		

It's a / spaceship	I hate / oysters
She's / bizarre	No, don't / please
Thank / you	A / new one
A / chocolate egg	A / liar and a cheat

Describe as many different ways as you can how the same word may be said, for example, "The boy jumped." Was it a high jump, a low jump, or a broad jump? "The car went by." Was it a racing car or a slow car? Let's try to think of all the different ways that "The car went by" might be said: As a question (Are you sure?), as a fact (Don't argue with me), telling where (It went *by*), telling it's gone (It *went* by), telling it was definitely a car and not a truck (The *car* went by), telling it was special (*The* car went by).

Choosing the word in the sentence to make the picture word is fun. It can change the meaning of the whole sentence. We can also choose more than one picture word sometimes. Or we can let our voices be a picture of our feelings for all of the words in the sentence. Listen while I say some words and tell me if I'm feeling pleased or upset.

"Oh, what a day!"

"I'll come now."

"That's my test."

I have some pictures and words written on these cards. Choose a card and decide whether you want to say it in a high or low voice. Then do it and let me guess which one you tried to do.

Here are some words with arrows beside them. Some of the arrows point down and some point up. Slide your voice on the word. Make it go the same way the arrow goes. Listen while I do one first.

Here is a rebus story. Every time you read a picture you must make a picture of that word with your voice.

Here are some words that are easy to let our feelings out on. Can you think of some more and show us how you say them?

Yuk!	Not me!
cool	No way!
disgusting	I forgot
Oh, no	That's mine
You think you're smart.	awesome

I'll be a "listening mirror," and after you say it, I'll tell you what I think you were feeling.

Let's read from your reading book. Use a voice picture in every sentence.

Treatment Approach 2: Giving Production Goals Initial Priority

Occasionally we encounter a child who has a severely altered mechanism. When these alterations are permanent, we need to teach the child to adapt to the changed state, to avoid acquiring maladaptive compensations, and to deal with the interpersonal problems associated with having to adjust to being different from the peer group. We have said earlier that clinicians need to be cognizant of a child's medical history and to coordinate their intervention program with the other professionals involved in the treatment. In the case below, the importance of the child's medical history is especially apparent, since he had a tracheostomy.

The approach in therapy was one that immediately focused on production goals. In our previous discussions, we have consistently stressed the importance of beginning therapy with awareness goals. In the case of a child such as Jonathan, however, where an altered mechanism necessitated the learning of very individualized new behaviors, the most pressing need was that he practice new behaviors. Learning theorists might call this approach "behavioristic." As the new behaviors were habituated, the child was then able to gain insight into the reasons why the new behaviors were effective. In cases of a radically and noticeably different mechanism the child comes to therapy aware that he is different and that he has a problem. We need quickly to demonstrate to him that he can be helped. Thus, we immediately zero in on showing him what to do and how to do it.

Jonathan: Adaptation to a Permanent Tracheostomy Tube

Jonathan was referred to the speech–language clinician by his third-grade teacher. He had never received therapy and had been plagued throughout his life with severe respiratory tract problems. His physician had hoped that as Jonathan grew older his trach tube could be removed. Now, however, Jonathan's breathing difficulties, caused by the excessive production of secretions in the tract, would necessitate the presence of a stoma for some time because regular suction was needed to clear the airway. Until this point, the parents had focused primarily on his health problem, but Jonathan's disruptive behavior in class, the teacher's concern about his communication difficulties, and the physician's assessment that this condition would continue for some time led them to agree that some therapy might be valuable. During the case conference, the parents were cooperative; they agreed to work with school personnel to help Jonathan cope in school. The teacher reported that she was anxious about Jonathan's health because she had never before had a child in her class with "a hole in his neck." She said that Jonathan "made strange noises" through his stoma and that she wasn't sure whether he did it on purpose. The speech–language clinician evaluated Jonathan, consulted with his physician and the school psychologist, and observed him in class. The physician suggested the use of a Passy-Muir speaking valve as the best option for Jonathan and the clinician agreed with this recommendation. However, for some reason the parents were adamantly opposed to this alternative and could not be convinced to let Jonathan try the device even though it was explained to them that finger closure was a less sanitary as well as less effective method for Jonathan to use during speech.

It soon became clear that Jonathan was anxious and confused about his altered mechanism; like his parents, he had believed the problem was temporary. Now he was frightened by the prospect of "having the opening forever." He was embarrassed about being "freakish," and he compensated by clowning and making wheezing noises at inappropriate times to get his classmates to laugh. Only brief explanations had been given to him about the purpose of the opening, and no one had systematically worked with him to teach him how to coordinate using his finger to close the stoma with exhalation for speech. As a result, he intermittently tried to talk on both inhaled and exhaled air, used hyperfunctional behaviors to talk louder, and was inefficient at using his finger to close the stoma and reduce the noise of air leakage through it. His disruptive behavior seemed related partly to his lack of skill in using his altered mechanism and partly to a compensatory attempt to gain attention.

Jonathan needed help in all areas of vocal behavior. Because he was anxious and self-conscious about his vocal efforts, however, the clinician moved quickly to teach him production of more appropriate respiratory, phonatory, and resonance behaviors in the hope that some initial success at controlling his voice output would help Jonathan develop confidence and would build trust in the therapeutic relationship. This initial targeting of improved production in the areas of respiration, phonation, and resonance proved helpful. Later, as Jonathan developed a sense of control and his random unpredictable phonatory behaviors decreased, the interpersonal aspects of his behavior were emphasized more and more in therapy.

Goals

The clinician noted that Jonathan's negative vocal behavior could be grouped into four categories:

1. Respiration
   a. Lack of coordination of use of finger to close stoma and exhalation phase for voicing
2. Phonation
   a. Attempts to phonate on inspiration
   b. Attempts to phonate when stoma not closed during exhalation
   c. Voluntary and involuntary stoma noise
   d. Hyperfunctional muscle tone during phonatory activity (to compensate for inefficient use of airstream)
3. Resonance and Articulation
   a. Minimal use of supraglottal activity to amplify tone
   b. Minimal articulatory effort
4. Interpersonal Factors
   a. Attempts to gain attention and bolster self-esteem by maladaptive behaviors
   b. Attempts to "cover up" embarrassment of involuntary sounds activity by pretending it was intentional
   c. Avoidance of talking situations or distracting "acting out" because of fears of ability to control voicing appropriately

d. Confusion and fear about nature of handicap, its permanence, and others' reactions to it

Jonathan needed to achieve a better understanding of the trach tube and of his mechanism. He needed to become aware of his distracting behavior in class and of the effect this had on both himself and his classmates. The clinician felt that if she could show him more appropriate ways of coping with his differences, Jonathan would feel in control of himself and of his effect on others.

The clinician's first goal was to teach Jonathan the key concepts concerning the use of his airstream and to help him coordinate using his finger to close the stoma with exhaling to speak. It was important to monitor closely his correct and incorrect behaviors.

Once Jonathan understood these basic concepts of *respiration,* the clinician could begin to teach him easy, relaxed *phonation* during exhalation.

The next step would be to teach Jonathan increased *resonance* in supraglottal cavities and improved *articulatory* precision.

As Jonathan became technically more adept, the clinician would begin to address his interpersonal difficulties, helping him to verbalize the effects of his contrasting patterns of behavior on himself and others. She would help him devise strategies to eliminate the "old" behaviors and adopt more appropriate patterns of interacting.

Sample Strategies

Respiration. Look at these pictures. The air comes from your lungs and can go two ways. It can go straight out of your stoma or it can go up your throat, through your vocal folds, and out of your mouth or nose. When you want to use the air for talking, you must be sure to take a deep breath first. Then, as you let the air out, you cover the stoma with your finger. You must be sure the stoma is completely covered.

On these diagrams I want you to draw lines to show which way the air should go when you breathe in, when you breathe out and don't want to talk, or when you want to use the air for talking. Now tell me where your finger should be when you breathe out and don't want to talk (finger away from stoma) and when you breathe out for talking (finger on stoma).

Let's think of some rules:

Always remember to wash your hands after you go to the bathroom, after recess, or if they get dirty.

Always talk as the air is going out.

Never talk when you are breathing in.

When you want to talk, cover the stoma with your finger.

When you need more air, open the stoma (move finger).

Make sure your finger completely covers the stoma (no leakage of air).

Keep your neck and shoulders relaxed.

Phonation. When you get ready to talk you must remember to:

Take in plenty of air.

Put your finger on the stoma before you start to breathe out.

Keep your throat relaxed.

Begin the sound gently.

Let's practice some long easy sounds, like this: /ha/. Keep it going as long as your air lasts. I'll say, "Get ready," and then, "Go." When I say, "Get ready," breathe in and have your finger near the stoma. When I say, "Go," close the stoma, breathe out, and make the easy voice as the air vibrates your folds gently. The airstream, your finger, and your vocal folds are a team—they all work together.

Now let's practice stopping and starting the sound during the time the air is coming out. We'll do it in only one breath.

ha—ha—ha (gradually increase number)
Let's see how many you can do in one breath.

Now I want you to use that same easy sound saying, "Hey." Let's practice it. This time I want you to be ready to say it whenever I stop talking. Like this:

"I saw Joe and I called to him, 'Hey.'"

"Cats like milk, but horses like . . . 'hay.'"

"I said [hey!] when the boy knocked into me. He did it again, so I said [hey!] again. Because I said [hey!] he stopped it."

Resonance and Articulation. You can use your lips to do some of the work for you. Let's practice prolonging [h m m m]. Feel the vibrations on your face. Make your lips tickle. "Hum" is a good word because the [h] helps get the air started and the [m] helps you get lots of extra sound vibrating on the bones of your face and teeth. Hear how strong and rich the sound is.

Hum mm my

Hum mm me

Hum mm moo

Keep the sound going as you link the words:

Hum—my name

Hum—my mom

Hum—me me

Let's pretend we are a strange chiming clock:

Hum—bong—bong

bong—bong—bong—bong [different pitches]

bing—bong—ding—dong [move lips well]

Let's alternate the chimes; I'll do one, and then you do one (match pitch and length).

Interpersonal. Let's think about some reasons why people talk:

To ask for things they want

To share their feelings or let off steam

To make friends

To have fun

To show how much they know

Can you think of some reasons why people sometimes choose *not* to talk?

When they don't know something

When they want to listen

When they are afraid they'll sound funny or different

When they are embarrassed

When they are angry or sulking

When they don't want to

When others make fun of them

Nobody likes to feel embarrassed or to have their feelings hurt. Most people like to feel respected and understood. What are some things that make people feel others understand them?

When others listen to them

When others don't name-call

When others don't purposely hurt them, their body, their feelings, their things

When others notice good things they do or say

What can people do to help others understand them better?

Tell them about themselves: what they like, what they want, and how they feel

Tell them to stop doing things they don't like

Explain things about themselves that are special

Stop pretending things

Listen to this story about a boy called Jay. Jay fell off his bike and knocked out his two front teeth. They were not his baby teeth, but his permanent ones. His mother was very upset because now Jay had a big gap in his mouth. Jay was upset, too, because the dentist said it would be a long time before he could fix it so that Jay had teeth in front again. He looked funny when he smiled, and when he talked, some of the words sounded strange. Jay was embarrassed and tried to keep his mouth closed and not talk much at first. He felt very bad about it but tried to hide his feelings from the other children, who, of course, didn't know how he felt inside. One girl in his class was mean to him and laughed at how he looked. Instead of telling her to quit it or ignoring her until she got tired of it, Jay made a face at her. He stuck his tongue through the gap in his teeth, pulled down his lower eyelids, and screwed up his face like a monster. The girl shrieked and yelled, "The toothless monster!" Jay kept on doing monster faces a lot after that. He always got a reaction of some kind when he did it. But he often felt bad inside. Although he wished people would notice him, being called "monster mouth" all the time didn't help him feel respected. But he kept doing it anyway.

1. What did Jay do to deal with his sadness about the way he looked?
2. What did he do about helping others understand his problem?
3. Did it work?
4. What else could he have done?
5. What would have made him feel better?

Let's redo this story. Let's pretend Jay decided to choose a different way of handling his problem. He could have done some of these things:

1. Tell the teacher about his problem and ask her to tell the class.
2. Explain to his friends that he felt bad about his teeth but was trying not to worry about it too much.
3. Decide not to let other people make him do stupid things.
4. Decide "sticks and stones can break my bones but words can never hurt me."
5. Tell the girl that he had had an accident, and it surprised him that she felt like laughing.
6. Ignore the girl (which was what she wouldn't want).

Remember, the way people choose to handle things that happen to them affects how others understand them and how others act toward them. It also affects how they feel about themselves: if they are hiding their real feelings or if they can explain. If they can explain their feelings, then others often forget it more quickly.

Some ways that people can explain about things are to say:

1. "Look, this is different but this is how I handle it—it's no big deal."
2. "Would you like me to tell you what happened? It is interesting to learn about things like this."
3. "I know you are giggling because you're embarrassed, but that's okay, I understand your feelings. I used to feel embarrassed about it, too."

What other ways are there to cope? Think of what would work best for someone like Jay.

1. Walk away.
2. Look someone right in the eyes and say, "That's a mean thing to do."
3. Talk over the problem with an adult.

I'm asking you for some suggestions because I know you've had a lot of experience in coping with the problem of having the trach tube in your neck. What have been the hardest things for you to deal with? What has worked best for you? What has not worked well? Can you help me make up a list of suggestions for other children who have this problem?

Learning New Compensatory Behaviors

1. I can demonstrate (at will) the "old" way of using voice-distracting associated behaviors.
2. I can describe how it looks and sounds to others.
3. I can describe how it feels to me.
4. I can describe why it doesn't work well for me.
5. I can demonstrate new ways of talking
   a. with a model, cues, and instructions.
   b. with cues and instructions.
   c. with instructions.
   d. at will some of the time.
   e. at will most of the time.
6. I can eliminate distracting associated behaviors
   a. with a model, cues, and instructions.
   b. with cues and instructions.
   c. with instructions.
   d. sometimes.
   e. often.
   f. always.
7. I can explain the rules of good voice use.
8. I can use my new voice/patterns of behavior
   a. when I'm in the speech room.
   b. when I'm in the classroom.
   c. when I'm on the playground.
   d. when I'm at home.
   e. when I'm calm and think about it.
   f. when I'm excited.
   g. when I want to (usually).
   h. when I want to (always).
9. I can explain the effects of the old and new patterns
   a. on myself.
   b. on others.
   c. on getting what I want.
10. I can analyze a situation (and change what I'm doing)
   a. after it has happened.
   b. while it is occurring.
   c. before it occurs.

Treatment Approach 3: Associating Semantic Dictates With Respiratory Control

With all children, but with older children especially, it is usually efficacious to present a logical rationale that helps them understand the precise reasons for the needed changes in their behavior. This is particularly so in cases where there are a number of subtle differences that together contribute to an unusual pattern of voice use. At such times, motivation can be enhanced by associating, or making explicit connections between, relevant aspects of the behavior and specific effects on the listener. In many cases, we can tie together a group of important supporting behaviors and show their effect on the message that is transmitted. A listener's ability to comprehend what is said is a key concept to which children can readily relate. When we begin with an explicit need (i.e., helping listeners understand our thoughts) and then proceed to demonstrate how what we do helps us achieve this, the therapy seems more relevant to the child. In the case study that follows, the clinician could have merely told the child she needed to improve her breathing. Nonetheless, the clinician decided to approach treatment by creating an awareness of the way the durational characteristics of the voice pattern shape the way others perceive the meaning. Once this was achieved, the child developed considerable interest in shaping respiratory behavior in response to semantic demands.

Donna: Uneven Voicing Related to Respiratory Inefficiency

Donna was 10 years 7 months and was enrolled in the fifth grade. She had received speech therapy for misarticulation of sibilant consonants and had made good progress with her sounds. Her voice pattern seemed inappropriate, however; it was characterized by poor phrasing and erratic rate changes that seemed unrelated to the meaning. The clinician hypothesized that the inappropriate timing of pauses and the resultant lack of smoothness in voicing during connected utterances were related to inconsistent respiratory support during connected speech. Donna could sustain vowel sounds for approximately 12 seconds on repeated trials. During her reading of a paragraph, however, the clinician noted that phrases were usually approximately two to three words in length and that volume consistently faded at the ends of sentences. Her spontaneous speech sounded sporadic and jerky, and the listener was left with an impression of a pattern of voicing that seemed disorganized. Diadochokinetic rates were within normal limits, and there was no indication of neurologic involvement.

Goals

Donna was an excellent reader. The clinician designed a therapy to capitalize on this skill and also to coordinate with classroom activities. Her classroom teacher was cooperative and agreed to help Donna practice her new behaviors daily in the course of classroom activities. She also gave Donna opportunities to share with others in her reading group some of the new information she learned in therapy.

The clinician made a list of Donna's negative vocal behaviors:

1. Insufficient depth of initial inhalation
2. Inadequate "chunking" of exhaled air during connected utterance
3. Inappropriate use of replenishing breaths
4. Frequent and inappropriate pauses between word groups
5. Pauses not used to reflect meaning
6. Inappropriate variation of rate
7. Voice faded at end of sentences

The three general targets during the treatment would be for Donna to verbalize the relationship between durational changes and the transmission of meaning and feeling, to demonstrate appropriate breath support for connected utterances, and to use appropriate durational patterns during voice production. It was important that Donna first learn to identify appropriate and inappropriate durational changes during reading and connected speech, so that she could then use breathing and voicing patterns to convey meaning and feeling more effectively.

Sample Strategies

Let's look at this sentence and find ways that the words can be grouped to suggest different meanings: "Oh George Henry said Mary is not interested." Let's punctuate it.

"Oh, George Henry said Mary is not interested."

"Oh George, Henry said Mary is not interested."

"Oh George Henry," said Mary, "is not interested."

Where we choose to pause changes the meaning.

Sometimes we pause before and after a parenthetical statement, one that is not absolutely essential to the sentence but adds extra information. Make slashes to separate the parenthetical parts of the sentences from the rest of the sentence. After you have marked the page, we'll put my transparency over it and see if our slashes agree.

1. Mary / she is Bill's cousin / was bridesmaid at the wedding.
2. Uncle Dick / who must be at least one hundred years old / is a millionaire.
3. On Tuesday I'll know if I passed the test the hardest one I've ever done.
4. I own my very own horse a bay mare with a white blaze.
5. Last winter Dad and I went ice fishing something I'd certainly like to do again.
6. One day Mom and I visited an art gallery not too far from here in a quaint old building.
7. Betty Josephine and Deborah will live in Washington one of the most interesting cities in the USA.
8. By Tuesday June 30th I'll be told if I'm going to Chicago the windy city capital of Illinois.
9. Glenda an excellent typist loves to ski and is very good at it.
10. Allen and Paul both tall for their age are friends of mine but not really close friends.

As well as using pauses to show the meaning, we sometimes say some parts of sentences faster or slower than other parts. Sometimes we say the essential part of the sentence slower to be sure the listener gets the main idea, then the extra information is said faster because it's not as critical.

Let's take two colored magic markers and underline parts of the sentences above. Use one color for important parts to be said slowly and the other color for extra pieces of information that can be said more quickly.

The meaning of the words also helps us decide whether to say them fast or slow. Underline word groups in the following sentences that could be lengthened or shortened to suggest the meaning.

1. Jill is as slow as molasses.
2. My new Trans Am can go ninety miles an hour.
3. The farmer plodded behind his plow.
4. Mom said that getting my brother to do the dishes is like pulling teeth.
5. "I'll get you for that," said the boy, suddenly darting across the room.
6. The car sped by, and then all was still.

Feelings also can be expressed by using pauses and rate changes. Think of different feelings for these words. Say how a rate change, a pause, or both could change the feeling.

"Oh it's you is it."

"No I won't and you can't make me."

"I wonder if she knows we saw her do it."

Listen while I read these sentences from your reading book, and you tell me where I used pauses and rate changes and why I said them the way I did. How could I have said them differently?

Sometimes groups of words have to be said together to make the meaning clear. Take, for example, "Rae, she is my best friend, is very pretty." There are five words together that must be said in one breath. Let's practice taking in plenty of air and counting to five so we get used to making the breath last for five words. Don't run out before the end. Now say a b c d e in one breath. Now, "She is my best friend." Do you think you could stretch the breath long enough to say, "Rae, she is my best friend"?

Sometimes we can add to our air supply as we go along. We take a deep breath to start and then little "catch breaths" at pauses. Let's try taking a "catch breath" after "friend" and then finishing the whole sentence. Remember "catch breaths" must be quick so that the smoothness of the sentence is not interrupted. Mark places for "catch breaths" in the sentences in this book.

Smoothness is also very important, especially if a mood or feeling would be changed if our speech was jerky. Practice smooth pauses and phrases in the sentences that follow. Mark the pauses first.

1. Slowly and silently the river flows to the deep blue ocean.
2. Without a sound or even a flicker of recognition the man glided by them all.
3. In her dreams she floated gently away up up and over the tree tops to be gone forever from the earth.

Quotation marks show us the direct speech, and after it we must pause long enough so the listener knows where the quote ends. Sometimes it helps to change our voice after a pause to signal to the listener that a different person is speaking. Mark the breath pauses in the passage in this book and practice reading the paragraph so the meaning and feeling comes through clearly. Let's record your reading and play it back.

Did you take in plenty of air to start?

Did you make the air last for the whole group of words?

Did you let your voice fade at the end of words?

Did you pause after important thoughts so the listener could digest the meaning?

Did you use enough catch breaths?

Did you use catch breaths in the right places?

Did you use catch breaths without interrupting the flow?

Did you vary the rate?

Did you sound jerky at any time?

It is harder to remember to ration our air when we are talking instead of reading from a page. Let's gradually increase the number of words per breath as we take turns saying the following, adding only words that start with /b/.

"I went on a picnic."

"I went on a picnic and I took bread."

"I went on a picnic and I took bread, butter, etc."

Now I want you to think about using your air supply correctly as you explain some things to me. Pause and take catch breaths as you need them.

1. Name all the children in your class.
2. Name all the families who live on your street.
3. Name all the months of the year, making one parenthetical statement about each, for example, "The first month is January—usually it's snowy. The second month is February—Valentine's Day comes then." And so on.
4. Describe the plan of your house, going through each room in order and stating one piece of information about each. Remember the breath! For example, "You go into the hall, and the coats are kept there. Then there's the kitchen, and we cook in there." And so on.
5. I'll give you some riddles and jokes. Then you tell them to me, making sure the pauses illustrate the punchlines. For homework, practice a new joke to tell me

next time. See Appendix B for jokes and riddles to practice.

Treatment Approach 4: Treating Hypernasality

Because of the complex pattern of voicing during speech production, children with resonance problems are often unaware of the specific aspect of their behavior that warrants attention. When we deal with a hypernasal child who has a functioning velopharyngeal mechanism, it is important to teach the behavioral characteristics of orality and nasality. Andrews Tardy, and Pasternak (1984) have suggested that this can be accomplished during the awareness phase of a treatment program by grouping all the speech sounds into two basic categories. In this way, commonalities in the observable cues and feeling states can be related to the auditorially perceived resonance patterns. It is also important to teach the associations between the auditory targets and the obligatory modifications in the vocal tract. Self-regulatory speech, in the form of concrete verbal descriptions, should be modeled for the child. These verbal patterns become an integral part of self-monitoring and self-evaluation in the production phase of therapy.

The oral–nasal dichotomy in voice resonance is difficult for a child to perceive, since in running speech the modifications of the vocal tract occur in rapid succession and the resonance characteristics are only part of the fleeting auditory events. Before any awareness of the appropriate sequencing and interplay of oral and nasal voicing can be learned, the behaviors have to be reduced to static states. Later, the transitions between the two states can be taught in slow motion and then, gradually, production of dynamic movements and sequences can be habituated.

The case study that follows illustrates ways of teaching a child the basic distinction between orality and nasality during the awareness phase. During the production phase, ideas from sources such as Cooper (1973), Fisher (1975), Hanley and Thurman (1970), and Moncur and Brackett (1974) are verbalized in language consistent with the child's developmental stage. Some techniques are described as "tricks" the child can use to facilitate oral resonance. Because some children who have (or have had) velopharyngeal valving difficulties use hard glottal attacks (Wilson, 1979), /h/ was frequently used to precede vowel sounds during early production tasks.

Virginia: Hypernasality That Remained After an Adequate Velopharyngeal Closure Mechanism Was Achieved

Virginia was 7 years 11 months, was in the second grade, and was above average in her classroom work. She had been treated at a university medical center for a congenitally short palate. A year earlier, she had undergone pharyngeal flap surgery. When she was referred to her school's speech–language clinician, the report indicated that she had had 2 years of articulation therapy, and it was recommended that she now receive therapy at school, while continuing regular evaluations by the medical center craniofacial team every 6 months. Testing revealed that Virginia produced all speech sounds correctly with the exception of the /r/ phoneme, which was inconsistently correct in connected speech. Her voice quality, however, was still hypernasal in connected utterances, although she could produce sustained vowels with appropriate resonance when cued.

The clinician decided that she would continue therapy to habituate correct production of the /r/ phoneme in reading and spontaneous speech. In addition, she planned a treatment approach that would capitalize on Virginia's academic strengths. Because Virginia could read and knew the letters of the alphabet and the sounds those symbols represented, the sounds were divided into two categories: the sounds made with the mouth voice and the sounds made with the nose voice. Once the child learned to categorize the nasal sounds (e.g., m, n, ŋ) contrasted with vowels and all nonnasal consonants, the clinician would then teach the specific behavioral characteristics of the two categories. For example, "How do you know it is a sound where the voice comes out of my nose or mouth?"

Mouth Sounds	Nose Sounds
1. The mouth is open.	**1.** I can feel the vibrations in my nose.
2. The air comes out of my mouth.	**2.** My mouth is closed or blocked in some way.
3. It is a vowel, and all vowels come out of my mouth.	**3.** I can't make it if I hold my nose.
4. I can make it, even if I hold my nose.	**4.** Some air comes out of my nose.

Because Virginia needed to learn to associate proprioceptive feedback from the velopharyngeal area with the auditory characteristics of orality and nasality, the therapist decided to use the concept of a "door" at the back of her mouth. When the door is open, the air comes out of the nose. When it is closed, the air comes out of the mouth. The See-Scape, a piece of equipment that provides visual feedback when air is emitted nasally, would be used to operationalize this concept. The See-Scape is available from C.C. Publications, P.O. Box 23699, Tigard, OR 97223. A tube is placed in the nostril, and when nasal emission occurs, a small balloon rises in a plastic tube on the table in front of the child. When working with Virginia, the clinician decided to describe the velopharyngeal closure mechanism as similar to a door. However, to emphasize the part played by the pharyngeal muscles in closing the apertures on either side of the pharyngeal flap, the clinician would also use a drawstring and show how an opening can be closed when the drawstring is tightened. The clinician would link these demonstrations of tightening to the feeling at the back of the throat when the muscles help close off the opening (or door).

Goals

Because Virginia used a hypernasal voice in connected speech, she needed to learn to produce appropriate oral–nasal resonance in simple, self-generated sentences. The clinician would achieve this by first making Virginia aware of the two categories of sounds: sounds made with the "mouth voice" and sounds made with the "nose voice." She would work with Virginia to verbalize the connection between pharyngeal movement, air emission, and type of voicing, and to identify sound sequences coded as "mouth, mouth, nose" or "door closed, door closed, door open." Virginia would then be ready to learn production of sequences of all oral sounds (syllables, words, sentences); production of transitions between oral–nasal and nasal–oral sound sequences in "slow motion"; and production and evaluations of strategies used (e.g., "I opened the door too soon/too late"). Virginia would then be able to verbalize and apply "rules" to increase perception of orality.

Sample Strategies

Let's work with these cards. I'll say the sound of the letter printed on each card. If the sound comes out of my nose, then it's a "nose sound," and it goes in this box. Remember, m, n, and ŋ are the only nose sounds. All of the other consonants and all of the vowels are "mouth sounds," and they go in the other "mouth box." Let's begin. I'll pick up the card and say the sound. Then you decide if it's a nose or a mouth sound and put the card in the correct box.

Here is a picture of a side view of the top half of the human body and head. It looks as if the poor person has been sliced in half! We can see from this drawing how air travels from the lungs, through the vocal folds into the pharynx and then goes out of either the mouth *or* the nose. Trace with your finger the direction of the airstream as I make some different mouth and nose sounds.

Remember we can use muscles at the back of our mouth (in the pharynx) to close off the door to the nose. When I make a mouth sound such as /a/, I close the door to the nose and send the air and the sound out of my mouth. When I say /m/, though, it is a nose sound, so I leave the door open. Describe the next sound I make and tell me whether the door is open or closed. (Clinician says ŋ; child says, "It's a nose sound, so the door is open.")

Now I'm going to say a series of sounds slowly (e.g., /p/, /æ/, /m/). They are mouth sound, mouth sound, nose sound, or, if I describe the position of the door I could say, "door closed, door closed, door opened." Are you ready to try one?

Sometimes we make mistakes and send mouth sounds out the nose because we forget to close the door properly. If air leaks out of the nose during a mouth sound, that's a sure sign that we forgot to close the door tightly enough. Today I brought the See-Scape. I'll say a vowel and you watch to see if any air comes out of my nose. The balloon will move up if it does. Tell me how you know that was a correct mouth sound? Did the balloon stay down? (If the See-Scape is not available, simpler materials, such as feathers and facial tissues can be used to illustrate direction of air emission [Wilson, 1979].)

Now you make some mouth sounds. Watch and listen and say them after me. We'll make them long (vowels and continuant consonants). Feel the door squeezing shut at the back of your mouth. Feel the sound vibrating on your teeth and in your mouth. Be sure no air comes out of your nose. We'll check with the See-Scape if we think we hear some air coming through the nose.

Now let's try some strings of sounds in slow motion. We'll use both mouth and nose sounds this time. (Clinician contrasts and produces the sounds and the child imitates.)

	(h)	æ	m
Prolong the sound	(h)	ɪ	m
Feel the vibrations	(h)	ei	ŋ

Here are some more strings of sounds to try. We'll read from the letters printed on these cards. These are all mouth sounds, so I've drawn a mouth on the card. I'll do each one and then hand the card to you and you have a turn. (Child imitates CV's and is encouraged to describe the characteristics and to self-monitor. Visual, auditory, and graphic cues are provided throughout.)

Now we'll play a card game. We'll take turns taking a card. If we say the sounds correctly we keep the card. We'll see who ends up with the biggest pile. (Child produces CVV syllables and then CVC syllables, first with a model and cues and then spontaneously.)

Here's a word list:

book	baby
take	hot
set	fat
say	doll
lady	bug

Let's say these words in a sentence: "I have a ____________."

Now pick an object from this secret box and say its name. (Box can include a toy horse, a toy truck, a toy car, a doll, a ruler, a vase, a shoelace, a book, a feather, a leaf, a piece of chalk, etc.)

Here are some pictures of words with all mouth sounds. Make a sentence, for example, "At the store I bought ____________," with the words:

eggs peppers bread
juice radishes butter
apples peaches chocolate
pears cottage cheese

Use your lips and open your mouth well to send *all* of the mouth sounds through your mouth. Say these sentences after me. Then we'll play them back, and you tell me any words that sounded as if they came out of your nose.

1. Peter picked peppers quickly.
2. Charley Chadwick liked the toys.
3. Here, Harry, that's a good dog.
4. There are pretty leaves in October.
5. March is cold and gray.
6. The lovely doll has clothes to wear.

I'll say some sounds slowly, and you say whether they are mouth or nose sounds. Then we'll switch, and you say them in slow motion. Remember to separate each sound.

(oral–oral–nasal):

same hem ham pan
fang song Sam fame

(nasal–oral–oral):

meat nose news
moat neat knees

(oral–nasal–oral):

Amy ant end
any ink eeny

Now instead of separating all the sounds in the words, let's make the vowel sound long and end with a short nose sound.

(prolonged vowel–pause–short nasal):

Ben hem
sang pan
fine Tim

Now let's make a short nose sound to start and then stretch out the rest of the mouth sounds in these words:

Maze niece Noddy
Neal mess meaty

Color all the nose sounds red in the words on these cards. Then say them after the phrase, "I have a." Don't open the door before you get to the red letter.

I have a balloon.

I have a pen.

I have a song.

I have a ring.

I have a ham.

Did you send all the sounds through your mouth except the red letters? Let's play the tape recording of those sentences and listen. Circle any words you think you could do better.

Let's practice these pairs of words:

hat ham
fad fan
seed seen
oat own

Did you open the door too soon?

me	he
meal	seal
neat	feet
no	toe

Did you close the door too late?

Can we think of some tricks to help us?

1. Find the nose sounds before starting to read the words.
2. Make the nose sounds shorter.
3. Make the vowel sounds longer.
4. Make sure the door doesn't open too soon or close too late.
5. Feel a "squeeze" as the door closes well.
6. Open mouth well.
7. Use lips and tongue well.
8. Read slowly at first.

Read these sentences and then we'll play them back and see if you used some of those tricks.

I need a pen.

I need a gong.

I need a dress.

I need a book.

I need a pear.

I need a fan.

Now you think of some ways to finish this sentence. Say the whole sentence. We'll take turns.

"I know ___________."

Here are some things in a bag. Put your hand into the bag and feel one of them. Then describe how it feels.

"It feels small and has wheels."

"It feels thin and long."

Treatment Approach 5: Improving Supraglottal Behaviors

We have noted that all children do not always need to exhibit optimal behaviors in every area relating to voice production. Adequate skills and the absence of maladaptive behavior are realistic in most instances. When there are limitations in one area, however, the overall vocal effect can usually be improved by enhancing activity in other areas. If, for example, a child has a permanent structural constraint in the phonatory system, improved respiratory activity, better resonance, and more precise articulation may help the child compensate for the laryngeal defect. In fact, teaching the child to use other parts of the vocal mechanism optimally may also be a way of preventing the development of less appropriate compensatory behaviors.

In our next case study, we describe a treatment plan devised to optimize supraglottal activity. During our discussion, we shall be using the term *forward tone focus,* meaning a concentration of attention, energy, and activity in the front of the oral cavity. With young children, it may sometimes be helpful to contrast "front of the mouth" voice with "neck voice." We can then link the sound and the feel of the voice to specific anatomic sites.

Robbie: Phonatory Behavior Limited by Structural Deviation

Robbie, aged 10 years, had a paralyzed right vocal fold, fixed in the abducted position. He previously had been enrolled in therapy in another school district and had worked on techniques to encourage compensatory movement of the left vocal fold during adduction. Strategies to achieve closure, such as pushing while phonating, had been used with some success. Robbie's vocal quality during cued and prolonged phonation of vowels was appropriate, but in his connected speech there was reduced loudness and considerable breathiness. Robbie's voice was weak and did not carry well, and he had difficulty being heard in noisy environments. It was noted that although Robbie did not exhibit any negative behaviors in terms of resonance, neither was he maximizing his full potential in that area to compensate for his reduced phonatory power. Robbie demonstrated appropriate respiratory behavior and had hearing sensitivity that was within the normal range bilaterally. His interpersonal skills also seemed to be within normal limits.

The speech–language clinician hypothesized that Robbie needed to develop more optimal use of resonance and improved mouth-opening and articulatory precision to enhance his vocal effectiveness. She felt that Robbie needed to improve the carrying power of his voice, particularly during projected speech. She decided that she would continue to work on improving Robbie's phonatory adjustment, moving systematically from sustained vowels, CVs and VCs and CVCs (voiced continuant consonants) to words, phrases, and sentences. She decided to add some new objectives as well, however.

Goals

Robbie's negative vocal behaviors included

1. Reduced loudness in connected speech
2. Breathy quality
3. Lack of projection

The clinician's target areas during treatment would be to improve Robbie's use of resonance to compensate for weak and breathy laryngeal tone during connected utterances and conversational levels and to improve his vocal power during projected speech. She established six goals for the therapy:

1. Identification of techniques to enhance audibility during connected speech
2. Increased mouth opening
3. Improved forward tone focus
4. Increased durations of vowels and voiced continuants
5. Increased reverberation in supraglottal cavities
6. Increased precision of articulatory contacts to maximize intelligibility

Sample Strategies

Listen to the following sounds. Some carry more sound than do others. In fact, some (like f, θ, and s) are just breath. The sounds that carry the vibrations (like v, ð, and z) can help us get more power in our voice if we make the most of them. Listen while I prolong some sound-carrying consonants. Feel the vibrations on the front of my face as I make them [m n v ð z ʒ]. These consonants can help put more "oomph" and "carrying power" in our voice. Let's look at this list of consonants, and we'll circle all the ones that are the best "sound carriers."

The vowel sounds can be a great help to us also because all vowel sounds are voiced. When we open our mouths well and linger on the vowels, we can help to make our voice carry better. You underline the vowel sounds in the following words, and then I'll say each word, making sure I open my mouth well so that the sound waves vibrate on the bones of my face. Which ones sounded richest? Which ones sounded muffled? Why? Sometimes people say vowels too far back in their mouth. The back of the mouth is soft tissue. The front of the mouth has more hard surfaces. Listen while I make the /a/ sound in the back of my mouth. Now listen while I throw the sound /a/ forward so that it "rings" against the hard roof of my mouth and my teeth. Listen, too, while I say it just in my throat, with not much mouth opening for it to come out. The vowel had a muffled, "deadened" sound with no "ring" to it.

Using "sound carrying" consonants well and opening the mouth and throwing the sound forward is sometimes called "focusing" the voice in the front of the mouth. A lot of our voice energy is then at the front. I will say some words, and you tell me whether the voice was a "front of the mouth" voice or a "muffled" voice (e.g., too much in the throat only or stuck in the back of the mouth).

Bobby	arrive
little	brave
lazy	pleasure
vase	range

When we take photographs, the picture is sometimes blurred if our camera is not focused well. Our voices also can sound blurred and fuzzy if we don't focus the voice forward in our mouth. Tell me which of these words are focused forward and which are not. (*Hint*: Watch to see if I am using my lips and tongue well to help the focus.)

Tell me what I did wrong, and I'll do it again; for example: Was my mouth open enough? Did I make the bones of my face vibrate? Did I use the sound-carrying consonants?

Let's look at the words that follow and decide some things we could do to help focus them forward. Underline the sounds that could help.

able	Maisie	easy
tunnel	dime	revise

Some ways we can focus forward on the above words are:

1. Prolong the vowels
2. Prolong the voiced continuants
3. Use lips and tongue well
4. Open mouth well

I'll use some of the hints, and you guess which ones I'm using. (Chant letters of the alphabet prolonging vowels; count using emphasized mouth opening; say "Bob, Bill, Ben, Boris" using vigorous lip movement; say "running, jumping, going, coming" prolonging voiced continuants, etc.)

In the words that follow, underline the vowels in red and the helpful sound-carrying consonants in green and then say the words, prolonging the red and green sounds.

Come on	Mommy	lizards
go now	lazy boys	ending

Pretend you are chanting in a big cathedral or synagogue. Throw the sound to hit the back walls of the church.

Sing a new song.	God of our Fathers
Away in a manger.	Hear the music
Monday morning.	Sing songs of praise
Have some more honey.	Ring the bells

Let's listen to a tape recording and note which words sounded strongest. Why? Redo the ones that could be made to sound better.

I am going to tell you a short story. Every time I pause I want you to say, *"Tell me more"* or *"maybe"* or *"never mind."* (Make sure your voice is well focused and that the "sound carriers" vibrate.)

M is a good sound carrier because the bones of the face (and nose) vibrate when *m* is prolonged with forward tone focus. Let's make up as many words as we can with *m* in them. Make sentences with those words (e.g., Mary Manning made Mervyn mad). Let's play a game where we add *m* words, for example,

*M*ay motored to *M*aine and met ___________ (Mabel; Mabel and Mary, Mabel, Mary, and Millie; Mabel, Mary, Millie, and Mort; Mabel, Mary, Millie, Mort, and Melissa; etc.) Think of all the foods (cities, games, movies, etc.) that have *m* in their names.

A good way to practice prolonging the vowel sounds in words is to play a rhyming game. (Make sure you prolong the vowels.) For example, "I'm thinking of a word that rhymes with 'tree.'" Take turns rhyming until you run out of ideas.

Sea rhymes with tree.

Bee rhymes with tree.

Now that you are really good at focusing the sounds, let's make the rhyming game harder.

Person 1: I'm thinking of a word that rhymes with hole.
2: Is it a horse's baby?
1: No, it's not foal.
2: Is it something you eat cereal in?
1: No, it's not bowl.
2: Is it a small animal?
1: No, it's not mole.

Mark all the sound-carrying consonants in the following readings. Hum *m* before you start each line to get your tone focus. Whenever your tone focus slips as you are reading, hum *m* again to get it back.

In this poem, there are lots of sounds at the ends of words that can be prolonged. Circle them. Now chant the poem. When you are good at chanting it, then try to say it in a normal conversational way, keeping the tone focused forward throughout.

Anna Banana chews bubble gum

Anna Banana "Give me some"

Anna Banana's gum is green

"Anna Banana, don't be mean!"

Treatment Approach 6: Modifying Pitch

In this plan, we focus on some strategies that are useful for children with pitch problems. When a child exhibits an habitual pitch that is inappropriate for age and gender, the clinician's first task is to obtain information concerning the condition of the folds. Congenital anatomic constraints, such as the presence of a laryngeal web, can limit a child's laryngeal function. Additive lesions, such as nodules, also may result in a pitch level that is inappropriate. If there is no anatomic constraint present and if there is no medical condition that causes swelling of the folds (consistently or intermittently), it may be that the child has habituated a pattern of misuse. Wilson (1979) has noted that faulty learning may be a factor in the inappropriate use of pitch. It is important for the clinician to consider relevant case history information carefully, including the possible influence of vocal models in the child's family and peer group.

Before treatment was planned for Cynthia, the child to be discussed in the case history that follows, the clinician ascertained that the problem was functional and that no laryngeal pathology existed.

Cynthia: A Conversational Pitch Range That Was Inappropriately Low

Cynthia, aged 10 years, was referred by her fifth-grade teacher because her voice sounded "too low and gravelly for a female student of her age." Reports indicated that Cynthia had hearing thresholds in the normal range bilaterally and had no indications of laryngeal pathology, gastroesophageal reflux, or allergic or infectious conditions. Cynthia's mother reported that the girl had always been a tomboy, who had tried to emulate her older brothers in the past but now became upset when she was mistaken for her brothers on the telephone. Cynthia told the speech clinician that she would like to sound "more like a girl" at times when she was not trying to "clown around" with the boys. She said, "I used to try to talk in a rough voice, but now I don't seem to be able to talk any other way, even when I want to."

Cynthia seemed to be at a stage in her life where she wanted to increase her vocal options. After years of trying to be "one of the boys," she had habituated a pattern of pitch use that now made her feel different from the girls in her peer group. She had habituated a conversational pitch range that was limited to the lower end of her overall available pitch range. Vocal testing revealed that she spoke at a pitch level that was so close to her basal pitch level that she frequently lasped into vocal fry. She used few rising intonation patterns, with the result that her variability was minimal. Most often, when her pitch changed, the movement was downward. The perception of her voice as "gravelly" was related to the frequent episodes of vocal fry during connected speech. Cynthia was stimulable and could produce more appropriate pitch levels when she was cued. The most useful cues seemed to be words and phrases that evoked an upward movement of the voice. The clinician decided to present visual cues (diagrams and patterns depicting the desired range of pitches and sequences of inflections) and words and phrases whose meaning evoked rising inflections. Cynthia was quick to see the relationship between meaning and voice patterns. The selection of materials for Cynthia seemed a critical component of the treatment plan. It made sense to her to explore different methods of varying her voice in response to specific word images and cognitive cues.

Goals

Cynthia's negative vocal behaviors included

1. An inappropriately low habitual pitch level
2. Restricted conversational pitch range
3. Limited use of upward inflections
4. Frequent episodes of vocal fry

The clinician decided to target in on developing in Cynthia an appropriate habitual pitch level and an increased use of inflection. Her goals were

1. To orient the child to the area to be addressed in therapy
2. To develop concepts that are basic to learning in the area
3. To elicit the target behaviors
   a. in isolation
   b. in simple linguistic contexts
   c. in complex linguistic contexts
4. To describe the child's responses in terms meaningful to the child:
   a. how
   b. why
   c. when
5. To provide techniques to shape consistency and accuracy of responses:
   a. imitation
   b. extensive cueing
   c. minimal cueing
6. To encourage the child's self-monitoring of responses.

Sample Strategies

Think of your voice as similar to a multilevel house or apartment building (show diagram). The basement voice sounds like this (demonstrate and explain vocal fry). The first floor contains a number of different and useful clear pitches, as does the second floor. Then there is an attic, which contains high notes that we use mainly for singing. When we talk, the best notes to use are the ones from the first and second floors. The voice moves around most effectively in the main part of the house. Your conversational pitch range is located in the "main living areas" of the house. If you begin to talk on a note that is too low, it's far too easy to slide on down into the basement. But if you try to aim for a level somewhere in between the first and second floors, you'll find that you can vary your voice quite comfortably. It would be helpful if you'd try to keep your voice away from the basement. On this diagram mark an X every time you hear me use my "basement" voice. Describe the way it sounds.

Now take the pencil and mark the Xs in the "living areas" of the house. Mark the X on the first floor when I use a low, clear pitch and on the second floor when I use a higher, clear pitch. Now draw arrows down and up between floors as I slide my voice in different directions.

There's a word that is sometimes used to describe words that sound like the idea they are expressing. That word is *onomatopoeia.* For example, "squeak" can be said so it reminds one of a "squeak." "Shush" is another; it makes one feel like being quiet. Here are some words that make us think of high and low sounds:

shriek–growl	yelp–moan
eek–groan	yip–bark
shrill–grovel	whistle–boom
creak–thump	ding–dong
meow–moo	leap–crash

Below is a list of words. Which of these would be easy to say in a high-pitched voice? Which would be hard to say in a high voice? Thinking of the meaning of the words helps us decide.

shriek	bump
whine	crash
valley	kite
thin	cave
down	fly
zip	peak
eek	sad
bang	glum
tip	glee

Sometimes the sounds the letters make (especially the vowels) suggest the pitch level. For example, [i] vowels in words are easier to say in a high voice that are [ʌ] vowels. Some of the letters in words can be helpful as we practice different pitches.

Sometimes what the words stand for suggests something high in space; for example, "peak" is easier to say on a high note than "cave."

A movement or action suggested by a word, for example, "fly," or "zip," sometimes helps the voice move in the same direction. Of course you can "zip" a "zipper" in two directions. Listen to me say the word and tell me which direction I am "zipping." Feelings can also suggest the way a voice can move. Generally, happy excited feelings are said with an upward movement of the voice; unpleasant feelings (and the words that express them) tend to drag the pitch of the voice down. Consider "sad," "excited," "laugh," and "cry."

Not only single words but also groups of words can be said at different pitches. Look at the sentences that follow and start them in the voice you normally use, and then let your voice go up as the meaning suggests.

The rainbow in the sky.

The chairlift on the top.

The balloon floated up.

The bird soared away.

The plane flew off.

The hawk circling.

That girl stand up.

The arrow shot up.

Oh, a surprise.

Gee whiz.

Oh gosh.

The fish jumped.

Oh no.

The siren shrieked.

Now let's reverse some of these sentences. We'll start off with the high part and then say the low part. But start high enough so that the low part is low and clear. Let's not dip down into the basement if at all possible.

In the sky, the rainbow.

On the top, the chairlift.

A surprise, oh!

Circling, the hawk.

Stand up, that girl.

This time I'll ask you a question, and you reply with just the high part of each of our word groups.

Where is the rainbow?

Where is the chairlift?

Where is the hawk?

What did the girl do?

Here are some words and phrases that have "up" feelings. See if you can use pitch changes to show those feelings.

"Oh boy"

"Right on"

"Yes, sir"

"Happy day"

"Good morning"

"Fun time"

When we are uncertain or questioning, we let a word drift or slide upwards: Who? What? When? Sometimes the same words can be said with different meanings depending on the direction of our voice. Read the following words that can sound as if we mean "Yes, for sure" or "Yes, maybe." As you say them, I'll try to describe what I think you mean.

yes	me	Dad	you're kidding
good	mine	food	for sure
tomorrow	yours	dirty	right now

Here is a short reading passage. Underline any words or phrases that may be helpful in varying your pitch. A good rule is to remember that new ideas often need a new pitch. Also punctuation can help when you are reading. A comma signals that more is to follow, so the pitch signals this by staying up. A period usually indicates that there is an end to the last idea, so the pitch goes down to show the listener. Question marks always mean that the voice goes up to signal that we need an answer to our question.

> The siren shrieked, and the girls exclaimed, "Yippee." The adults laughed at the young people's joy. The air raid was over. Mary looked up in the sky. Some white clouds floated by. The bombers were gone. "Oh, happy day," she said. All over London

people came up out of bomb shelters, happy that the danger was past.

Now we'll replay our tape recording of your reading. Use this red pencil and mark the places where your voice goes into the basement (fry). Circle words that you think you can do better when we try it again. Here is another reading to practice. Note the punctuation.

> Many girls like to jump rope. Do you? I have many friends, Caitlin, Madison, MacKenzie, Liz and Sarah, to name just a few. All these friends jump rope with me, as well as doing other fun things, when we get together at each other's houses.

Treatment Approach 7: Using a Hero and an Antihero

It is traditional in voice therapy to focus on individual maladaptive behaviors in a sequential fashion. This case study, however, illustrates a gestalt approach. In a gestalt approach, desirable and undesirable behaviors are presented as sets associated with characters in a narrative framework; there is a storybook hero and an antihero. The child's identification with the hero character enhances his motivation to change his abusive practices and negative behaviors. During the general awareness phase of therapy, the child gains an understanding of the effects of certain patterns of behavior first and then is more willing to focus on individual perceptual attributes. The meaningful context facilitates discussion of intangible vocal events. This use of a meaningful context is one way of organizing a program so that it meshes with a young child's developmental stage.

To begin our discussion we shall look at a treatment approach that was designed for Freddie, a kindergarten child who was demonstrating a pattern of excessive muscular tension but who did not exhibit any tissue change in the larynx. Freddie is a dramatic example of a hyperfunctional voice user, yet many of his negative behaviors are typical of vocal abusers. The severity of his problem was somewhat unusual for his age.

Some young children gain attention from their peers because of their ability to produce atypical voice patterns. Freddie's entry behaviors included maladaptive voice use as a way to seek and hold attention. Because of his age, the satisfactions he was deriving from his behavior, and the difficulty in focusing his attention on individual vocal parameters, the storybook approach was adopted.

Freddie: Hyperfunctional Voice Use

Freddie, aged 5 years 6 months, was referred by his kindergarten teacher because the other children in his class told him he sounded like a frog when he talked. The otolaryngologic report noted that the child had a normal larynx but that there was observable tension in the vocal tract during phonation and some intermittent dysphonia plicae verticularis.

During the initial diagnostic interview the parents reported that their son had begun using his "frog voice" following recurrent episodes of laryngitis during his preschool years. His general health at the time of the interview was described as "excellent." The parents were concerned about the excessive amount of loud strained talking that the child engaged in and his attempts to gain attention and amuse his peers by using his strange voice. They described him as "a bit of a clown" and said he "got very uptight if he wasn't the center of attention." They had attempted to modify his behavior by telling him not to talk so much. They said he was aggressive at play and that he tried very hard to make friends.

Voice testing revealed that when Freddie was asked to prolong vowel sounds he had difficulty sustaining phonation for longer than four seconds. He prolonged the consonant sounds /s/ and /z/ for approximately 5 seconds each (Eckel & Boone, 1981). When he counted to 10 loudly, he demonstrated hard glottal attack on 8, and his voice sounded strained and diplophonic. When he was asked to count to 10 softly, he demonstrated no observable tension in the neck, jaw, and shoulder areas and improved vocal quality up to the number 5; thereafter, he appeared to have run out of air and attempted to complete the sequence using residual air with a recurrence of observable tension. Inspiration appeared to be shallow with no lower chest movements, and he appeared to have little control over the expiration phase. Replenishing breaths were rarely used during connected speech. An analysis of his pitch level and range, using the Kay Elemetrics Visi-Pitch, resulted in findings that were within normal limits for age and gender. To analyze his pattern of usage of hard glottal attacks on words beginning with vowels, the clinician asked Freddie to repeat the sentence "Uncle Eddie eats eggs" at varying loudness levels as she moved farther away from him across the room. He consistently initiated phonation with hard attacks on every word during every trial; however, the consistency of the diplophonic production seemed related to the increase in loudness. During conversational speech, the child spoke rapidly and eagerly and seemed anxious to maintain the clinician's attention on him at all times. When the clinician looked down at her notes, the child responded immediately by interjecting a loud statement or by suddenly becoming diplophonic. His attempts at vocal variety during conversation were restricted to increasing the loudness level or increasing the amount of diplophonia. To see if the child was aware of other, less abusive methods of varying his voice, the clinician asked him to make "pictures" with his voice. She presented him with nouns and adjectives selected for the purpose of eliciting pitch and duration changes. Visual and auditory stimuli were provided, and the child was stimulable when given a model (e.g., worms *crawl*, reach *high*, a *deep* hole, a *fat* man, warm and *snuggly*). Audiologic testing revealed that hearing sensitivity was within normal limits bilaterally.

Freddie was enrolled in therapy for two 20-minute sessions each week for individual voice therapy. In addition, his parents agreed to participate in a parent program designed to help them provide additional modification of the vocal behavior in the home environment. Conferences were arranged with Freddie's classroom teacher and a school psychologist to gather information and ensure cooperation and understanding of therapy strategies.

The parents, teacher, and voice clinician agreed to coordinate their efforts to find ways in which Freddie could be rewarded for using an easy phonatory pattern. They decided to ignore the boy's attempts to gain attention by using the diplophonic voice and to give him a great deal of attention whenever he was *not* using a forced production. They identified methods of describing the characteristics of the vocal behavior and the general behavior that was targeted. For example, they described their own reactions to the sound of his voice when he spoke at an optimal loudness level or with an absence of diplophonia by saying, "You make me feel so calm when you use your easy voice"; I like to sit and talk with you—your smooth voice sounds so good to me"; "I love the feeling of sitting close to you and talking quietly together"; "When you talk to me like that, my ears feel so good"; "Children know you are a friendly boy when you use that voice to talk to them."

The clinician adopted two characters to personify the behavioral characteristics associated with the "old" vocal pattern and the "new" vocal behavior. To achieve worthwhile results and because Freddie was an energetic, assertive boy, the character chosen to personify the easy laryngeal production needed to be a high-status, masculine figure who illustrated efficient and economic use of vocal power. Superman was selected to fulfill those expectations. It was essential that the character personifying the less acceptable vocal behaviors be a less enviable personage and one with whom the child might be less inclined to identify. This character needed to be noisy yet inefficient in the use of his vocal energy and unsuccessful in achieving meaningful relationships and personal goals. The Tin Soldier was chosen for this role.

In the awareness sessions the clinician told Freddie stories about the exploits of the two central characters, emphasizing the consequences of their total behaviors. Later, specific behaviors were discussed, and Freddie was encouraged to predict possible outcomes. This nonthreatening framework offered frequent opportunities for him to practice identifying appropriate and inappropriate behaviors at the interpersonal level. Later, the clinician and Freddie decided on behavioral objectives together. They agreed that certain behaviors were worth copying because they worked. Freddie discovered that both Superman and the Tin Soldier had similar personal needs but used different strategies to try to meet those needs. He verbalized insights such as, "The Tin Soldier wants people to like him but he makes too much noise. His friends get tired of listening to him" "Superman helps people. They listen to him when he talks. The baddies are scared of him, too." The child was especially impressed by one situation in a story, which he paraphrased by saying, "That Tin Soldier just yelled and screamed at the bad guy, but he wasn't even scared. Then Superman talked in a deadly voice—real quiet but it sure scared that guy."

The following reasons for talking and listening emerged and were summarized on a chart in the therapy room.

Why People Talk

To tell others what they want

To share feelings

To find out things

To get adults to help them

To make friends

To scare enemies

To show off

To make people laugh

To hear how good they sound

Why People Listen

To find out things

To show they like you

To think what they'll say next

To share with you

To rest their voices

To get clues to mysteries

It seemed unrealistic to tell Freddie that he could never talk loudly. The environmental and emotional demands relating to loudness were discussed and some conclusions were drawn.

Times People Talk Loudly

When playing outdoors

When listeners are a long way away

When lots of people are making a noise

When they are talking to lots of people

When grandparents can't hear you

When they are in a big place:

When cheering at a game

When they are angry

As therapy progressed, the stories focused more on specific vocal strategies that were productive and nonstressful. It became possible to help the boy state his own goals for changing his behavior.

Superman's Super Voice Rules

1. Always take plenty of air deep into your lungs before you start to talk (use lower chest breathing).
2. Make sure you have a lot of air before you talk loudly (use deeper inspiration for projected speech).
3. Always "top off" your air supply before you start to run out of air (use replenishing breaths).
4. Start your voice motor gently (use easy initiation of phonation).
5. Use a smooth voice to talk (elimination of diplophonia).
6. Never talk with a tight neck (avoid tension in laryngeal area).
7. Let your mouth and tongue do more work when you throw your voice a long way (use improved resonance and articulation to help voice carry).
8. Think of ways to save your voice so that it doesn't get tired (use alternative nonvocal behaviors).

By the end of the first semester, Freddie was able to use appropriate respiratory patterns in the therapy situation during the production of prolonged vowels and consonants. His respiratory behavior on both an inter- and intrapersonal level was advanced to the stage that it was possible for him to give a presentation during Show and Tell in his kindergarten classroom about the best way to breathe. During the second semester of therapy, he extended his skills in the appropriate use of speech breathing so that he was able to use the correct methods most of the time. After approximately 2 years of therapy, there was complete habituation of the use of the target vocal production. Intermittent diplophonia still occurred occasionally during the second year, when he was excited or anxious about maintaining the clinician's attention. Dismissal with periodic follow-up checks occurred when the parents reported that they were no longer hearing the "old" voice used at home during animated play sessions with peers.

The initial grouping of the behaviors as constellations associated with the hero and antihero reduced the level of abstraction and enhanced the child's motivation throughout the course of therapy. This approach appears to be a fruitful one to use with young children with limited motivation to change their abusive vocal behaviors. The selection of the two major characters is, of course, a key factor in the process. The characters need to be chosen with care and developed in a manner consistent with the child's interests and needs.

Goals

The clinician grouped Freddie's negative vocal behaviors into three categories:

1. Respiration
   a. Shallow inspiration
   b. Tension in shoulders, neck, and jaw
   c. Short, inefficient exhalation
   d. Inefficient use of replenishing breaths
2. Phonation
   a. Hard initiation of phonation
   b. Inefficient coordination of respiration and phonation
   c. Diplophonia
   d. Weak resonance on voiced continuants
   e. Little mouth opening or articulatory movement
   f. Effortful laryngeal tone
3. Interpersonal
   a. Excessive bids for attention and excessive talking
   b. Poor listening skills
   c. Lack of awareness of other's feedback and needs
   d. Little adaptation to situational constraints

The targets for treatment would be Freddie's use of appropriate respiratory patterns for sustained voicing, use of easy laryngeal tone, and use of appropriate attention-getting behaviors. The clinician decided to structure the therapy goals in three general areas.

1. Respiration
   a. Describe appropriate respiratory patterns.
   b. Achieve deep, quick inhalation.
   c. Sustain long controlled exhalation (15 seconds).
   d. Use replenishing breaths.
2. Phonation
   a. Describe appropriate phonatory patterns.
   b. Initiate easy phonation.
   c. Use appropriate loudness level during phonation in conversational and projected speech.
   d. Use vocal variety through pitch and duration changes.
   e. Maintain a "smooth" quality during phonation.
3. Interpersonal
   a. Describe purposes of talking.
   b. Discuss or role play varied communication strategies.
   c. Improve ratio of talking and listening time.
   d. Improve question-asking skills.

Sample Strategies

The Story of Superman and the Tin Soldier. Superman came out of the phone booth and looked at the crowd. He stood with his head high; his cape floated behind him in the wind. He took a deep breath and his lower chest and rib cage swelled with air. Suddenly he swirled around, called, "I'm off and away," in a strong clear voice, and flew off as the startled crowd watched.

The Tin Soldier rattled around yelling, "Did you see that? That was Superman. He can fly. I can fly, but I won't do it now. I'll do it later. I am as strong as he is, you know. I can do anything I want to."

Someone in the crowd said, "Oh, shut up, you stupid soldier. Stop making such a fool of yourself. We're sick of listening to you. Your voice is so creaky and rough it hurts our ears!"

The Tin Soldier shook with embarrassment and anger, and so he tried even harder to be important. "Look at me, look at me," he screeched. "Watch me fly." He tried to take a deep breath and jerked his arms, but he couldn't move his chest at all because he was so stiff and rusty. Instead he pushed his shoulders up, tightened his neck and tensed his creaky jaw. He screeched, "Look at me fly." He twirled around, tripped over his feet, and fell with a crash in a heap on the sidewalk.

The crowd roared with laughter. "What a jerk," someone said. "He thinks he can fly like Superman, and all he can do is fall on his face!"

"I can so, too—fly," said the Tin Soldier. But no one heard him, because he ran out of air before he could say all the words.

Later that day Superman came back to see some of the boys on the block. He asked them all about themselves and listened to their answers. The Tin Soldier rushed up to the group later on while they were playing ball. "I want to show you how good I am," he said, grabbing the ball. "Look at me, I'm really something. Watch me, watch me, I can do it better."

"Oh, get out of here," the boys said. "You butt in all the time, and we're sick of the sight of you."

Guess whether I am breathing like Superman or the Tin Soldier.

Tell me what the Tin Soldier is doing.

His shoulders are raised.

His neck is tight.

His arms are tight.

His jaw is clenched.

His chest isn't full of air.

He runs out of air before he's finished.

He doesn't top off his air tank.

He looks uncomfortable.

Tell me how Superman gets his air supply.

He fills the bottom of his chest.

He holds lots of air in his air tank.

He lets it out slowly (15 seconds).

His shoulders are down.

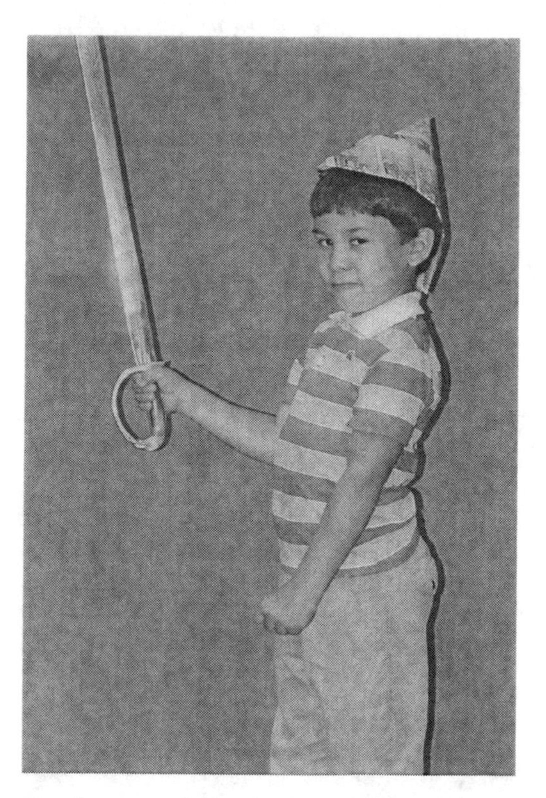

Simple props help the Tin Soldier demonstrate overall tension.

His neck is relaxed.

His jaw is not stiff.

Guess who is talking—Superman or the Tin Soldier.

Superman starts his voice motor easily. Describe how he does this.

He first takes in plenty of air.

He begins with /h/.

He doesn't jerk or click.

His neck is relaxed.

What are the Tin Soldier's mistakes? Tell him what he is doing wrong.

He doesn't take in enough air.

He is too tight all over.

He grunts as he starts.

He is jerky and creaky.

Let's analyze people's reactions to Superman and the Tin Soldier. Why does the Tin Soldier talk all the time? Do people like him? Describe how they feel when he makes so much noise.

Why do people like Superman?

He listens to them.

He asks good questions to find clues.

He praises others when they help him.

He sounds good—easy and relaxed.

What could the Tin Soldier do to get what he wants? Think of another ending for the story, for example: The Tin Soldier could play quietly with the boys and then ask them about their game. Before, when he just butted in and kept talking about himself, it made the other boys angry with him.

Let's copy the way Superman breathes in. How long can he make his air last? (Prolong continuant consonant 15 seconds.) Let's both count to 10 in one breath. Now let's both count to 10, take in air, and count to 10 again. I'll go first, then you do it.

See if you can be Superman saying /ha/. Walk around the room saying /ha/ like Superman. Now say /ha/ like the Tin Soldier. Who lasted the longest? Describe how you felt.

Superman has some tricks to get extra power without tiring himself. Copy the ways he gets extra power by working his mouth not his neck. Feel the vibration (*m, n, z, z,* etc.; CVs; chant phrases loaded with vowels and voiced continuants). Stretch out the words; give them Superman's easy power. (Prolong vowels and voiced continuants.)

I'm Superman.

I'm flying high.

My, oh my, I'm so high.

Baddies, beware—if you're there!

How do you know you sound like Superman?

smooth

easy

not tight

can go on longer

not ever jerky

easy to listen to

Show the Tin Soldier how Superman would do it. Let's go through our Tin Soldier story again and find the places where he could have paused to be sure he was understood. Now speak the words he said, showing him how Superman would have done it. What does he do instead of shouting? When he uses a quiet but "deadly" voice, the baddies know he means it all right! Why did the pauses help?

He could use them to get more air.

He made the pauses before important words.

During pauses, he could receive feedback from his listeners.

Treatment Approach 8: Using a Storybook Character

Our next case history illustrates a different symptom pattern. The otolaryngology report noted the presence of bilateral voice nodules, which meant we were dealing with a child who has an altered mechanism. In such cases, until the nodules subside, it is unrealistic to suggest that the child use a normally smooth and clear tone. Thus, the target voice, at first, is an easy breathy voice that allows the child to learn a less forceful adduction pattern. With older children this type of voice pattern could be described as a "confidential" voice.

Amanda: Repetitive Abusive Practices

Amanda, aged 6 years, 4 months, was referred by the school nurse, who noticed that she sounded "more like a man than a young girl." According to the medical report, Amanda had a history of severe allergic reactions of the upper respiratory tract, but the situation was now controlled by desensitization shots. Bilateral nodules were observed under direct laryngoscopy; redness and edema of the laryngeal mucosa were also noted. The parents reported that Amanda had always had a "low-pitched, gruff-sounding voice" and that people used to think it was "cute" that she had such a deep voice when she was a little girl. Lately, however, they had become concerned because they felt her voice made her self-conscious and prohibited her from joining a children's choir. She took ballet lessons but had not been given a speaking part in a recent recital because the teacher said, "She dances like a fairy but doesn't sound like one." They said Amanda coughed and cleared her throat a lot, even though she no longer seemed to have problems with excessive mucus. The physician had also ruled out the possibility of gastroesophageal reflux as a factor related to Amanda's voice problem.

Voice testing revealed that Amanda demonstrated adequate respiratory support; she could prolong /s/ for 25 seconds on repeated trials. Amanda said her dancing teacher stressed good breathing habits. Sustained phonation of /z/ was approximately 11 seconds and was characterized by low-pitch, uneven voicing, breaks, and severe hoarseness. The quality improved when she phonated loudly. During sentences there were frequent episodes of aphonia on unstressed syllables and some hard glottal attacks. Audiologic testing revealed that hearing sensitivity was within normal limits bilaterally. Frequent nonproductive coughing and throat clearing were observed; Amanda also filled pauses ("ahs," "ers") with hard glottal attacks while she appeared to be thinking of what to say next. She listened attentively, used appropriate eye contact and facial expression and appeared to be eager to have help with her voice. She said, "My granny says I should sound more like a lady."

Amanda was enrolled in therapy for two, 20-minute sessions each week. In addition, the parents agreed to help Amanda at home. It seemed that Amanda's frequent use of abusive behaviors (e.g., throat clearing and coughing) stemmed from earlier attempts to deal with excessive mucus in the vocal tract. Now that her allergies were under control she continued to habituate behaviors that were irrelevant and irritating. The use of hard glottal attacks had probably also developed as a compensatory device.

The clinician adopted two characters to personify the behavioral characteristics associated with the clusters of inappropriate and appropriate behaviors. Because Amanda was interested in pretty visual effects, ballet, and fairies, the clinician decided that the heroine character would be "Princess Amanda"—a feminine and beautiful woman who spoke in a gentle, easy voice and sighed (a breathy, easy sigh!) happily every time the prince rode by her castle window. The inappropriate behaviors were associated with "Wendy the Witch," a most unenviable character, who could not dance or sing or use an easy breathy voice at all! The noises Wendy made in her throat were irritating to everyone, and the prince even said that they gave him a headache and startled his white charger.

Amanda eagerly identified with the beautiful princess. During the awareness phase of therapy, stories about the princess and the witch focused on the effects their behaviors had on others (especially the prince). Amanda quickly identified the distracting mannerisms exhibited by the witch and described the specific characteristics of her behavior. She also analyzed why the witch was making so many noises and identified some things that the witch could do instead.

Why Wendy the Witch Makes Noises in Her Throat

To scare people

Because she doesn't realize she's doing it

To be silly

To stop other people from talking

To show she is thinking of what to say next

Because her throat tickles

To try to clear her voice

What Wendy Could Do Instead

Be more pleasant

Try to relax

Notice what she's doing

Use more quiet pauses

Swallow when her throat tickles

Drink more water

Use a gentle voice

Copy the beautiful princess

As therapy progressed, the stories focused more on specific vocal strategies that were nonstressful to the mechanism. Amanda stated some goals in her own words to describe how the princess behaved.

Princess Amanda's Beautiful Voice Hints

1. Always sound relaxed and easy.
2. An "airy," gentle voice is nice.
3. Start each word gently.
4. "Mmm" is better than "ah," "er," or "um" (because your lips work, not your throat).
5. Don't make noises during pauses if you can help it. Just listen and nod or smile.
6. Think of ways to save your throat from getting tired (use alternative nonvocal behaviors).

Amanda quickly adapted her behavior and was dismissed after one year in therapy. Her voice notebook included pictures of her characters and lists of their "special" habits. She also kept lists of celebrities on television who did not use their voices well and became expert at describing what they were doing incorrectly.

Goals

The clinician noted the following negative vocal behaviors, all having to do with phonation:

1. Hard initition of phonation
2. Weak resonance
3. Laryngeal tone focus
4. Habituated nonproductive coughing
5. Habituated nonproductive throat clearing
6. Filled pauses (hard glottal attacks on fillers)
7. Low pitch level (related to size and mass of folds, i.e., nodules, edema)
8. Limited pitch variability (related to size and mass)
9. Restricted pitch range (related to size and mass)
10. Hoarseness (related to size and mass)
11. Intermittent aphonia (related to size and mass)

The target areas for treatment would be to teach Amanda to use easy breathy phonation and to reduce her abusive practices.

The clinician established the following goals:

1. Easy initiation of phonation
2. Gentle, easy approximation of folds
3. Substitution of alternative behaviors (e.g., swallowing, quiet pauses, nonvocal signals)
4. Verbalization of key concepts of voice conservation
5. Verbalization of key concepts of effects of negative behaviors on others
6. Increased resonance and forward focus to improve tone

Sample Strategies

Story of Princess Amanda and Wendy the Witch. Wendy the Witch got very excited every time she saw the handsome prince. She was so excited, she talked all the time. When she didn't know what to say next, she said "ah," "um," or "er" very loudly so that no one else would start to talk until she thought of what to say. The prince never seemed to notice her, because he was too busy smiling at Princess Amanda. The witch tried dancing and hopping and skipping. She tried coughing and throat clearing and cackling. She tried talking and singing louder and louder. But the harder she tried, the worse she sounded and the more the prince frowned and ignored her. All her noises made his head hurt. And the more anxious Wendy got, and the more she tried to impress the prince, the more awful her screeching voice sounded. She even tried hiding behind a curtain in the prince's palace, just so she could be near him. But nothing she did seemed to work. He only wanted to talk to Princess Amanda. Poor Wendy felt terrible. She so much wanted him to notice her.

How do you know Wendy is behind that curtain?

What exactly did she do to make that noise in her throat (sensory awareness)?

What else made the prince annoyed with Wendy?

What did the princess tell Wendy to do to help her voice?

How does the princess start to say her name? (*A*manda); the Prince's name? (*A*lbert); the horse's name? (*A*lphonse). How is that different from the way Wendy says those names?

Listen to the poem Wendy says and count her mistakes and tell me what they are:

I'm *a*ngry and *a*nxious

Because *e*veryone's *a*ware

that my voice is *a*wful

and *a*t me they stare

(cough, throat clearing, cough!)

Tell poor Wendy about the Princess's beautiful voice hints. How could they help her?

You copy the princess and say her words after me as I read the story:

The Princess was at her window as the Prince rode by. She waved her scarf at him and called happily, "Hello, Albert."

"How gentle and soft and pretty your voice is, Princess," said the Prince.

*"Oh, A*lbert," said the princess in an excited (but gentle) voice. "May I ride your horse later today?"

Let's listen to the tape recording of the princess reading words. We'll put a purple tiara over every word that sounds just right. Did we both put tiaras over the same words, I wonder? Why do you think I didn't have one on that word?

Our case studies of Freddie and Amanda illustrate a Gestalt approach and how to use storybook characters to establish behavioral associations. This approach is useful because it allows liberal opportunity to use visual cues and images that are so necessary in therapy with very young children. In both cases, the purposes and effects of voice use were defined in simple, direct language to help the children develop personal rationales for change. In both cases the children created dialogue for their characters and adopted appropriate vocal behaviors when speaking as the person with whom they identified. Since reading Kolbenschlag (1981), our clinicians are careful to encourage "princesses" to be action-oriented rather than submissive when they talk to "princes." Although the princess character appealed to Amanda, our clinicians advocate the use of strong female characters, such as Wonder Woman and the avoidance of characters that suggest stereotypical nonassertive feminine characteristics.

Here is a list of some additional examples that may be useful in therapy with very young children.

Star Wars. Characters are appealing as hero figures for many children; however, it is sometimes difficult to identify an antihero who is not perceived as powerful. Other characters suitable for older children are Tiger Woods (other locally and nationally well-known sports figures), Tom Brokaw

Suggested Characters	*Possible Sets of Vocal Characteristics*
Inspector Clear Tone	1. Adequate respiration for speech 2. Appropriate loudness level for varied situations 3. Use of vocal variety 4. Appropriate listening skills 5. Easy initiation of phonation
Sergeant Sore Throat	1. Inadequate respiration for speech 2. Inappropriate use of loudness levels for varied situations 3. Limited vocal variety 4. Underdeveloped listening skills 5. Strained quality 6. Hard glottal attacks
Raggedy Anne or Andy	1. Relaxed posture 2. Flexible jaw and neck 3. Lower chest expansion during speech breathing 4. Relaxed vocal production
Rusty Ruth or Randy	1. Tense posture 2. Tight jaw and neck 3. Clavicular breathing 4. "Creaky" strained vocal production
Luke Skywalker	1. Smooth, easy quality 2. Direct eye contact and facial expressions 3. Honest expression of feelings 4. Effective results
Jabba the Hutt	1. Rough, "crackly" quality 2. Erratic eye movements and facial expressions 3. Manipulative, angry, or unpleasant feelings 4. Ineffective results
Batman	1. Appropriate tone focus (opens mouth well) 2. Appropriate breath support for projected speech 3. Maximizes loudness by increasing articulatory contacts 4. Appropriate balance of oral and nasal resonance
Mumbles Morgan	1. Pharyngeal tone focus 2. Inappropriate breath support for projected speech 3. Increasing loudness with laryngeal effort 4. Cul-de-sac resonance
Wonder Woman	1. Appropriate posture during inhalation 2. Use of mouth opening and tone focus 3. Clear articulation 4. Clear, pleasant vocal quality 5. Authoritative inflectional patterns
Shy Sue	1. Inappropriate posture during inhalation 2. Minimal mouth opening 3. Slurred articulation 4. Soft, breathy vocal quality 5. Timid, questioning inflectional patterns

(other locally and nationally well-known television or radio personalities), Brad Pitt (other locally and nationally well-known television or film personalities), and Katie Couric.

Treatment Approach 9: Addressing Interpersonal Behavior

Before adopting a particular approach to treatment for any child it is helpful to review all the negative behaviors and decide which should be translated into therapy objectives. In the cases of Freddie and Amanda, objectives were selected from more than one area of behavior, and sets of negative behaviors were contrasted with sets of positive behaviors. Thus, the approach involved a substitution of a whole new set of respiratory, phonatory, and interpersonal behaviors.

Although this approach worked well with Freddie and Amanda, other approaches need to be considered. In this section, we describe a treatment plan designed to meet the needs of children who were exhibiting severe problems in interpersonal behavior. Their negative vocal behaviors were only one aspect of a general pattern of aggression. Thus, although negative behaviors in the areas of respiration and phonation were observed, the area of interpersonal behavior was targeted as the priority area for treatment. This case study therefore demonstrates an approach predicated on the assumption that improvement in interpersonal behavior is a prerequisite in some cases to improvement in other areas.

Joe, Bill, and Howie: Aggressive Vocal Behavior Related to Reduced Emotional Control

Children who habitually respond by shouting and yelling and acting aggressively rarely get what they want. Sometimes, as they become more frustrated in achieving their needs, they may increase the frequency of unproductive vocal strategies and act out more belligerent physical behaviors.

Clinical psychologists, such as Spivack and Shure (1974), have shown that there is a relationship between the cognitive ability to generate a variety of solutions to interpersonal problems and behavioral deviance in young children. In particular, deficiencies in cognitive skills, such as role playing, have been identified by some (see Chandler, 1973) as possible explanations of aggressive behavior. Dodge (May, 1981) believes that, since an aggressive child does not always behave aggressively, the relationship between cognitive skills and social behavior must be assessed within situations. To perform competently in a social situation, a child may need to process cues in an orderly manner. Dodge (May, 1981) suggests that aggressive boys carry in their memory an expectancy that peers will be hostile; then they act aggressively and encounter more retaliatory aggression that confirms their expectations. It is possible that training them to attend to a greater number of social cues and to process social information more carefully may improve their social interactions. Richard and Dodge (1982b) have shown that the deviant boys in their study had particular deficits in the ability to generate alternative solutions during problem-solving tasks.

Aggression is an acquired strategy for dealing with strong feelings such as anger and anxiety. In an interesting study done by Seymour Feshback (in Mallick and McCandless, 1966), third-grade children were presented with three alternative strategies for handling their anger, frustration, and irritation caused by the behavior of another child. The three strategies presented were

1. Talking out the anger with an adult.
2. Getting even with the other child, or releasing the feelings by role playing.

3. Receiving reasonable explanations from an adult for the child's annoying behavior (i.e., the child was not feeling well, was upset).

The most effective strategy was found to be the reasonable explanation of the classmate's behavior.

Fixsen, Phillips, Baron, Coughlin, Daly, and Daly (1978), in a discussion of strategies for teaching the peaceful settlement of disputes and the nonviolent resolution of angry feelings in a program that was successful at Boys Town, highlighted the importance of teaching problem solving. They maintained that more effective problem-solving techniques than aggressive and abusive behavior could be learned. They stressed the importance of differentiating between aggressive actions and controlled, understood anger.

Some children need to learn about their emotions, how those emotions are reflected in actions and voices and how one assumes responsibility for one's actions. When an awareness of the effects of one's behavior is created, it becomes easier to develop a rationale to promote change.

Joe, Bill, and Howie were all in different fourth-grade rooms in a large elementary school, and the clinician decided to work with them as a group for 30 minutes once a week. All three boys used combative styles of interaction, were of average intelligence, and had normal hearing. They were referred by their teachers, who complained about loud and constant talking, strain and effort in speech, and difficulties with peer interactions. Bill had been labeled a "behavior problem" for some years and had a long history of visits to the principal's office because of fighting on the playground. His mother described him as "difficult to manage, mouthy, and destructive." Joe was heavy for his age and talked in a low-pitched, "gruff" voice; he was described by his parents as "belligerent, sullen, and moody at times." Howie was small and wiry in appearance, and his mother reported that he was "always wound up and tense" and that he teased his younger siblings constantly. The medical reports indicated that Bill and Howie had vocal nodules and that Joe's folds were edematous and red. Joe's physician suspected "chronic nonspecific laryngitis" related to hyperfunctional use. The speech–language clinician observed that all the boys used too much effort and tension when talking, seemed unaware of the effect of their behavior on others, and exhibited poor impulse control in dealing with aggressive feelings. He suspected that the frustrations and tensions of their interpersonal relationships precipitated and maintained the loud and strained patterns of their voice use.

During the initial case conferences, the school psychologist and the speech–language clinician explained to the parents that the priority objective in therapy should be to demonstrate the effects of aggressive behaviors on self and others. All participants in the conferences agreed that the current strategies the boys used were not helping them achieve acceptance by their peers, positive recognition from teachers and family members, or solutions to their everyday problems. It did not seem likely that the boys could change their abusive vocal patterns until some amelioration of the maintaining factors was achieved. The classroom teacher, the parents, the psychologist, and the speech–language clinician decided to give consistent rewards for desirable interpersonal behaviors. The parents agreed to cooperate with the school personnel by implementing a home program. They observed therapy periodically, met with the psychologist to discuss strategies to manage the aggressive behavior at home, and helped the boys with worksheet assignments.

The boys attended group therapy for $2\frac{1}{2}$ years. During that time, they developed insight concerning their emotions (specifically their anger, anxieties, fears, and satisfactions), their available options to express or inhibit emotional reactions, and the effects of a variety of their interpersonal strategies. A framework of analysis and evaluation was initially applied to general interpersonal behaviors (e.g., fighting) and then was applied to specific vocal practices.

In the treatment plan that follows, only the therapist's work on the boys' interpersonal behavior is outlined in detail. The clinician drew on previously published materials to formulate strategies specifically designed to eliminate vocal abuses and substitute improved phonatory behaviors. (For example, the Drudge and Philips, 1976, program, originally designed for college students, was adapted to eliminate hard glottal attacks. Ideas for elimination of phonatory abuses and the substitution of alternative behaviors were drawn from Blonigen's 1978 excellent article; Deal, McClain, and Sudderth's 1976 comprehensive approach to the rehabilitation of children with vocal nodules also provided valuable suggestions that were implemented.)

Goals

The clinician grouped the boys' negative behaviors into three categories:

1. Immature Understanding of Feelings
   a. How to describe them
   b. Ways they are communicated
   c. Effects on others
   d. How feelings are controlled
   e. Relationship to goal achievement
   f. Effect on physical and psychological state
2. Poor Self-Esteem
   a. How actions affect self-concept
   b. How others see us
   c. How we decide what we want and why
   d. How we can choose how to react
3. Ineffective Vocal Practices to Satisfy Needs
   a. Level of tension
   b. Amount of listening
   c. Adaptation to feedback
   d. Limited, unproductive strategies to gain attention (e.g., talking too much, too loudly)

The targets in treatment would be for the children to describe their emotional expression and response patterns and to analyze the effects of their behaviors on themselves and others. The clinician also needed to help them adopt more productive interpersonal strategies. Specifically, the goals would include

1. Defining emotional states (e.g., anger, anxiety, fear, and satisfaction)
2. Expressing anger, anxiety, fear, and satisfaction appropriately
3. Deciding when and how to deal with anger, anxiety, fear, and satisfaction
4. Practicing methods of dealing with the emotions of anger, anxiety, fear, and satisfaction
5. Evaluating effects (on self and others) of these new methods

Sample Strategies

Guess how everyone feels in the following three stories. Are the feelings the same or different? Why?

1. Henry was sitting next to George during a math lesson. George kept trying to see Henry's paper. Finally, Henry yelled, "Don't look at my paper or I'll break your face." The teacher, seeing Henry talking, came over and said, "You'll stay in during recess, Henry. I told you not to talk during math." Henry was upset and said, "It's not my fault. George is the one that was cheating." The teacher said, "I've had enough of this. See me at recess, both of you."

How did Henry feel? Why?

How did George feel? Why?

How did the teacher feel? Why?

2. Blair was drinking at the water fountain when Jack and Greg ran by. Greg accidentally knocked Blair's elbow, and the jolt caused water to spray over Blair's shirt. Blair immediately grabbed Greg and hit him. Jack, turning, saw Blair hit Greg and screamed at him, "Hey—leave Greg alone or I'll smash your face in."

How did Blair feel? Why?

How did Greg feel? Why?

How did Jack feel? Why?

3. Mario's young brother, Ramon, was doing his homework at the kitchen table. Mario passed by and said to him, "Mom said I can go to the pool for an hour before we eat, but you can't come." Ramon let out a yell and screamed, "I *can* go. Mom said I could go as soon as I finish." Mario laughed and yelled, "But you're *not* finished, and I'm not waiting for you anyway—so there!" Mario ran out the door laughing as Ramon started crying loudly. Their mother, hearing the noise, came in and said to Ramon, "Why are you crying? I thought you'd be pleased that I told Mario to tell you that you both could go to the pool now and that you could finish that work later."

How did Ramon feel—why?

How did Mario feel—why?

How did their Mom feel—why?

How can a person tell when someone else is angry? What does he or she do (e.g., yell, scream, punch, kick, scowl, bite, sulk, get red in the face, fight, pout, clench teeth, curse, bully, frown, complain)?

How can people hide their feelings when they are angry (e.g., clench fists under table, choke back angry words, take deep breaths, think of something else, pretend not to be angry, walk away, ignore the cause, it's not possible to hide it if you're really angry)?

What makes people feel angry?

When something isn't fair.

When people get in their way.

When someone hurts them on purpose.

When someone takes their things without asking.

When someone damages their possessions.

When they are teased.

When someone puts them down.

When someone ignores them.

When someone insults them.

When they do something "stupid" themselves.

When something won't work properly.

When someone is mean or cruel.

When a lot of things go wrong at once.

When they think someone is out to get them.

What do people want when they act out anger?

They want to feel better.

They want to let off steam.

They want to get what they want.

They want to punish someone or get even.

They want to tell their side of it.

They want an apology.

They want another person to stop doing something.

They want another person to change.

They want to hurt or get back.

They want attention.

They want their rights.

They want to stop an injustice or a meanness.

Do people always get what they want when they act out their anger? Listen to the following two stories.

1. David saw Kevin working on a science project during a free period in class the week before the science fair. David walked up to Kevin's table, stumbled, and knocked Kevin's project onto the floor. Kevin was angry because . . . . Think of some reasons why Kevin was angry.

He thought David did it on purpose.

He thought David was clumsy.

He thought his project was ruined.

He thought David didn't like him.

He thought the teacher would be mad at him.

He thought David should help him pick it up.

He thought David should apologize.

David felt ___________ because . . .

He wanted to ruin Kevin's project.

He accidentally knocked the project.

He was clumsy and he felt foolish.

He was afraid of what the teacher would say.

He wanted to be friends with Kevin.

He tried to get even with Kevin for something that happened earlier.

He wanted to make sure his project was the best in the class.

He wanted the other children to notice him.

He didn't know why he had done it.

2. Bob saw Hugh had a new bike. He watched Hugh ride up and down the street for a while but pretended not to be looking. Then he yelled out to Hugh, "Hey, you stupid idiot, you're going to get run over."

Bob felt ___________ because . . .

He thought Hugh was showing off.

He was concerned about Hugh's safety.

He wished he had a new bike, too.

He was thinking of something Hugh did earlier.

He wanted Hugh to let him ride it.

He felt bad about himself.

He wanted to hurt Hugh's feelings.

He wanted to be friends with Hugh.

He was afraid Hugh didn't like him.

He knew Hugh wanted him to be impressed.

He wanted to show he didn't care.

Hugh felt ___________ because . . .

He thought Bob was putting him down.

He was sensitive about his safety skills.

He wanted Bob to be impressed.

He wanted Bob to like him.

He thought he was stupid to ride by Bob's house.

He thought his new bike was just great.

He thought Bob was jealous.

He thought Bob was just kidding him.

Feelings are messages. Sometimes people misunderstand the messages they are sending and receiving. Sometimes they send messages that don't help them get what they want. Describe some of the messages sent in the previous examples. Then describe another way those messages could have been sent.

Different people sometimes feel differently about the same situation or event. The way they feel depends on

1. What they want to get
2. What they think should happen
3. How they feel generally about themselves
4. What happens before an event

Describe how the boys in the following three stories deal with their feelings.

1. Kenneth broke the point on his pencil just before the spelling test. He wanted to do well on the test because he'd have to stay in at recess if the words weren't well written. He had done badly on the test the week before because his writing was messy. He knew he was a bad writer, and the teacher was always telling him he was careless. He was sure the broken point on the pencil would ruin his chances on the test. He swore loudly and felt himself get tense all over. He kept thinking how unlucky he was and how everything was against him. He sat at his desk brooding until the test began.

How could Kenneth have dealt with his feelings in a different way? What actions or thoughts might have helped? Do you think he did well on the test?

2. Russ saw Ed knock some papers off the teacher's desk. He wanted to feel important so:

He told the teacher quietly that Ed did it.

He told Ed he saw him but wouldn't tell.

He told Ed he'd help him pick them up.

He told Ed he was always doing stupid things.

He told the other boys Ed was in trouble again.

He waited until recess and made fun of Ed.

He minded his own business and got on with his work.

He yelled out loudly, "Look what Ed's done!"

3. Isaiah was playing ball with James. Isaiah accidentally knocked James over, and James was angry. James had a difficult choice to make. He could choose to interpret the event a number of different ways. Which ways would make him feel best? Which ways would make Isaiah feel best? Why? What penalities are there for himself and others?

James retaliates

He yells, "I'll get you for this!"

He screams, "I'll never play with you again."

He punches Isaiah.

He insults Isaiah.

He complains to the teacher.

He sulks and broods.

James denies his anger

He pretends it's OK.

He blames Isaiah.

He swears at the "dumb ball."

He blames himself for his clumsiness.

James acknowledges his feelings but keeps them specific to the situation

He says, "That hurt, you know."

He asks Isaiah to be more careful.

He cries for a while but then tries to forget it.

He says, "I know it was an accident, but it really hurt me."

He asks Isaiah to apologize.

He says he's "had enough" for now.

He suggests they both go and get a drink.

Discuss penalties with respect to self-esteem and the relationship.

List some ways feelings are redirected or transformed.

By describing them

By taking them out on inanimate objects

Through physical exercise

By writing them down

By thinking about something pleasant

By counting to 10

By breathing deeply

Discuss some situations when you might choose not to reveal the full force of your feelings.

When the penalty is too great

When it makes you feel worse

When the person couldn't help hurting you

When you can understand why the person behaved badly

When you're angry with someone in authority over you

People make choices about what they do. Things don't always just happen to them. Think about some of the ways people make choices.

1. How to act
2. When and how to talk
3. Whether to show real feelings
4. Whether to let a tense situation get worse
5. Whether a relationship with a friend over the long term is more important than a specific incident

Let's talk about each of these choices.

Sometimes when we are upset we just blurt out things. Sometimes expressing strong feelings without thinking much about it is helpful to us, and sometimes it isn't. Think of as many reasons as you can why people yell at others when they are angry. I'll write them on the blackboard.

1. To get even
2. To get revenge
3. To improve things
4. To make someone stop or change
5. To get fair treatment
6. To blow off steam

Let's role-play as many different endings to this story as we can:

> Lamont came out of school to discover his bike had a flat tire. He saw Pete and Mike not far off, grinning. . . .
>
> Describe the effect of what Lamont said. How did it make him feel? How did it make the other boys feel? Did Lamont act in a hostile way? Do you think the flat tire was an accident? Did Lamont? Could it have been? Do you think that if Lamont immediately felt someone had done something to him on purpose, he might have overlooked other possibilities? Solving problems involves thinking about all of the possible alternatives—not jumping to just one conclusion. Let's make up some rules for solving problems. A solution to a problem should make us feel better, not get us into a worse mess.

1. Take time to think about all the possibilities.
2. Don't automatically suspect the worst possible outcome.
3. Don't try to get even without thinking first. You might attack an innocent person.
4. Assert your rights in a way that does not violate the rights of others.

5. Don't do anything that will later make you feel bad about yourself.
6. Never hurt someone else's feelings, body, or property.
7. Remember that if you lose control you often feel worse.
8. Remember that yelling, screaming, and fighting cause tension in your body.
9. Choose the best thing for you and not just the easiest.

Look in the mirror and say the following sentences with both an angry feeling and a good, satisfied feeling.

I knew that all the time.

My mom saw me do it.

My father is a policeman.

Now look in the mirror and say the following sentences with both a scared, anxious feeling and a satisfied, confident feeling.

Is anyone coming with me?

I think I can do that!

It wasn't me, Mr. Anderson.

Note what your face and body looked like and how your voice sounded when you expressed anger. Think of some alternative ways to tell people how you feel and how to avoid problems in the next stories.

> Jason was playing with his Legos and left them on the floor of the family room. His young brother, Jeremy, messed up the space station Jason had made and scattered all the pieces. When Jason came back, he grabbed Jeremy and shoved him aside. He yelled, "I hate you! You're always messing up my things, you brat!" Jeremy cried, and their mom was angry at Jason for hurting his brother.

What did Jason want? Let's see how many ideas we can think of:

1. He wanted his brother not to touch his things.
2. He wanted to punish his brother for ruining the space station.
3. He wanted to make sure his brother never did it again.

Do you think he got what he wanted? What effects did his actions have? What could he have done differently?

1. Put his Legos away in a safe place
2. Told his brother, in advance, not to touch his things without asking
3. Asked his mom, in advance, if it was OK to leave the Legos on the floor, and if so, if she'd tell Jeremy to leave them alone
4. Told Jeremy he was angry because he'd worked a long time on that space station
5. Told Jeremy he had to help pick up the pieces
6. Avoided name calling and "put downs"
7. Told Jeremy he'd let him play with the Legos if only he'd ask first
8. Told their mom that Jeremy had done it
9. Remembered not ever to hurt another person's body or feelings
10. Tried to think why Jeremy might have done it (e.g., to get attention, to make Jason mad, to get Jason into trouble, to get back at Jason for not letting him play, because he felt upset or angry about something else)

Discuss the effects of the following ways of expressing anger:

1. Name calling
2. Put-downs
3. Yelling and screaming
4. Talking quietly
5. Tenseness and strain

6. Calm discussion
7. Repeating oneself
8. Saying something once and waiting for an answer

For homework, find some definitions of the following words:

proof	circumstantial
evidence	suspect
hearsay	victim
retaliation	rights

Imagine you are a detective assigned to the following case. Read the facts and decide (a) how to proceed, (b) whose rights need to be protected, and (c) what advice you would give.

> Tony's grandmother was mugged. Her purse was later found in a trash can, and her money and credit cards were missing. Two teenagers had been seen loitering on a nearby corner after the incident. The grandmother reported that she did not see the assailants who came up behind her and knocked her to the ground as her purse was grabbed. She was hospitalized for a broken hip. Tony says he won't rest until he finds those two teenagers and breaks *their* hips!

Note that emphasis is placed on the universality of the feelings before specific discussion of an individual child's own feelings is attempted. The task sequence that follows is a useful guide for clinicians. It shows a progression of steps in which feelings are first described and then related to specific vocal behaviors. It can be adapted for use with a variety of emotions and vocal symptoms.

Task Sequence: Interpersonal Behavior–Vocal Behavior

A. *General Awareness*

1. I can identify feelings people have.
   anger — fear
   frustration — guilt
   joy — anxiety
   boredom — embarrassment
   sadness
2. I can describe how people express these feelings.
   facial expressions — words
   gestures and actions — postures
   voice
3. I can describe how feelings can be hidden.
   withdrawal — lies
   pretense — defiance/boasting
   aggressive/destructiveness — distractions
   humor

B. *Specific Awareness*

1. I can identify negative behaviors exhibited by others when they are in different moods.
   angry
   frustrated
   happy
   embarrassed
2. I can identify positive behaviors exhibited by others when they are in different moods.
   angry
   frustrated
   happy
   embarrassed
3. I can suggest some reasons why people act/or react in different ways.
   self-image
   role (e.g., power or authority)
   peer pressure
   fear of consequences
4. I can suggest some ways others can avoid or change inappropriate behaviors.
   voice
   posture
   actions
   words
5. I can describe how feelings can be expressed by changes in people's voices.
   pitch level — loudness level

pitch inflection	loudness changes
pauses/rate	tension/hard attacks on words
breathing	amount of talking/silence

6. I can describe how other people use their voices incorrectly in certain emotional states.

angry	excited or satisfied
anxious	dissatisfied
frightened	disappointed

7. I can describe how listeners react to some of these vocal characteristics.
   feel uncomfortable
   withdraw/don't listen
   become aggressive
   cooperate
   feel sympathetic/friendly/put down
8. I can describe the specific behaviors associated with incorrect vocal use.
   talking too loudly/too softly
   not using enough variety
   using a strained/tense/unpleasant voice
   using a hard sound to get started
   not taking in enough air to get started
   not pausing enough to replenish air supply
   talking too fast/too slow
   not responding to listener's feedback
   talking only about self
9. I can describe alternative behaviors people could use in certain emotional states.

angry	dissatisfied
anxious	excited
afraid	disappointed
satisfied	

10. I can describe ways to use the voice correctly.
    take in enough air to begin talking
    pause enough to refull air supply
    use an easy sound to get started
    use an easy/relaxed voice
    use an appropriate loudness level
    share talking time
    use more variety
    use gestures, questions, etc.

C. *Production*

1. I can demonstrate alternative nonvocal behaviors to use in certain emotional states.
   frightened
   satisfied
   anxious
   excited
   dissatisfied
   disappointed
2. I can demonstrate how to use my voice correctly in role playing certain emotional states.
   angry
   frightened
   satisfied
   anxious
   excited
   dissatisfied
   disappointed
3. I can evaluate the effects of my vocal behavior during role playing.
   on my body
   on my feelings
   on achieving what I want
   on others' reactions to me

D. *Carryover*

1. I can describe the times in my everyday life when it is hardest for me to use and maintain appropriate vocal behavior.

emotional state	background noise
size of group	physical state
type of activity	specific person spoken to
time of day	purpose of interaction
location of the talking	

2. I can develop strategies for correct behavior in my difficult emotional states and situations.
   alternative vocal strategies
   alternative nonvocal strategies
3. I can use correct vocal and nonvocal behaviors in difficult emotional states and situations I have preplanned.
   sometimes

most of the time
all of the time

4. I can evaluate the results of my preplanned vocal and nonvocal behaviors.
   on myself
   on others
   on achieving my goal
5. I can use correct vocal and nonvocal strategies in difficult emotional states and situations spontaneously.
   some of the time
   most of the time
   all of the time

In the treatment plan just discussed, extensive use was made of self-regulating speech. The various interpretations of some of the situations were modeled first by the clinician and gradually were picked up and used spontaneously by the boys as new examples were analyzed. It became clear that the boys' expectations concerning the intent of others' actions were frequently that the action was purposeful rather than accidental. The clinician noted this and included more frequent examples of aggressive reactions to "accidental" happenings so that the boys could see that accidents frequently occur. The use of discussion of situations and analyses of events concerning other children proved extremely helpful. The boys delighted in identifying what others did wrong and competed with one another in the group to be the first to find better solutions. The group interaction was stimulating. Nevertheless, the clinician found it necessary to establish and enforce certain ground rules:

1. No two people talk at once; take turns.
2. No solutions can involve lying, physical abuse, or the hurting of another's feeling or property.
3. Talk at a moderate level or forfeit your turn.

The clinician praised the boys liberally when they obeyed the rules and awarded points for appropriate participation in activities. The group kept and reviewed weekly a running total of points, and rewards were given each month for the highest number of points. The boys' self-esteem was bolstered by the way the clinician praised their participation (e.g., "Howie is always good at thinking of this kind of solution—I bet he'll know what the boy could try," or, "Now, Joe had trouble with interrupting too much last week, but I can tell he's got that under control today"). The boys responded well to the clinician's reiteration of his confidence in their ability to control their impulses and seek creative solutions to their problems. Their expectations that they could handle tough situations in acceptable (and more profitable) ways seemed to increase as a result of the way the clinician reflected his positive view of their abilities.

One of the most important insights that the boys developed was the need to analyze the purpose of an interaction before discussing alternative strategies. For example, once they clarified that their purpose was to make the listener understand their point of view rather than react angrily to them, they then could see the advantages of adopting a quieter, more reasonable vocal style as opposed to a loud, defiant, or belligerent tone of voice.

In this approach, the clinician plays an important role in helping the child understand his or her goal in each interaction. The clinician's questioning and prompting during discussions helps children strip away the emotional components in an interaction to focus on what they wish to achieve (e.g., to explain their position, to defend their actions, to persuade another to change).

Richard and Dodge (1982) suggested that the generation of many solutions to hypothetical persuasive tasks does significantly increase the number of actual persuasive attempts made by children in behavioral situations. The number of solutions generated does not necessarily predict the competence or success of those attempts. They say that clinicians who wish to train these skills must remember that generating many solutions and generating competent solutions to hypothetical persuasive tasks are independent cognitive skills. Our clinicial experience suggests that group treatment aimed at addressing interpersonal difficulties underlying negative vocal behaviors is a useful approach. It is a format that allows the clinician to capitalize on opportunities to demonstrate how different people see things differently and thus to teach perspective-taking. It also allows for role-playing activities to practice and evaluate the use of competent solutions.

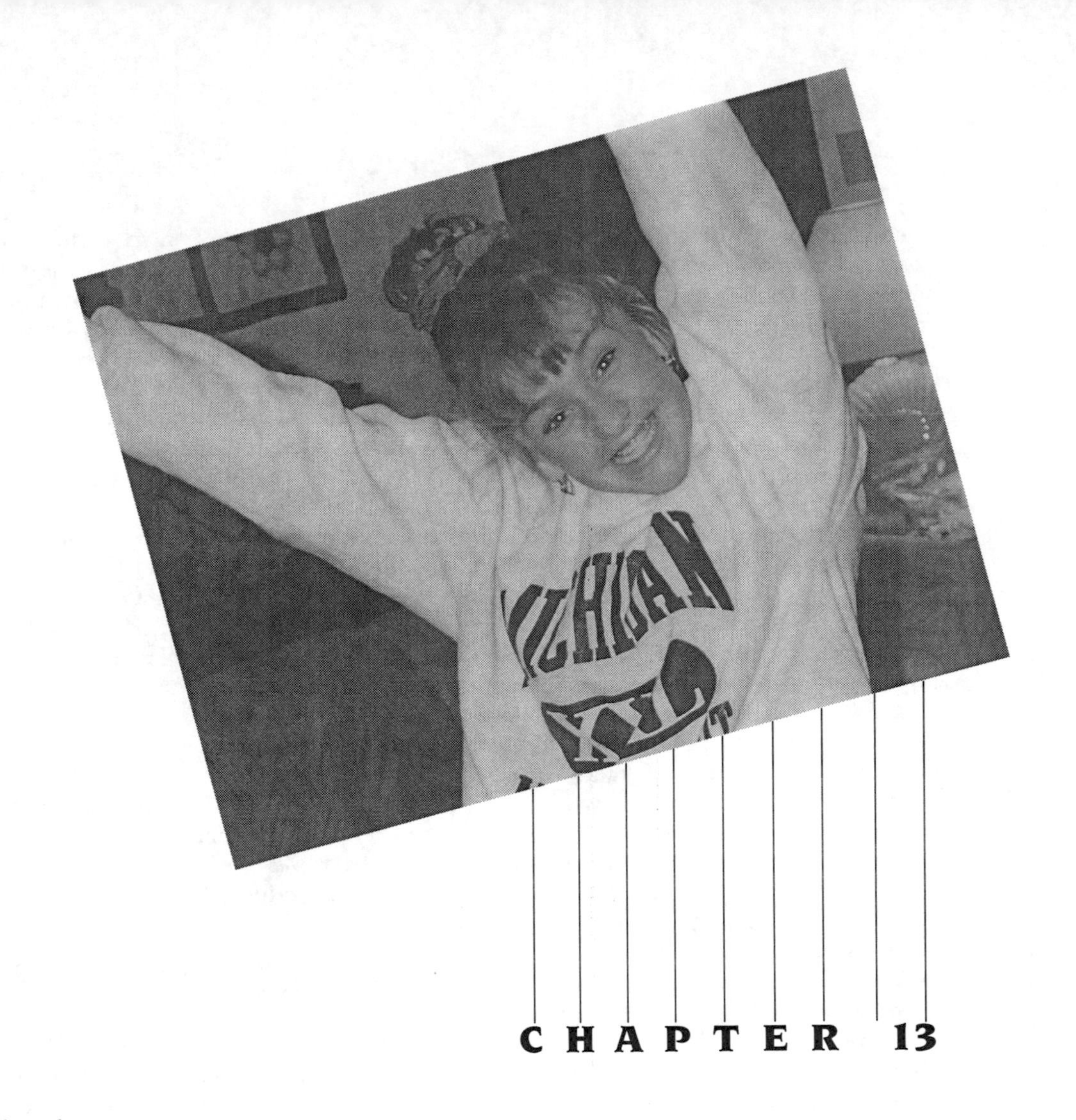

CHAPTER 13

Adolescence: A Time for Change

The treatment of middle and high school students with voice disorders has been underemphasized by both training institutions and speech–language pathologists working in the field (Wilson, 1987). One possible explanation for this neglect is the assumption that the treatment of younger children is more productive because problems are less habituated and therefore more responsive to intervention.

The passage of PL 105-17, the Individuals with Disabilities Education Act Amendments of 1997 (IDEA '97), mandated free and appropriate services for all infants, toddlers, children, and youth with disabilities, including communication impairment. Nonetheless, although speech–language pathologists now recognize their responsibility to service the adolescent population, many clinicians express a lack of confidence in working with this age group. Most have clinical experience primarily with younger children or with adults. Consequently, when faced with adolescents to treat, they often are forced to make adaptations of strategies previously used with different age groups.

Frequently, too, speech–language pathologists may be frustrated by what they perceive to be a lack of motivation on the part of the adolescent. Yet it has been suggested that during puberty, many students become motivated to make vocal changes because of an increased need for social acceptance (Wilson, 1985). A clinician's own knowledge, attitudes, and expectations concerning the efficacy of intervention with this population probably has a dramatic effect on the outcome. To meet the needs of the adolescent population, speech–language pathologists need to have adequate information and resources. Access to specific information relevant to the needs of these students enables speech–language pathologists to design and implement viable intervention programs.

Most voice disorders seen in adolescents (with the possible exception of mutational falsetto) also are seen in younger children and adults. Our central thesis is not that a specific disorder is unique to any population, but rather that an individual's needs, interests, and motivation are different at different stages of development. Thus, voice therapy programs should be designed specifically for adolescents. It is particularly important to recognize the interactive nature of adolescent development. Physical development occurs simultaneously with emotional and cognitive changes, all of which affect each other as well as identity formation. Of course, the timing, sequence, and relative emphasis of the changes are unique to each individual.

The adolescent is neither a child nor an adult. Although some authorities refer to distinct stages during adolescent development and note the diverse needs of the age range, it is probably safe to generalize that all adolescents are in transition. They experience dramatic changes in their bodies, social interactions, and lifestyles.

Physical and Hormonal Changes

Most obvious in adolescence are the physical changes. They influence, to some extent, the emotional and sociologic changes that occur as the individual redefines the self-concept. Changes include growth in height, growth of the sex organs leading to the capacity for reproduction, appearance of body hair, increased activity of sweat glands, increased secretion of skin oil, increased muscle mass and strength, and growth of the larynx, particularly an increase in the length of the vocal folds.

The predominant physical change that is of interest to voice clinicians working with adolescents is maturation of the laryngeal mechanism. Sometime during the middle and high school years, boys and girls experience the hormonal changes that result in the physical manifestations of puberty. The time of onset and duration of puberty vary, but generally puberty occurs earlier in girls. Nonetheless, vocal mutation, or the voice change that takes place as one manifestation of puberty, is more dramatic in boys than in girls. According to Aronson (1973), complete mutation of voice takes place within 3 to 6 months. During this time, the neck lengthens, and the larynx increases in size and descends. The male vocal folds increase about 10 mm in length and become thicker. This increase in the size and mass of the folds influences the modal frequency of the voice, and a boy's pitch level lowers about an octave. Girls' vocal folds increase about 4 mm, and their pitch levels lower about 3 to 4 semitones (Zemlin, 1968).

Most boys and girls go through voice change uneventfully. Generally, the changes in a girl's voice are not noticed. The majority of boys also proceed through vocal mutation without the extreme vocal fluctuations and pitch breaks that society associates with the stereotypical pubertal boy. Nonetheless, a boy may experience embarrassment when his increased laryngeal growth is not synchronized with neurological control of the changed structures and unpredictable vocal behaviors occur, such as unexpected pitch breaks. To keep this in perspective, one study (Pedry, 1945) reported only four breaks in a total reading time of 84 hours for 1,014 adolescent boys. When Pedry questioned his subjects, 674 boys reported experiencing vocal breaks at some time and, of these, less than half remembered some feelings of embarrassment. Only six boys reported extreme embarrassment.

Derived from the Greek word *hormon*, meaning "to set in motion," hormones govern every aspect of growth and development as well as reproduction, metabolism, and emotional states. Hormones are secreted by the endocrine glands (thyroid, pituitary, adrenals, ovaries, and testes) and interact in a complex manner. In adolescence, there is a sudden flooding of hormones into the bloodstream. The process starts with the master hormone, gonadotropin-releasing hormone (GRH), released in the hypothalamus. This signals the pituitary to secrete the gonadotropic hormones FSH (follicle-stimulating hormone) and LH (luteinizing hormone). These are called gonadotropic hormones because their targets are the gonads, or sex glands (ovaries in girls and testes in boys). FSH and LH cause the ovaries to produce estrogen and the testes to make testosterone. These sex hormones exert an additional influence on the brain, liver, salivary glands, skin, and muscles.

The human growth hormone (GH), produced by the pituitary, controls growth during childhood and puberty. The genders appear to differ widely in the timing of the adolescent growth spurt, more so than in the age at which secondary sex characteristics appear. The growth spurt usually is the first overt sign of the onset of puberty, and longitudinal studies provide the most accurate information concerning the approximate range of ages at which each stage of puberty is reached. Boys develop, on the average, 2 years later than girls. The growth spurt occurs in American boys, on the average, at 14 years with the standard deviation of 0.9 years (Tanner, 1971). This peak velocity of height averages about 10.5 cm/year in boys. Children who have their peak early reach a height that is often somewhat higher than those who experience it late.

Changes in Boys

The adolescent growth spurt affects nearly all skeletal and muscular dimensions, but to different degrees. Leg length usually reaches its peak first, followed by body breadth and shoulder width. Increase in the muscle mass of the limbs and heart coincides with skeletal changes and with loss in fat. Boys also develop larger lungs relative to their overall size, which increases their respiratory capacity. Power, athletic skill, and physical endurance all increase rapidly throughout adolescence. Boys experience a greater increase in both muscle size and strength than do girls, and this results in the ability to perform heavier tasks. Boys' physical endurance also increases.

Boys have greater increase in the length of their bones. Skeletal maturity, or "bone age," is frequently measured to ascertain developmental age. Skeletal maturity is closely related to the age at which adolescence (maturity measured by secondary sex characteristics) occurs. The physiologic processes controlling skeletal development seem closely linked with those that initiate sexual maturation. Tempo of growth and maturation is biologically rooted but depends somewhat on an interaction of genetic and environmental factors (Tanner, 1971).

In boys, the earliest hormonal alterations of pubertal maturation involve secretion of the adrenal androgens, dehydroepilandrosterone and dehydroepiandrosterone sulfate. (Androgens are any substances that produce masculinizing effects. Others include androsterone and testosterone.) Plasma levels of these two hormones begin to rise between 6 and 10 years of age. Testosterone concentrations increase slightly by 11 years of age, whereas levels of pituitary gonadotropins, FSH and LH, increase slowly after age 8 to 10.

Although the timing of the onset of puberty varies, the sequence of events is usually strikingly similar between individuals. The first sign of puberty in boys is most often growth of the testes (Tanner, 1971). Male genital development, according to Marshall and Tanner (1970), is considered normal if it occurs between ages 9 and 15; however, male pubic hair growth in the absence of genital enlargement is sufficiently unusual to arouse suspicion of abnormality.

Growth of pubic hair (appearing about 18 months later in boys than in girls), height spurts, and penis growth usually begin approximately 1 year following the changes in the testes. The seminal vesicles and the prostate and bulbourethral glands develop and enlarge at the same time as penis growth occurs. About a year after penis development begins, there is the first ejaculation of seminal fluid.

Sebaceous and apocrine sweat glands develop rapidly in boys' skin, and enlargement of the pores gives a coarser appearance to the skin, especially on the nose and limbs. Acne seems more common in boys than in girls because skin changes are related to androgenic activity. Male breast changes include an increase in the diameter of the areola and some temporary enlargement of breast tissue in some boys.

Axillary hair and facial hair do not generally appear until about 2 years after the onset of pubic hair growth. Although this is variable, there seems to be a definite pattern in the way the hairs of the mustache and beard occur. First, hair is seen at the corners, and then all over the upper lip. Next, hair is seen on the upper part of the cheeks, in the midline below the lower lip, and then along the sides and lower border of the chin. The amount of hair a boy finally acquires on his body seems to be related to heredity.

Because the appearance of facial hair in boys occurs toward the end of the sequence of physiological changes (e.g., genital development; height spurt; growth of pubic, axillary, and facial hair), it is a useful reference point for the speech–language pathologist. Facial hair observed during a diagnostic session can indicate that the male student has reached the latter stages of pubertal maturation. Indeed, the speech–language pathologist who remembers the individual differences in boys' tempo of growth yet is aware that the sequence of events remains consistent would not be alarmed to note a high-pitched voice in a boy who obviously has not undergone a growth spurt or a low-pitched voice in a boy who obviously has. Between the ages of 9 and 14, boys begin the sequence of pubertal changes, and the speech–language pathologist can expect greater variability. The diagnostician must have the flexibility to observe indications of skeletal and maturational levels.

Enlargement of the larynx and lengthening of the vocal folds usually occur relatively late in the maturational process (e.g., after the onset of genital changes). This is caused by the action of testosterone on the laryngeal cartilages (Tanner, 1971) and affects pitch level and variability. Quality changes in the male voice are related to increased respiratory capacity and enlargement of the resonating cavities above the larynx. The increased resonance capacity is related to adolescent enlargement of the nose, mouth, and maxilla. The observant speech–language pathologist may detect, for example, "adolescent facies" that are associated with the structural growth of the oronasal areas.

Changes in Girls

Girls complete the adolescent growth spurt earlier than boys (at about age 11 to 13 for girls, versus as late as about 15 for boys). The peak velocity of height (PHV, which is used extensively in growth studies) averages about 9 cm/year (Tanner, 1971). The velocity over the whole year encompassing the 6 months before and after the peak is somewhat less. During this year, girls usually grow between 6 and 11 cm (in contrast to boys who grow between 7 and 12 cm). Nearly all skeletal and muscular dimensions are involved in the dramatic growth spurt, though not, of course, to the same degree. The earliest structures to reach their adult size are the head, hands, and feet. Many adolescent girls complain about having big hands and feet, and many parents note that in fights with siblings, adolescents do not always realize their hand strength. Leg length usually reaches its peak next, followed by body breadth and shoulder width. Most of the spurt in height is due to acceleration of trunk length rather than leg length. The increase in muscle mass coincides with skeletal growth. There may be a period when girls' muscles are larger than those of their male contemporaries because they experience their spurt earlier. Once the growth spurt has occurred in boys, however, they become stronger than girls. They have larger muscles, hearts, and lungs and a higher systolic blood pressure. Boys lose fat during the growth spurt, whereas it merely decelerates in girls.

Although the sebaceous and apocrine sweat glands develop rapidly during puberty, this is usually less marked in girls than in boys. In girls, the appearance of the "breast bud" is usually the first sign of puberty, though the appearance of pubic hair may precede it in about one third of the adolescent female population. Both the uterus and vagina develop at the same time as the breast, and the labia and clitoris also enlarge. These developments precede menarche (the first menstruation), which occurs relatively late in the maturation sequence and rarely begins before the height spurt has been achieved. On the average, girls grow only about 6 cm more after menarche (Tanner, 1971). During the adolescent growth spurt, a girl's body composition shows a ratio of lean to fat tissue of 5:1. At menarche, this ratio has reached 3:1. At the average age of menarche (between the 12th and 13th birthdays), 24% of a girl's body composition is fat, and her critical weight is between 94 and 103 pounds (Frisch & Revelle, 1971a). Naturally, there is tremendous normal variation that occurs in the interval from the appearance of the first sign of puberty to complete maturity (from 18 months to 6 years). Marshall and Tanner (1969) provided an excellent summary of the limits of what may be considered normal.

The sequence of biologic changes that occurs at adolescence has not changed over centuries, but the time of onset has changed markedly. Improved social conditions and improved nutrition across socioeconomic levels have resulted in less variation in onset as a function of class status. Much of the variation that still exists could probably be attributed to genetic factors. Nonetheless, it frequently has been observed that girls in warmer climates (e.g., Mediterranean cultures) mature earlier than those in less temperate climates. Modern writers relate these differences to dietary practices rather than to geographic influences such as temperature and light exposure.

Since the publication of Frisch's (1972) studies on critical weights, attention has been focused on the role of exercise on the biologic development of the female adolescent. Legislation that mandated equal opportunity for female high school students has, in many instances, improved the physical education programs available for girls. In view of the earlier age of onset of menarche in present-day society and concerns about high pregnancy rates among teenagers, many experts feel that sedentary lifestyles, in combination with rich diets, could be responsible for the shift toward fertility at earlier ages. To combat this trend, some educators are committed to providing courses in nutrition and regular exercise for all female students in the middle and high schools. When female athletes and dancers exercise to the point where critical body ratios are jeopardized or in cases of anorexia or bulimia, however, cessation of menstrual periods can occur.

A widespread concern of middle and high school girls is learning to deal with the discomfort associated with managing their early menstrual cycles while maintaining active teenage lifestyles. Some girls experience severe menstrual pain, cramping, and irregular, unpredictable cycles. Increased anxiety, irritability, and mood swings can occur in the week or so preceding the onset of the menstrual flow. A cluster of symptoms associated with this time in the female cycle has been categorized as premenstrual syndrome (PMS; Dalton, 1977).

It is documented that as many as 95% of women experience some symptoms of PMS (e.g., depression, fatigue, irritability, anxiety, edema of laryngeal and nasal mucosa, acne, breast soreness, or bloating) in the week or so preceding their menstrual flow. The intensity of discomfort during the menstrual cycle may be influenced by the circumstances in which it is experienced. Some physicians have postulated that PMS is due to the tension of modern life, but studies of cultures throughout the world dispute this hypothesis, and definitive evidence concerning the exact cause of PMS still eludes researchers.

Occasionally, the speech–language pathologist may encounter female students with cyclical vocal symptoms that may be related to the menstrual cycle—lowered pitch, hoarseness, vocal instability, voice "breaks," huskiness, sinus or nasal congestion, and decreased flexibility in the upper part of the singing range. It is possible also that some individuals may be especially sensitive to the effects of synthetic hormones (such as those in birth control pills) on the phonatory system. Many professional voice users avoid use of contraceptive pills, which are made up of synthetic estrogen and progestin, because they believe the changes that occur in the vocal mechanism seriously affect vocal quality and artistic performance. It is also interesting to note that it has long been the custom in European opera houses for female singers to have the option of not performing during those times in the menstrual cycle when their voices are adversely affected. Usually, however, the effects of the menstrual cycle on the voice are subtle and may not be significant unless the young woman has a great investment in activities involving aesthetic vocal performance.

There is some evidence that premenstrual swelling of the laryngeal and nasal membranes contributes to voice quality deviations. Women who experience severe vocal problems will require a comprehensive medical evaluation by a physician who is knowledgeable concerning PMS. They may also need assistance in monitoring fluctuations in specific symptoms. Lifestyle changes (e.g., stress reduction techniques, dietary modifications to reduce fluid retention in tissues, and exercise) are frequently suggested as management strategies. Each individual needs to monitor her own reactions and learn optimum ways of managing symptoms. For example, avoiding vocally abusive activities when laryngeal edema is present may be especially important for students who aspire to professional voice use.

Hormonal Therapy

Reiter (1981) reported that delayed adolescence occurs in 25 of every 1,000 children; in 2 to 5% of boys, sexual development will be delayed more than 2 years, and in 0 to 1% more than 3 years. Unless the physical growth spurt has occurred, however, physicians frequently may not think about delayed sexual maturation.

If the adult stage of genital development has not occurred by the age of 17, physicians usually consider the possibility of systemic or endocrinologic disease. There also can be a familial pattern of constitutional delay where the timing of pubertal events is shifted to a later time. Sometimes this may be related to nutritional deprivation or psychologic aberrations within the family.

Physicians use hormonal therapy to treat adolescents with delayed or disturbed growth and sexual development. There seems to be some evidence that stress hormones can suppress growth and may be linked to depression, upper respiratory infections, cancers, and memory loss. Some researchers believe that teenagers who mature late and have adjustment problems may have higher levels of cortisol (an adrenal cortical hormone).

Close medical supervision is required in all instances of hormonal therapy because of the vast array of side effects that can occur. Currently, the major reasons for hormone usage in the adolescent age group include treatment of medical conditions, birth control, and improved athletic performance.

Testosterone is classified as a steroid (which resembles cholesterol compounds) rather than as a protein hormone. The functions of testosterone are (a) the androgenic, or masculinizing effect; (b) the anabolic, or protein-building effect; and (c) an inhibitory effect on the hypophysis (pituitary gland; Witzmann, 1977). When the body does not produce enough male hormone, such as in children with chromosomal abnormalities, testosterone replacement therapy is frequently the only means of clinical intervention designed to stimulate sexual development and the emergence of the male secondary sex characteristics. In cases such as kidney disorders and slow-healing fractures, the protein-building effect may be used therapeutically. With these patients, however, the body is already producing testosterone at the appropriate level for the individual. Therefore, the added steroid hormone almost always produces some adverse effects directly proportional to the dosage and length of treatment. Occasionally, testosterone is administered clinically to produce an inhibitory effect on hormone production. This occurs because the hypophysis is part of the body's mechanism for regulating hormone production and, in the presence of increased hormones, the hypophysis will send the message for the body to reduce production of that hormone.

It is impossible to completely separate the three functions of testosterone. Almost all testosterone recipients experience the hormone's androgenic, anabolic, and inhibitory effects, as well as the substance's adverse side effects. There is general agreement that prolonged ingestion of very large doses of testosterone does increase lean body mass and total body weight. Thus, for the athlete, this may appear to be an easy way to increase overall athletic strength. When a male ingests large doses of synthetic testosterone, however, the testes stop producing their own testosterone. Paradoxically, even though a large amount of synthetic testosterone is present in the blood, a cessation of natural testosterone results in a feminizing effect.

If high doses of testosterone are given to a prepubescent boy (e.g., a junior high football player who is under pressure to gain weight and muscle mass quickly), the results may be disastrous. The physical changes (appearance of facial and pubic hair, increase in height, increase in vocal fold size resulting in a deepening of the voice, and the production of testosterone) may occur only partially, if at all. This is because the hypothalamus monitors the level of testosterone in the body rather than specific physical changes. Thus, in the presence of high levels of exogenous testosterone, the hypothalamus sends messages to the target organs saying, "OK, puberty is over. You can stop growing facial and pubic hair, close the growth plates, and stop lengthening the vocal folds." The boy may be only 12 years old, 5 feet tall, and not yet through puberty, but the hypothalamus has done its job. As a result, the boy will probably grow up to be several inches shorter than he would have been if he had not taken testosterone. He may not develop facial and pubic hair, and he will probably go through voice change (vocal mutation) at a late age, if at all.

Androgenic (masculinizing and virilizing) effects of testosterone on girls may include menstrual disturbances, coarsening of the skin, male hair-growth patterns or baldness, and a deepening of the voice.

Some of the signs of steroid use include impatience, hostility, increased sex drive, less sleep, aging skin, head hair loss, increased body hair, darker colored genitals, and collection of cholesterol globules on the underside of the eyeballs (Jerome, 1980; Todd, 1983). Possible side effects from steroid use include sterility, liver problems, and atherosclerosis (Todd, 1983).

Jerome (1980) stated that birth control pills are, in themselves, steroids. Oral contraceptives contain synthetic forms of estrogen and progesterone. These externally supplied hormones assume some of the functions of the internally produced hormones but block others. For example, the synthetic estrogen and progesterone in oral contraceptives build up the uterine lining but suppress ovulation. They have been used not only to control fertility, but also to ameliorate menstrual pain.

Vocal Mutation

Aristotle was probably the first writer who definitely connected voice change with puberty. Prepubertal male and female larynges are the same size. At puberty, the larynx descends, and the dimensions of the infraglottal sagittal and transverse planes increase. The anterioposterior dimensions also increase, with greater increases in the male larynx than in the female larynx. The angle of the male thyroid lamina decreases to 90° compared with the female angle of 120° (Aronson, 1980). The vocal folds increase in length, the mucosa becomes stronger, and the epiglottis increases in size.

Kahane (1978) reported measurements he made from 10 White male and 10 White female cadaveric larynges, ranging in age from 9 to 18 years at death. He compared his findings with the relatively few other studies of the human circumpubertal larynx reported in the literature. When Kahane compared his prepubertal and pubertal groups, he consistently observed several morphologic relationships:

- Pubertal cartilage and soft tissue measurements were significantly larger than prepubertal measurements for both genders, although within-sex differences were greater among boys than girls.

- Gender differences were not present before puberty (first noted by Klock, 1968). Some of the differences noted included:
  1. Length of vocal folds and weights of laryngeal cartilages were significantly larger in pubertal boys than in pubertal girls.
  2. Thyroid eminence in pubertal boys was more prominent than in pubertal girls.

  Kahane believed that his measurements of the cricoid, arytenoid, and soft tissues also supported the notion that there is significantly greater growth in the larynx of the boy than in the larynx of the girl from prepuberty to puberty.
- Pubertal laryngeal measurements in both genders, however, were still clearly different from adults in seven dimensions:
  1. The weights of all laryngeal cartilages
  2. The angle of the thyroid laminae (regional growth in the male thyroid cartilage appeared to take place in the anterior aspect)
  3. The height of the cricoid arch, anteriorly at midline
  4. Distance between the cricoid facets
  5. Midsagittal length of the cricoid lumen
  6. Superiolateral length of the cricoid
  7. Anterior ridge height of the arytenoid cartilages

Because the prepubertal female dimensions more clearly approximate adult size and weight, Kahane (1978) extrapolated that the pubertal girl requires less laryngeal growth per unit of time to mature than does the prepubertal boy. Sizable differences found in the weights of adult and pubertal cartilages led to the conclusion that differences were probably related to ossification that may begin as early as 20 years of age (Hately, Evison, & Samuel, 1965). In contrast, the length of both male and female vocal folds at puberty was not significantly different from that of adults (measurements of vocal fold length were "total or inclusive," not merely the membranous portion). The amount of increase in vocal fold length in the boy was 10.87 mm and 4.16 mm in the girl. Kahane noted that the greater growth in the length of the male folds is probably accompanied by increases in width, although this dimension was not explored in this study. The greater structural changes in the male larynx correlate with the greater drop in fundamental frequency of the male voice during puberty.

Weiss (1950), in his classic study, listed several changes within the organs of phonation during pubertal development of boys:

- The lungs undergo a large increase in breathing capacity. Both the circumference and length of the chest cavity increase rapidly.
- The neck increases in length and width. When the neck lengthens, the larynx descends relative to this growth. This increases the length and width of the pharyngeal tube. Weiss claimed a widening of the oral pharynx during this time, coupled with the change of length in the pharyngeal cavity, causes the change of vocal timbre.
- There is relatively little material available in regard to the pubertal development of the nasal sinuses. Some sinuses do not appear until this time, especially the frontal sinuses. The addition of these sinuses gives more resonance and a distinct quality to the voice.
- The larynx enlarges considerably due to the influence of sex hormones. The concept that the larynx increases to double its size is false. This idea was derived from the belief that the pitch of the voice depends upon the length of the vocal folds, and because male voices generally descend one octave, the folds must double in size. The length of the vocal lips within the larynx grow by about 1 cm in boys and about 3 to 4 mm in girls.

Weiss (1950) determined that the main difference between pubertal development in boys and girls concerned the main direction of the growth of the larynx. Until puberty, they are essentially the same size, but during pubertal growth, the male larynx grows especially fast in the anterioposterior direction. This results in the "protrusion of what is known as the 'pommmum Adami' (Adam's Apple), the distinct lengthening of the vocal cords, and the narrowing of the angle formed by both plates of the thyroid cartilage. All these features are more pronounced in individuals with deep voices and may appear even in females in that same category" (p. 131). Generally, the female larynx grows more in height than in width or depth at this stage and becomes distinctly different from the male larynx.

Weiss (1950) claimed an overall increase in the size of all organs of phonation. This results in a deepening of the voice and an increase in breath and resonance with more vocal power. The range of descent averages an octave for boys and 3 to 4 notes for girls. Weiss mentioned further physical transformation that takes place during this mutation: "The mucosa of the larynx becomes stronger and less transparent. The tonsils and adenoids atrophy (decrease in size) to a certain degree. The cavernous tissue of the nasal turbinates develops. The epiglottis increases in size, flattens out, and assumes a more elevated position" (p. 132).

Weiss (1950) felt that there were certain "premutational" changes, including some loss of voice, a slight lowering of pitch, and problems controlling the voice. The "huskiness" has been noted by many writers and may be due to incomplete closure of the glottis (posterior glottal chink) before the folds complete the thickening and lengthening process. It is generally believed that the speaking voice completes mutation within about 3 to 6 months, but that the singing voice may take 1 to 2 years to completely mature.

Tosi, Postan, and Bianculli (1976) studied boys in Buenos Aires over an 8-month period. They found that at mean age 13.3 years, their subjects showed maximal change of fundamental frequency and minimal value of standard deviation (17 Hz).

A study of pitch changes by McGlone and Hollien (1963) demonstrated that female voices lowered 2.4 semitones during puberty. At completion of vocal mutation, the female average fundamental frequencies found by Mischel et al. (1966) were 277 Hz. Hollien and Malcik (1967) reported the median fundamental frequency of 18-year-old men was 126 Hz. In an earlier study by Curry (1940), 10-year-old boys had a median fundamental frequency of 269 Hz, and 14-year-old boys had a median of 241 Hz, with 18-year-olds dropping to 137 Hz. Hollien and Malcik (1967) and Hollien, Malcik, and Hollien (1965) studied Southern male subjects and reported lower median fundamental frequency levels for adolescent Black subjects.

Andrews (1982) tested 740 Australian school children aged 5 to 13 years and analyzed vocal frequency measurements in relation to age, gender, weight, height, and neck circumference. A significant difference between boys' and girls' measurements appeared at age 9.5 years. When the children were divided into two groups (i.e., 5 to 9.5 years old and 9.5 to 13 years old), an analysis of variance indicated that with respect to habitual levels of the younger group, height, weight, neck circumference, gender, and age (and the interaction between gender and age) were not significant. Weight was significant ($F = 6.030$, $p < .015$), however. For the older group, gender was highly significant ($F = 23.280$, $p < .001$) as was height ($F = 4.548$, $p < .034$). These results underscore the relationship between habitual frequency level, gender, and height as the child matures. As children grow older, height may be a more useful index of vocal maturity than chronologic age. Neck circumference did not correlate with frequency measurements in this study.

Two methods of eliciting measurements of basal frequency were compared in Andrews' (1982) study. One method involved sliding down to the lowest possible pitch (visual feedback was provided on the Visi-Pitch screen), and the other method was the traditional approach of asking children to produce their lowest pitch (visual feedback was also provided). Three trials were given for each approach. It is interesting to note that for all age groups, the sliding method of obtaining basal frequency resulted in measurements that averaged 20 Hz lower than those obtained using the traditional method of elicitation. For example, the 12- to 13-year-old children produced an average basal frequency of 208 Hz when asked to produce their lowest note, yet "slid down" to an average basal pitch of 187 Hz. It seemed as if it was easier for these students to "descend" to their basal pitch than to "land" on it. One is reminded of how untrained singers sometimes seem to "slide down" to the lower notes in their range.

When basal frequency measurements were compared with habitual frequency levels for all children in the study, there was an average of 43 Hz difference between the two measures, whereas the lowest limit of the conversational pitch range they used averaged 23 Hz below the habitual average level. A summary of the habitual and basal levels of the students aged 9 to 13 years appears in Table 13–1. It may be that basal pitch measures reflect laryngeal change earlier than do habitual pitch measures because lower notes may be added to the available range before the adoption of a lower habitual level.

A technique that is sometimes helpful in facilitating production of basal pitch is to ask students to "slide down" into vocal fry, the lowest frequency register characterized by a rough vocal quality. Some high school choir directors may at times even encourage male students to sing low notes with fry. The technique is referred to as the "Russian" method because Russian bass voices are noted for depth and richness of tone. Teachers of

Table 13–1. Averaged measurements of habitual and basal frequency levels during early adolescence.

Age	*No.*	*Habitual Level* (Hz)	*Basal Level* (Hz)
Boys			
9 years	68	237	192
10 years	67	226	191
11 years	92	227	186
12 years	30	225	182
13 years	32	221	180
Girls			
9 years	55	236	199
10 years	49	237	196
11 years	70	237	196
12 years	26	236	192
13 years	31	227	191

singing also use the term *low terminal pitch* when referring to the basal or lowest musical note in an individual's range of available pitches.

During the 19th century in Italy, castration was frequently practiced to maintain the childlike soprano voice in male singers. The castrati had pure high-pitched voices because of their immature laryngeal development, combined with the respiratory capacity of an adult male. Today, rather than attempting to prevent voice change in male singers, choir directors and teachers of singing work to ensure a careful transition from the child's singing voice to mature male voice. There has been a great deal of controversy concerning whether adolescent boys should sing during their period of voice change, and the type of singing that should be encouraged. Writers such as Cooper (1970), McKenzie (1956), and Swanson (1960), have presented differing views concerning the way the singing voices of adolescent boys should be treated. Whereas the speaking voice has a mutational duration of 3 to 6 months, the singing voice can take longer, perhaps up to 2 years. This vocal mutation generally follows a predictable pattern during puberty: from soprano to alto (11 to 12 years of age), to a cross between alto and baritone (13 to 14 years of age), to light baritone (14 to 15 years of age), and, finally, to a more settled baritone, bass, or tenor (16 to 19 years of age).

Joseph (1963) studied 200 adolescent boys (aged 11 years 10 months to 16 years 9 months) and tape recorded them once monthly for 8 consecutive months. The average low terminal pitch at the start of the study was around C to C# on the bass staff. This average lowered to a low A on the bass staff, or by about a third, during the 8-month test. The average boy's range at the beginning of the study was $1\frac{1}{3}$ octaves, whereas the median range was $1\frac{1}{5}$ octaves. The aver-age range at the end of the study was $2\frac{1}{3}$ octaves, whereas the median range was 2 octaves and 1 second.

Naidr, Zobril, and Sevcik (1965) in Czechoslovakia performed a longitudinal study of male adolescent voice mutation. On the average, the most significant changes took place during ages 13 and 14. The lower limit of the singing range lowered 8 semitones, and the upper limit lowered 13 semitones. Cooksey (1977) provides a detailed summary of changes in the singing voice of the adolescent male. Also see Spiegel, Sataloff, and Emerich (1997) for a description of the young adult voice.

Psychosocial Factors Related to Physical Maturation

Teenagers are in the process of acquiring new body images. Pubescent boys and girls are busy "trying out" new social roles and their attention, quite naturally, is focused on comparisons of their own bodies with those of others. Their degree of physical maturation affects the perceptions adults, as well as peers, have of them, so environmental reinforcers interact with somatic changes. Money and Clopper (1974) break down "psychosocial" age into academic, recreational, and psychosexual age. These usually correlate with chronological and physique age. When deviations from the usual timetable of pubertal development occur, the predictable psychosocial adjustments of adolescence are more difficult.

Physical changes and the wide variability that exists among individuals when these changes occur affect the adolescent's body image, which is closely related to self-esteem. It is important to note that body image is not objective. It is affected by how the individual perceives others' reactions and by society's concept of the "ideal body." Adolescent anxiety is generated by real or imagined defects and differences in physical characteristics. A number of studies have reported how boys and girls are affected differently by early or late maturation (Grinder, 1973; Hamachek, 1973; McCandless & Coop, 1979; Miller, 1974; Mussen & Jones, 1957; Tanner, 1971). Boys who approach adult height and muscle power early tend to be more successful in sports (Espenschade & Eckert, 1967). They are more likely to be accepted and treated by peers and adults as more psychologically and socially mature. Early maturing boys are more often chosen as leaders and as dates (Jones, 1958). Adults also may thrust responsibility onto a boy whose physical appearance is mature and expect mature social and emotional responses before those facets of the child's development are complete. Although adolescents who mature early are likely to be given opportunities to learn responsibility, late-maturing adolescents may be given fewer opportunities to demonstrate mature behaviors. The late-maturing boy may feel insecure and inferior and may be perceived as more dependent and rebellious (Mussen & Jones, 1957). Early maturers may seem more independent and mature in interpersonal relations. There is some evidence to suggest that these personality and behavioral differences may persist into adulthood (Grinder, 1973; Jones, 1965).

Differences between early and late-maturing girls, although similar to those noted in boys, seem neither as dramatic nor as long lasting (Hamacheck, 1973; Jones & Mussen, 1958). An early maturing girl may be disadvantaged, initially, if her peer group is less mature and her parents treat her as a "little girl" (Kiell, 1964). As her peers catch up with her, however, this disadvantage disappears, and she may, in fact, be admired by them. A late-maturing girl may develop problems with interpersonal relations and may develop a negative self-concept, but, again, these disadvantages dissipate as she, too, matures and shares experiences and interests. Girls are sometimes perceived to be less stigmatized by deviant rates of development than are boys in our culture because the female sex role has been less clearly defined (Hamachek, 1973; McCandless & Coop, 1979). Although girls are judged more frequently on their appearance, they also have the advantage of being able to modify appearance with the help of cosmetics and foundation garments.

Dobson (1984) stated that feelings of inferiority plague the majority of adolescents. He believed that there are three things that cause great anxiety and depression for teenagers: physical attractiveness, intelligence, and money. Most teenagers also have difficulties with the jumble of emotions they sometimes experience at the same moment. For example, they may have difficulties with special occasions when expectations collide with disappointments or fears.

Teenagers face a wide array of adult experiences and problems for the first time, and many of them have trouble dealing with mistakes. It is hard to hold on to self-esteem in the face of what seems like miserable failure. Their reaction to accumulated frustrations is frequently a feeling of powerlessness. Problems and decisions take on major proportions not always commensurate with reality. To assuage the frightening feelings of inadequacy that engulf them at such times, teenagers need a tremendous amount of encouragement and understanding from adults to "shore up" their shaky self-images. It's imperative that they have helpful, supportive adults to talk to and learn from. This enables them to hear some "good things" about themselves and to build self-confidence.

One of the major tasks of adolescence is to learn to experience intense feelings and to express them appropriately. Adolescents need adult models, structure, and opportunities for trial and error as they develop coping strategies. They need reassurance that in their confusion and moodiness, they are not alone.

Depression

A healthy adolescence is characterized by variability in emotional state, and balance between activity and privacy. Although the vast majority of adolescents develop methods for coping with stress through trial and error, some, unfortunately, do not. Serious depression affects 1 person in 5 at some time (Zehr, 1983). This is not the same as ordinary unhappiness, but a persistent mood that affects a person's basic emotional disposition.

Acute or "reactive" depression is precipitated by an event that occurs in the normal course of life. A loss of a loved one or loss of possessions or opportunities are predictable triggers of acute depression. Adolescents who "break up" with friends, fail exams, or don't make the team experience forms of acute depression, which is intense and painful, but short lived. It is frequently a strengthening experience that leaves the individual with greater insight and flexibility. Usually within 6 months to 1 year after the event, an individual is able to place it in perspective. The loss may still be felt, but its effect is no longer debilitating.

Chronic depression is harder to explain than depression related to a specific event or loss and often is associated with a person's mood or temperament. A chronically depressed person may deny the effects of a traumatic event and block out the experience. It is common in chronic depression for there to be a delay between an event responsible for it and the first signs of mood change. Young women who have been raped or sexually harassed sometimes appear to handle the aftermath "calmly" and are proud of their ability to do so. Later, other difficulties (such as examinations or financial problems) may appear to create major depression and help may then be sought for a problem that postdates the real cause of the depression.

Chronic depression may be related to family problems, such as divorce or alcoholism, where the adolescent feels responsibility for another person's pain and self-destructiveness. Children of alcoholics or of other substance abusers frequently exhibit coping strategies that are related to their dysfunctional family lives (Wegscheider-Gruse, 1983). Because in our culture families afflicted with alcoholism tend to conceal or deny it, adolescent children of alcoholic parents frequently do not receive the assistance they need. This occurs at a time in the adolescent's life when support and emotional stability at home are vital to emotional growth and development.

Divorce, the adjustments required in families combined by new marriages, violence in the home, and rape (especially date rape in this age group) all constitute major emotional traumas that threaten the very core of the adolescent's self-esteem. All will engender some degree of loss and grief. Loss and grief are complex processes involving many emotions and coping strategies. The adolescent personality, which is already unstable, is particularly vulnerable to the effect of loss. For example, recent violent events in schools, reported in the media, indicate that adolescents may feel the school environment is more threatening than it once was. Educators (Begley, 2000) have written about the effect of violence on students' sense of security and comfort in educational settings. Loss of security may be felt by an adolescent who moves to a new school or community or who loses some function or ability through accident or illness. Any aspect of the lifestyle that is curtailed can be the impetus for depression. Loss of sources of satisfaction and stability threaten a student's overall feelings of security and worth. Individuals deal with loss and grief in different ways; however, Kubler-Ross (1969) listed five stages that she believed were consistently seen: denial, anger, bargaining, depression, and acceptance.

An adolescent's inability to cope with normal developmental stresses (gender-role definition, emerging independence, the inability to tolerate temporary frustration to gain long-term satisfaction) may result in serious depression. The statistics on teenage suicide in the United States indicate that this is a problem that cannot be ignored. The U.S. Census Bureau (1999) reports that the suicide rate in the 15–24 year old range is 20 males and 3.6 females per 100,000.

A suicide attempt is usually a cry for help (Bell, 1980). Eight out of 10 people who commit suicide tell someone that they're thinking about suicide before they actually attempt it. When a student talks about suicide, it is important not to change the subject. A person who mentions suicide should be taken seriously and given a chance to express his or her feelings. Warning signs of severe depression include

- A noticeable change in eating and sleeping habits
- A loss of interest in friends
- Feelings of hopelessness and self-hate
- Constant restlessness and hyperactivity
- Significant change in school performance
- Verbalization of a plan for suicide
- Possession of a weapon or pills
- Giving away of prized possessions
- A long and deep reaction to a breakup or death

When the speech–language pathologist sees warning signs of severe depression in a student in voice therapy, it is wise to refer the student to a mental-health professional.

When to Refer to a Mental Health Professional

Questions for the voice clinician to ask when trying to determine if a referral is appropriate:

1. How longstanding is this problem/issue?
   If the client has been struggling with anxiety, depression, dysfunctional family patterns, and so on for a prolonged period of time (months or even years), the issues may be deep rooted enough to benefit from more intense psychotherapy than can be provided within voice therapy.
2. What is the intensity of the problem or issue?
   If the client's difficulties are so severe that they impair his or her functioning in several areas of life, counseling or psychotherapy might be appropriate.
3. Does the client seem to be requiring directive feedback about emotional issues? Do you find yourself going well beyond active, empathic listening, and problem-solving with your client?
   An example of this might be a client who is continually requesting corrective feedback about his or her thoughts or feelings. Additionally, if you observe irrational thoughts, feelings, or behaviors that seem to be interfering with the person's healthy functioning, and which seem beyond the scope of voice therapy, it may be appropriate to consider a counseling referral.
4. Has therapy progress stalled?
   If you are not making progress with this client, it becomes necessary to assess why therapy has not been moving forward. Unresolved psychological issues may serve as barriers to voice-therapy progress.
5. Are you feeling competent at providing the level of counseling skills required to work with this client?
   If your answer is no, obviously, it is time to either obtain consultation or supervision or to make an appropriate referral. If you are unsure, it becomes important to listen to your "third ear." What is your intuition telling you about working with this client? A second opinion from a colleague may also be helpful.

Cognitive and Psychosocial Factors

Adolescents are ideal candidates for voice therapy because they have the cognitive development to deal with the ideas and concepts related to modification of behavior. Adolescents have the ability to think abstractly, to develop hypothetical solutions to problems, and to test solutions against the evidence. They are able to consider not only what is, but what might be. The behavior and beliefs of adolescents are influenced by many factors, including the socioeconomic status of their families, the quality of schooling, individual personality characteristics, psychosocial factors, and emerging independence from parents. Naturally, there are some adolescents who do not achieve the more advanced levels of cognitive functioning because of intellectual, cultural, or experiential constraints. Cognitive development significantly influences how adolescents think about themselves, their families, peers, and society.

Emerging cognitive abilities may cause friction between adolescents and significant adults. Once an adolescent has the cognitive ability to consider things "as they might be," impatience and criticism of reality result. Parents, school, therapy, home life, and societal values frequently are the targets of criticism when they differ from what the adolescent considers to be the ideal.

Many adolescents with well-developed cognitive skills are idealists critical of the existing social order. They propose solutions that may be unrealistic and question authority without always having the responsibility for implementing their ideas. The capability to examine a number of ideas simultaneously and to point out inconsistencies is characteristic of the adolescent's maturing cognitive abilities. Because adolescents can conceive of and consider many alternative solutions to a problem, they are capable of perceiving a variety of options to behavioral and interpersonal skills. Generating a variety of options enhances student participation in the voice therapy process.

Defense Mechanisms

Defense mechanisms are unconscious means for dealing with anxiety (Laughlin, 1970). Two defense mechanisms that first appear in adolescence are intellectualization and asceticism (Conger, 1973; Muuss, 1975). Intellectualization involves dealing with emotional matters on an intellectual plane so that instinctual drives can be consciously controlled. Asceticism is an attempt to deny instinctual drives, such as sex and hunger, and it sometimes provides group support for self-denial. Some writers consider asceticism to be a negative strategy because it prevents adolescents from coming to terms with their instinctual drives. Intellectualization, when carried to excess, may result in social isolation and may serve as a way to avoid coping directly with needs and conflicts. On the other hand, intellectualizing problems provides useful experience in hypothetical and abstract thinking. It may also help an adolescent deal with instinctual drives realistically.

Egocentrism

Eklund (1967) believed that because an adolescent's thoughts are mainly self-centered, he or she therefore assumes that other people are equally obsessed with his or her behavior and appearance. Adolescents feel they are the focus of everyone's attention, which increases feelings of self-consciousness. This may result at times in a fear of exposure to the criticism of others, which leads to an increased desire for privacy. Eklund also believed that an adolescent's egocentric cognitive processes may lead to overdifferentiation concerning feelings. The adolescent may believe that no one else has felt such important or special agony or rapture. Adolescent egocentrism is broken down as the young person observes, listens, and talks to others and discovers that peers share similar feelings and concerns. Some adolescents' sense of uniqueness extends beyond the feeling domain to other areas, however, and may result in dangerous activities. For example, if a girl feels that her feelings, her person, and, indeed, her fate are unique to the extent that accidents, rape, pregnancy, and death happen only to others, the consequences may be very unfortunate. Some adolescents, however, assume instead that the world is indifferent. Consequently, bids for attention may be made to shore up feelings of inadequacy. Kagan (1971) believed that adolescents are anxious about living up to, and not violating, the standards of society.

Moral Development

Kohlberg (1975) stated that there are three levels of morality: the preconventional, the conventional, and the postconventional. He expanded on Piaget's work (1974) and related moral development to Piaget's cognitive theory.

The preconventional level of morality corresponds to Piaget's stage of concrete thought and is generally seen in middle-class children from 4 to 10 years of age. At this stage, goodness and badness are considered in terms of physical consequences and the physical power of authority figures. The child behaves because of fear of punishment and desire for reward. Conventional morality initially appears and then dominates moral judgment during preadolescence; morality is equated with social approval and the maintenance of law and order to avoid guilt and penalties. The postconventional level does not appear until adolescence and corresponds to a higher level in Piaget's stage of formal thought. Here, morality does not rely on obedience, conformity, and social approval, but rather on universal principles of justice. It is probably true that the need for peer acceptance, as well as increased sexual and aggressive urges, however, often influence the decision making more strongly than do moral values. At age 12 or 13, a young person usually moves from a protected elementary school environment to a middle or junior high school, where an increasing number of moral dilemmas are encountered.

The Role of Peers

In Western cultures, the peer group is an important factor in the maturation process during adolescence. Peers help support a young person's growing autonomy by allowing experimentation with new roles and providing reassurance and psychological security.

Peer groups tend to be chosen because of similarities, rather than differences, and help define identity. Adolescents receive more comfort from peers who are simultaneously experiencing the same anxieties and concerns, and, in this sense, the peer group can be therapeutic (Begley, 2000). The intimacy of the peer group allows the expression of hostile, guilty, and resentful feelings associated with school, sexuality, disobedience, parental restrictions, and the ambiguous future that cannot be shared with significant adults (Osterrieth, 1969). Comfort from peers, although important for all adolescents, is especially critical for those who have inadequate support in the family environment. Although concerned, supportive parents are primary sources of high self-esteem, acceptance and admiration by peers provide objective sources for feelings of self-worth. Peer evaluation may be especially important in the young person's self-perception because the roles played at this vulnerable stage of development may have long-term ramifications.

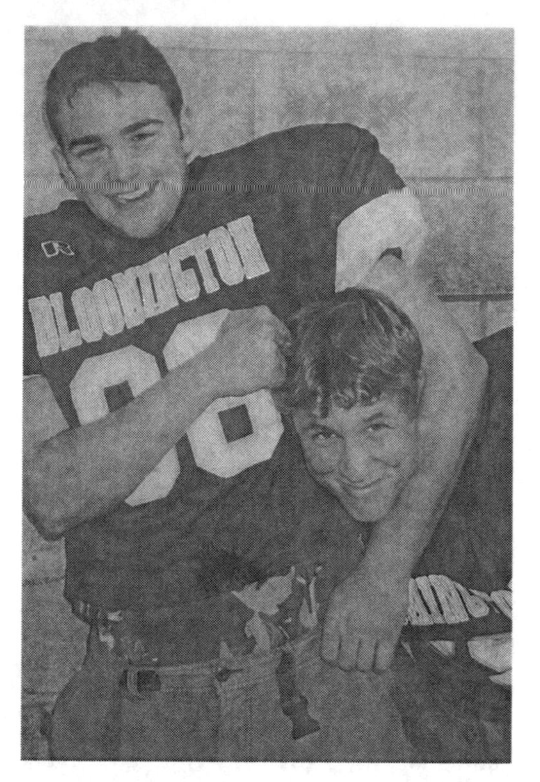

Interaction with peers is an important factor in the maturation process during adolescence.

Material benefits, such as a car, money, or clothes, may contribute to an individual's sense of power within the group. In addition, personality characteristics and physical and mental skill have an effect on perceived power within groups.

The peer group allows the adolescent to learn more mature ways of relating to both genders (Winder, 1974). Gender role identity, although learned in the context of the family, is reinforced within the context of peer group (Mischel, 1970). Intense friendships develop during adolescence. During childhood, the choice of friends is influenced most by proximity and the focus is on activity, whereas during adolescence, the focus is on interpersonal involvement (Douvan & Adelson, 1966). Although both boys and girls have intimate friendships, these relationships are more intense among girls because boys are usually socialized toward achievement, action, and the attainment of power.

Because the adolescent's values tend to be learned within the family, the peer group chosen will often reflect the socioeconomic class, values, and morality of the family.

Styles of Parenting

It is important for the speech–language pathologist to understand parenting styles for three reasons: (a) the dynamics existing within an adolescent's family frequently affect the student's reactions to other adults; (b) teachers and counselors frequently adopt recognizable parenting styles during interactions with students; and (c) frequently it is necessary for the speech–language pathologist to monitor his or her style and adapt it to the needs of individual students.

Parenting styles may exist on a continuum. At one extreme is the authoritarian parent and at the other is the permissive parent. Authoritarian parenting thwarts self-mastery and decision-making ability, encouraging conformity to external demands. Permissive parents, on the other hand, carry acceptance to an extreme, making few demands of any sort on the child. This attitude may hinder development of self-esteem and decision-making ability. At the midpoint in the continuum is the "authoritative" parent. Many researchers believe the authoritative parent tends to be most prevalent in middle-class families, where young people's feelings are considered and the development of self-control and self-direction is valued. The authoritative parent retains ultimate responsibility, but is willing to discuss relevant issues, allow adolescents to voice their opinions, and work toward compromise where possible. Authoritative parents, who are warm, accepting, and respectful of the young person's physical and psychologic privacy, enhance the young person's self-esteem and provide confidence in the possibility of affecting change and compromise through self-assertion (Coopersmith, 1967).

The Influence of Significant Adults

The ability to develop autonomy and competence is highly influenced by the relationships adolescents have with their parents. Nonetheless, adolescents are also influenced by other significant adults who provide a variety of interactions from which the adolescent may make decisions on adult levels and, therefore, develop self-sufficiency and decision-making skills. Family therapists report that in cases of dysfunctional families, "community anchors" (significant adults outside the family) are particularly important to emotional development.

Stereotypical Attitudes

In our culture, it is sometimes assumed that boys and girls will behave in certain ways because certain traits are inherent or biologically determined. More often, however, different social expectations and behaviors for boys and girls (as well as for students with different racial backgrounds or handicapping conditions) are learned. The evidence suggests that many stereotypes persist because they appear to be verified or because they seem desirable. For example, boys may try to be rational, unemotional, ambitious, and independent because those traits are congruent with "true masculinity" or with society's ideal image of it.

Many studies have investigated how children learn their gender role identities, and social learning researchers (e.g., Mischel, 1970) believe that parents, teachers, and peers reward children for activities consistent with society's view of their gender. Maccoby and Jacklin (1974) reviewed 9,000 empirical studies and found that there is support for a biological basis for only two areas of gender differences in behavior: (a) physical aggression and dominance in males (apparently related to prenatal hormones) and (b) a female advantage in verbal skills emerging early and a male advantage in visual–spatial skills emerging at adolescence. The effect of training and learning is more important on human development than it is on other animals and seems to modify the effects of biology. Although there may be biologically determined differences by gender, they do not preclude development of skills through environmental influences. The range of individual differences is great.

Expectations seem to play a dramatic role in the way teachers respond to students' endeavors. Representatives of minority groups or female students may sometimes be perceived by adults as "not likely to achieve" and this may, in actuality, become a self-fulfilling prophecy.

Perceptual bias refers to the influence of attitudes and values on what is actually observed. Recognition of the fact that perceptual bias and invisible discrimination do not usually indicate conscious prejudice or ill will is often helpful. Authority figures involved with adolescents may sometimes expect them to be "difficult," and, indeed, sometimes they are! By reviewing the information available in the literature, however, we can remind ourselves of the wide range of individual differences that exist and identify aspects of behavior patterns that may trigger certain perceptual biases of our own.

The speech–language pathologist is often called on to deal with unpredictable adolescent behavior. One way to try to understand this behavior is to identify the reasons for some adolescent coping strategies. It is probable that many students are, at times, confused about what they believe and how they should behave. Therefore, they have mixed reactions in certain situations and may exhibit negativism (e.g., saying they don't want to do something that really interests them) as a means of coping with their ambivalent mixture of excitement and anxiety.

Adolescents have difficulty maintaining continuity between the child and the emerging adult within themselves. This is demonstrated by fluctuations in levels of responsibility and reactions to disappointments, as well as by exaggerated concern for physical appearance. It is also difficult for adolescents to wrestle with the task of transforming esteemed adults from examples of perfection into ordinary people with faults and weaknesses. Many of the reactions of adolescents that adults find most perplexing are based on attempts to find coping strategies congruent with peer pressures. For the adolescent, group membership and peer acceptance is critical. The most acute difficulties for the adolescent come from the conflict between the priorities of adults and the perspectives of the peer group.

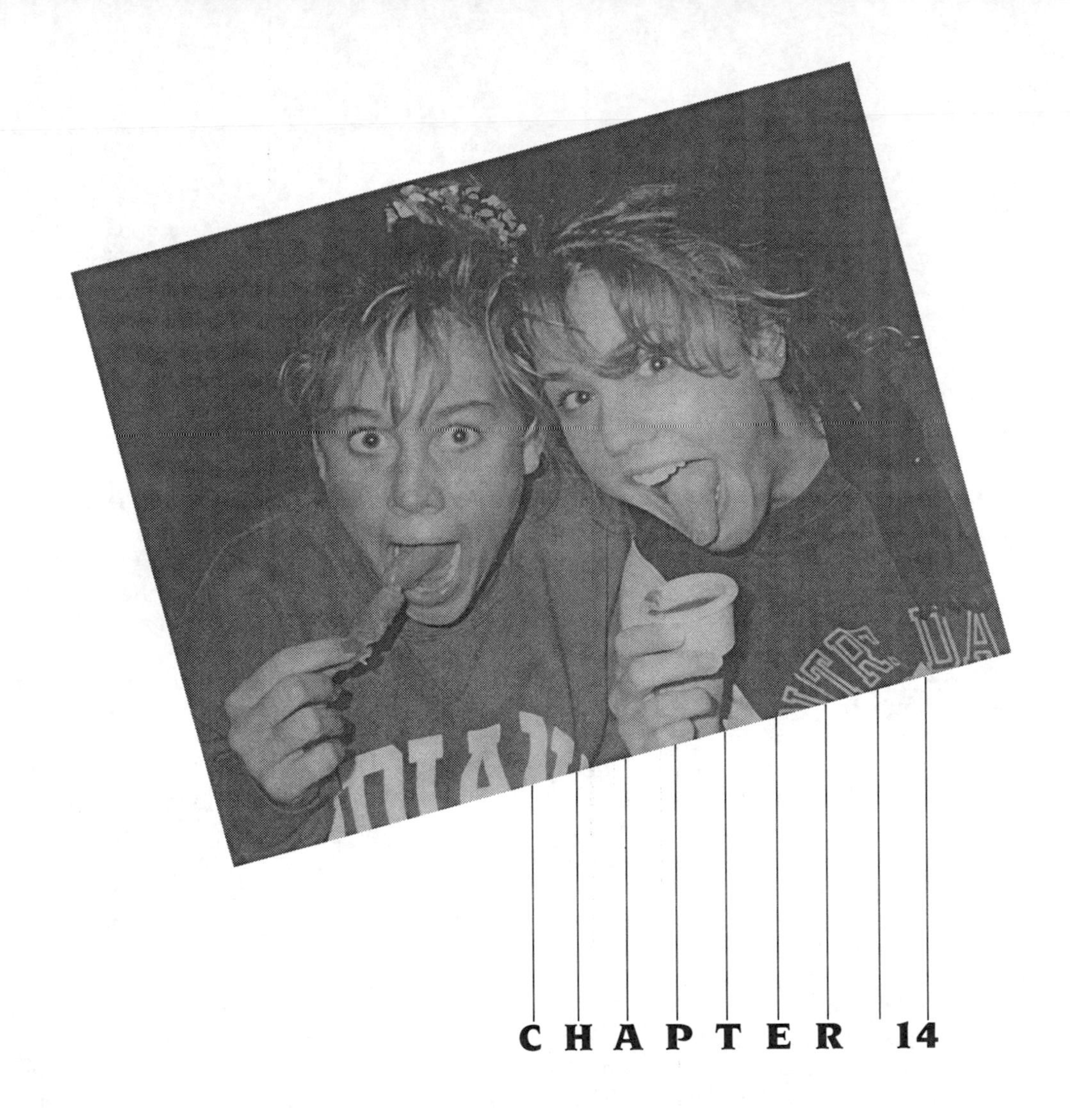

CHAPTER 14

Conditions That Affect Vocal Behavior During Adolescence

It is sometimes difficult to isolate the primary factor causing a voice disorder. Vocal symptoms, however, are frequently seen in conjunction with conditions that may predispose an individual to acquire a voice problem. Theoretically, any disorder (anatomic, medical, endocrinologic, psychogenic, sensory, cognitive, or muscular tension) that has the potential to alter the structure or function of the upper respiratory tract or alter affective behavior may contribute to the development of a voice disorder. Some individuals, however, may produce an unusual voice in the absence of any easily identifiable constraint on the system. Others may exhibit a whole array of conditions that could contribute to a voice disorder but have voices that sound perfectly healthy.

Some conditions occur frequently enough in association with voice problems for clinicians to suspect a causal relationship. This is especially true with some organic and sensory impairments. However, the coexistence of a condition and a vocal symptom does not necessarily imply a relationship between the two. For example, some children with learning disabilities who have voice disorders also have inappropriate interpersonal skills. The cause of the voice problem in such cases may or may not be related to the interpersonal difficulties. Nonetheless, the learning disability is a significant factor to be considered when designing a treatment program. The interpersonal difficulties need to be addressed because most students with voice disorders need interpersonal insight and skill to make the personal adjustments necessary to protect the vocal mechanism.

A wide variety of conditions may predispose an adolescent to develop vocal problems (see High Risk Inventory in Appendix B). Frequently, many factors in combination interact to increase susceptibility to voice disorders. The adolescent years are characterized by considerable vocal activity. Both the amount and type of voice use are significant. Teenagers are typically involved in many academic, sporting, and social pursuits that involve loud talking, cheering, singing, yelling, and laughing. Telephone conversations are often protracted, emotional outbursts are intense and frequent, and group interactions often seem overexuberant to adult ears.

At the same time when the laryngeal mechanism is undergoing structural maturation, the demands on it seem to peak. Healthy laryngeal structures, however, seem capable of withstanding a wide variety of vocal demands, although resilience of tissues in relation to severity of insult varies among individuals.

Listed below are some of the most common symptoms associated with vocal problems.

- **Hoarseness**—This symptom includes aperiodicity of fundamental frequency, random fundamental frequency variation, escape of air, and noise. Some clinicians define hoarseness as a combination of breathiness and harshness. It varies in severity and is sometimes described as mild, moderate, or severe. Hoarseness is the most prevalent symptom associated with vocal problems and may be caused by a variety of conditions, including local and systemic diseases, disorders of motor nerves, abuse and misuse, lesions that increase size and mass of folds, inflammation, and injury.
- **Breathiness**—In a breathy voice, medial compression and longitudinal tension of the folds is lessened so that air leakage creates turbulence during vocal fold closure. The audible escape of air through lax glottal closure is perceived as aspirate noise. In its most severe form, it sounds like a whisper. Lesions that affect the margins of the folds, edema, and paralysis may give rise to this symptom.
- **Harshness**—Hanley and Thurman (1970) defined harshness as an unpleasant and rough quality. There is considerable laryn-

geal tension and constriction and frequent hard glottal attacks. Laver (1980) observed irregular pertubations of fundamental frequency (jitter) and intensity (shimmer).

- **Vocal fry**—Zemlin (1981) described vocal fry as being produced with the vocal folds relaxed so that the sound is emitted in discrete bursts. It is produced at the bottom of the pitch range and has been likened to the sound of popcorn popping or "creaky-door" voice.
- **Diplophonia**—This term is used to describe a "two-toned" voice or a situation in which one fold vibrates at a different rate from the other (Perkins, 1977). Some individuals can produce this at will, but in most cases it is pathologic.
- **Ventricular phonation** (dysphonia plicae ventricularis)—When the false vocal folds vibrate, the sound perceived is usually harsh, low pitched, and tense.
- **Aphonia**—This is the absence of sound during intentional phonation. It may be consistent or sporadic, acute, or chronic. Time of onset may provide clues concerning etiology, for example, upper respiratory tract infection, emotional or physical trauma, inhalation of irritants, allergic reaction, postintubation, and so forth.
- **Syllabic aphonia**—This symptom is the absence of sound on unstressed syllables, which may occur because of difficulty adducting folds that are swollen because of allergic reactions, nodules, and so forth. It may occur randomly or consistently. When it occurs consistently at the ends of breath groups, syllabic aphonia may be related to inefficient use of replenishing breaths.
- **Dysphonia**—This disturbed phonation is perceived auditorially as breathiness, harshness, or hoarseness. Changes in normal vibratory patterns are related to size, mass, tension, or the even approximation of folds.
- **Hard glottal attack**—Abrupt forceful onset of phonation is frequently associated with excessive laryngeal tension, and/or lack of coordination of aerodynamic and myoelastic features during initiation of phonation, or both. It may be perceived as a grunt or click and is frequently heard on stressed vowels in initial positions in words.
- **Restricted pitch range**—This may occur in the singing voice only or in the speaking voice as well. It may indicate the presence of a nodule or polyp, the onset of neurological disease (e.g., myasthenia gravis), hearing loss, or a psychogenic disorder.
- **"Tickle" in the throat**—This symptom may be associated with dryness or strain, allergic reactions, or lesions (e.g., nodules and polyps). Swallowing may temporarily relax the tension, whereas throat clearing exacerbates it.
- **Dry throat**—This may be related to lack of humidity and may be helped by a vaporizer at night. Mouth breathing, allergic reactions, dusty open-air environment, limited fluid intake, decongestants and antihistamines, excessive alcohol and smoking, and early diabetes may be factors.
- **Burning sensation in the throat**—So-called "scratchy" or "raw" throat may be caused by irritants (such as inhaled chemicals or other pollutants) or by acidic secretions from the digestive tract, as happens in gastroesophageal reflux.
- **Aching throat**—Muscle tension in strap muscles of the neck may cause this, especially if the anterior part of the neck is involved. Movement of the swallowing muscles when phonating may indicate muscular hyperfunction.
- **Tightness in throat**—This may indicate hyperfunction, tension in pharyngeal muscles, retracted tongue position, or edema of vocal folds (e.g., allergic reaction).
- **Lump in throat**—This sensation can occur in association with extreme stress, hiatal hernia, or thyroid enlargement.
- **Pain**—Disorders of the temporomandibular joint, contact ulcers, intubation, trauma,

prolonged vocal abuse, inflammatory conditions, or referred pain from the ear may cause complaints.

- **Mucus strand**—A strand of mucus at the junction of the anterior and mid-third portions of the folds may be noted during laryngeal examination. It seems to appear at the point of maximum excursion of the folds and is associated with nodule and polyp formation and with vocal abuse and strain.
- **Fatigue after voice use**—Vocal abuse, polyps, and neoplasms (rare in adolescence), early paresis, and neurologic disease may cause this symptom. "Vocal endurance" may be measured in a diagnostic session.
- **Throat clearing**—Throat clearing may be (a) an attempt to clear secretions related to allergic conditions, (b) a nervous habit or "starter," (c) the residual of an earlier respiratory tract problem now resolved, (d) related to a hiatal hernia. Frequently, the individual does not realize that throat clearing has become habitual.
- **Inappropriate pitch variability**—When an individual uses limited pitch variability it may be due to sensory deficits (e.g., hearing loss), intellectual impairment, depression, or paralysis of folds. Occasionally, lesions of the folds may also preclude the use of higher pitches (because of increased size and mass), thus affecting general pitch variability. Sometimes, too, a vocal abuser may restrict voice change to loudness changes. In such cases, it may be beneficial to teach the abuser some other methods of varying the voice.
- **Inappropriately high pitch level**—An abnormally high pitch for age and gender may be related to delayed or incongruous pubertal development, a small web, mutational falsetto, or learned behavior.
- **Inappropriately low pitch level**—An abnormally low pitch may be habituated through choice by some individuals who prefer a "deep" or "throaty" voice. A person's "vocal image" (Cooper, 1973) may need to be explored. Other factors to be considered include contact ulcers, virilization, edema, tumors, nodules (or any lesion increasing size and mass of folds), or paralysis that decreases elasticity of folds.
- **Weak volume level**—A weak or thin voice may be due to respiratory limitations, lack of resonance, reduced valving capacity of the larynx, or psychosocial factors.

It is useful to review conditions that heighten an adolescent's susceptibility to voice problems and to identify constraints on the voice system that may influence etiology, maintenance of disorders, and treatment. Therapy programs will be designed more appropriately and implemented more effectively if all pertinent factors have been considered. Recognizing factors that can trigger behavioral compensations helps a speech–language pathologist to identify the behaviors and to help students recognize and extinguish or shape these behaviors.

The vulnerability of the laryngeal structures to abuse and misuse seems to be heightened by factors that irritate the mucosa. Irritated tissues react more readily to insult, and chronic irritation in combination with chronic vocal abuse is particularly significant in the etiology of voice disorders. An individual with irritated and swollen folds often adopts compensatory vocal practices (e.g., forceful adduction, louder level, throat clearing) that exacerbate the original problem. An overlay of secondary abusive practices may be misguided attempts to compensate for structural changes that were caused by primary irritants.

Sore Throat

Sore throat is a symptom of many different illnesses, and its cause may be hard to diagnose. Illnesses responsible for sore throats may be as serious as leukemia or as relatively harmless as a common cold.

The upper respiratory tract is lined with mucous membrane, which feels moist and slippery (the inside of the mouth is lined with mucous membrane). Infections, allergic reactions, and irritation can cause inflammation of these tissues. Infections that can cause sore throats may be bacterial, viral, or fungal. Fungal infections are the least common cause of sore throat, and viral infections are the most common causes (the common cold is caused by a virus). A sore throat is usually accompanied by a runny nose and a generally miserable feeling. Because antibiotics are not used to treat viral infections, a physician usually recommends rest (to help the body fight infection), fluids (to keep tissues moist and to thin mucus secretions so they can be expelled), and aspirin (to reduce feelings of discomfort).

Bacterial infections, on the other hand, are usually treated with antibiotics prescribed by a physician. An example of a bacterial infection is strep throat, which is caused by streptococcal germs. Symptoms of strep throat include fever, white or yellow spots on the throat lining, and pain when swallowing. The illness is potentially dangerous because it may lead to rheumatic fever or to kidney infection if not accurately diagnosed and treated by a physician. The most accurate way to diagnose strep throat is by taking a throat culture or by use of rapid diagnostic devices designed to detect the bacterium.

Tonsillitis is another common cause of sore throat and may be due to either viral or bacterial infection. It is a painful inflammation of the tonsils, bulges of lymph tissue on either side of the back of the mouth. Although it is not known why, these infections most often occur in children aged 3 to 7 and 12 to 13. Adults who still have their tonsils may also suffer from tonsillitis, however. Forty years ago, tonsillectomies were recommended by physicians for almost all children. Today, however, the operation is recommended only when there is a high frequency of recurrence (e.g., four to seven episodes per year) or when the tonsils are so swollen that breathing is affected. Another viral illness, mononucleosis, often strikes teenagers and adults and causes uncomfortable sore throat and other debilitating symptoms.

Allergies can cause sore throat if the sufferer is allergic to airborne substances (such as dust, pollen, animal dander, or mold) or ingested substances that cause changes in the upper respiratory tract (such as foods or drugs that affect tissues lining the tract). Excessive dryness or overproduction of secretions are typical reactions to allergens. Sometimes an allergic condition may be exacerbated by a secondary infection or by overuse of an irritated mechanism.

Irritation of the delicate tissues of the throat may be caused by smoking, drinking alcohol (which results in dryness of the tissues), and by digestive problems, which can result in the backing-up of stomach contents into the esophagus and pharynx. Airway irritation resulting from gastroesophageal reflux disease (GERD) is also seen in adolescents. Symptoms such as frequent cough, wheezing, nasal congestion, hoarseness, throat clearing, globus sensation, sore throat, halitosis, and emesis (vomiting) have been noted (Carr et al., 1999). Gastroesophageal reflux is characterized by the retrograde movement of stomach acid into the esophagus. In most patients the condition is caused by episodic relaxation of the sphincter that keeps the lower end of the esophagus closed when a person is not swallowing liquids or food. Although most people experience occasional acid refluxing into the esophagus, it is only considered chronic when it severely impacts an individual's life or damages the tissues of the esophagus or trachea. Laryngeal redness in the posterior section of the larynx (e.g., arytenoid area) is symptomatic of GERD. Adolescents' eating habits and their tendency to drink carbonated beverages lying down may also exacerbate this condition. Reflux of acids may occur at night, when an individual is lying down and may be responsible for chronic morning sore throat. Antacids can often soothe sore throats caused by stomach acids. Some clinical evidence suggests that repeated vomiting (such as in girls with bulimia) can be damaging to throat tissues.

Sore throats often seem more prevalent during winter months, when people tend to congregate indoors. Because infectious agents may be spread by air and touch, it is important to wash hands frequently and to avoid rubbing the eyes and nose or touching the mouth. Good nutrition and adequate rest also help the body resist infection. A dry atmosphere, without adequate humidity, dries out throat membranes, and nasal stuffiness increases mouth breathing. Because dryness increases susceptibility to infection, drinking liquids and using a humidifier are frequently helpful. People who are susceptible to allergies should check for molds and fungi in damp basements and on objects such as plants, books, and shower curtains. Dust-harboring objects should be removed from sleeping areas, and the head should be elevated during sleep. Inhalation of steam may also help dislodge excess mucus.

If a sore throat is the result of a cold, a visit to a physician is probably not necessary. A doctor should be consulted if there is a possibility of strep throat or if a sore throat is accompanied by difficulty in breathing, earache, rash, fever greater than 103°F, inability to swallow saliva, and difficulty opening the mouth. If a sore throat has not gone away within 2 or 3 weeks, an appointment with an otolaryngologist (ear, nose, and throat specialist) is recommended.

Asthma

Symptoms of asthma include shortness of breath, wheezing, and the production of excess mucus in the passages leading to the lungs. Attacks can be terrifying if the patient cannot breathe easily. Exhalation is usually affected by obstructed or constricted airways. Asthma attacks may be triggered by respiratory infections; cold air; exercise; allergens such as pollens; and molds, chemicals, and pollutants. Occasionally, the attacks may be exacerbated by emotional upset.

Treatment of Asthma

Histamine is a chemical in the body that is released in response to allergens if a person's immune system is extra sensitive to a substance. Histamine causes blood vessels to dilate and leak fluids, which cause tissues to become red and itchy. Antihistamines are drugs that slow down the action of histamine and help control allergic symptoms. Oral decongestants are used in association with antihistamines. Decongestants reduce fluid buildup and ease nasal congestion. Allergy shots are sometimes prescribed to desensitize the immune system to specific allergens. Nebulizers and sprays are also used to treat asthma and allergy symptoms. It is best to seek medical advice rather than to use nonprescription medications for persistent symptoms involving the ears, nose, throat, or breathing system.

Allergies

Allergy may be defined as a condition of unusual sensitivity to foreign substances or environmental conditions. The substance an individual is allergic to is known as an allergen or antigen. Allergens may be inhaled, digested, touched, or injected, and responses to them vary. Inhaling a certain substance could produce a rash in one person, whereas eating the same substance could produce breathing difficulties in another. Reactions to allergens may be immediate or delayed. Hives, bronchial asthma, hay fever, drug reactions, and reactions to insect bites are usually apparent immediately after exposure, whereas skin reactions to chemicals (e.g., poison ivy or cosmetics) and diarrhea are delayed.

When an allergen such as pollen enters blood vessels in the lining of the nose, a variety of allergic reactions may take place in the vocal tract. The muscles surrounding breathing passages contract and cause spasms that restrict air flow. Additionally, large amounts of mucus may be discharged into the air tubes, which further hinders free breathing. Dilation of blood vessels causes swelling in adjoining tissues lining nasal cavities and bronchial tubes.

Allergens in combination appear to have a cumulative effect. If, for example, an individual is exposed to two allergens simultaneously (e.g., inhaling pollen and eating nuts), the interaction of the two allergens may result in an allergic response that would not occur if the exposure was limited to only one of the substances.

It is common for allergic patterns to change at puberty. Sometimes manifestations take different forms or disappear during adolescence. Some girls, for example, experience relief from asthma when they begin to menstruate. In other cases, adolescence may be a time when allergic symptoms are noted for the first time. The onset of hypersensitivity to weeds, grasses, trees, or mold spores may be associated with relocation to a different geographic area or may be related to increased outdoor activity. Seasonal variations may also affect symptoms. For example, molds are parasitic plants that grow on corn, wheat, and oats, and mold spores are blown through the air during the summer, especially in grain-growing regions. Molds also are found in stored grain, straw, and hay. Unlike the pollens from weeds and grasses, spores are not killed by freezing weather. Perennial allergic rhinitis (inflammation of the mucous membranes of the nose) occurs year round from unseasonal substances such as mold (on houseplants, in paper products, in damp basements), house dust, and animal dander. Seasonal rhinitis (e.g., ragweed) is more transitory, depending on pollinating seasons in various areas. Weather may exacerbate allergic reactions (e.g., cool rainy days or humid conditions may increase the effects of molds and chemical pollutants in the air), and hot, sunny, windy conditions may alleviate suffering temporarily.

Drug allergies are particularly important in relation to the adolescent population. Drugs may be sniffed, sprayed, rubbed on the skin, or taken orally or by injection. Tranquilizers, aspirin, and a variety of "recreational" drugs cause adverse allergic effects in some individuals. Penicillin is well known as a drug that can be potentially life-threatening to some sensitive people. Nonprescription drugs, however, pose the greatest threat to adolescents. Allergic reactions to drugs range from mild rashes to death, and include hives, wheezing, sneezing, swelling of lips and tongue, pain from an inflamed intestinal tract, dizziness from circulatory disturbances, and pallor related to anemia. The lymph nodes may enlarge, the kidneys may slow down, and the heart may become inflamed. A distorted response to medication may include a lowering of the white blood cell count, resulting in a lowered resistance to infection. Liver damage may also occur with prolonged drug use (Joseph & Mills, 1983).

Treatment of Allergies

Because respiration and phonation, and thus, the quality of an individual's voice, can be greatly affected by allergic reactions, a speech–language pathologist should carefully explore with the student the possibility of unidentified allergies. It is not unusual for a therapy plan to consist of environmental and medical control of an allergy in conjunction with a program of vocal hygiene. A vocal hygiene program is important for teaching a student ways to avoid stressing an already "at-risk" mechanism.

Medications may be used to control hay fever or upper respiratory tract problems.

They are given orally or inhaled. The "drying" effect of antihistamines is useful in controlling symptoms such as sneezing and runny nose. Antihistamines are never recommended for an asthmatic because they hamper the ability to cough up sputum and intensify the asthmatic's difficulties. One side effect of antihistamines includes loss of alertness. Coordination problems may occur when antihistamines are combined with decongestants. Students who use over-the-counter antihistamines to alleviate nasal secretions may also suffer from dryness throughout the laryngeal mucosa. Excessively dry tissues are particularly at risk for vocal abuse. There are now a variety of perscription medications, and new varieties are being introduced, that minimize side effects, so consultation with a physician is recommended.

Desensitizing injections are used to treat severe allergic reactions, particularly to pollen and molds. This treatment, of course, requires expert medical consultation. Very severe allergic conditions, and especially incapacitating asthma attacks, are treated with hormone drugs (e.g., cortisone), but physicians use these cautiously because the side effects are sometimes quite dangerous.

Chemically Induced Irritation

Individuals vary in their reactions to chemical substances. For example, some people are highly sensitive to cigarette smoke, whereas others are barely affected by it. The possibility for irritation of tissues from smoke inhalation should be considered during the diagnostic process because many middle and high school students smoke cigarettes. Mouthwashes and gargles, if used excessively, can also cause mucosal irritation. Gastroesophageal reflux has been identified as causing severe dental, pharyngeal, and laryngeal irritation in adolescents who are bulimic (especially girls). Mild reflux may occur in many individuals during sleep. The inhalation of noxious fumes, either intentionally or because of environmental pollution, also occurs with deleterious effects on the laryngeal structures of some adolescents. Sometimes, exposure to industrial pollution or dust results in excessive dryness of the respiratory tract, and this lack of lubrication creates a high-risk environment for vocal abuse (Punt, 1979). Similarly, however, exposure to airborne irritants can cause excessive mucus to be produced in the tract, and post-nasal drip and laryngeal secretions can lead to increased frequency of abusive throat clearing and coughing. Over-the-counter medications, such as antihistamines and decongestants, are sometimes used excessively by teenagers who are trying to control high levels of vocal tract congestion. Pharmacologically induced dryness can occur as a result. Recreational drugs and birth control pills may cause swelling of the nasal or laryngeal mucosa.

A speech–language pathologist should obtain a complete history of exposure to chemical agents during voice evaluation. Because many adolescents are reluctant to provide specific information, the speech–language pathologist should word questions concerning drug use in a nonjudgmental way: "How often do you use ___________?" "Which of the following best fits *your* pattern of smoking? More than a pack a day, a pack a day, less than a pack a day." "Have you noticed an increase in nasal congestion with some drugs more than others?"

Vocally Demanding Activities

The type and amount of vocalization and the vocal adjustments the individual makes during sustained vocalization, especially against background noise, are significant with respect to susceptibility to voice disorders.

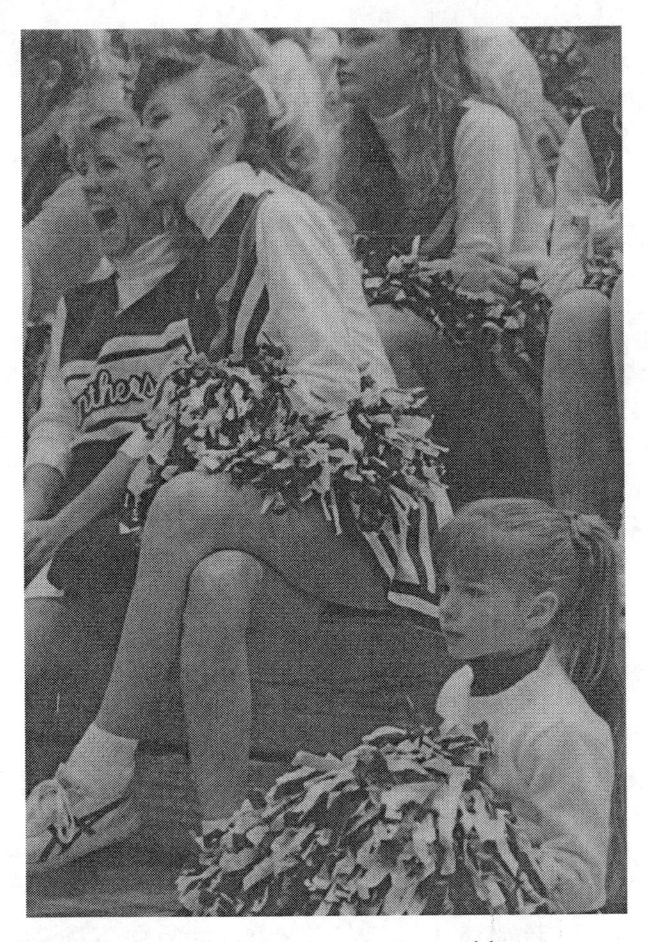

Cheerleaders often experience voice problems.

Susceptibility may also be affected by the individual's general level of health and fatigue.

Types of extracurricular activities, the balance between quiet and noisy activities, and the manner of voice production during sustained or projected vocalization are important considerations when evaluating predisposition toward voice problems. Many factors interrelate in placing an individual at risk. For example, the student who sings a great deal but uses voice inappropriately is obviously more vulnerable than one who naturally uses an appropriate technique or is studying with a qualified voice teacher. Members of athletic teams whose voices are used constantly in the open air, students who abuse alcohol and engage in rowdy parties, and character actors who use a variety of distorted phonatory patterns may run the risk of subjecting their mechanisms to unusual levels of stress.

Jensen (1964) found that 12% of 377 high school cheerleaders studied had hoarse voice quality. Andrews and Shank (1983) studied 102 females aged 13 to 17 years and found that 37% reported a history of voice problems.

Older girls with more years of cheerleading experience reported more voice difficulties than did girls with less cheerleading experience. In a questionnaire (Reich, McHenry, & Keaton, 1986) administered to 146 cheerleaders, it was found that episodes of "tired voice" and "sore throat" increased significantly following cheerleading events. The evidence suggests that both acute and chronic laryngeal changes (aphonia, aphonic syllables, diplophonia, and pitch breaks) occur more frequently among cheerleaders than among noncheerleaders. Laryngeal changes due to abuse, misuse, and overuse of the vocal mechanism are referred to as phonotrauma.

Respiratory Disorders

Any condition that makes it difficult for a student to inhale deeply or to prolong and control the exhalation phase of speech breathing can limit vocal performance. Tracheal stenosis (narrowing of the airway) or pulmonary obstruction is usually significant in these cases. Stenosis of subglottal structures frequently results from birth defects, trauma, inflammatory conditions, or intubation injuries and their sequelae. Severe problems (e.g., congenital malformations) are usually identified early in life and are not likely to be seen in untreated form in teenagers. Mild-to-moderate stenosis may occur for a variety of reasons and is usually characterized by stridor with deep and rapid breathing, especially during exercise and physical exertion. Dyspnea during exertion, cough, or intermittent wheezing related to excessive or thickened secretions may also be observed and occasionally misdiagnosed as asthma. In asthma, constriction and spasms of the airway generally cause wheezing only during the exhalation phase of breathing.

Sleep apnea, the transient cessation of breathing during sleeping, affects some adolescents. Tonsillar tissue and craniofacial anomalies (e.g., Treacher Collins syndrome, Stickler syndrome, hemifacial microsmia) may make individuals prone to obstructive sleep apnea. Micrognathia (e.g., Pierre Robin syndrome) seems to heighten the risk of sleep apnea because the tongue moves back and blocks the pharyngeal cavity during sleep. Symptoms that may be associated with sleep apnea include snoring, restless sleep, interrupted respiration cycles during sleep, fluctuations in weight, hyperactive gag reflex, and speech problems. Obstructive sleep apnea does not have a direct effect on the voice; however, it may occur together with mouth breathing, resulting in dry mucosal tissues and hoarseness. Chronic fatigue may lead to lowered immunity to infection and increase susceptibility to voice problems.

Sleep deprivation in teenagers is common and is thought to be biologically linked. Adolescents need sleep sufficient to handle the great physical changes occurring in their bodies at this time. There is an adjustment in their internal clock after puberty causing them to want to stay up later, but they need sleep to grow. The American Sleep Disorders Association says that teenagers need between 8½ and 9¼ hours of sleep per night, but that they average 7 to 7½ hours on school nights nationally. A small percentage suffer from "delayed sleep phase syndrome" in which their internal clocks prevent them from falling asleep before 3 or 4 A.M.

Respiratory obstruction or excessive secretions result in coughing that may also irritate laryngeal mucosa. Many serious illnesses (e.g., cystic fibrosis), inflammatory conditions (e.g., infections, allergies), growths (e.g., papillomatosis of the bronchi or trachea), and systemic diseases may limit respiratory function. Obesity may also contribute to some respiratory difficulties. The checklist in Table 14–1 (which is not exhaustive) may be helpful during history taking.

Treatment of Respiratory Disorders

Exercise is helpful for some types of respiratory disease. Physicians, physical therapists, and respiratory therapists frequently provide guidelines for individuals with chronic respiratory problems, and a speech–language pathologist should never implement a program of breathing exercises (Table 14–2) before obtaining appropriate information concerning medical status. The following suggestions, however, may be useful with some students. Students who complain of breathlessness should be encouraged to relax, breathe in slowly, and purse the lips in a whistling position and blow out slowly and evenly, attempting to increase the length of the exhalation phase. Pursed-lip breathing may be used whenever a student feels short of breath. It should be explained to students that this technique maintains air pressure in the airway so that more stale air can be breathed out. Sometimes clogged or narrowed airways or damaged air sacs in the lungs trap stale air.

Table 14–1. Respiratory conditions affecting breathing efficiency.

Paresis/paralysis of respiratory muscles
Congenital abnormalities
Trauma/stenosis
Tracheal amyloidosis
Bronchial/tracheal papillomatosis
Immotile cilia syndrome
Chronic infections (e.g., bronchitis)
Asthma
Allergies
Smoke inhalation/pollution
Iatrogenic respiratory disease
Chemical reactions (e.g., drugs, alcohol)
Cystic fibrosis
Foreign bodies
Obstructive sleep apnea
Tumor

Coughing spells are frightening, embarrassing, and tiring. The cough reflex is useful when it expels mucus and clears the airway. Productive coughing (Table 14–3) comes from deep in the lungs, and students may need to be taught the difference between a cough that expels mucus and one that is nonproductive. A nonproductive cough may be habituated and cause unnecessary irritation of laryngeal structures. Swallowing or a "silent" cough are less irritating substitutes.

When dryness is a problem, it is important that students increase hydration by fluid intake (usually eight glasses of water a day) and use humidifiers or vaporizers to moisturize the air. Fluids and moisturized air help to soften mucus so that it can be more easily expectorated. Humidifiers and vaporizers must be carefully cleaned on a regular basis because they can harbor and breed germs. Sometimes postural drainage is recommended to help drain mucus from the lungs. Postural drainage (Table 14–4) tilts the body so that mucus moves from the lungs into the upper airway where it is more easily expelled. (There are many possible positions, and a physician will usually recommend one that is appropriate for the individual.)

Physicians may prescribe medications for people with respiratory disease. The speech–language pathologist should ask about medications that adolescents may be using on doctor's orders, as well as those they may be taking without medical advice.

- *Bronchodilators* come in various forms, including pills, liquids, and sprays. Side effects include insomnia, nervousness, and upset stomach.
- *Nebulizers* are sprayers that deliver a mist that can be breathed into the lungs. They should be used carefully under a doctor's direction.
- *Expectorants* are used to make mucus thinner and easier to expel.

Table 14–2. Exercising breathing muscles.

1. Place hands on sides of lower chest.
2. Breathe in slowly, observing movement of the lower chest.
3. Keep shoulders and upper chest relaxed.
4. Breath out slowly through pursed lips, trying to extend the length of the exhalation and timing each successive trial.
5. Practice several times a day and rest or hold breath if dizziness occurs.

Table 14–3. Controlled coughing.

1. Sit in a chair with feet on floor and head slightly forward.
2. Take a deep breath.
3. Hold breath for a few seconds.
4. Cough twice (once to loosen mucus and once to bring it up).
5. Breath in by sniffing gently.
6. Spit out the mucus into tissue (do not swallow mucus because this can upset the stomach).

- *Sedatives and tranquilizers* are occasionally prescribed to promote relaxation or to help a person sleep. They can dangerously slow breathing if too many are taken, however.
- *Steroids* are strong medications that are sometimes prescribed to reduce swelling in the airways and to ease breathing. They also increase energy. If used for a long time, steroids can have the following side effects: fullness in the face, stomach ulcers, weakened skin and bones, tendency to bruise easily, and decreased immunity to infection. Because they slow down the adrenal glands, they must be tapered off gradually. New topical steroids are available that do not have the same side effects as systemic steroids.
- *Antibiotics* are used only for treating bacterial infections because viruses do not respond to them. Side effects include stomach upset and skin rashes.
- *Diuretics* are sometimes called "water pills" and are used to rid the body of extra fluid. Reduced salt intake is also recommended in such cases. Use of diuretics is linked to potassium loss, which can cause weakness and muscle cramps.

Phonation

Any change in tissue that interferes with vocal fold approximation, equal distribution of vocal fold weight, size, or mass may disturb normal laryngeal vibration.

By the time students reach the middle and high school years, most congenital anomalies of the laryngeal structures have been identified; however, small laryngeal webs are occasionally undetected before puberty if they do not significantly obstruct the airway. (The majority of congenital laryngeal webs occur at the vocal fold level, and only approximately 25% occur in the supraglottal and infraglottal areas.) In the case of a small web, the voice of a prepubertal child may not sound significantly different from those of peers. At the time of vocal mutation, however, when the peer group demonstrates more mature vocal characteristics, a higher pitched voice, for example, may finally draw attention to a

Table 14–4. Exercises and positions to open airways.

Postural Drainage*

- Place a pillow under the hips (so that chest is lower) and lie prone on the floor or lie on back with pillow under hips and knees raised.
- Clap or vibrate the chest to help loosen mucus.

Other Postural Exercises to Open Airway

- Raise arms during inhalation and lower arms during exhalation.
- Sit in a straight chair with shoulders relaxed and breathe in. During exhalation, turn trunk to left, reach arms over left shoulder, and bounce. Repeat on right side.
- Lie down, place hands behind head, and breathe in. Breathe out while raising head and shoulders as high as possible. Feel the stomach muscles tighten but don't sit up completely.
- Lie down and raise the right knee toward chest while breathing out. Breathe in as leg is lowered. Repeat with left knee and then both knees. Switch and breathe in while raising knees and breathe out while lowering them.
- Lie down and tilt pelvis during deep breathing. Relax during inspiration. Tighten muscles of stomach and buttocks during expiration.
- Sit in a chair, lean back, and raise arms during inspiration. Then lean forward slowly until chest lies on legs and head falls to knees (chin tucked under chest). Exhale slowly, feeling the movement on legs.

*Often best when done early in the morning to clear mucus that has built up during the night. In the evening it should be done at least an hour before bedtime.

student with a small web. Students who have been treated surgically for removal of webs during infancy may occasionally demonstrate residual effects of earlier intervention during later life. Careful history taking is critical to identify vocal symptoms related to early trauma, surgeries, and intubation. Questions concerning any conditions related to airway obstruction, for example, should routinely be asked when the speech pathologist interviews students and parents.

Some teenagers who had multiple surgeries for papillomatosis as children may exhibit hoarseness, compensatory hyperfunctional vocal behavior, or overly protective vocal patterns such as extreme breathiness and minimal loudness. Laryngeal edema and posterior commissure narrowing may occur as a result of previous intubation. Postsurgically, patients often use the same pattern of laryngeal control that they developed to compensate for lesions before surgery. Scar tissue at the site of a lesion may reduce the pliable mucosal covering and, therefore, the vibration at that part of the fold. Iatrogenic injury subsequent to surgical removal of benign lesions near the anterior commissure may also result in web formation.

Penetrating neck trauma may sometimes result in hematoma that compresses the airway and produces symptoms of stridor and dysphonia. Trauma may also result in lacerated mucosa, fractured cartilage, or displaced arytenoids. Signs of laryngeal trauma include palpable fracture, stridor, dyspnea, dysphagia, laryngeal pain or tenderness, hemoptysis, hoarseness, and aphonia or dysphonia.

Systemic diseases, such as leukemia and anemia, and infectious diseases, such as diphtheria, may affect laryngeal function and are frequently associated with lowered resistance to respiratory tract infections. Endocrine disorders (e.g., thyroid dysfunction) may produce symptoms of hoarseness, as can nodules, polyps, papilloma, and hyperkeratosis.

Benign neoplasms (neurofibromas, hemangiomas, lymphangiomas), cysts, and laryngoceles may occur infrequently and disrupt phonation, depending on the site of the lesion. Ulcers and granulomas sometimes occur and are thought to be residuals of intubation trauma.

Occasionally, an acute episode of hoarseness may be triggered in a healthy larynx by excessive vocal abuse (and may be referred to as phonotrauma), such as cheering for prolonged periods of time. More common, however, is chronic hoarseness that results from vocal abuse in association with other factors that irritate tissues in the airway and, specifically, in the larynx. Irritated (i.e., red or swollen) folds are particularly susceptible to long periods of use, misuse, sudden overexertion, and compensatory attempts at forceful adduction. Allergic reactions affecting the mucous membranes of the folds frequently result in inflammation and edema. Approximation of the folds is inhibited, and vocal fold vibration is impaired.

Vocal Pathologies

Vocal nodules are small noncancerous growths that occur on the vocal folds. They are caused by irritation of the delicate membranes covering the muscles and are one of the most common disorders of the larynx. Nodules appear as small bumps on the vibrating edge of one or both folds. Because "lateral" means "side," they are described as "unilateral" if there is only one, and "bilateral" if they occur on both sides (i.e., one on each of the vocal folds). When the vocal folds come together during speaking or singing, the free edges of the folds must approximate evenly for a clear voice to be produced. When vocal nodules are present, the folds are unable to meet evenly along their entire length and leakage of air occurs when voice is produced. The weight of the nodules may also cause the vocal folds to vibrate unevenly during voice production, causing diplophonia. People with vocal nodules speak with a hoarse voice quality. Other symptoms of vocal nodules include voice breaks, restricted pitch range, lower pitch level, and observable tension in the muscles of the neck. When nodules are small, the voice may sound clearest when a person is speaking loudly or on a high pitch. Throat clearing and coughing may also be noted. Treatments include surgery, voice rest, and the elimination of abusive vocal practices. Speech–language therapy to encourage appropriate vocal hygiene and nonstressful vocal production is recommended so that nodules do not recur.

Vocal nodules, polyps, and hyperkeratosis are frequently seen in "performance-oriented" young adults. Among singers, nodules seem most common in sopranos (Brodnitz, 1971; Punt, 1979). Young adults, particularly young women, who are talkative or active in dramatics, musicals, cheerleading, or other performance-related activities seem especially susceptible to developing nodules.

Signs of vocal pathology include lack of stability of vocal behaviors and atypical pitch range, loudness, or quality. Pitch level is considered in relation to age, gender, and pubertal development. Judgments of appropriateness of pitch levels can be correlated with acoustic measures. Perkins (1977) found that in nine studies 27 different terms were used to describe quality defects. This illustrates one of the problems of describing quality in perceptual terms. However, individuals with sudden onset of voice problems usually report that their voices have changed significantly. When quality deviations cause an adolescent embarrassment or frustration, the problem is real, despite professional difficulty with descriptive terminology. A weak voice, in which loudness cannot be sustained without difficulty, frequently causes fatigue from the strain of talking. Hyperfunctional muscle involvement is a common compensation in such cases and may compound the original problem. Problems of organic etiology are frequently characterized by difficulties with appropriate loudness. Sometimes an individual with vocal nodules can produce a clear voice only when speaking loudly. By overadducting the folds, the effect of the lesion is minimized until the nodules increase significantly in size. Speaking loudly or at a higher pitch to "clear" the voice quality is not an effective long-term strategy. This hyperfunctional pattern exacerbates the lesion further. Excessive throat clearing, a strategy used by some speakers with conditions that increase the size and mass of the folds, is also deterimental. Usually, it is more sensible to substitute swallowing for throat clearing.

The fact that such a variety of medical problems may be accompanied by hoarseness underscores the need for medical referral and evaluation of teenagers who exhibit chronically hoarse voices. A speech–language pathologist should be vigilant in ensuring that students and parents are alerted to the importance of a medical examination in diagnosis and management. In fact, a medical report before the initiation of voice therapy is required by most speech–language pathologists. Table 14–5 is a list of suggestions for decreasing vocal strain.

Mutational Falsetto

If a boy has completed the process of puberty (i.e., genital growth, skeletal growth, and secondary sex changes) but maintains a childlike vocal pattern, the condition is called *mutational falsetto.* Medical examination is necessary to ensure that endocrinological or structural problems are not present. Greene (1972) said that the larynx is usually pulled up high in the throat and the musculature is tense. Frequently, demonstration of the availability of a lower pitch results in habituation of more adult pitch levels. Partial mutation may be observed in some boys. Aronson (1973) described voice therapy for mutational falsetto and stressed the need to ensure that a boy is comfortable with his newly acquired voice. Many clinicians have hypothesized that the retention of a high-pitched voice by a postpubertal boy is related to underlying psychosocial conflicts and that psychologic counseling may be needed (Aronson). Wilson (1987) noted that an effective test for mutational falsetto is to ask a boy to breathe deeply and to cough or say a vowel with an abrupt glottal attack. Other techniques include using other vegetative functions such as sighing or laughing. Gutzman's pressure tests (Luchsinger & Arnold, 1965) or other digital manipulations of the larynx may be used to demonstrate the availability of a lower pitch level. Symptoms associated with mutational falsetto include high pitch level, pitch breaks, minimal vocal variety, thin breathy or hoarse quality, shallow breathing, muscle tension, reduced loudness, and reticence and embarrassment in conversational interactions.

Speech–language pathologists should also be aware that an apparent absence of pubertal vocal change may be related to a nutritional or medical problem delaying puberty. Undernutrition due to anorexia nervosa or bulimia, a systemic disease resulting in malabsorption of nutrients, and obesity can all inhibit puberty. Maturational delays may also be caused by collagen diseases, anemias, cardiac disorders, severe renal diseases, and diseases of the respiratory tract. When questions concerning pubertal development occur, medical evaluation is warranted.

Paradoxical Vocal Fold Dysfunction

Trudeau (1998) reported on a sample of 65 juveniles and adolescents aged 3.5 to 20.5 years who demonstrated a respiratory pattern where the individual constricts the larynx when breathing in so that inhalation is noisy and effortful. The constrictions may be related to at least three etiologies: psychogenic, reflexive

Table 14–5. Ways to decrease vocal strain.

- Use nonverbal "attention getters" such as clapping, waving, and hand signals rather than the voice whenever possible.
- Make use of "mouthing" during unison singing or cheering.
- Increase listening time and quiet activities.
- Reduce the distance between yourself and the listener so there will be no need to shout.
- Avoid hard glottal attacks when you speak.
- Maintain good posture and relax your neck, jaw, and shoulders.
- Avoid repeated throat clearing and nonproductive coughing.
- Avoid talking in the presence of loud noise.
- Avoid talking during periods of upper respiratory problems.
- Avoid smoking.
- Drink lots of water to improve lubrication of the throat.
- Learn to be a good questioner and encourage others to talk. Increase the ratio of listening versus talking.
- Use pitch and rate changes rather than loudness changes in order to get and hold attention.
- Always use plenty of air when you speak and breathe frequently.

closure associated with irritation such as in GERD, and neurologic such as a form of laryngeal dystonia. Asthma has also been associated with PVCD in the literature. In fact, episodic paroxysmal laryngospasm has also been referred to as factitious asthma when seen in the absence of specific organic etiology. Sometimes both true and false folds are adducted, and stridor is heard during both inhalation and exhalation. Between episodes, the function of the larynx appears to be normal. Kaufman (1995) and Blager, Brugman, Howell, Mahler, and Rosenberg (1998) advocated nasal sniffing, and Treole and Trudeau (1997) suggested nasal inhalation followed by exhalation through pursed lips. Exercise-induced laryngospasm has been discussed by Gracco, Jones-Bryant, Fahey, DeStephens, and Naito (1995). Although laryngeal behavior of this type does not usually result in any voice quality deviations, patients with such problems can be treated successfully by speech–language pathologists skilled in voice treatment approaches and respiratory and laryngeal dynamics.

Clinical Information: Tourette's Syndrome

This condition was first described and named for Georges Gilles de la Tourette more than a century ago. It is a disorder that is poorly recognized by health professionals and by the general public, involving involuntary movements and vocalizations, which are exhibited sporadically. Consequently, many individuals who suffer from it are not diagnosed. The Tourette Syndrome Association, since it began in 1976, has promoted research and improved recognition of this neglected disorder. The national office can be reached by calling (800) 237-0717. A copy of an award-winning hour-long video, "Twitch and Shout," produced and directed by Laurel Chiten, is available through New Day Films, phone: (201) 652-6590 or fax: (201) 652-1973.

Researchers have traced the cause of the condition to a single abnormal gene that seems to cause abnormalities in dopamine and, perhaps, other neurotransmitters. A person with the gene has a 50% likelihood of passing it on to an offspring. The gene can cause a wide array of symptoms ranging in severity, with occasionally no symptoms appearing at all in affected individuals. Of those, 99% of boys but only 70% of girls are likely to exhibit at least one sign; 31% might not know they have it but could still transmit it to their children. Prenatal environmental factors, such as low birth weight, can influence severity adversely.

Intermittent episodes of symptoms such as repetitive blinking, head jerking, grimacing, barking, sniffing, compulsive behaviors, personality traits, and perfectionism are sometimes observed in affected individuals. Only about 15% demonstrate copralalia (periodic outbursts of foul language). Some echolalia and mimicking of what others say also may be observed. Sometimes there is a compulsion to keep doing something until it is right. School children with Tourette's frequently may seem to have attention deficit disorder and may be diagnosed as hyperactive. Physicians and caregivers may assume a child has an emotionally based disorder or "psychological problems" rather than a neurologically based genetic condition. Dr. Oliver Sacks has written a book of case studies of neurological disorders, including a Canadian surgeon, Dr. Carl Bennett, whose condition was not accurately diagnosed until he was 37 years old. The book, *An Anthropologist on Mars* (1995), is published by Alfred A. Knopf.

People with Tourette's syndrome are usually able to suppress their symptoms for varying lengths of time, and the symptoms are not apparent during sleep, sexual activity, and periods of intense concentration. Sometimes, symptoms can totally disappear for weeks or months at a time. Of children who are affected, 20 to 30% can be expected to outgrow the condition in their teens or early twenties. When a person has continuing symptoms, efforts to suppress the symptoms are often followed by uncontrollable bursts of the tics. When tics disrupt an individual's lifestyle because of severity and frequency, a physician may prescribe drugs that affect the chemistry of the brain. These drugs include haloperidol (Haldol), clonidine (Catapres), pimozide (Orap), fluphenazine (Prolixin), climipramine (Anafranil), and fluoxetine (Prozac). Medications have side effects such as weight gain that make some clients feel that the symptoms may be less troubling than the effects of the drugs, however.

A student with Tourette's syndrome exhibiting mild symptoms such as spontaneous vocalizations caused by vocal fold tics may occasionally be referred to the voice clinician. When such a student is seen for assessment, a prompt neurologic referral is indicated.

Resonance

Craniofacial anomalies of serious proportion are usually identified during childhood and are rarely encountered in the teenage population without a treatment history. When a severe organic abnormality is present, a medical history is usually available for the speech–language pathologist. Sequelae of earlier trauma (e.g., scar tissue, reconstructive procedures, and surgical aftermaths) occasionally present unusual symptoms during adolescence, but again case history information can generally be obtained and current symptoms can be analyzed with respect to pertinent medical information. A speech–language pathologist may also need to obtain information from orthodontists because many adolescents receive orthodontic treatment.

Acute pharyngitis refers to all acute infections of the pharynx, including the tonsils and adenoids. Systemic diseases that cause pharyngitis include infectious hepatitis, toxoplasmosis, infectious mononucleosis, and herpangina. Infectious mononucleosis is a viral disease that frequently occurs in teenagers. Although rarely life threatening, "mono," which can recur, causes extreme fatigue and discomfort in swallowing. Occasionally, a teenager may also contract a fungal infection affecting the upper respiratory tract, but this is much less common than bacterial or viral infections. Occasionally, a lateral pharyngeal abcess occurs during adolescence. Generally, speech–language pathologists are not concerned with acute conditions due to infection. It is chronic conditions that tend to be related to voice problems.

Chronic rhinitis and chronic sinusitis may create symptoms of hyponasality because of partial or complete nasal obstruction. Nasal polyps and septal defects may also cause hyponasality. Hyponasality (also called "denasality") is perceived as "blocked nose" voice. Any obstruction (partial or complete) of the nasal cavities may cause this resonance pattern. In adolescents, sports injuries, allergic rhinitis, chronic sinusitis, growths, adenoiditis, premenstrual edema of nasal mucosa, and drug use (e.g., cocaine) should be considered as causes of hyponasality. Habitual mouth breathing, often in association with dryness of laryngeal structures, is frequently seen.

The tonsils and adenoids regress during adolescence, but episodes of adenotonsillitis are frequent and occasionally occur as part of systemic diseases, such as gonorrhea and immunodeficiencies. Neoplasms of the nose and paranasal sinuses may also occur and show symptoms of hyponasality. Angiofibromas occur in male adolescents. These are vascular lesions occurring in the posterior nasal or nasopharyngeal areas.

Trauma to the face may result in frontal sinus fracture; nasal septum damage; or maxillary, mandibular, or soft tissue injury. Residuals of past trauma may affect mouth opening, the resonating cavities, and neurologic function. Penetrating wounds to the skull base, for example, may affect both the glossopharyngeal and vagus nerves, resulting in both dysphagia and vocal fold paralysis. Handler and Wetmore (1982) described sports-related injuries that can occur in childhood and adolescence and advocated the use of protective masks.

Videofluoroscopy and flexible fiber-optic nasopharyngoscopy techniques have made it possible for clinicians to observe movement of the velopharyngeal sphincter during speech. Such studies yield valuable information concerning function of the sphincter and changes with age. Sadewitz and Shprintzen (1985) found significant change in the morphology of the oropharynx and nasopharynx. As children develop through adolescence, the relationship of the velum to the pharynx changes, producing a shift in angulation of the orifice. The relative anterioposterior dimensions of the velopharyngeal movement had decreased in most of Sadewitz and Shprintzen's subjects who were retested after 10 years. The actual point at which the velum contacted the pharyngeal wall had changed in all subjects, and the relationship between the planes of lateral wall movement and velar elevation had also changed. Passavant's pad was present in only two subjects when the original testing occurred in childhood, but was present in five subjects when retesting occurred during the teenage years.

Children with obstructed airways due to enlarged tonsils or adenoids frequently have trouble eating because they are mouth breathers. Thus, they eat slowly and eat less. Removal of the lymphatic tissue results in improved eating habits and weight gain (Potsic, Miller, & Corso (1983). Removal of tonsils and adenoids in the presence of velopharyngeal insufficiency or submucous clefts can result in symptoms of hypernasality and nasal emission, however. Hypernasality may be observed in adolescents with normal velopharyngeal mechanisms for about 6 weeks following removal of tonsils and adenoids. This is a temporary condition related to learning new speech and voice patterns with an altered mechanism.

Hypernasality, sometimes called "nasal" voice, may be accompanied by nasal emission and incorrect production of consonants requiring oral breath pressure (e.g., if velopharyngeal inadequacy is present). Hypernasality that is inconsistent, especially when it occurs only when the system is fatigued, is considered a possible early sign of neurological disease (e.g., myasthenia gravis or multiple sclerosis). When hypernasality occurs only on vowels, it may be referred to as "assimilated" nasality and may be due to the influence of nasal consonants (e.g., *pãn*). Word pairs such as (*pat, pan*) can be used to ascertain whether nasal production of the vowel is indeed the result of the adjacent nasal consonant. Nasal production of vowel sounds is frequent in some regional speech patterns (e.g., *Indiãna*) and may be due to faulty learning or may be habituated as a result of certain emotional states (e.g., whining). It is not usually considered a problem unless an individual aspires to professional use of voice (e.g., broadcasting, acting, singing).

Postsurgical alterations in the vocal tract (e.g., repaired clefts, secondary procedures such as pharyngeal flaps, reduced tissue subsequent to tonsillectomy and adenoidectomy, and scar tissue) should be documented through interviews, histories, and medical reports. Compensatory behaviors may be intricately related to such alterations. A mixed pattern of both hypernasality and hyponasality may be present.

Faulty learning, regional dialects, and psychosocial factors may also affect the development and maintenance of appropriate resonance behavior. Lack of self-esteem is often characterized by minimal mouth opening, reduced articulatory precision and vocal projection, and inappropriate resonance. Extreme tension in the mechanism, especially in the pharyngeal area, retracted tongue posture, and the substitution of laryngeal movements to compensate for inadequate velopharyngeal activity may be observed in adolescents with faulty learning, hearing impairment, or mild velopharyngeal inadequacy. Muffled (cul-de-sac) resonance, articulatory imprecision, and an inappropriate balance of nasal and oral resonance is frequently heard in speakers with moderate to severe hearing impairment.

An appropriate balance of nasal and oral resonance may be affected by the degree of mouth opening and by lip and tongue movement. Any condition that constrains mouth and tongue movement (e.g., Bell's palsy, depression, orthodontic appliances, or glossitis) may be pertinent to the resonance characteristics of the voice.

Psychosocial Factors

Voice is the most direct channel through which thoughts and feelings are shared. The way others react to the voice influences the way individuals think and feel about themselves. Human communication is dynamic and circular, and vocal behavior is an intrinsic and critical component of interpersonal interactions.

Sound self-esteem and satisfying interpersonal relationships correlate highly with vocal well-being. When vocal behavior causes difficulties, there is always some deleterious effect on self-concept and relationships (both intimate and casual). The degree of disruption will vary, but some disruption will always occur. That is why clinicians always need to address the social and emotional effects of any vocal disorder. No problem exists in a discrete form. Any problem that affects the ability to communicate creates social and emotional difficulties. Similarly, social and emotional problems can themselves create or exacerbate communication disorders. These interrelationships are what make differential diagnosis so challenging.

Sometimes, an individual's ego development, personality structure, or coping strategies give rise to atypical vocal behaviors. For example, voice symptoms may be indicative of internal distress, disorientation, or disintegration. Personality disorders can be the root cause of absent or distorted phonation, as can psychosexual conflicts. Thus, withdrawal of the self can be demonstrated through muteness, aphonia, or dysphonia. The lack or distortion of voice is then a symptom of the internal distress of the individual, and volitional control is absent or diminished.

Life stresses that an individual cannot confront directly are sometimes dealt with by using the voice as a defense to ward off pain or to protect and shield the ego. Conversion reactions are an extreme example of this, and in such instances the person is aphonic or severely dysphonic. Aronson (1980) defined a psychogenic voice disorder as the manifestation of one or more types of psychological disequilibrium where normal volitional control is suspended or disrupted.

The degree and type of interference with volitional control influences the number, type, and severity of the symptoms. There is a continuum of psychogenic disorders ranging from acute, short-term reactions to interpersonal conflicts or environmental stress, to chronically debilitating psychotic disorders.

Sometimes, abuse and misuse of the voice, musculoskeletal states, and hyperfunction or hypofunction of muscle patterns result in structural changes in the vocal mechanism. What began as maladaptive behavior due to psychological disequilibrium develops into a problem with organic components. Conversely, an organically based problem may be compounded by psychosocial overlays. In some instances, precipitating and maintaining factors (e.g., secondary gains) interweave in complex patterns, proliferating defense mechanisms, anxieties, learned behaviors, and compensations.

When vocal problems are part of a cluster of psychosocial difficulties, the speech–language pathologist may play a major role in helping adolescents learn more adult behaviors as a result of working through their difficulties. Vocal psychotherapy (Cooper, 1973) is frequently useful with adolescents. Adolescents often adopt roles or act inappropriately as a means of communication or as a way of testing whether adults can be trusted. They also experiment to test limits that are set by significant adults. Troubled adolescents may relate to a "neutral" adult (such as a speech–language pathologist) more easily and comfortably than to teachers or counselors. "Working on speech and voice" may seem less threatening and stigmatizing than seeking psychologic counseling. A speech–language pathologist is often perceived as a professional who has no direct responsibility for grading academic performance. This can help students feel more open and less defensive. They may also feel more comfortable in revealing the general disequilibrium underlying their vocal symptoms. Speech–language pathologists are usually skilled communicators who can give support and direction and accept ambivalence and inconsistency with a certain amount of tolerance. Because their students are usually seen in individual or small group settings, they can relate to each student in a more personal way than a busy classroom teacher can. This individualized attention is what so many adolescents seem to crave. Thus, speech–language pathologists are sometimes in unique positions to intervene with adolescents who have adjustment difficulties related to self-concept and interpersonal relationships. Such students are frequently receptive to "trying out" new communication styles and testing and analyzing new strategies. Participation in situationally based activities is often seen as particularly "relevant" by adolescents. Mild-to-moderate psychosocial problems in combination with communication disorders can usually be dealt with most effectively by a skilled speech–language pathologist.

When a speech–language pathologist finds that a communication problem is related to a severe or global personality disorder (i.e., when the student is consistently unable to control behavior), more specialized assistance will be needed. Referrals for psychologic or medical evaluation may be necessary, and a team approach to treatment may be needed. Even in cases of severe psychosocial dysfunction, the speech–language pathologist is usually part of the intervention team and collaborates closely with other professionals during the implementation of treatment programs.

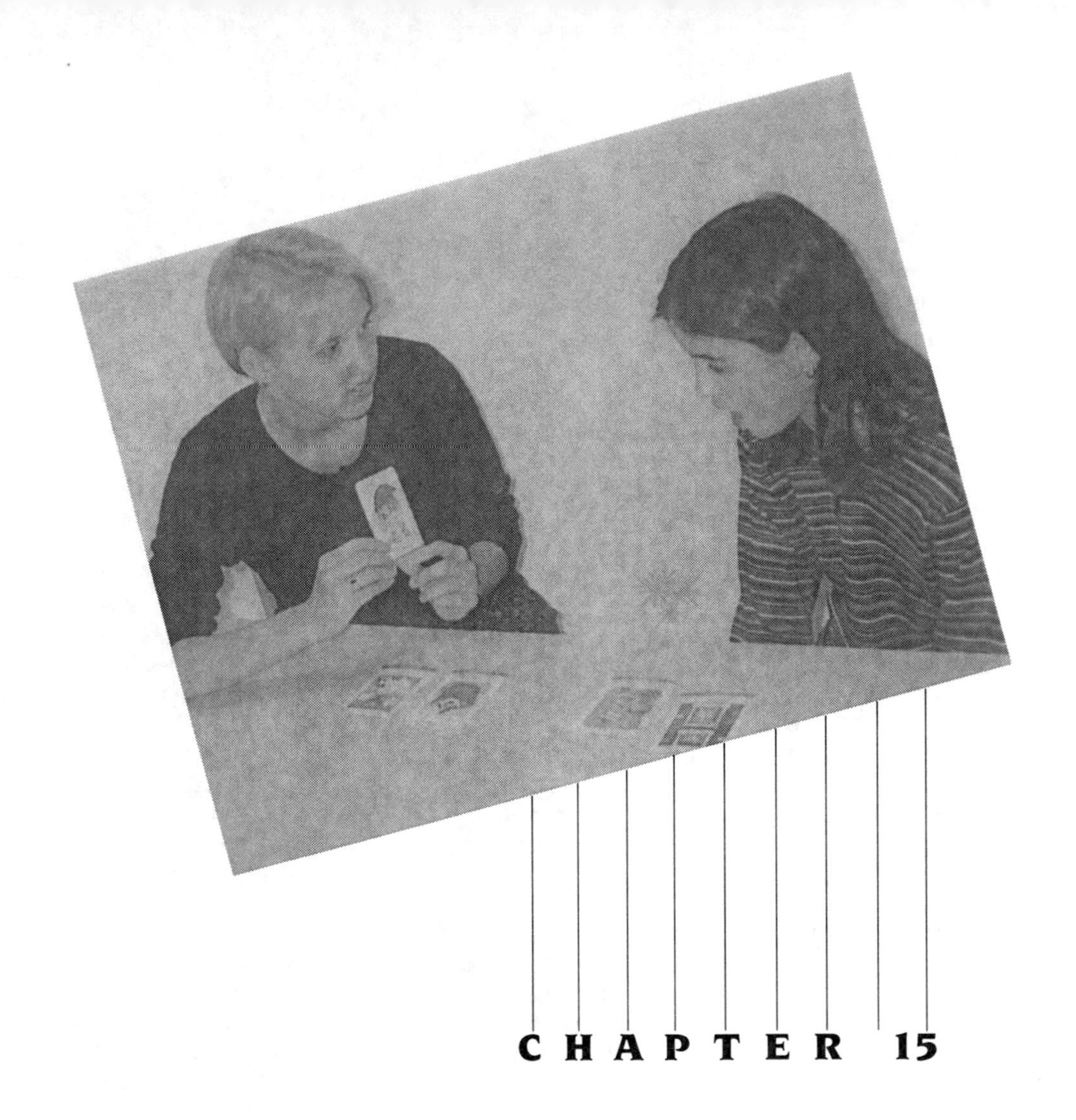

CHAPTER 15

Evaluation

In the absence of standardized tests, clinicians frequently develop a series of tasks designed to elicit samples of relevant behaviors. From these samples, the appropriateness of the voice is determined. Such subjective impressions are often difficult to record and classify systematically. Pannbacker (1984) reviewed classification systems of voice disorders. She stated that classifications need to be used in ways that facilitate communication with other professionals, as well as in ways that are useful in making management decisions. This is especially true for the school speech–language pathologist, who must communicate with parents and other professionals, as well as be the major designer of the voice managment plan.

A speech–language pathologist faces other decisions when structuring the voice evaluation. These include selecting appropriate diagnostic procedures, an efficient system of recording and synthesizing data, and an effective way of translating diagnostic information into meaningful therapy objectives. Although excellent descriptions of assessment methods appear in texts such as Wilson (1979), Boone (1983), Aronson (1980), and Fox (1978), clinicians frequently want additional assistance in adapting these procedures for use with adolescents.

Speech–language pathologists need to collect and assimilate as much pertinent information as possible. The case conferencing procedure requires a succinct yet thorough presentation of diagnostic information. Nonetheless, time constraints demand that a speech–language pathologist collect and summarize diagnostic information as efficiently as possible.

A convenient way to organize the vocal diagnostic process is to consider three general areas of behavior relevant to voice production: respiration, phonation, and resonance. Nonetheless, it must be remembered that these three general areas are neither discrete nor all-inclusive. A student's behavior during diagnostic sessions provides only part of the information necessary to determine appropriate referrals and management strategies. A student's problem must be seen in a wider context, and information from additional sources must be integrated with data on respiration, phonation, and resonance.

Certain physical, psychological, and sociological factors, individually or in combination, can heighten susceptibility to the development and maintenance of a vocal disorder. For example, conditions of the upper respiratory tract, such as chronic infections or allergic reactions, may place a vocally active student, such as a cheerleader, at greater risk than a student with a less vocally demanding lifestyle. High-risk factors relating specifically to the adolescent lifestyle must be identified and considered.

A speech–language pathologist needs to observe a student and gain supplementary information from school personnel concerning the student's patterns of interaction, coping strategies, and favored activities. During the vocally active middle and high school years, students engage in many activities (e.g., cheerleading, athletics, debate, dramatic productions, choral activities, lengthy telephone conversations) that place unusual demands on the vocal mechanism. The transition from childhood to adulthood results in physiological changes of the mechanism and psychologic stress. In an effort to cope with stressful situations, some students engage in crying jags, alcohol and drug abuse, and loud attention-getting behaviors. There is some evidence that eating disorders, such as anorexia nervosa (which lowers the body's resistance to infection) and bulimia (with frequent spasmodic contractions of the trachea and esophagus combined with acidic secretions) may heighten the risk of vocal problems.

Evaluating vocal risk is often challenging because there are so many pertinent risk factors to be considered in relation to a student's medical history, family situation, lifestyle demands, and interpersonal relationships. The most important aspects of this task are (a) considering all relevant risk factors, (b) condensing information into a manageable format, and (c) integrating information concerning the relationship of risk factors to each other and to data collected from traditional areas of evaluation (respiration, phonation, and resonance). When this is accomplished successfully, the collected information results in a comprehensive picture of a student's voice problem presented in a manageable format. The speech–language pathologist can then easily retrieve pertinent information and identify appropriate management strategies.

The organizational system outlined in this chapter is presented so that therapy planning arises naturally from collected data. The evaluation form contains traditional questions on respiration, phonation, and resonance, as well as sample tasks designed to target critical behaviors that are prerequisites for appropriate vocal production (Figures 15–1 through 15–3). The evaluation also covers high-risk factors: physical conditions, abusive practices, demands inherent in lifestyle and environment, and interpersonal behaviors (Figure 15–4). A "skipping option" is provided in each section to shorten the in-depth evaluation for students who demonstrate appropriate behavior in certain areas of performance. For example, a student who demonstrates appropriate behaviors in a general area, such as resonance, need only be checked as "appropriate." Demographic information, a summary of areas to be considered in therapy, recommendations, and referrals should also be recorded. This facilitates the easy retrieval of pertinent information for case conferences and therapy planning.

Respiration

If there are indications that respiration may be inappropriate for speech, the speech–language pathologist completes six items designed to record characteristics of a student's breathing pattern (Figure 15–1). Information for items A and B may be obtained by observing a student during a spontaneous speech sample involving connected speech for approximately 2 minutes.

Because voicing occurs during the exhalation phase of speech breathing, it is helpful to determine the length of the exhalation and maximum phonation time (item C). Typically, prepubertal children prolong consonants (Tait, Michel, & Carpenter, 1980) and vowels (Wilson, 1979) of approximately 10-second duration. In the adolescent age range, 10 seconds should be regarded as a minimal proficiency level. Higher levels (i.e., adult levels of 20 to 25 seconds) would be necessary for students with vocally demanding lifestyles (Ptacek & Sander, 1963).

It is critical to observe the relationship between the prolongation of /s/ and /z/ (Eckel & Boone, 1981). A student who prolongs the unvoiced /s/ for a significantly longer time than the voiced /z/ obviously has adequate available air supply and can sustain flow but is experiencing difficulty at the laryngeal valving level. A student who demonstrates an s/z ratio of 2:1 should be referred for laryngeal examination. Prater and Swift (1984) recommended that a cutoff ratio of 1.20:1 be used to determine the need for laryngeal evaluation. This means that a student who, on repeated trials, sustains /s/ for 18 seconds and /z/ for 15 seconds should be referred for medical evaluation, even though the length of the exhalation falls within normal limits.

After a student has been given clear instructions, a model, and practice trials, an averaged performance on prolongation of /a/ that falls below 10 seconds could suggest inadequate respiration, inadequate laryngeal valving (laryngeal pathology, such as nodules), neurologic involvement, or faulty learning of the coordination of airflow with voicing.

Because running speech involves segmentation of airflow during the exhalation phase,

Figure 15–1. Evaluation form: Respiration.

Respiration for speech appears appropriate ____ inappropriate ____.
A. Inspiration: appropriate ____ shallow ____ audible breathing ____
B. Tension sites: none ____ upper chest ____ neck ____
C. Length of exhalation
1. Counts on one breath to ____ (note number)
2. Sustains s-s-s ____ secs. } Ratio of s/z = ____ *
3. Sustains z-z-z ____ secs. }
4. Sustains /a/ ____ secs.
Average maximum phonation time: ____
D. Control of exhalation (segments exhalation into equal thirds)
yes ____ no ____
E. Use of replenishing breaths
1. Number of breaths taken while counting to 100 ____
2. Number of breaths taken while reading (100 words at reading level) ____
F. Coordination of respiration with phonatory demands in spontaneous speech is
rhythmical ____ arrhythmical ____.

*Is the s/z ratio noted above greater than or equal to 1.20:1? yes ____ no ____. If yes, the possibility of laryngeal pathology exists and medical referral should be made.

it is helpful to observe a student's ability to interrupt the continuity of airflow. The task in item D (Figure 15–1) involves the production of the unvoiced phoneme /h/. This is to ensure that respiratory activity can be observed in the absence of laryngeal valving or articulatory interruption of airflow. Space for three trials is provided to ensure that a student is comfortable with the task and is given an opportunity to improve performance with practice. Instructions and a model should be provided.

To produce smooth, connected utterances, a student must be able to use replenishing breaths in ways that do not detract from the content of a message (items E and F, Figure 15–1). Therefore, the frequency, obtrusiveness, and timing of these breaths must be observed in both automatic and spontaneous speech samples, as well as in a predetermined linguistic pattern (e.g., reading a passage). The advantage of including a predetermined linguistic pattern is that it can also be used as a posttest later in the therapy program.

Phonation

If phonatory behavior appears inappropriate in quality, onset, loudness, pitch, or rate, the speech–language pathologist should evaluate the inappropriate dimensions (Figure 15–2). Nonetheless, it is usually advantageous to evaluate all dimensions of phonation to obtain comprehensive information.

To observe the quality of a student's voice, the speech–language pathologist should elicit prolongations and then a spontaneous speech sample of at least 2 minutes in duration. It is important to have the student prolong the consonants /s/ and /z/ because the *s/z* ratio provides informa-tion concerning vocal fold pathology (Eckel & Boone, 1981). The prolongation of /a/ provides an oppor-

Figure 15–2. Evaluation form: Phonation.

Rate the following dimensions of phonatory behavior:

	Quality	*Onset*	*Loudness*	*Pitch*	*Rate*
Appropriate	____	____	____	____	____
Inappropriate	____	____	____	____	____

A. Quality in sustained phonation
1. Sustains s-s-s ____ secs. } Ratio of s/z = ____*
2. Sustains z-z-z ____ secs. }
3. Sustains /a/ ____ secs.
   (Note quality, continuity)

B. Quality in spontaneous speech sample
1. Breathy ____ mild ____ moderate ____ severe ____
2. Harsh ____ mild ____ moderate ____ severe ____
3. Hoarse ____ mild ____ moderate ____ severe ____
4. Related observations: pitch breaks ____ phonation breaks ____
   aphonia ____ glottal fry ____ diplophonia ____ tremor ____
   other ________________
5. How does a higher pitch affect quality? Improves ____ worsens ____ no change ____
6. How does a louder level affect quality? Improves ____ worsens ____ no change ____
7. Is quality affected by menstrual cycle? yes ____ no ____

C. Onset of phonation

In single words	*Appropriate*	*Breathy*	*Hard glottal*
1. arm /a/	____	____	____
2. eggs /e/	____	____	____
3. umpire /ʌ/	____	____	____
4. out /au/	____	____	____
5. ooze /u/	____	____	____
6. eight /el/	____	____	____
7. apple /æ/	____	____	____
In sentences (to be said loudly)			
8. Allen Edwards is engaged to Erica Underwood.	____	____	____
9. Is everyone awfully angry?	____	____	____
10. Amy Anderson always understands.	____	____	____
11. Extra actors are out at the entrance.	____	____	____
In spontaneous speech (conversational level)	____	____	____

D. Loudness
1. Prolonged vowel loudly ____ sec.
2. Prolonged vowel softly ____ sec.
3. Sustained vowels gradually increasing and decreasing loudness
   Ability to control loudness: yes ____ no ____

*Is the s/z ratio noted above greater than or equal to 1.20:1? yes ____ no ____ If yes, the possibility of laryngeal pathology exists and medical referral should be made.

(continued)

Figure 15–2. *(continued)*

Limited loudness range: yes _____ no _____
Tension present: yes_____ no _____ when _____
4. Counting from soft to loud, loud to soft
Ability to control variation: yes _____ no _____
Limited range: yes _____ no _____
Tension present: yes _____ no _____ when _____
5. Level during reading passage: overstrong _____ weak _____
fading _____ lacking in variety _____ inappropriate to meaning _____
tension present _____
6. Level during spontaneous speech: overstrong _____ weak _____
fading _____ lacking in variety _____ inappropriate to meaning _____
tension present _____

E. Pitch observed during reading _____ spontaneous speech _____ both _____
1. Habitual level
a. Appropriate to age and gender _____ too low _____ too high _____
b. Does the student's age and physical development indicate the possibility of pubertal voice changes? yes _____ no _____
2. Voice breaks to higher pitch _____ lower pitch _____
3. Variability
a. Amount: appropriate _____ limited _____ monotone _____ exaggerated _____
b. Consistency of use of pitch changes to reflect meaning:
always _____ sometimes _____ never _____
4. Ability to produce extremes of pitch range (isolated vowels):
good _____ fair _____ poor _____
5. Ability to discriminate pitch differences (isolated tones, series of tones):
good _____ fair _____ poor _____
6. Ability to imitate a given pitch (isolated vowels):
good _____ fair _____ poor _____
7. Ability to imitate sequential pitch patterns (series of vowels):
good _____ fair _____ poor _____
8. Ability to imitate pitch inflections (phrases, e.g., It's mine? vs. It's mine!):
good _____ fair _____ poor _____

F. High–quiet singing (quality and continuity)
appropriate _____ inappropriate _____

G. Rate (in spontaneous speech):
too fast _____ too slow _____ arrhythmical _____ appropriate _____*

H. Phrasing errors during reading.
insufficient replenishing breaths _____ lack of smoothness _____
inappropriate to meaning _____ inappropriate pause lengths _____
limited variety _____ dysfluencies _____

*165 syllables per minute (Peters & Guitar, 1991)

tunity to evaluate characteristics such as pitch breaks, aphonic episodes, and diplophonia. A reading passage is also useful because some people adopt a different phonatory style during reading. Students with vocal nodules frequently produce a clearer voice quality during higher pitched or louder speech, and this can be observed by asking the student to recite the months of the year, first in a higher voice, then in a louder voice. Hormonal fluctuations during the menstrual cycle may result in swelling of the laryngeal or nasal mucosa, so female students should be questioned to ascertain possible changes in voice quality before and during menstruation.

The appropriate timing and coordination of airflow with the onset of phonation (item C) is a prerequisite for effective vocal production. When the relationship between airflow and onset is disturbed, the appropriate initiation of phonation should become a therapy goal.

A vocally abusive practice frequently seen in students with voice disorders is the hard glottal attack. Items C1–C7 provide opportunities to observe the type of onset during the production of stressed syllables beginning with vowels because this is the context in which hard attacks are most likely to occur. Examples of sentences to be repeated in a loud voice are included in the evaluation form to identify the frequency of occurrence of hard attacks in relation to loudness level (items 8–11, Figure 15–2). Finally, the type of onset most frequently occurring during spontaneous speech should be noted.

Many people with voice disorders, especially those whose disorders are related to vocal abuse, may habituate excessively loud vocal behavior and limited control and variability of loudness patterns (item D). The ability to produce a clear phonation at a soft level is often difficult for the student with vocal pathology. The presence or absence of observable tension can indicate the relationship between effort and output. The pattern of habitual loudness level may also be significant. For example, if a student's voice consistently fades at the end of sentences, it may suggest a relationship between available air supply and loudness.

Precise adjustments of the laryngeal musculature in association with control of airflow are necessary to produce appropriate pitch patterns. Conditions of the vocal folds, such as edema, inflammation, growths, or neurological deficits, interfere with these adjustments. Because nodules are a frequently occurring vocal pathology, it is important to note that the resulting changes in the mass of the folds may be reflected in inappropriate pitch behavior. High–quiet singing is often more difficult than singing in the mid-range at normal or loud levels when there is increased vocal fold mass. The quality and evenness of the singing may be observed during the singing of "Happy Birthday" (item F). See Bastian, Keidar, and Verdolini–Marston (1990).

It is important to note the influence age or physical maturity may exert on vocal characteristics and to note the direction of voice breaks because clinical observation suggests that a voice breaks in the direction it wishes to go (Figure 15–2). Variability of the voice may be affected by such factors as environmental models, neurological or cognitive deficits, emotional state, and hearing acuity. If a student's variability of pitch is limited, items 4 and 5 (Figure 15–2) can be used to assess available pitch range and pitch discrimination ability. When a student is able to imitate both isolated and sequenced pitches but does not employ meaningful variation spontaneously, the use of pitch changes to reflect thoughts and feelings could be an appropriate therapy goal. Lack of vocal variation in adolescents may indicate depression, however. A student's general demeanor and facial expression are further indicators of emotional state.

Resonance

An appropriate resonance pattern is the result of a balance of direct nasal resonance (on /m/, /n/, and /ŋ/), indirect nasal resonance, and oral resonance (all vowels and nonnasal consonants). Hypernasality, or an excess of direct nasal resonance on sounds other than /m/, /n/, and /ŋ/, may indicate velopharyngeal inadequacy, whereas hyponasality, or an absence of direct nasal resonance on /m/, /n/, and /ŋ/, may indicate acute or chronic nasal congestion or other obstruction. It is important to emphasize the need for medical referral if hyponasality or hypernasality is noted. Although inappropriate resonance may be the result of faulty learning, the presence of organic impairment must always be carefully explored before attempting behavioral modification. Fluctuations in resonance patterns may also indicate the early onset of neurologic disease or, in girls, intermittent swelling of the nasal mucosa related to menstrual cycles.

If resonance appears inappropriate for speech, the speech–language pathologist completes eight items designed to record a student's resonance characteristics (Figure 15–3). Items A, B, and C (Figure 15–3) allow the speech–language pathologist to explore the possibility of hyponasality. It may be valuable to occlude the nares one at a time while the student is humming to determine the presence of a nostril obstruction (item A). Occluding the nares in item B can help the speech–language pathologist determine if an obstruction is total or partial. In the absence of an obstruction, direct nasal resonance will be normal when the nares are not occluded. Characteristics that are indicative of adenoidal enlargement, tissue changes in the nasal cavity, or upper respiratory conditions should be noted in item C.

Items D, E, and F (Figure 15–3) allow the speech–language pathologist to explore the possibility of hypernasalsity. Inadequate velopharyngeal closure may be indicated if the sentences in item E sound more appropriate when spoken with both nares occluded than with both nares open. Characteristics frequently associated with velopharyngeal inadequacy are listed in item F. The Iowa Pressure Test, a subtest of the Templin-Darley (Morris, Spriesterbach, & Darley, 1961), may be used to explore further the articulation of pressure consonants.

Items G and H (Figure 15–3) focus on the ability to valve appropriately on sequences of oral and nasal sounds. Contrasting word pairs allow the clinician to observe changes related to the effect of nasal consonants on vowels. The conversation and reading sample can show the overall effect of the resonance pattern in connected speech. The influence of associated articulatory behaviors on resonance during conversational and projected speech should be noted in item J.

High-Risk Factors

It is clear that certain physical and emotional factors, as well as learned or habituated behaviors, may (a) increase susceptibility to developing a voice disorder (e.g., upper respiratory conditions), (b) maintain or reinforce inappropriate vocal use (e.g., cheerleading, throat clearing), (c) provide secondary gains for an individual (e.g., attention-getting behaviors such as impersonations), or (d) result in compensatory behaviors that compound the original problem (e.g., hyperextended jaw coughing). Noting the risk factors during an evaluation (Figure 15–4) helps a speech–language pathologist to determine the need for referral to other professionals and to determine the influence risk factors have on the therapy prognosis. Recognizing risk factors facilitates the design of a voice therapy program that is relevant to a student, that

Figure 15–3. Evaluation form: Resonance.

Overall resonance in reading and conversation: appropriate ____ inappropriate ____

A. Nasal resonance while sustaining a hum: weak ____ absent ____ appropriate ____

B. Nasal sentences (to check for hyponasality):
Mary Morgan's money. (nares open)
Mary Morgan's money. (nares occluded) } same ____ different ____
Neal Neville knows. (nares open)
Neal Neville knows. (nares occluded) } same ____ different ____

C. Observed characteristics of nasal obstruction:
swelling/dark circles under eyes ____ noisy breathing ____ mouth breathing ____
swelling of nasal bridge ____ discharge ____ congestion ____
enlarged tonsils ____ snoring ____ deviated septum ____
Comments: ____________________

D. Prolonged /a/: nasal emission is absent ____ present ____

E. Oral sentences (to check for hypernasality):
She eats sweet peas. (nares open)
She eats sweet peas. (nares occluded) } same ____ different ____
Charley chews potato chips. (nares open)
Charley chews potato chips. (nares occluded) } same ____ different ____

F. Observed characteristics of velopharyngeal inadequacy:
snorts ____ grimaces ____ nares constriction ____ nasal emission ____
palatal deviations ____ distortion of pressure consonants ____
Comments: ____________________

G. Word pairs (vowels in nonnasal vs. nasal contexts):

	Appropriate	*Hypernasal*	*Hyponasal*	*Assimil. nasality on vowels only*
hat/ham	____	____	____	____
pat/mat	____	____	____	____
bat/man	____	____	____	____
towel/town	____	____	____	____
how/now	____	____	____	____
pout/noun	____	____	____	____

H. Oral–nasal balance (during conversation and/or reading):
appropriate ____ hypernasal ____ hyponasal ____ mixed ____
cul-de-sac (muffled) ____

I. Tone focus (when counting):

	Seated near clinician		*Projecting voice across room*	
	Adequate	*Inadequate*	*Adequate*	*Inadequate*
mouth opening	____	____	____	____
lip movement	____	____	____	____
tongue movement (retracted?)	____	____	____	____
supraglottal tension	____	____	____	____

Figure 15–4. Evaluation form: High-Risk Factors.

High-risk factors appear to be present ______ absent ______.

A. **Physical conditions that may be pertinent:**

hearing loss ______ craniofacial anomalies ______ hyperextended jaw ______
allergies ______ deviated septum surgery intubation
frequent upper respiratory infections ______ medications ______ PVCM ______
trauma to face/neck ______ postnasal drip ______ bifid uvula ______
neurological symptoms ______ excessive mucus ______ hormonal problem ______
cerebral palsy ______ mouth breathing ______ developmental delay ______
enlarged tonsils/adenoids ______ GERD ______ atypical tongue carriage ______
learning disability______ anorexia/nervosa ______ premenstrual syndrome ______
dentition/orthodontia ______ dehydration ______
Other: ______
Comments: ______

B. **Abusive practices:**

throat clearing ______ crying ______ excessive talking ______ strained laughing ______
screaming ______ impersonations ______ coughing ______ smoking ______
competing with background noise ______ yodeling ______ grunting ______ bulimia ______
sings along with records/tapes/radio ______ cheering ______
Other: ______
Comments: ______

C. **Factors inherent in lifestyle/environment:**

voice models ______ noisy environment ______ cheerleading ______ sports ______
choir/singing ______ poor sleep/poor eating habits______ dramatics ______ debate ______
stress ______ family communication style ______ air pollution ______
Other: ______
Comments: ______

D. **Interpersonal behaviors:**

talking too much ______ ignoring feedback ______ not seeking feedback ______
ignoring differences between people ______ ignoring differences in situations ______
ignoring needs and interests of others ______ poor self-esteem ______ depression ______
aggressive behavior ______ competing for attention ______ emotional lability ______
Other: ______
Comments: ______

incorporates factors in the student's physical environment that should be modified (e.g., television/music level at home), and that isolates factors that can be addressed through consultation with parents and teachers.

Item D (Figure 15–4) focuses attention on the important area of interpersonal behavior. Self-esteem and relations with others affect vocal effectiveness. Although research does not indicate that students with voice disorders also exhibit interpersonal problems, clinical experience suggests that voice problems may be exacerbated by poor interpersonal skills. It is often necessary for speech–language pathologists to incorporate therapy goals designed to restructure patterns of interpersonal interaction. For example, a student who talks incessantly in a loud voice may be unaware of the effect this behavior has on others and may need to learn to observe others' reactions to communicate more effectively. In addition, the student may need to learn that getting louder is not the most effective way to hold a listener's attention. A therapy goal for such a person might be to use various vocal options (pitch, rate, inflection) to increase communication effectiveness.

Because most public school speech–language pathologists do not have access to sophisticated laboratory equipment, this evaluation system does not require the use of any instrumentation. See chapter 9 for a review of approaches to evaluation using instrumental analyses.

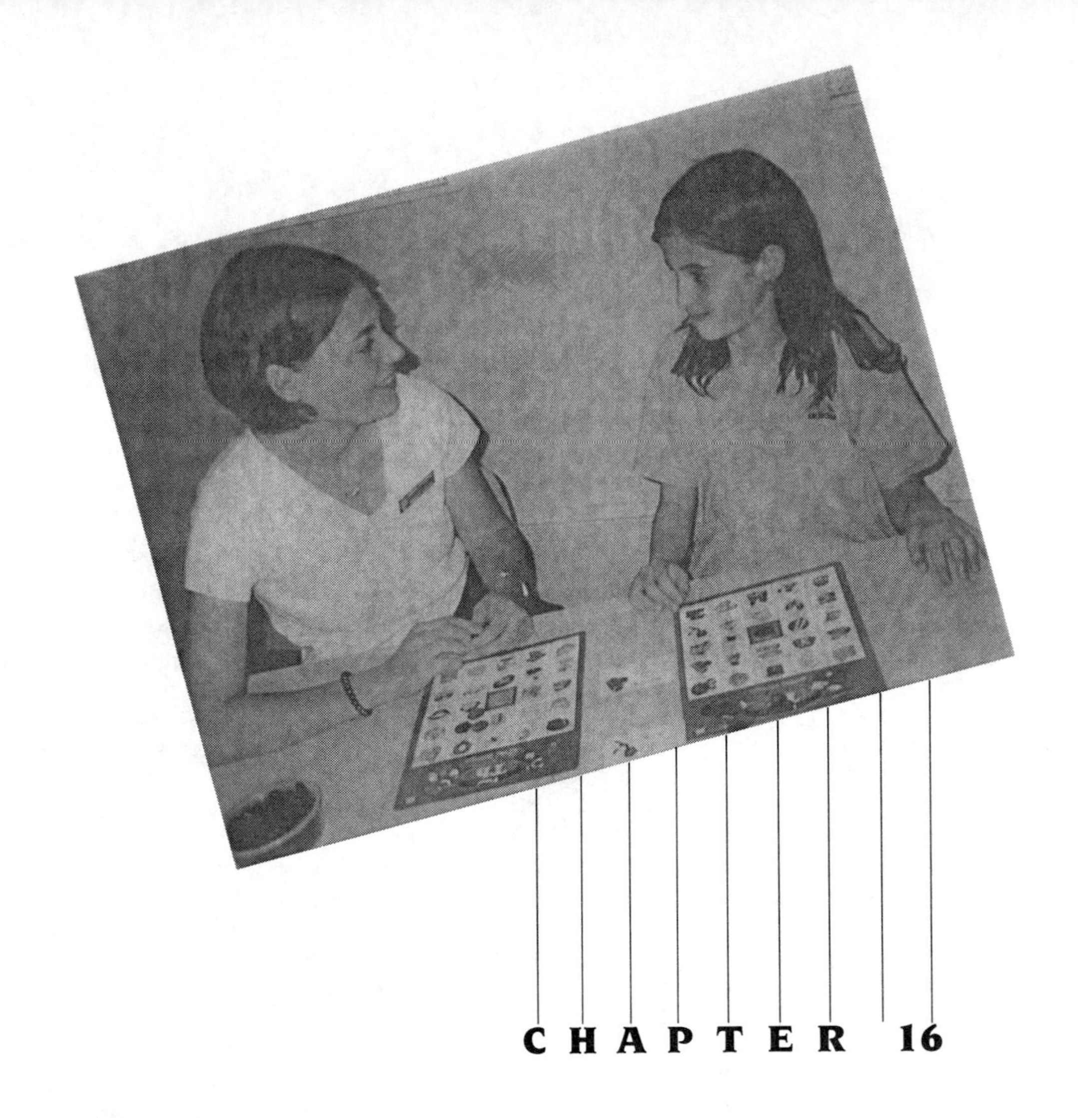

CHAPTER 16

Establishing a Therapeutic Partnership

Voice therapy is a process that begins with the initial meeting and covers a series of stages, including the following:

- growth of the therapeutic relationship
- exploration of the client's concerns and vocal symptoms
- determination of goals
- development of an individualized approach to achieving goals (contract negotiation, when appropriate)
- implementation of an individualized approach to achieving goals
- evaluation of results
- termination and follow-up

Before their initial contact, the speech–language pathologist and the student are usually strangers. They bring vastly different orientations, perspectives, and expectations to their first meeting. Each may have heard about the other by reputation, but neither is likely to know much about the other as an individual. For success to be achieved, they must learn to interact as partners. The quality of the therapeutic partnership is of great significance. It undergirds the predictable stages of the intervention process and is crucial to its outcome. That is not to say that students and clinicians must become close friends. There is a difference between a professional partnership and a personal relationship, and it is usually counterproductive for an adult to try to interact with an adolescent as if they were peers.

It is imperative that a speech–language pathologist be concerned with the adolescent as an individual—that is, as a person rather than as a person with a voice defect. If the speech–language pathologist allows sufficient time at the outset of the intervention process to learn about the student as a whole person (rather than as just a set of disordered symptoms), a useful framework for the intervention program will evolve.

Before a speech–language pathologist and student can develop a shared sense of their mission, they must have a clear definition of their roles. Many students approach voice therapy believing that the speech–language pathologist will "fix" their voice. They may not understand the interactive nature of the therapy process. Speech–language pathologists, on the other hand, may believe that a student should enter the relationship with an understanding of the problem, a commitment to change, and an unconditional trust in the therapist's expertise.

It is important to remember that adolescents enter voice therapy at different levels of readiness. Many students "test" speech–language pathologists to be sure that they can be trusted and have the ability to help. Some students approach voice therapy hoping to hold the speech–language pathologist responsible for its outcome. Students who have been pressured to seek help may be uncomfortable, defensive, or hostile. Their hostility can be expressed openly (as in the case of defiant behavior) or in more subtle ways. Some of the passive ways in which hostility may be expressed are digressions, reticence, substituting another issue for the real issue, pretending to cooperate, joking or avoiding the real issue, and minimizing the problem.

All speech–language pathologists should be sensitive to the inevitable differences between their own and the student's views of roles and expectations in the voice therapy process. A major task in voice therapy is to mesh perceptions and expectations to build a workable partnership.

Equality in an interaction is communicated in many ways, both verbal and nonverbal. Speaking and listening time should be roughly equal, and disagreements should be seen as predictable means of solving problems rather than as power plays. Equality does not mean never challenging another's behavior, but it does mean accepting another's rights. Equal relationships are generally supportive relationships because no one is attempting to win or prove superiority. The way questions are asked is often an indication of the way one person feels about another. Questions asked in a demanding way presume compliance and frequently result in defensive or resentful responses. Consider, for example, how "Have you forgotten to do your assignment again? Why don't you write it down next time?" communicates superiority. The clinician is not presenting a cooperative approach to problem solving, and the questions reflect it.

If a student has had previous experience in a speech or voice therapy program, an exploration of reactions and feelings to what occurred is in order. If the speech–language pathologist is accepting of the student's negative, as well as positive, reactions, this information sharing can enhance their relationship and provide valuable insights for future programming.

A speech–language pathologist may find students reluctant to share information for numerous reasons. Students will feel inhibited if information they divulge can be used against them or if they are criticized or made to feel foolish. Many students are reluctant to divulge information that violates the privacy of events occurring within the family. Adolescents often find it difficult to express painful feelings and may try to repress feelings such as guilt, embarrassment, and anger because these feelings seem less painful if ignored. Feelings that diminish an individual's sense of adequacy are especially threatening to the self-concept. For example, a male adolescent may be reluctant to report information about situations in which his voice was perceived as "unmanly." Divulging such information could come in conflict with the emerging masculinity he is trying so hard to project.

The clinician must listen to the literal meaning of a student's communication and be sensitive to other levels of meaning. Nonverbal communication may provide critical information concerning the student, and frequently, the style of communication is significant. For example, the student who continually challenges content may not merely be debating the issues. Such a student may be signalling objections to the clinician's authoritarian approach. On the other hand, such a student may have a more general problem in relating to adults. Indeed, some teenagers seem to go from the submissiveness of childhood to an aggressive "question authority" mode of operation without ever exploring the value and pleasure of a cooperative, interactive style.

The active listener considers both verbal and nonverbal signals and is sensitive to the underlying as well as literal meanings of messages. When students express disappointments, the sensitive listener responds in ways that accept the validity of their feelings. When a listener uses strategies that acknowledge negative feelings, more open communication follows.

When barriers, such as defensiveness or an unwillingness to trust the clinician, interfere with the growth of the therapeutic relationship, the clinician may adopt an indirect approach. Some clinicians prefer not to "press" too hard, fearing that a defensive client will become more intimidated and less open. If a clinician feels that a student's sense of self is particularly fragile, an indirect approach in which the student's unwillingness to share information is not challenged may be adopted. The clinician may observe the student's indirect refusal to deal with the central problem in behaviors such as evasion of significant issues during discussion, emphasis on peripheral information, or denial of negative feelings. A student who repeatedly states that others are overreacting to the voice problem or who denies concern about a voice problem is exhibiting a lack of readiness to deal with the central problem.

In an indirect approach, the speech–language pathologist focuses attention on general information and allows students to internalize at their own pace. In the direct approach, the speech–language pathologist challenges students in a supportive, nonthreatening manner, to apply specific insights to their own particular situations. For example, "During our discussions I have noticed that you have been saying very little. I know it might be difficult for you, but it would help me to understand how you really feel if you could give me some examples of times when you feel your voice has let you down."

A speech–language pathologist must always be concerned with the development of a trusting relationship when working with the adolescent. A student needs to feel free to talk about personal concerns and feelings in a nonthreatening environment and must be aware that confidences will not be betrayed. Rogers (1961) and Truax and Carkhuff (1967) stated that empathy, genuineness, and positive regard on the part of a counselor helps to facilitate a sense of trust and open communication.

Encouraging Self-Disclosure and Participation

Self-disclosure helps adolescents gain a new sense of themselves and a deeper understanding of their own behavior. Self-acceptance is difficult without self-disclosure. Frequently, it is not the clinician who identifies salient issues, but students who see new aspects of their behavior. The following guidelines can help a speech–language pathologist encourage self-disclosure:

- Be an effective and active listener (give verbal and nonverbal responses).
- Listen for different levels of meaning.
- Listen with empathy.
- Listen with an open mind.
- Paraphrase the student to check understanding.
- Express understanding of the student's feelings.
- Ask questions to check understanding and to indicate interest.
- Provide support for the student. (Refrain from evaluations during disclosures, allow the student to set the pace, and signal support through verbal and nonverbal responses.)
- Maintain a climate of trust. (Keep information confidential, reinforce self-disclosing behaviors, show positive attitudes toward the student and the disclosures, maintain appropriate eye contact, don't use disclosed information against a student at a later date.)
- Avoid burdensome reciprocal disclosure. (Lengthy anecdotes from the speech–language pathologist may shift the focus away from the student.)

When a student begins the process of sharing personal information, it is important for the clinician to respond in ways that facilitate the continuation of productive dialogue. Some of the techniques frequently used to achieve this goal include the following:

- Paraphrasing (e.g., "You said you were nervous before speaking to the teacher.")
- Reflecting statements (e.g., "It seems that you are angry that she wanted you to come to voice therapy.")
- Clarifying information (e.g., "Could you tell me more about what you were doing when you lost your voice?")
- Clarifying feelings (e.g., "How do you feel when you anticipate giving a report before the class?")
- Making tentative inferences (e.g., "I have a hunch that it was a very difficult situation for you.")
- Sending "I" messages (e.g., "I am confused. Could you explain it once more?"

The clinician assumes responsibility for not understanding.)
- Affirming (e.g., "You're giving me a good picture of the situation.")

Empathetic probes can clarify the feelings associated with a student's description of events and circumstances. These statements are especially useful when a clinician senses a disparity between what a student is saying and how the student may actually have been feeling. The use of emphathetic probes can provide support for what the student has said as well as further clarify what actual feelings were projected. Such probes should be used cautiously early in therapy, before trust and open communication have been fully developed. It can be intimidating to a student if a clinician seems to be inferring and interpreting too much too soon.

Carkhuff (1969) talked about additive empathy responses of this kind. He defines them as responses that "add significantly to the feeling and meaning of the expressions of the client . . . The counselor responds with accuracy to all of the client's deeper as well as surface feelings" (p. 175). He contrasted these additive empathy responses with interchangeable empathy responses. Interchangeable empathy responses merely capture and reflect back to the client the essential part of the message. We have called Carkhuff's additive empathy responses "empathy probes" because they probe beyond the student's stated message.

Carkhuff (1969) stated that counseling is effective when a client experiences a developmental process of exploration leading to awareness, which leads to new actions. In voice therapy, as a student begins to explore feelings and underlying assumptions, an open relationship with the clinician allows for clarification of vague or confusing issues, the application of different ideas and information, and increased understanding of the motivations for behavior. Through continued examination, the student develops new insights and can decide how to practice new vocal behaviors in a variety of contexts.

The intervention process should proceed to a discussion of specific vocal behaviors only after a speech–language pathologist has become familiar with a student's interests, needs, social interaction, communication style, and aspirations. The clinician projects that the student is interesting as a person by not rushing in and pinpointing problems before understanding the student as a whole. In other words, the intervention process begins with due consideration of the person, not the problem. This assures the student that the clinician has adequate information and does not jump to conclusions or make suggestions without understanding the whole situation.

Too often, an experienced clinician concerned with the most efficient use of time feels compelled to "zero in" on vocal problems, describe them succinctly to the student, and prescribe appropriate strategies for behavior modification. This approach, although time saving, may result in costly long-term consequences. Motivation is rarely encouraged by a clinician telling an adolescent what is wrong and what needs to be done to fix it. An adolescent's self-esteem is not enhanced by adult authority figures presenting ready-made solutions to problems. Rather than applauding the skill of the clinician who diagnoses a voice problem in 10 minutes, an adolescent may react with resentment, feeling that the clinician could not possibly understand the problem in so brief a time. The student may feel threatened and may resist the therapy plan to assert autonomy.

It is difficult for adolescents to become part of something as anxiety provoking as behavioral change. They first need to feel that they are accepted and understood as unique human beings and that they are involved in the change process. Anyone affected by change must "buy into" or "invest" in the project before change can truly be accepted. Rosabeth Kantner (1983), in her book *The Change Masters,* called this stage "tin cupping," that is, giving those most affected by change the opportunity to throw "their two-cents worth" into the cup. The speech–language pathologist gives students this opportunity by allowing them adequate time to describe themselves, their aspirations, and their priorities. Feelings of self-worth are enhanced as students perceive that a clinician values the information they have to offer. Their shared insights can become intrinsic parts of a cooperative approach to problem solving.

Adolescents are frequently difficult to motivate in situations in which they feel adults are forcing change on them. They frequently feel ambivalent about authority figures and may resent being singled out for specialized help. An adolescent may react against a parent or teacher's suggestion that voice therapy will be helpful. Because many teenagers need feelings of independence, extrinsic factors such as parental involvement in a therapy program may detract from the therapy outcome.

Involving students in the decision-making process assures them that a clinician has confidence in their abilities to control and chart their own futures. If some initial success can be achieved, it provides evidence that therapy is, indeed, worthwhile and creates additional momentum and enthusiasm.

Writing a Contract

Because voice therapy with adolescents assumes a level of independence and self-determination on the part of the student, explicit contracts are methods for formalizing mutually agreed-on goals and expectations. Contracts can take various forms as long as they are mutually determined and not forced on a student. It is generally not a good idea to present a preplanned contractual agreement to a student. That is not to say an agreement should not be written, but rather the written format should evolve as a result of interaction between a speech–language pathologist and a student. Negotiations concerning the agreement are then an integral part of the learning process.

It is sometimes helpful, particularly with reticent students, for both the clinician and student to complete a set of open-ended questions independently and then discuss these documents together. At other times, it may be helpful for the student to answer selected questions to increase the clinician's understanding of the student's perspective, expectations, and commitment (Figure 16–1).

Typically, a contract includes not only long-term objectives but also such requirements as attendance, division of responsibility, frequency of contacts with the clinician, and termination criteria. A contract should also include dates for progress reviews and for termination, extension, or revision of the treatment plan, and a list of those who will receive copies of progress reports. It is helpful to add statements concerning the voice therapy approach and format. This is done to maximize a student's investment in the program and to exploit the student's self-knowledge about preferred learning style.

In some middle and high school settings, the contract has been incorporated into the language arts curriculum so that a student in a speech–language pathology program can earn credit toward the language arts requirement. In such cases, requirements for a grade must be stipulated in the contract. Some speech–language pathologists offer an independent studies option in which the clinician serves as a resource teacher and assists the student with self-directed programming. In such cases, a standard school form is generally used. Clinicians interested in this type of programming should work with school administrators to refine or develop procedures consistent with school policy.

Figure 16–1. Student questionnaire.

1. My purpose in therapy is ________________________________.
2. I am prepared to commit the following amount of time each day: ________________________________
________________________________.
3. I am prepared to commit the following amount of time each week: ________________________________
________________________________.
4. I expect this program to last approximately ________________________________.
5. I will discontinue therapy when ________________________________.
6. For my therapy, I feel that being grouped with other students
   ______ is desirable.
   ______ is undesirable.
   ______ is desirable on a limited basis.
7. For my therapy, I feel that working individually with the pathologist is desirable
   ______ on a regular basis.
   ______ on a limited basis.
8. Where homework is concerned I feel that ________________________________.
9. The home assignment(s) I would most enjoy is/are ________________________________.
10. One type of home assignment I do not enjoy is ________________________________.
11. My parents' attitude to my problem is ________________________________.
12. My family should be involved in the following way: ________________________________.
13. Significant others in my life view my problem as ________________________________.
14. My reaction to their help with my therapy program would be ________________________________.
15. When someone makes a recommendation to me I prefer that ________________________________
________________________________.
16. I respond best to criticism when ________________________________.
17. Generally, I absorb new ideas best when ________________________________.
18. When I read a self-help book I am most likely to pay attention to ________________________________
____
________________________________.
19. When I am tested, I prefer ________________________________.
20. To solve problems, I am likely to ________________________________.
21. I prefer therapy to be ______% with the pathologist, ______% with a group of other students, and ______% on my own.
22. When it comes to identifying errors, I prefer to
   ______ check myself.
   ______ have other students help check me.
   ______ have the speech–language pathologist check me.
   ______ have significant others check me.

(continued)

Figure 16–1. *(continued)*

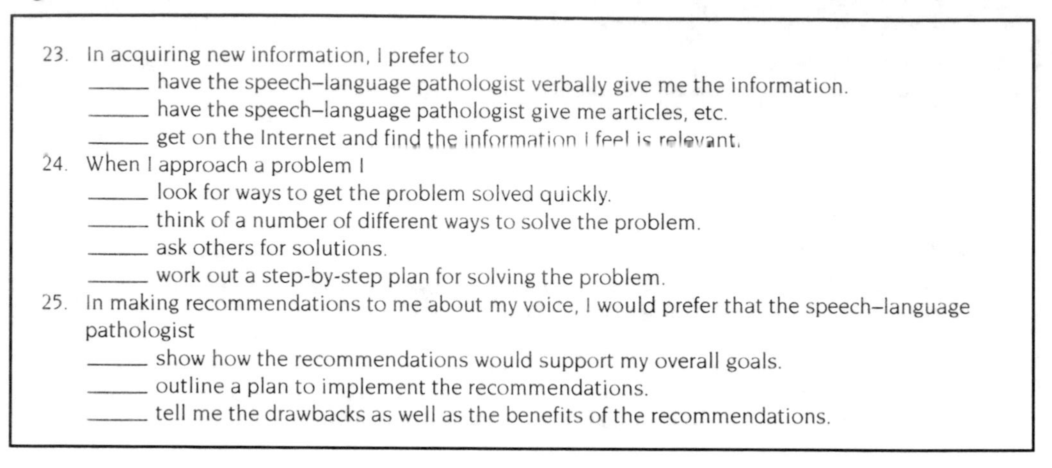

23. In acquiring new information, I prefer to
    _____ have the speech–language pathologist verbally give me the information.
    _____ have the speech–language pathologist give me articles, etc.
    _____ get on the Internet and find the information I feel is relevant.
24. When I approach a problem I
    _____ look for ways to get the problem solved quickly.
    _____ think of a number of different ways to solve the problem.
    _____ ask others for solutions.
    _____ work out a step-by-step plan for solving the problem.
25. In making recommendations to me about my voice, I would prefer that the speech–language pathologist
    _____ show how the recommendations would support my overall goals.
    _____ outline a plan to implement the recommendations.
    _____ tell me the drawbacks as well as the benefits of the recommendations.

Steps in Negotiating a Contract

Identifying Areas for Modification

The clinician and student together decide which of the areas relevant to voice need attention: respiration, phonation, resonance, interpersonal and psychological factors, lifestyle, and high-risk factors. Initially, the results of the diagnostic evaluation are presented in a factual manner by the clinician, who necessarily assumes the leadership role in interpreting assessment data. Because this is observable data and conclusions can be supported by evaluation results, targets usually emerge logically and with mutual acceptance by both parties.

Ordering Targets

Open discussion that results in reciprocal, rather than asymmetrical, input is critical at this stage of contract negotiation. The clinician, who will have professional insights drawn from experience and specialized training, may be predisposed to select a particular hierarchy of targets. Nonetheless, the student's self-knowledge must be allowed equal weight in the negotiation process. The clinician can benefit from thoroughly exploring the student's perceptions and priorities and, in so doing, can encourage the student's participation in the therapy process.

It is imperative that a speech–language pathologist explain each of the targets and what is required in modifying each behavior. This should be done in a way that does not coerce a student to select a predetermined target. The speech–language pathologist should avoid using technical language that might confuse or intimidate a student and should avoid leading the student to "feed back" the clinician's own biases. Because the targets were mutually agreed on in the previous step of contract negotiation, a speech–language pathologist should be comfortable with allowing a student to sequence them.

Matching Targets and Approaches

Concurrent or Sequential

As the clinician and student observe the number and sequence of targets, patterns for attacking the modification process emerge.

Some targets may form the basis for modification of future targets, whereas other targets may lend themselves to a concurrent approach. It is important to negotiate with the student how many targets will be undertaken at one time. Frequently, a student may be motivated to attack a large number of targets. However, if the student's semester schedule is heavy, as in seasonal sports participation, it may be judicious to contract the heavy commitment for the following semester and limit targets for the present semester. Frustration and failure may be inevitable for the student who is allowed to contract an unrealistic number of goals.

Acquisition of Facts and Information

At this stage of contract negotiations, the clinician presents a list of resources and techniques available for acquiring information, and the student selects those that are most appealing (Table 16–1). For example, some students may prefer approaches that require little interpersonal communication (e.g., Internet searches, computer projects), whereas others may enjoy approaches that require more interaction (e.g., discussions, interviews, observations). Of course, interpersonal interaction will be a prime ingredient of later voice therapy stages, but at this stage, allowing a student to express preferences builds momentum by enhancing early learning.

Table 16–1 contains a list of resources and techniques that could be used by a student as a preferential checklist. It may be necessary for the speech–language pathologist to describe the application of some of these resources so that a student can make informed choices.

Format for Implementation

Special problems arise with scheduling at the secondary school level. Students at the middle and high school levels usually have inflexible schedules. Homer (2000) provided a variety of creative scheduling suggestions, including consideration of regularly scheduled speech–language classes as part of the academic curriculum, and advises clinicians to be creative and flexible with students and teachers.

Van Hattum (1969) stated that scheduling at the middle and high school levels is usually best accomplished on a two-visits-per-week basis. Battle and Van Hattum (1982) noted that problems with scheduling during the school day included students' unwillingness to miss classes. Frequently, the length of a voice therapy session does not coincide with the length of an academic class. Neidecker (1980) said, "High school students who may be able to assume more responsibility for themselves may need only one 1-hour-session per week" (p. 119). Little research has been conducted concerning the effect of scheduling in the secondary schools, however.

The American Speech–Language Hearing Association Task Force report (Jones, Austin, MacLean, & Warkomski, 1973) suggested that when there are severe scheduling conflicts, intensive services can be provided during the

Table 16–1. Resources and techniques for acquiring information.

• readings	• library searches	• projects
• models (e.g., larynx)	• Internet	• discussions
• observations	• group reports	• presentations
• tapes or films	• experiments	• field trips
• interviews	• lectures	

summer. Offering services in the late afternoons, evenings, or on Saturdays has also been suggested (O'Toole & Zaslow, 1969). For instance, some school corporations have included extended-hour services for secondary school students. Such programming may involve speech–language pathologists' work days being rearranged to include four 10-hour-days rather than five 8-hour-days. Speech–language pathologists may need to work with school administrators to develop flexible scheduling alternatives to traditional models.

Discussing available time and scheduling preferences with a student is usually valuable. For example, some students prefer intensive, short-term commitments. An all-day workshop, perhaps held on a Saturday or on an in-service day, combined with periodic follow-up, may be an appropriate format to adopt. Other adaptations include brown-bag lunch meetings once a week, evening tutorials, or after-school scheduling.

When therapy is conducted after school hours, the speech–language pathologist will need to negotiate the issue of "comp time" with school administrators. Of course, the speech–language pathologist working at the secondary school level should discuss the feasibility of adopting alternative scheduling models with school administrators before suggesting such variations to a student.

When voice therapy is conducted during the academic day, there are variations that can make the scheduling more meaningful for the adolescent. McKinley and Lord-Larson (1985) strongly advocated the use of course credit, because students invest at least as much time and energy in communication retraining as they do in other courses. A contract may provide useful documentation if a school system elects to offer an academic grade and course credit upon successful competition of the contract. The voluntary nature of this system often seems to contribute to its success.

Another option for scheduling is to provide voice modification or professional voice training as an elective at the beginning of a school semester. Such a system involves considerable planning on the part of the speech–language pathologist. In-service training for school guidance counselors and advisors is particularly important because they may be helpful in identifying students who might profit from a speech–language elective. This format is similar to a delivery of service model presented by Albritton (1984), who described the development of middle school language classes that were alternatives to the traditional "pull out of class" method of scheduling speech–language therapy.

It is especially important for a student to participate in setting up attendance criteria so that the expectations concerning attendance are explicitly stated and mutually agreed on. The contract might include a specific number of sessions or hours of programming. In such cases, absences would extend the duration of therapy so that the total number of sessions or hours would be completed. To avoid infrequent attendance, a percentage attendance criterion could be set in advance. Failure to achieve criterion (without adequate excuse) would result in termination or renegotiation of the contract.

Designing the implementation format involves a great deal of flexibility and creativity on the part of the student and speech–language pathologist. Areas that should be addressed include frequency and length of contacts with the speech–language pathologist, type of contact (e.g., individual therapy, group therapy, consultation, and monitoring), course credit or noncredit, setting for therapy meetings, and attendance criteria.

Establishing Methods for Monitoring and Evaluating Progress

It is beneficial for students to realize the importance of monitoring vocal behaviors on a continuing basis and to understand milestones that indicate progress. The process of selecting evaluation procedures helps students gain a realistic perspective of what lies ahead. Discussions of these procedures also helps a clinician understand more about a student's personal style. Nonetheless, a clinician should encourage students to try as many ways of monitoring and evaluating as possible. Some of the strategies that can provide feedback to students include tapes, videos, logs, diaries, checklists, graphs, percentages, reports from other sources, and oral self-reports. Although continual monitoring and evaluation are integral parts of the voice therapy process, scheduled documentation of progress can focus both the clinician and student on what has been accomplished and what tasks still lie ahead.

The reader is referred to Brodnitz's (1963) categories for determining the outcome of vocal rehabilitation, Boone's (1974) five dismissal criteria for voice patients, and Cooper's (1977) criteria for completing voice therapy. Cooper suggested using the laryngologist's report on visual impressions, the student and pathologist's evaluation of auditory characteristics, and the student's own sensory judgments. Depending on the lifestyle and aspirations of the individual, the standard for dismissal may not be complete rehabilitation. For instance, one student may be satisfied if most undesirable features (both attitudinal and behavioral) have been eliminated. Another student who has a high investment in vocal performance (e.g., drama or choir) may strive for higher levels of proficiency.

A time limit for voice therapy can increase the efficient use of both the student and clinician's time and allay the fears of students who feel that enrollment in therapy is a "life sentence." Berryman (1986) stated that voice therapy is typically of shorter duration than therapy for other speech–language problems. She noted that the time needed to change one vocal parameter is roughly equivalent to the time needed to change one speech sound. Voice therapy can proceed rapidly with a highly motivated adolescent because much can be accomplished by the student independently. Nonetheless, some students require a great deal of help with attitudinal and behavioral modification of vocal symptoms.

We have found that approximately 15 hours is a realistic amount of intervention time for an initial contract. This timeline prevents a student from thinking that change can occur without effort and allows sufficient time for in-depth programming. The contract can be renegotiated after 15 hours for complicated problems. In the case of less complicated vocal problems, dismissal before the contracted time results in positive attitudes toward the speech–language program. Andrews (2000) provides methods for measuring outcomes of therapy and determining the criteria for dismissal.

The final phase of contract negotiation is determining the method for follow-up after direct intervention ceases. An advantage of discussing maintenance procedures is that a student gains a realistic understanding of the various stages of the rehabilitation process and an understanding that responsibilities continue, although in different form, after an acceptable level of proficiency has been reached. Techniques for follow-up and the dates and frequency of posttherapy checks should be addressed during this phase. Follow-up techniques include the clinician's evaluation of spontaneous speech (face-to-face, tape recordings, telephone calls), the student's self-evaluation, voice evaluation by peers and significant adults (casual or structured), and progress notes, E-mails, and checklists from the student and from teachers, parents, and peers. (Peers who have been part of the student's therapy group provide especially good trained listeners.)

It should be remembered that behavioral changes of any kind are difficult to achieve. An individual's readiness to change is related to self-concept, to knowledge about what is involved, and to scheduling demands. Sometimes a clinician expects all students with voice problems to enroll in voice therapy and follow through until their problems are solved. A clinician must be flexible enough to alter expectations according to a student's input, however. Rather than being frustrated by a limitation imposed by the client, a clinician should be challenged to focus on achievable goals. It is important to realize that the process of self-knowledge can continue even during times when there is no direct intervention. A short therapy segment may be a springboard for increased determination and commitment. Dismissal does not always have to be tied to total rehabilitation.

The therapeutic relationship may be marked by periods of intense interaction interspersed with periods during which a student deals with problems independently. This type of model can foster independence and self-growth and can enhance a student's motivation. It cannot be assumed that a student who "drops out" for a while is unmotivated. The priorities of a speech–language pathologist and an adolescent may not coincide in the short run but may converge in the long run. The ability to adapt to changing needs and lifestyle demands can be demonstrated by a willingness to accept the student's right to self-determination.

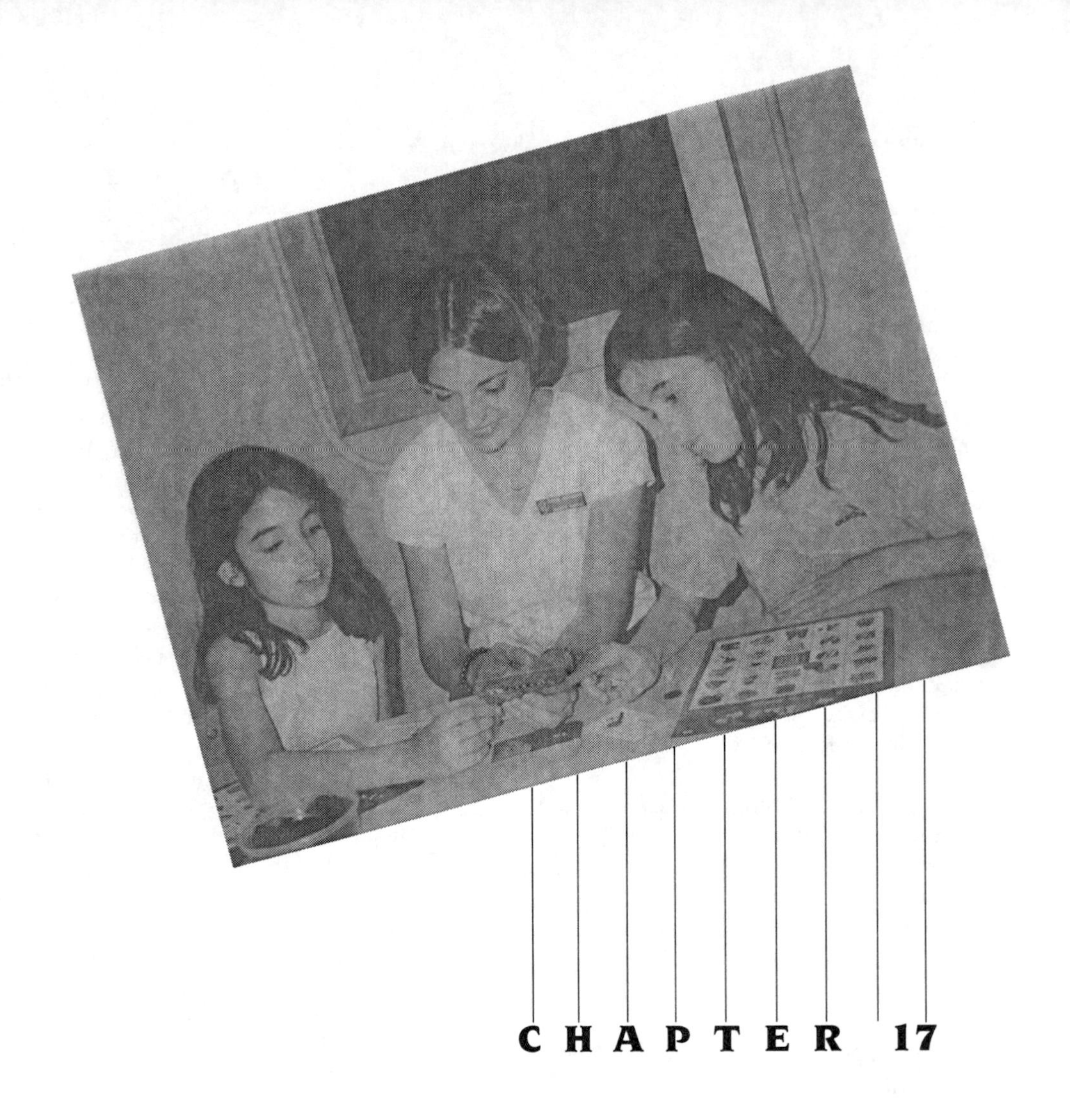

CHAPTER 17

The Therapeutic Process

In voice therapy, long-term goals (the expected outcome) and short-term goals (the prerequisite steps leading to the long-term goal) are usually written in behavioral terms. Nonetheless, the establishment of a trusting therapeutic relationship is the foundation on which modification of vocal behavior is built, even though it cannot be defined precisely in behavioral terms.

Establishing a trusting relationship with an adolescent is sometimes a challenging task. Students are frequently uneasy with authority figures or adults who they think may seek to change their behavior. Frequently, an adolescent may come to voice therapy with negative expectations or feelings that seem to put the speech–language pathologist at an immediate disadvantage. To dispel these preconceived mental sets, the speech–language pathologist must consider factors that contribute to the development of a warm, trusting relationship. Many of these factors are, of course, relevant to all relationships; others have particular significance to working with adolescents.

Personal Adjustments by the Clinician

The clinician working with adolescents must make conscious personal adjustments in attitudes (communicated both verbally and nonverbally), in the environment, and in the choice of materials. Attitudes toward the teenager can be conveyed through the use of posture, eye contact, intonation patterns, and vocabulary. Assuming a relaxed attitude that promotes a nonauthoritarian, friendly climate (such as placing both the clinician and student's chairs on the same side of a table) is usually helpful. Direct eye contact and a balance of clinician–student talking and listening times can promote an atmosphere of equality. It is sometimes difficult for a speech–language pathologist who has been working with young children to switch to more adult patterns. It is degrading, however, for a young adult to hear exaggerated intonation patterns, such as are frequently used with young children. The use of plural pronouns, such as, "Now what did we do for homework this week?" and the excessive use of "should" statements ("You should do this or that") are also perceived negatively by older students. Because of their greater cognitive skills, adolescents can understand advanced terminology and explanations. Because the adolescent is sensitive to immature approaches, the speech–language pathologist should allow a student to take a leadership role (e.g., record keeping, note taking) whenever possible.

The room in which voice therapy takes place should reflect the age and interests of the adolescent. If the room is used by a large number of students of different ages, it is important to have a corner that reflects more adult interests and is equipped with adult-sized furniture and decorations. Even the use of large-ruled lined paper such as that used in elementary school for note taking should be avoided.

Clinicians often try to adapt materials used with elementary children for use with middle and high school students. Experience suggests this is usually obvious to the older student, however. Designing new materials specific to the adolescent population can avoid inadvertently insulting the teenager's emerging sense of maturity. The extra effort required is more than offset by the stimulation that results from working on a higher cognitive and experiential level. For example, the higher reading levels of adolescent students make it possible to utilize a wider range of reading materials. Adolescents also possess the skills necessary to share responsibility in identifying available resources and using electronic equipment.

Advances in technology have made many pieces of electronic equipment readily available and within the budgets of both students and school system. Daily logs and record keeping are efficiently handled on computers. Graphics software is available to expedite the presentation of data, and students can use "Walkmans" to listen to voice therapy homework assignment tapes at their convenience. Adapting the classroom environment and materials to the adolescent can increase the student's motivation, the clinician's stimulation, and the sharing, creative atmosphere of the therapeutic interaction.

It might be helpful to remember some of the major differences between working with elementary-aged children and the adolescent population. Some of these differences are outlined in Table 17–1. Clinical experience suggests that the amount of voice therapy time devoted to behavior modification tasks is greater with younger children, whereas insight development requires a greater percentage of time with adolescents. Ideally, adolescent students assume greater responsibility for rehabilitation progress than younger children do. A therapy sequence designed for use with adolescents appears in Table 17–2.

Personal Adjustments by the Adolescent

Therapy with the adolescent requires a meshing of goals related to both skill acquisition and self-actualization. The process of self-actualization during adolescence includes goals such as

- Accepting responsibility for changing vocal behavior
- Understanding self in relation to authority figures, family, peers, institutions, and social groups
- Understanding the effect of emotions on the reactions of self and others
- Improving decision-making skills by recognizing and evaluating options and resources and by projecting short- and long-term consequences of decisions
- Refining and enhancing self-esteem by developing confidence through responsible problem solving

When adolescents habituate vocal behaviors that are self-defeating and counterproductive, they need to understand not only the situations and events that trigger negative behaviors but also their own cognitive coding. For example, Mary was so anxious in large group situations that she found it impossible to initiate conversations and spoke inaudibly when others approached her. She needed to understand her belief that others would not be interested in listening to her. Rather than telling herself that she had nothing to offer that was of interest to others, she had to learn to foster more positive internal statements concerning her own worth. Her sequence of insights proceeded in the following way:

1. Identify self-defeating behaviors and the situations in which they occur
2. Recognize erroneous assumptions and negative internal statements about self in high-risk situations
3. Understand how negative beliefs lead to self-defeating behaviors
4. Develop more positive assumptions
5. Practice (through trial, error, and analysis) new vocal behaviors consistent with positive assumptions concerning self
6. Practice conversational strategies for focusing attention on the interests and needs of others

Some students need guidance to understand that feelings may be suppressed and that even suppressed feelings can affect vocal behavior. They can then understand

Table 17–1. How voice therapy with adolescents is different from voice therapy with younger children.

Children	*Adolescents*
Wants to please teacher	Complicated, ambivalent feelings about authority figures
Influenced by parental support of therapy program	Wants independence from parents in therapy program
Extrinsic reinforcement usually effective (stickers, tokens, praise, treats)	Intrinsic reinforcement usually effective (individualized with reference to self-image, peer interactions, lifestyle activities)
Definition of goals: Major contributors: clinician, parents, teacher Minor contributor: student	Definition of goals: Major contributors: student, clinician Minor contributors: school personnel, parents
Homework assignments structured (speech books), tangible (worksheets); parents and teachers frequently involved.	Homework assignments relevant to a variety of situations, activities. Occasional involvement of school personnel, infrequent parental involvement
Group therapy frequently provides competition, reinforcements, stimulated discussion; clinician assumes major leadership role	Individual therapy provides effective format for counseling, contracting; group therapy provides important peer support, clinician assumes indirect leadership role
Referral to voice program: clinician, parent, classroom teacher, physician	Referral to voice program: counselors, advisors, nurse, physician, self-referrals
Scheduling: students seen as frequently as possible in relatively short sessions	Scheduling: students seen less frequently but for longer sessions; intensive sessions and independent work supplementary
Self-awareness and self-monitoring must be taught; reactions of others must be specifically defined	Self-consciousness and awareness of peer group provide framework for discussion and analysis
Concepts basic to voice program require significant therapy time	Concepts basic to voice program require less time because of higher cognitive level.*
Materials generally concrete, action-oriented, visually appealing	Complexity and scope of materials reflect social and cognitive development, age
Balance between counseling and skill development: major amount of time spent practicing skills	Balance between counseling and skill development: major amount of time spent in counseling or on insight producing tasks that are immediately applicable to situations, lifestyle

*Applies to children without developmental disabilities.

that awareness of feelings helps to gain control over them and that such control can enable a person to modify vocal behavior.

Self-examination (understanding of the student's attitudes toward and reactions to significant others) and situational and con-

Table 17–2. A sample therapy sequence for adolescents.

Developing the student's internal motivation
A. Elicit information about the student
B. Identify aspects of lifestyle where communication is important
C. Identify positive or satisfying aspects of current communication behavior

Defining the problem
A. Identify situations where vocal behavior has not met expectations
B. Review vocal behavior in terms of current needs and future goals
C. Review vocal behavior in terms of reactions of others (family, friends, teachers)
D. Target aspects of vocal behavior that student would or would not like to change
E. Interpret diagnostic results
F. Describe intervention options

Negotiating the contract (where applicable)

Analyzing the problem
A. Student acquires knowledge
   1. Scientific principles: normal vocal production, student's vocal production
   2. Interpersonal communication styles: general principles, analysis of others, self-analysis
   3. Lifestyle factors: general principles, self-analysis
B. Student demonstrates knowledge
   1. Describes vocal symptoms accurately
   2. Describes physiologic factors affecting voice
   3. Describes psychosocial factors affecting voice

Defining characteristics of new and old behaviors
A. Explain when, how, and why inappropriate behaviors are used
B. Determine ways to avoid or change inappropriate behaviors
C. Determine alternative strategies to substitute for inappropriate behaviors

Producing short utterances with facilitating techniques
A. Produces target behavior in isolation
   1. Instruction, cues, model
   2. Instruction, cues
   3. Instruction
B. Prolongs or repeats target behavior
C. Stops or starts target behavior at will
D. Demonstrates both appropriate and inappropriate behaviors
E. Produces target behavior, varying length of utterance
   1. Isolated sounds
   2. Syllables
   3. Words: lists, sentence completions, fill in the blanks, structured repertoire of responses, associations, responses to questions, word-generating activities
   4. Phrases: lists, salutations, expansion with adjectives and adverbs, rhymes, phrase completions, rewording (e.g., negatives, opposites)
F. Monitors and self-corrects each target level with accuracy
   1. Clinician identifies correct or incorrect production
   2. Clinician and student discuss characteristics of correct or incorrect production
   3. Student identifies specific techniques and cues that facilitate correct target production

(continued)

Table 17–2. (*continued*)

4. Student analyzes why and how these techniques and cues facilitate correct production
5. Clinician and student devise data-keeping methods to determine accuracy

Producing Long Utterances of Increasing Complexity

A. Written text materials
 1. Sentences
 2. Paragraphs: limericks/jokes, verses/poetry, personally relevant materials, narrations/characterizations, dramatic readings

B. Visually cued materials: sentences generated from pictures, sentence clusters generated from picture sequences

C. Verbally cued materials: definitions, story completions, paraphrases/summaries, supporting evidence, refutations, role-playing

D. Self-generated materials: jokes, anecdotes, moral dilemmas, minidebates, improvisations, extemporaneous speeches, recaps (sporting, social events), reviews/critiques (books, performances)

E. Monitors and self-corrects each target level (with standards)
 1. Clinician and student devise performance standards
 2. Clinician and student devise sampling techniques; percentage of session to analyze, tapes/videos/peers, interruption vs. post hoc analysis, independent vs. joint analysis of responses
 3. Clinician and student analyze effect of length and context on performance
 4. Clinician and student devise preparatory sets and cues to facilitate correct production
 5. Clinician devises method for checking reliability of student's monitoring skills
 6. Clinician and student devise short-term and long-term record keeping systems

Habituation

A. Identify situations in student's everyday life that student would like to target (e.g., academic, social, recreational, family)

B. Design a sequence of rehearsal and practice activities analogous to those encountered in student's everyday life

C. Role-play simulated situations in voice therapy room

D. Analyze factors impeding appropriate vocal behavior: emotional/physical state, size/type of group, location, background noise, time of day

E. Role-play difficult situations with distractions present: visual, auditory, physical/motor, social/emotional

F. Student uses appropriate behaviors in selected situations for short durations (outside therapy)

G. Student records and analyzes performance: anecdotal records, checklists, logs, charts

H. Student uses appropriate behaviors in complex situations for extended periods of time

I. Evaluate student's general performance level

J. Compare student's behavioral and attitudinal progress in terms of established timelines for treatment

K. Confer with student on progress and revise, renegotiate, or project dismissal accordingly

L. Identify techniques for maintenance of correct behaviors: coping strategies, self-reinforcements, insights, acceptance of help from supportive others, recognition of secondary gains

M. Student uses appropriate behaviors in nontargeted situations

N. Student monitors and adjusts behavior without support from others

textual awareness (understanding surrounding circumstances and reinforcing events that support present behaviors) provide the tools to monitor behavior.

Sometimes insights emerge gradually and at other times they are discovered suddenly. Insights that are most relevant to vocal behavior are those related to how one views oneself, how one is viewed by others, feelings experienced on occasions when vocal anxieties are highest, and how interpersonal behavioral patterns conform to expectations of self and others.

Factors Related to Successful Intervention

Neal's (1986) discussion of motivation and attendance underscores the clinical impression that these related factors seem to be of equal importance to the success of intervention with adolescents. Boone (1977) noted the advantage of working with self-referred adolescents, and Neidecker (1980) reported that vocational choice may provide incentives to change communication patterns. Goda (1970) referred to the social needs and interests of adolescents and commented that they seemed more likely to be self-motivated than younger students. It may be that increased maturity provides the perceptual and cognitive skills to analyze cause-and-effect relationships appropriately. Greater involvement in dating and social activities may also lead the adolescent to conclude that changes in vocal behavior will have a positive effect on social relationships.

Neal (1976) and Bradford, Hosea, and Neal (1977) identified the factors most important for intervention success at the secondary level as (a) consistent student attendance, (b) a student's motivation for self-improvement, and (c) a student's opinions of other people's attitudes toward the communication problem. Neal also discussed the decreasing role of parents and classroom teachers in therapy as a child grows older. He indicated, however, that their attitudes continue to influence the intervention process.

As children enter adolescence, the adult's perception of the student must change dramatically. This is fundamental both to the adult's understanding of the voice therapy program and to the roles the adult and student are assigned in the process. The speech–language pathologist's philosophy concerning intervention, the teacher's philosophy of education, and the parent's definition of the parent-child relationship must be markedly different with the teenage population than with younger children. The adolescent is in a stage of transition. The process of becoming an independent, responsible adult requires that the roles of authority figures be radically redefined. That is not to say that adult roles become less important, but that they are different.

According to Neal (1976), next to correction of a speech-language problem, the most frequently stated reason for dismissal from voice therapy is lack of motivation. Speech–language pathologists may wonder if poor motivation is sometimes the result of inappropriately designed therapy programs. The student's perception of the attitudes of others was ranked third in importance on Neal's survey and is highly relevant to both motivation and attendance. Fear or embarrassment at being singled out for help may trigger avoidance reactions, which include denial that a problem exists, rejection of the possibility that voice therapy could be helpful, and rebellion against suggestions that services be sought. School personnel and parents need to be aware of the way their actions and suggestions can communicate their attitudes toward a student and the use of resources. Well-meaning adults sometimes confront adolescents with statements such as, "I notice you've got something wrong with your voice. You should go see the speech–language pathologist to help you with your problem." This choice of language communicates negative feelings that will probably elicit embarrassment and defensiveness. It may be more advantageous to emphasize a student's own problem-solving abilities with statements such as, "What are your thoughts about taking advantage of some of the resources we have available here at school? For example, did you know we have a speech–language pathologist who knows a lot about voice? You might want to explore that opportunity."

Clinician–Student Interaction

A clinician's attitude toward a student is revealed through body language, such as posture, gesture, and eye contact, and through metalinguistic aspects, such as tone of voice, loudness level, and inflection. It may seem trite to say that if a clinician is relaxed, warm, and accepting, a student will be more at ease. Nonetheless, the ways in which a clinician attends, listens, encourages, and focuses on information can be critical to the success of voice therapy.

Attending behaviors encourage a student to verbalize ideas and feelings. Active listening has a strong reinforcing effect. It is often helpful if a clinician refrains from adding to the student's meaning. Confirming comments, such as "I can understand what you went through" or "That seems a helpful insight" may allow the student to explore further and to feel a sense of increased responsibility.

If, however, a student rambles or digresses, selective inattention may be a useful technique to return the student to a more productive track. Selective inattention strategies are usually nonverbal signs. For example, a student who is telling stories, when the clinician feels it may be more productive to discuss how the student feels now, may observe that the clinician seems attentive when the discussion is about feelings and seems inattentive when the discussion is about past events. Inattentive behaviors may include looking at the clock or looking out the window.

Verbal strategies that help a clinician guide productive verbalization include paraphrasing, clarifying, and perception-checking. Paraphrasing is used to test the clinician's perception of what has been said. Generally, the clinician rephrases and summarizes the student's message when there is a natural break in the conversation. When paraphrasing is used successfully, the student usually provides a confirming response or other cue indicating that the clinician's understanding is accurate.

If a message has been confusing, the speech–language pathologist may seek clarification by probing (e.g., "I'm not sure I understand. Can you tell me more?"). These remarks should be phrased to elicit clearer statements from a student without implying that the student is confused. It is important that the speech–language pathologist refrain from interpreting or explaining. Requests for illustrations or repetition are the best ways of clarifying the student's ideas and feelings.

Similarly, asking for feedback from a student is a technique used to check the accuracy of the clinician's listening skills. The technique of "perception-checking" involves both the giving and receiving of information concerning the accuracy of a perception. For example, statements such as "I want you to tell me if I'm understanding exactly what you mean" can lead into a paraphrase of what the clinician thinks the student has said. This allows the student to correct the clinician and suggests confidence in the student's abilities.

A clinician should be sensitive to a student's readiness to accept feedback; frequent unsolicited opinions may cause resistance, resentment, or denial. Feedback should not consist of personal judgments and should focus on behavior and issues an adolescent is capable of changing. Feedback should be a prompt response to specific behavior and should be given in small amounts so that attention can be fully focused on manageable items.

Developing skills to encourage a student to respond openly is important for clinicians working with adolescents. These skills are frequently referred to as "leading" and require anticipating the direction of a student's thoughts and responding with encouraging statements. The goals of leading are to help a student explore and elaborate on statements, to explore a variety of options and freely discuss alternatives, and to encourage a student to be involved in and maintain responsibility for decisions.

Indirect comments such as "Tell me why you are here" or "What do you think this means?" encourage a student to elaborate. Pauses or "expectant looks" can also serve as indirect leads. A speech–language pathologist should always have a clear purpose for a lead, make the lead general, and pause long enough for a student to respond.

A clinician tries to focus a discussion with direct leads. Statements such as "Can you give me an example of what happens to cause you to feel that way?" or "Tell me some more about how your friend reacted to your new voice" generally help a student to elaborate. A clinician can also help focus a discussion with leads such as "What word or words can best describe what you've been telling me?" and "What were your feelings as we talked?" It is important that a clinician clearly verbalize a lead.

Most leads are in question form, and it is important that they be open ended so that they cannot be answered merely with "yes" or "no" responses. Generally, questions beginning with "how," "what," or "why" will result in more elaborated responses.

"Reflecting" lets a student know that the clinician is perceiving an issue from the student's viewpoint. Successful reflecting requires identifying a student's feelings, reading nonverbal body language for implied feelings, and paraphrasing a student's message. The clinician should use language appropriate to the student's intellectual level and cultural experiences. Guard against using the same opening leads and include nonverbal responses, such as head-nodding, that can prevent segmenting a discussion with too many verbal responses.

When summarizing an interview, a clinician should leave the student with the feeling that progress has been made. The clinician may decide to state the summary or may ask the student to provide a summary. It is important that no new ideas or information be introduced during a summary so that an interview does not end with unexplored topics. Summarizing can also be used at the beginning of a therapy session, when a summary of the previous session can provide continuity for the new session.

Clinicians must understand their own emotional reactions during therapy sessions. They must decide if their responses are related to their own personal experiences or to what a student is saying. They must then decide if sharing their feelings with the student would be productive to the goals of the session.

Speech–language pathologists should be aware that they will not be capable of working with all of the issues or feelings that can surface during voice therapy sessions. Students may need to be referred to other specialists. Caution should be used in exploring the feelings of students who have personality problems, who are under pressure, or who have difficulty dealing with emotions. Speech–language pathologists may want to avoid emotional issues if they doubt their abilities to deal with such issues, if support services are inadequate or time is limited, or if the school or a student's parents discourage the exploration of feelings.

Recognition of Students' Learning Styles

An analysis of learning styles serves as a reminder that people think and learn in different ways. Content will make more sense to a student if it is presented in a manner consistent with the student's preferred style of learning. Speech–language pathologists who have thought about their own preferred learning styles are less likely to impose those styles on adolescents.

Bramson and Bramson (1985) proposed five categories of learning styles: synthetic, idealistic, pragmatic, analytic, and realistic. Their research showed that only about 15% of people use the five styles equally, 50% have a single preferred style, and the remaining 35% use a combination of styles. It is sometimes helpful for students to learn about differences in learning styles so that they can apply the information to themselves. See Appendix D for a sample worksheet.

Some students need to think and talk a great deal about different ways of solving problems. Bramson and Bramson (1985) would describe such individuals as "synthesist thinkers." It is ideas that make a difference to these students, not facts. In working with the synthesist, the speech–language pathologist should assume the role of the practical person without detracting from the student's enthusiasm and should remember that the synthesist sees arguments as fun, not as confrontations. The synthesist will probably enjoy the process of contrasting different treatment ideas. Although the speech–language pathologist may feel a need to encourage the synthesist to target concrete solutions, allowing the student time to develop insights may result in a greater commitment to the treatment program.

Idealists, on the other hand, are usually concerned with goals, ethics, and mutually agreed-on views. They enjoy focusing on similarities, pursuing agreement, and identifying with explanations involving what is good for them and others. These students would probably enjoy reading about links between nutrition and physical well-being, the effects of drugs on the mind and body, and the physiology of a well-functioning system. They may be ideal candidates for clear-cut definitions of behaviorial objectives linked to their overall vocational and educational goals. Because idealists often feel guilty about their imperfections, the speech–language pathologist should ensure that short-term rewards for gains are present as well as long-term rewards. Sufficient praise and careful documentation of progress can offset discouragement when larger goals are not met rapidly. An idealist can become so committed to the goals of good vocal hygiene that this commitment can be used as a positive force in peer support situations.

Pragmatists are concerned with getting things started immediately and not worrying too much about long-term planning. They are resourceful, innovative, and adaptable. Nonetheless, enthusiasm sometimes lags if a project takes very long. Pragmatists can easily understand that their voices can be changed and will be eager to get started, but they may not want to waste time discussing a detailed treatment approach. The speech–language pathologist should capitalize on the pragmatist's enthusiasm for moving ahead by providing action-oriented assignments immediately, demonstrating flexibility, and reinforcing the student's action, energy, and commitment. Growth may occur best in an experience-based format rather than one focusing on theoretical insight. The speech–language pathologist should maintain a clear focus on a single goal so that a student does not undertake more than can be accomplished successfully. Demonstrations of success, summaries of progress, and the relevance of present tasks to the next step in the sequence will help maintain the student's momentum. Role playing is an excellent strategy for this type of student, and motivation is highly correlated to the immediate demands of the student's lifestyle.

Analysts are concrete thinkers who give little weight to feelings. They believe in solving problems by patiently gathering data and carefully searching for the right solutions. They are concerned with thoroughness and accuracy and may seem obsessive about small details. A speech–language pathologist should be prepared to commit a significant amount of time to analyzing such a student's voice, discussing various remediation theories, providing additional readings, and developing a hierarchical sequence of goals. Praise from the speech–language pathologist may seem irrelevant to these students because reinforcement comes from grappling with issues. The speech–language pathologist should provide the analyst with information, careful referencing, and a variety of theoretical perspectives and should allow the student to assume a major role in organizing materials, summarizing information, and structuring the hierarchy of therapy goals. The evolution of a carefully orchestrated therapy program is rewarding in itself for the analyst. An analytical student may seem threatening to an inexperienced clinician, but exploiting the analyst's need for systemization can help the clinician work with these students.

Realists are most concerned about whether recommendations can be accomplished. They want to know, for example, how the voice can be changed and what recommendations can be implemented. They do not relate to fanciful or theoretical explanations or to too much detail, preferring facts, concrete examples of specific situations, and straightforward summaries. Such students distrust compromise, like to see their objectives clearly, and become impatient with soul searching and analysis. The speech–language pathologist will need to be assertive because realists have little respect for those they consider "soft," idealistic, or lacking in follow through. Realists are goal oriented, so expected results should be spelled out concisely and unequivocally. The realist is an excellent observer, and therapy activities should draw on those observational skills and on the realists' desire for factual evidence of progress. For example, imitation of a variety of vocal behaviors and facilitating techniques and data-keeping activities (charts, graphs, logs, workbooks, worksheets) would probably appeal to the realist. Realists are sensitive to inconsistency, appreciate a practical, no-nonsense approach to intervention, and value consistency and directness.

The categories used in the previous discussions are those of Bramson and Bramson (1985). This categorization system is simply a convenient method of highlighting the fact that diversity exists in the way people think and learn. Other writers have suggested equally useful designations for thinking and learning styles. It is important to remember that no one individual fits neatly into a single category. Nonetheless, clinicians should also remember that most students will have preferred learning styles and should be aware of how their own learning styles affect their expectations of student performance.

Students who feel they have some control over how and what they are learning develop an inner sense of satisfaction and mastery. They have the sense of pleasure that results from learning in a way that they help to determine rather than in a way that is forced on them. Choice, however, should not be equated with permissiveness. Permissiveness is allowing students to do whatever they want. Choice means combining structure and autonomy so that goals are clear, but the method for achieving the goals is flexible.

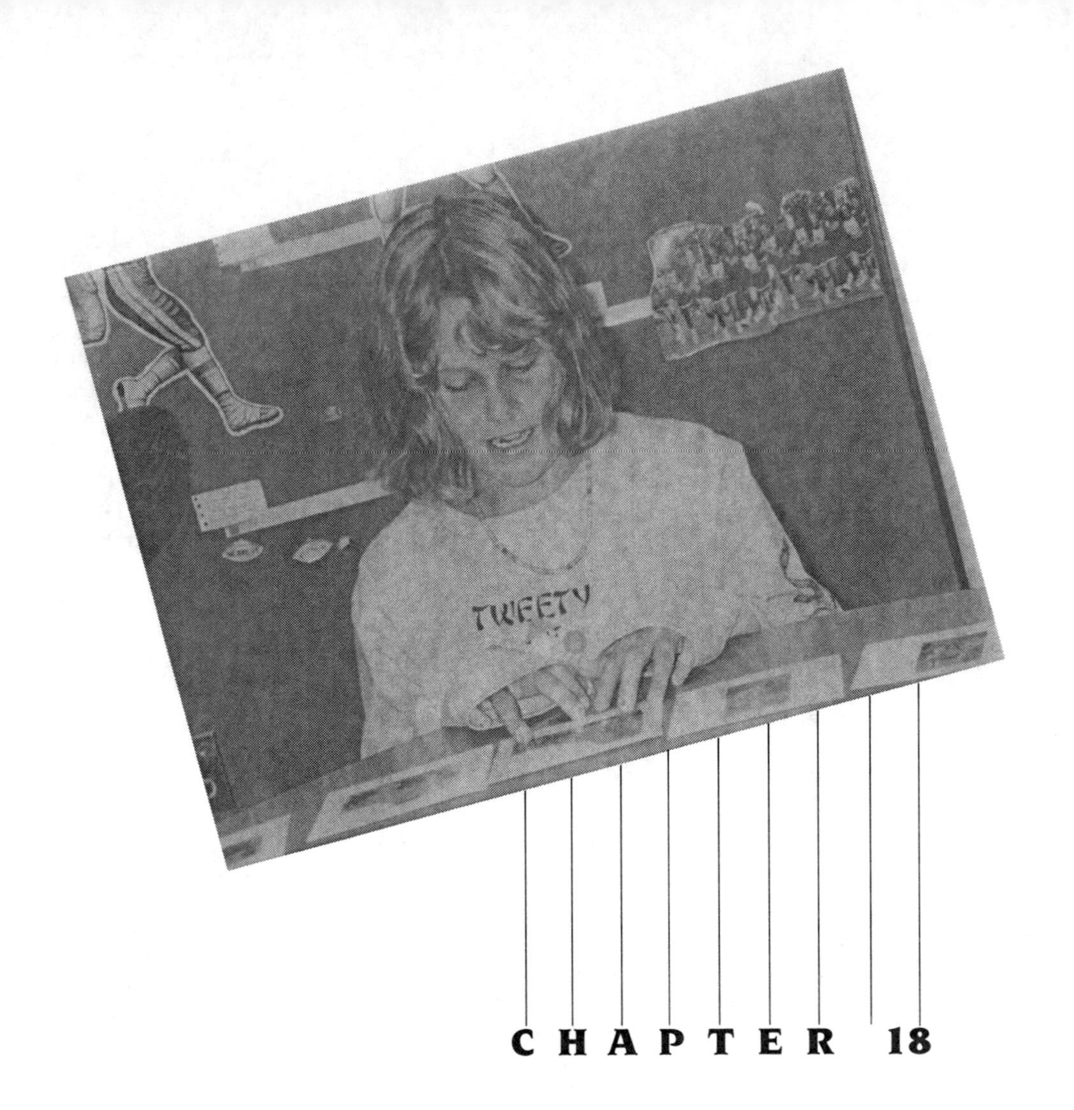

CHAPTER 18

Case Histories, Contracts, and Sample Program Plans

In a holistic approach to programming, the student's vocal symptoms are considered and dealt with in the context of the individual's own perspective and lifestyle. To illustrate ways in which holistic voice programs are designed and implemented, some examples of case histories, contracts, and program plans are presented in this chapter. The adolescents selected for inclusion in this chapter are typical of students seen in the public school setting. The programs, however, are not intended to be viewed as model programs that can be transferred and applied to other individuals. Rather, they are examples of how diagnostic information was translated into programs that were effective for the specific needs of these particular students.

Tammy: An Example of Vocal Abuse

Tammy, age 15, had been a member of the pompom squad for 2 years before earning a place on the varsity cheerleading squad of her high school. She was referred to the speech–language pathologist by the public speaking teacher because of frequent periods of hoarseness and occasional aphonia that made it difficult for her to participate in classroom speaking projects.

The teacher reported that Tammy seemed to find it difficult to control her urge to talk even when her voice was in "bad shape" and described her as an excitable, vivacious person. He observed that Tammy was constantly regaling her friends with stories and anecdotes and noted that she could always be heard above the others in a group. Tammy had responded to his suggestions that she rest her voice more by saying that she didn't want to be seen as a "boring, mousy person."

Initially, Tammy reacted negatively to being referred to the speech–language pathologist, saying that "was just the way she was," that she knew many cheerleaders who sounded hoarse, and that many people found her raspy voice attractive. Because the otolaryngology report showed the presence of bilateral vocal nodules, however, and because of her parent's concern, Tammy agreed to a trial period of voice therapy.

During subsequent discussions, it emerged that a significant part of Tammy's self-concept was tied to being "center stage." She viewed herself as being energetic, lively, and one who could lead and entertain. Because her grades were average, her recognition and status in school came not from academic achievement but from membership in groups that she perceived as having high social status.

Tammy engaged in a very demanding set of physical and vocal behaviors. Her schedule included enthusiastic participation in many physically exhausting activities, accompanied by loud talking, shrieking, and laughing. In the evenings, she spent hours on the telephone or invited friends to her home to work on homework assignments. Her CD player was in constant use, and she strained to talk over the background noise. She was frequently physically and emotionally "hyped-up" and rarely went to sleep before midnight. Late-night studying contributed to arguments with her parents that frequently ended in crying jags.

An outline and discussion of Tammy's voice therapy sequence follows.

Evaluation

I. Factors Precipitating Negative Behaviors
   A. Lifestyle
      1. Cheerleading and gymnastics practice after school
      2. Cheering at athletic events
      3. Loud singing and talking at social events
      4. Long telephone conversations with friends
      5. Late nights (fatigue)

II. Negative Behaviors Observed
   A. Chronic hoarseness and periodic aphonia

B. Excessive amounts of vocalization
C. Vocal impersonations
D. Loud vocal level
E. Hard glottal attacks
F. Neck and facial tension
G. Limited listening skills
H. Denial of vocal problem

III. Sample Target Behaviors for Therapy
A. Voice conservation techniques
B. Modification of lifestyle and self-image
C. Analysis of interpersonal skills, need satisfaction, and physical–emotional resources

Contract Negotiation

In negotiating a contract, the speech–language pathologist discussed with Tammy how her voice affects the successful achievement of her present and future goals. Tammy's only real concern was periodic aphonia. Therefore, voice conservation was of top priority. She agreed to analyze her interpersonal skills primarily, it seemed, because she wished to convince the speech–language pathologist that her personality and enthusiasm necessitated using her voice as she did. She vehemently refused to discuss significantly modifying her lifestyle because it "suited her just fine." Tammy's gregarious nature is reflected in her choice and ordering of the therapeutic goals.

I. Areas for Modification
A. Phonation
B. Interpersonal and psychological factors
C. Lifestyle

II. Ordering Targets
A. Conserve voice
B. Analyze interpersonal skills

III. Matching Targets and Approaches
A. Concurrent approach
B. Acquisition of facts and information
1. Discussions
2. Projects
3. Observations
4. Group reports
5. Interviews
6. Lectures
7. Experiments
8. Field trips
9. Models
10. Internet

IV. Format for Implementation
A. Frequency and length of contact with speech–language pathologist: once per week for 45 minutes
B. Type of contact: group
C. Twenty percent course credit in lieu of one public speaking class per week based on her performance in group therapy
D. Speech–language pathologist's office
E. Ninety percent attendance (not more than two absences)

Therapy Plan

Because Tammy was reluctant to attend voice therapy, the speech–language pathologist decided to create an informal, more social atmosphere by having soft drinks available during the first session and arranging the chairs around a circular table. Two other students who also exhibited vocally abusive practices were attending weekly therapy with Tammy. During the next three therapy sessions, one student attended a private discussion with the speech–language pathologist, while the other two students were assigned films or readings on vocal fold physiology in the library.

I. Developing the Student's Internal Motivation
A. Share biographic, academic, extracurricular, social, and recreational information
B. Students interview each other and develop lists of areas in their lives in

which communication is important to them

II. Defining the Problem
   A. Attend an individual session of 15 minutes with the speech–language pathologist to review diagnostic results and discuss the goals and options for intervention
      1. Prepare a randomly ordered list of positive and negative voice-use situations
      2. Compare perceptions of self and others on ranking task and discuss possible targets for change

III. Analyzing the Problem
   A. Share knowledge gained from Internet and readings about normal vocal fold physiology by demonstrating with a model of the larynx
   B. Speech–language pathologist explains and demonstrates effect of vocal abuse on larynx
   C. Videotape and replay group discussions of homework assignments to aid discussion and analysis of communication skills
   D. Speech–language pathologist discusses lifestyle factors and how they affect voice production
      1. "Brainstorming" session
      2. List lifestyle factors affecting members' own vocal behaviors
   E. Students present oral reports (midterm evaluation for progress report)
      1. Speech–language pathologist grades reports for accuracy and scope
      2. Group members provide feedback on oral presentation style

IV. Defining Characteristics of New Versus Old Behaviors
   A. Summarize findings of audiotapes and logs from homework assignment (see IV-C-6)
   B. Discuss environmental controls and alternative voice strategies
      1. Reset volume control on CD player
      2. Place timer near telephone and limit calls to 10 or 15 minutes
      3. Determine time in evening after which phone calls will not be accepted or made
      4. Allot quiet reading time before sleep
      5. Reduce length of homework sessions with friends
      6. Improve talking–listening ratio
      7. Reduce vocal impersonations
      8. Increase number of questions asked in social interactions
      9. Improve breath support for projected speech (e.g., cheerleading)
      10. Decrease tension in face and neck muscles
      11. Match loudness level to situational demands (increase soft talking)
      12. Identify times when it is pleasant to be alone (provide time for vocal rest)
   C. Outside assignments
      1. Identify four situations in which voice use is good
      2. Identify at least three situations in which voice use is poor
      3. Present a list of positive and negative voice use situations to one peer and one adult and ask each to rank-order the list according to their perceptions
      4. Read assigned information about interpersonal communication styles
      5. Observe communication styles and skills of television actors and admired adult friends
      6. Audiotape cheerleading practice session, telephone conversation, and homework session with friend
      7. Prepare daily log (including hours of sleep, bedtime, daily volume setting of CD player, number of telephone calls per day, number and length of friends' visits

V. Methods for Monitoring and Evaluating Progress
   A. Tapes
   B. Videos
   C. Diaries
   D. Checklists
   E. Reports from other sources
   F. Self-reports (oral)

VI. Timelines for Treatment Schedule and Dismissal Criteria
   A. Level of proficiency to be achieved in each target area
      1. Voice conservation techniques
         a. Eliminate neck and facial tension (100%)
         b. Eliminate hard glottal attacks (85%)
         c. Eliminate vocal impersonations (100%)
         d. Decrease amount of vocalization (20%)
         e. Understand principles of vocal hygiene (95%)
      2. Analysis of interpersonal skills
         a. Data keeping on listening skills (100% accuracy)
      3. Favorable report from physician
   B. Maximum duration of therapy: two semesters
   C. Progress review
      1. Dates for progress report: midsemester and end of semester
      2. Persons to receive progress reports: parents, public speaking teacher, physician
      3. Date for termination, extension, or revision of treatment plan: end of each semester
   D. Frequency and type of follow-up after cessation of therapy sessions
      1. Frequency: once a month for 3 months
      2. Techniques: evaluation of spontaneous speech in face-to-face or telephone interview
         a. Self-evaluation
         b. Public speaking teacher's evaluation of voice
         c. Physician's evaluation of status of vocal folds

Lamont: An Example of Allergic Reactions

Lamont, age 16, was referred to the speech–language pathologist by the school nurse who, while treating him for abrasions sustained during football practice, noticed that he exhibited audible wheezing and an extremely hoarse voice.

During questioning, Lamont stated that he was taking medication for hay fever. The case history revealed that Lamont had broken his nose as a child. Since then, he'd had difficulty breathing, especially during spring and fall, the hay fever seasons. His family reported that he breathed noisily during sleep. Lamont said he had used various over-the-counter preparations to try to "clear his head." He reported that his mouth was frequently dry, and his throat hurt during football practices. He also reported that he frequently lost his voice during football calisthenics. Because Lamont reported that he had not been seen by a physician for this problem, the speech–language pathologist requested a medical evaluation.

The evaluation by the speech–language pathologist revealed that Lamont's respiration for speech was characterized by adequate depth of inspiration but limited expiratory control. It was observed that Lamont habitually breathed through his mouth and assumed an open-mouth position at rest. Observation of the orofacial structures revealed a deviated nasal septum and puffiness and redness of the eyes. Redness of the faucial pillars was also observed. Lamont's voice was characterized by a raspy, hoarse quality with periodic aphonia on unstressed syllables. He said that his voice was "okay for an athlete," and it didn't bother him at all; he just wished he could breathe better. His vocalization pattern was characterized by short, tense phrases interrupted by labored inhalations, so that the continuity and flow of speech was disturbed. He used a low pitch level, infrequent use of inflections, and frequent throat clearing. Lamont's tonal focus appeared to be toward the back of the throat with minimal articulatory movement visible. The resonance pattern was predominately hyponasal and the oral consonants /b/, /d/, and /g/ were substituted for the nasal consonants /m/, /n/, and /ŋ/.

Results of the medical examination showed edema and redness of the vocal folds and entire vocal tract. The otolaryngologist made a subsequent referral to an allergist, who ascertained that Lamont was highly allergic to dust, mold, and pollen. Desensitization therapy was instituted by the allergist, and Lamont was advised to refrain from using nonprescription medication. The allergist explained that some of the preparations that Lamont had used had caused swelling of the nasal mucosa that had exacerbated rather than helped the narrowing of the airway caused by the deviated septum. Additionally, these preparations had contributed to dryness of the vocal tract. This dryness and irritation, as well as the vocal attempts Lamont had adopted to compensate for his swollen vocal mechanism, had compounded the original problem.

An outline and discussion of Lamont's voice therapy sequence follows.

Evaluation

I. Factors Precipitating Negative Behaviors
   A. Medical
      1. Deviated nasal septum
      2. Alterations in respiratory tract due to allegic reactions
      3. Alterations in respiratory tract due to self-medication
      4. Limited fluid intake
   B. Vocal Compensations and Habits
      1. Throat clearing
      2. Strained vocalization
      3. Short phrasing of utterances
      4. Substitution of oral consonants for nasal consonants
   C. Lifestyle
      1. Frequent exposure to airborne allergies during outdoor football practice
      2. Frequent, prolonged vocal demands accompanying physical exertion (calisthenic chants)
      3. Self-concept highly related to perception of the "macho athlete"

II. Negative Behaviors Observed
   A. Limited expiratory control
   B. Mouth breathing
   C. Raspy, hoarse voice quality
   D. Discontinuity of rate and phrasing
   E. Limited inflections
   F. Minimal articulatory movements
   G. Back tone focus
   H. Hyponasal resonance

III. Sample Target Behaviors for Therapy
   A. Analysis of medical factors and vocal compensations
   B. Modification of abusive behaviors:
      1. Strain during calisthenics
      2. Throat clearing
      3. Allergy management
   C. Improvement of respiratory patterns
   D. Improvement of balance of oral–nasal resonance
      1. Forward tone focus
      2. Increased mouth opening
      3. Articulatory precision
   E. Hydration Programs
      1. Increase water intake
      2. Humidifiers in room

Contract Negotiation

I. Areas for Modification
   A. Respiration

B. Resonance
C. Lifestyle and high-risk factors

II. Ordering Targets
A. Analyze medical factors and vocal compensations
B. Improve respiratory patterns
C. Eliminate abusive behaviors
D. Improve balance of oral–nasal resonance

III. Matching Targets and Approaches
A. Sequential approach
B. Acquisition of facts and information
1. Medical illustrations and models
2. Readings and medical references
3. Explanations by speech–language pathologist

IV. Format for Implementation
A. Frequency and length of contact with speech–language pathologist:
1. Consultation and monitoring during football season (two 30-minute consultations followed by one 15-minute monitoring session per month)
2. Two 20-minute sessions per week during spring semester
B. Type of contact: individual
C. No credit for therapy
D. Therapy in speech–language pathologist's office
E. Two mandatory initial consultations, 90% attendance during spring semester

Therapy Plan and Implementation

Because Lamont's schedule and priorities were heavily influenced by his participation in the football program, he supported the speech–language pathologist's suggestion that the major therapy commitment take place during the spring semester. By scheduling two consultations during the fall, however, the speech–language pathologist was able to provide Lamont with some basic information and to monitor the effects of the new medications throughout the first semester.

I. Developing the Student's Internal Motivation
A. Discuss effects of new medication on respiration and energy level, especially during participation in football and related activities
B. Describe breathing and vocal behaviors in terms of what is appropriate for an athlete (spring)
C. Present and discuss results of homework assignment (fall and spring)

II. Defining the Problem
A. Discuss situations where breathing and vocal behavior have not met expectations (fall)
B. Project plans for what Lamont would like to be doing in 10 years and how breathing and current vocal behaviors may influence achievement of those goals (spring)
C. Analyze tapes made in homework assignment (fall; see IV-C-3)
D. Review diagnostic results and student's perceptions of the problem (fall).

III. Analyzing the Problem
A. Review upper respiratory tract structure and function:
1. Types of obstruction
2. Compensations or adaptations
3. Effective medication
4. Mouth versus nose breathing (advantages and disadvantages)
5. Fluid intake and lubrication of the vocal tract
6. The influence of nasal obstruction on articulation, resonance, and respiration
7. Abusive practices and their effects
8. Environmental irritants
B. Present oral report on specific medical, chemical, environmental, and abusive factors influencing the consistency of breathing and vocal symptoms.

IV. Defining Characteristics of New Versus Old Behaviors
  A. Develop format for charting frequency and severity of inappropriate behaviors and precipitating factors
  B. Review patterns precipitating inappropriate behaviors and devise alternative strategies
  C. Outside assignments
    1. Make list of sportcasters on television and research to find out those who have been successful athletes (spring)
    2. Log times during football season and nonfootball season when respiration and voice do not interfere with performance (fall and spring)
    3. Record reading passage
      a. After football practice
      b. Immediately after awakening
      c. At a time when voice is "at its best" (fall)

V. Methods for Monitoring and Evaluating Progress
  A. Logs
  B. Checklists
  C. Graphs
  D. Self-reports (oral)
  E. Quizzes

VI. Timelines for Treatment Schedules and Dismissal Criteria
  A. Level of proficiency to be achieved in each target area
    1. Analyze medical factors and vocal compensations (90% on quiz)
    2. Improve respiratory patterns (85%)
    3. Eliminate abusive behaviors (85%)
    4. Improve balance of oral/nasal resonance (75%)
  B. Maximum duration of therapy: two semesters
  C. Progress review
    1. Dates for progress report: first and last sessions of the spring semester.
    2. Persons to receive progress report: physician, school nurse, parents
    3. Date for termination, extension, or revision of treatment plan: end of the spring semester
  D. Frequency and type of follow-up after cessation of therapy sessions
    1. Frequency: once per month during the football season
    2. Techniques
      a. clinician's evaluation of spontaneous speech in face-to-face interview
      b. student's self-evaluation of breathing patterns

Discussion

Prolongation of /n/, /m/, and /ŋ/ were practiced and timed to improve nasal resonance, forward tone focus, and the length and control of expiration. Cues included feeling vibrations on the bones of the face and the nasal emission of air. Lamont charted the number of repetitions on /n/, /m/, and /ŋ/ on one exhalation (goal = 30). A variation of this activity was to hum pitch patterns of football chants, cadences, or tunes using /m/. Oral–nasal word pairs (see Appendix C) were used to practice and contrast kinesthetic and auditory cues. (For example, Lamont described that the words *be/me* were identical in all aspects except for the direct nasal resonance and nasal emission of air felt on /m/). Chanting words, phrases, and sentences containing nasal consonants provided the opportunity to emphasize and prolong nasal reverberations. Initially, it was easier for Lamont to maintain continuity of voicing throughout an entire word when the words did not contain plosives, stops, and unvoiced continuants. As he progressed, more phonetic complexity was introduced (see Appendix C).

A sporting theme was used when Lamont practiced word lists and phrases to capitalize on his interest in football. Lamont generated word lists based on topics such as states and cities (with nasal consonants) that had good football teams and sports and sports-related terms ending in "ing." Practice materials at the "phrase" level included scores with numbers containing nasals, phrases heard at sporting events, and names of players and coaches containing nasal consonants. The sports theme was continued throughout the treatment plan. It had the advantage of encouraging some immediate carryover because many of the phrases and sentences practiced were used in Lamont's daily conversations and activities. Lamont reported that when he was watching television, he often had good ideas for words and phrases to use in his voice therapy program.

The sports theme also provided for integration of respiratory and resonance goals. For example, during the production of long, complex utterances involving descriptions of football plays, Lamont monitored not only the resonance characteristics but also the appropriateness of respiratory patterns. Elimination of abusive behaviors and correct respiratory support for projected speech were also rehearsed in chants and cadences used during football practice and game situations. Reading materials were drawn primarily from sports magazines, school newspapers, and the sporting sections of city newspapers. Lamont frequently brought articles to voice therapy that he wanted to share with the speech–language pathologist. He then used these articles to structure interviews to practice spontaneous speech.

Esther: An Example of PMS

Esther, age 16, requested an appointment with the speech–language pathologist. She was the captain of her high school debate team and described a problem with her voice that occasionally interfered with her performance in debate tournaments. She stated that her voice was usually clear and strong, but her voice had "really let her down" during some tournaments. Because as a debater she was very concerned about her record, she felt she could not afford being penalized by these voice fluctuations.

The speech–language pathologist could detect no problems in Esther's voice and suggested that Esther "drop in" to the office sometime when she perceived her voice as unacceptable.

When Esther returned 2 weeks later, the speech–language pathologist was startled by the extreme change in her voice quality. She exhibited severe hoarseness and hyponasality. The speech–language pathologist questioned Esther extensively concerning the possibility of the symptoms being related to a cold or allergic reaction. Esther's responses were intense. She said she definitely did not have a cold and that she had never had allergies in her life. When the speech–language pathologist gently indicated that it is sometimes difficult to identify the "trigger mechanisms" for allergic reactions, Esther became agitated and stated that her "chances of winning the upcoming debate were practically zero." Esther seemed so agitated and upset during the discussion, that the speech–language pathologist wondered if the problem was the result of emotional tension. Nonetheless, the speech–language pathologist remembered that she had been impressed by Esther's calm and rational manner during their initial interview.

The speech–language pathologist hypothesized that Esther's intermittent symptoms might be related to reactions to allergens or reactions to stress (i.e., pressures surrounding debate tournaments) and asked Esther to keep a log of her activities. She was to note details concerning her daily routine, diet, moods, and voice symptoms. She was to return in 2 months for another conference with the speech–language pathologist. Esther was counseled in the interim concerning general principles of vocal hygiene and cautioned to avoid vocally abusive behaviors when symptoms were present.

When Esther's log was examined at the end of 8 weeks, the speech–language pathologist was surprised by the cyclical pattern of symptoms. For 3 days following the conference, Esther's log showed the presence of the following conditions: hoarseness, nasal stuffiness and congestion, sneezing, coughing, irritability, increased food consumption, fatigue, and eye irritations (unable to wear contact lenses to read debate notes). For the next 3 weeks, none of these symptoms were recorded; however, symptoms recorded during the fourth week were very similar to those noted above. The second month of the log reflected a pattern similar to that of the first month: three symptom-free weeks followed by a recurrence of symptoms.

The speech–language pathologist suspected a correlation between the vocal symptoms and Esther's menstrual cycle. She thought that Esther might be affected by premenstrual syndrome (PMS). To verify her impressions, the speech–language pathologist suggested that Esther consult a local medical authority with special interest in PMS. The speech–language pathologist told Esther to be sure to take her log and her calendar to show to the physician.

Results of the physician's report indicated that Esther's pattern of vocal symptoms was compatible with patterns associated with PMS. He explained that changes in the laryngeal and nasal mucosa are sometimes related to hormonal fluctuations. Therefore, the hoarse voice quality that occurred the week before the onset of menstruation was due to edema of the vocal folds. The hyponasality that occurred concurrently was the result of obstruction of the nasal passages by similarly swollen tissue. The physician outlined several possible treatment strategies including changes in diet and medication. He also advocated continued consultation with the speech–language pathologist to ensure appropriate vocal hygiene during times when Esther's speech mechanism was vulnerable to vocal abuse.

An outline and discussion of Esther's voice therapy sequence follows.

Evaluation

I. Factors Precipitating Negative Behaviors
   A. Medical
      1. Cyclical swelling of nasal and laryngeal mucosa
   B. Lifestyle
      1. High expectations for personal performance
      2. Exacerbated anxiety and emotional lability during week preceding menstruation
      3. Prolonged, sustained speaking situations (debate tournaments and practice sessions)
   C. Interpersonal
      1. Premenstrual fatigue, irritability, and tension reduced effectiveness in interactions with debate team members

II. Negative Behaviors Observed
   A. Hyponasal resonance
   B. Hoarse laryngeal quality
   C. Effortful speaking style
   D. Vocal variety limited to loudness and pitch increase
   E. Lack of awareness of principles of vocal hygiene
   F. Vocally abusive behaviors (crying jags, loud emotional outbursts)

III. Sample Target Behaviors for Therapy
   A. Awareness of premenstrual changes and effects on voice
   B. Identification of physical symptoms associated with PMS
   C. Adaptation of lifestyle, where possible, to correlate with cyclical physical changes of premenstruum
   D. Awareness of general principles of vocal hygiene

E. Identification of vocally abusive practices during premenstruum
F. Elimination of vocally abusive practices

Contract Negotiation

Esther's level of commitment to improving her vocal behavior was so strong that the speech–language pathologist did not feel a contractual agreement was necessary. The decision was based on the fact that Esther was experiencing an acute, inconsistent pattern of symptoms rather than a chronic problem with severe symptomatology. Lifestyle factors are especially significant in such cases. If Esther had not been so involved with debating, she might not have noticed the intermittent changes in her vocal behavior.

The speech pathologist must be sensitive to the way in which an individual perceives and reacts to changes in voice. When reactions are intense and troublesome, they need to be addressed. Severity of symptoms, therefore, is not the only yardstick for defining a voice problem.

Therapy Plan

The consultation model seemed the most appropriate intervention strategy for Esther. Her high motivation and experience in researching topics for debate made her an excellent candidate for independent research and study on the topic of PMS and the voice. Esther met with the speech–language pathologist for 15-minute sessions during five study hall periods to learn about vocal hygiene. On each occasion, she received reading materials, assignments, and brief instruction. Because she was already evaluating her debate presentations on a tape recorder, this format for self-evaluation was continued.

Esther was so highly motivated that it was not necessary to develop programming to increase her internal motivation. Her problem was defined during discussions of vocal symptoms and during consultations with the medical specialist on PMS. Esther's voice program centered around analysis of the problem through knowledge acquisition and knowledge demonstration. As a result of her reading, Esther developed a list of PMS symptoms that specifically affected vocal interaction and a list of vocal hygiene rules for debaters.

Carlos: An Example of Mutational Falsetto

Carlos, age 17, was referred to the speech–language pathologist by his family doctor. He and his mother had consulted the physician concerning Carlos' high-pitched voice, which he found embarrassing. The medical report stated that Carlos was physically mature, there was no endocrine imbalance, and the laryngeal mechanism was within normal limits.

In the initial interview with the speech–language pathologist, Carlos appeared highly motivated and eager to pursue therapy. He stated that he had hoped that his voice would deepen as he grew older, but that didn't seem to be happening. He could produce a lower voice when he concentrated on it. When he was tense or excited, however, his pitch was extremely high, and pitch breaks occurred frequently. He said this affected his social life because he avoided situations involving a lot of talking, and was especially shy when he was around girls.

The speech–language pathologist administered a pure tone hearing test and ascertained that Carlos' hearing was within normal limits bilaterally. The voice evaluation indicated that respiratory patterns for speech appeared to be within normal limits. Carlos spoke with reduced phonatory power at a habitually high pitch of approximately 163 Hz (with a conversational range of 132 to 177 Hz as measured on the Visi-Pitch) and used minimal pitch inflections; however, pitch breaks were noted when tension increased. At such times, phonation ceased temporarily and reappeared at a lower pitch level. When Carlos reacted negatively to these pitch breaks, his overall tension increased, and his pitch resumed its higher level. He could produce loudness variations within normal limits during testing, although volume was habitually soft. Resonance patterns were appropriate, and no quality deviations were noted.

In discussions with Carlos, it emerged that he had a particularly close relationship with his mother, whom he perceived as supportive and understanding. He voiced some ambivalence regarding his relationship with his father, whom he admired for his professional success but whose passion for hunting and aggressive activities were contrary to Carlos' more sensitive nature.

The speech–language pathologist hypothesized that Carlos may have been unable to habituate an adult male pitch because he was unconsciously equating it with those masculine qualities personified by his father, with whom he was unable to identify. The speech–language pathologist decided that voice therapy should include opportunities for Carlos to explore a variety of ways to express adult masculinity consistent with his own values and personality characteristics.

An outline and discussion of Carlos' voice therapy sequence follows.

Evaluation

I. Factors Precipitating Negative Behaviors
   A. Psychosocial
      1. Equating adult male pitch level with personality characteristics personified by the father
      2. Lack of awareness of the range of acceptable adult masculine characteristics

II. Negative Behaviors Observed
   A. Reduced loudness
   B. Limited inflection
   C. Immature pitch level
   D. Pitch breaks
   E. Anxiety reactions to pitch breaks

III. Sample Target Behaviors for Therapy
   A. Analysis of relationship between pitch and perceptions of masculinity
   B. Lowered pitch level
   C. Increased use of inflectional patterns
   D. Increased loudness
   E. Reduction of anxiety in response to vocal behavior

Contract Negotiation

I. Areas for Modification
   A. Phonation
   B. Respiration
   C. Interpersonal

II. Ordering Targets
   A. Lowered pitch level
   B. Increased use of inflectional patterns
   C. Reduction of anxiety in response to vocal behavior
   D. Analysis of relationship between pitch and perceptions of masculinity
   E. Increased loudness

III. Matching Targets and Approaches
   A. Concurrent approach
   B. Acquisition of facts and information
      1. Readings
      2. Diagrams
      3. Discussions
      4. Instrumentation (Visi-Pitch, tuning fork, pitch pipe)
      5. Laryngeal model
      6. Written reports
      7. Observations

IV. Format for Implementation
   A. Frequency and length of contact with speech–language pathologist: twice per week for 45 minutes per session

B. Type of contact: individual
C. Noncredit (sessions scheduled during study hall)
D. Speech–language pathologist's office
E. Ninety percent attendance (not more than four absences)

Therapy Plan

Carlos was highly motivated and eager to pursue voice therapy because of embarrassment caused by his high vocal pitch. He was able to describe his problem and provide examples of how his voice limited his social interactions. Carlos was taught the relationships between air flow and vocal fold adjustments and the resulting pitch and loudness changes through the use of readings, diagrams, and models.

As an assignment, Carlos read Dr. Morton Cooper's *Change Your Voice, Change Your Life* (1984), which provided an introduction to a general discussion of vocal and speaking styles. Although the speech–language pathologist felt that Carlos was confusing his stereotype of masculinity and his negative reactions to his father's speaking styles, the point was not addressed directly. Rather, the speech–language pathologist discussed how speakers sometimes cause listeners to react negatively because of sentence structure and tone of voice. Carlos listed the "hidden message" in statements such as

- "I don't care how you feel about it, just do it." (*ordering*)
- "When I was your age . . ." (*preaching*)
- "You always look untidy. You kids are all alike." (*overgeneralizing*)
- "You probably feel that way because . . ." (*diagnosing*)

I. Methods for Monitoring and Evaluating Progress
   A. Tuning fork (auditory)
   B. Visi-Pitch (visual)
   C. Logs
   D. Graphs
   E. Self-reports
   F. Video and audio tapes
II. Timelines for Treatment Schedule and Dismissal Criteria
   A. Level of proficiency to be achieved in each target area
      1. Lowered pitch level: habitual pitch level between 120 to 128 Hz (100%)
      2. Increased use of inflectional patterns: conversational range of 90 to 156 Hz (80%)
      3. Reduction of anxiety in response to vocal behavior (50% increase in self-reported initiation of social interactions)
      4. Analysis of relationship between pitch and perceptions of masculinity (B or above grade on written report summarizing data collected by personal observations)
      5. Increased loudness (demonstration of 90 to 100 dB level on (VU) meter, with microphone 2 inches from mouth, during 50-word reading passage
   B. Maximum duration of therapy: one semester
   C. Progress review
      1. Dates for progress report: midsemester and end of semester
      2. Persons to receive progress report: physician, mother
      3. Date for termination, extension, or revision of treatment plan: end of each semester
   D. Frequency and type of follow-up after cessation of therapy sessions
      1. Frequency: once bimonthly for one semester
      2. Techniques: face-to-face or telephone interview

a. self-evaluation
b. evaluation of others

Annette: An Example of Reaction to Emotional Trauma

Annette, age 17, a senior in a large metropolitan high school, was referred to the speech–language pathologist by the music teacher, who was directing the annual school musical. The production was "Auntie Mame," and Annette was cast in the leading role.

The music teacher was concerned because of abrupt changes that had occurred in Annette's performance during rehearsals. He said that he had worked with Annette during previous productions with outstanding results but that recently both her concentration and vocal skill had deteriorated markedly. He noted that her singing voice was characterized by restricted range and intermittent pitch breaks, she seemed unable to project her voice in speaking parts, and she seemed much less enthusiastic than in previous productions. He felt Annette was committed to the role, but her fears of "losing her high notes" and not being able to predict when her voice would break were reducing her overall confidence. He hoped that the speech–language pathologist could help Annette with her vocal problems because he would have to recast the part if her performance did not improve significantly.

The speech–language pathologist had attended previous school musicals and had been impressed by Annette's strong vocal technique and vibrant stage personality. Because Annette's problems appeared to be related specifically to her onstage vocal behavior, the speech–language pathologist decided to observe part of the next rehearsal period to see if the problem warranted intervention.

While watching part of the next rehearsal, the speech–language pathologist observed that Annette seemed generally subdued: Her gestures and facial expressions were restricted, eye contact was poor, her voice was frequently inaudible, and pitch breaks occurred in the upper part of her singing range. She thought that Annette seemed depressed and withdrawn, but felt that short-term coaching on vocal projection techniques and eye contact awareness could improve Annette's performance.

The speech–language pathologist met with Annette and reviewed basic information concerning respiration and more precise articulation. Annette demonstrated that she understood the basic principles and was able to apply them during all of the exercises. She also demonstrated appropriate eye contact.

The speech–language pathologist decided that the difficulty must be related to Annette's inability to apply these principles while onstage. She arranged for another member of the cast to meet with her and Annette in the auditorium. She wanted to see if Annette could transfer her fine performance in the speech room to the larger setting. Again, Annette's performance was flawless.

The speech–language pathologist believed that Annette's problem had been solved. However, 2 days later Annette reappeared in the speech–language pathologist's office in tears. She said that rehearsal the night before had been a disaster. She seemed utterly despondent and kept repeating, "I just can't go on with it!" She felt the only thing she could do was to withdraw from the production.

Lengthy discussion revealed that Annette froze onstage during every rehearsal because she was always aware that a member of the stage crew was staring at her from the wings. She said, "He watches me all the time, and I can't stand it! When I know he's there, I feel paralyzed." Amidst a flood of tears, Annette revealed that shortly after rehearsals for "Auntie Mame" began, she accepted a ride home from the young man. Instead of driving her home, however, he had driven her to a secluded area and forcibly raped her. She was afraid to tell anyone about this because she felt it was her fault that she had unknowingly given him the impression that she was interested in him. She said he had told her it was her fault for leading him on. Although Annette felt she had treated him in the same manner as she had treated everyone else in the cast, she now questioned whether her outgoing personality could be misinterpreted. She had not told anyone about the incident because she wanted to forget it. She feared that her reputation would be ruined if anyone knew. Nonetheless, she was filled with terror everytime she saw this boy.

The speech–language pathologist assured Annette that her feelings and reactions were typical of the reactions of the victims of rape. She said she could understand why Annette did not want others to know, but that she had done the correct thing by finally telling someone. The speech–language pathologist assured Annette that she understood the problems with rehearsals and advised Annette not to resign from the cast until they spoke again the next day.

An outline and discussion of Annette's voice therapy sequence follows.

Evaluation

I. Factors Precipitating Negative Behaviors
  A. Lifestyle
    1. Failure in situations that formerly held high value and reward
    2. Negative feedback from music director
    3. Demanding rehearsal schedule
  B. Interpersonal
    1. Rape by member of the stage crew
    2. Attempts to repress the traumatic event
    3. Fear that others may find out about the rape
    4. Guilt associated with her perception that she may have provoked the rape

II. Negative Behavior Observed
  A. Inability to perform onstage
    1. Poor eye contact
    2. Limited facial expression
    3. Restricted gestures
    4. Insufficient volume and breath support
    5. Inadequate oral movement
    6. Pitch breaks on high notes
    7. Limited pitch variation in speaking segments

III. Sample Target Behaviors for Therapy
  A. Awareness of typical reactions of rape victims
  B. Awareness of the need to inform and involve police and family
  C. Referral to support group for rape victims
  D. Awareness of relationship between emotional state and vocal behaviors
  E. Awareness of the need to consult with the music director
    1. Explanation of the problem
    2. Removal of rapist from the stage crew
    3. Referral of rapist for counseling
    4. Negotiations for mutual expectations regarding continued participation in the cast

Discussion

Although Annette's problem was not one with which the speech–language pathologist would normally be involved, the fact that Annette had confided in her meant that the speech–language pathologist felt a responsibility to assist Annette in dealing with a very difficult situation. The speech–language pathologist realized that a case conference would have to be called as quickly as possible, but she also realized that she needed to talk more with Annette so that Annette would see the need to involve others. At their next meeting, the speech–language pathologist gave Annette readings to help her understand that her reactions were typical of others who had experienced similar trauma. Annette found *Top Secret* (Fay & Fletcher, 1982) especially helpful. The speech–language pathologist also discussed some of the myths that exist about rape.

Following another meeting with the speech–language pathologist, Annette agreed to talk the problem over with her parents and asked that the speech–language pathologist talk to the music teacher and school principal. The parents, speech–language pathologist, music teacher, and principal discussed the management of the problem with an emphasis on the maintenance of confidentiality. Management strategies included the following:

- Referral to a community rape support group for ongoing counseling
- Medical evaluation by the family physician (because there is always the risk of internal injury, disease, or pregnancy)
- The principal agreed to assume responsibility for
  1. Discussing the situation with both the boy and his parents
  2. Informing the boy and his parents that the police would be notified and contacting the police
  3. Informing the boy that he was being removed from the production's stage crew and could not participate in or attend any segment of the production
  4. Investigating and recommending appropriate resources (e.g., counseling) to assist the boy
  5. Seeking reports and follow-up from counseling agencies
- The music teacher assumed responsibility for
  1. Ensuring that the boy was not present at rehearsals or performances
  2. Monitoring Annette's vocal behavior and updating the speech–language pathologist
  3. Maintaining confidentiality concerning the problem with respect to the rest of the cast

The speech–language pathologist assumed responsibility for helping Annette become aware of the relationship between emotional state and vocal behavior and helping her practice techniques to reduce vocal tension. The speech–language pathologist and Annette agreed to meet once a week after school for 45 minutes. A 6-week duration was agreed on.

The parents agreed to maintain contact with the music director, speech–language pathologist, and school principal, as well as follow the suggestions of personnel in charge of the rape support group. They also volunteered to supervise car-pooling arrangements for Annette and her friends to and from extracurricular activities.

At adolescence, more than at any other life stage, new physical and psychosocial factors exert a profound influence on the individual. It is critical that all factors relevant to a voice problem be addressed. The case histories in this chapter illustrate a holistic approach to the modification of vocal symptoms that actively engages the students in the process of change.

References

Albritton, T. P. (1984, November). *Secondary speech-language programs: Strategies for a new delivery system.* Paper presented at the annual convention of the American-Speech-Language-Hearing Association, San Francisco.

Alpert, S. E., Dearborn, D. G., & Kercsmar, C. M. (1991). To the editor: On vocal cord dysfunction in wheezy children. *Pediatric Pulmonology, 10,* 142–143.

American Psychiatric Association. (1994). *Diagnostic and statistical manual of mental disorders* (4th ed.). Washington, DC: American Psychiatric Assoc.

American Speech and Hearing Association. (1974). Prevention of communication problems. *Asha,* 16, 141–142.

Anderson, G., & Nelson, N. (1988). Integrating language intervention and education in an alternate adolescent language classroom. *Seminars in Speech and Language, 9,* 341–353.

Anderson, V. A., & Newby, H. A. (1973). *Improving the child's speech* (2nd ed.). New York: Oxford University Press.

Andreassen, M. L., Leeper, H. A., & Macrae, D. L. (1991). Changes in vocal resonance and nasalization following adenoidectomy in normal children: Preliminary findings. *Journal of Otolaryngology, 20,* 237–242.

Andrews, M. L. (1975). Communication problems encountered in voice therapy with children. *Language, Speech and Hearing Services in Schools,* 6, 183–187.

Andrews, M. L. (1982). *Frequency characteristics of the voices of 740 Australian school children.* Unpublished manuscript, Indiana University, Bloomington.

Andrews, M. L. (1991). *Voice therapy for children: The elementary school years.* San Diego, CA: Singular Publishing Group.

Andrews, M. L. (1992). Management of vocal hyperfunction: Psycho-social aspects of children's behavior. In J. Stemple (Ed.), *Voice therapy: Clinical studies* (pp. 26–33). St. Louis, MO: Mosby.

Andrews, M. L. (1993). *Your best voice.* Tucson, AZ: Communication Skills Builders.

Andrews, M. L. (1997). The singing/acting child: A speech-language pathologist's perspective. *Journal of Voice, 11,* 130–135.

Andrews, M. L. (1999). *Manual of voice treatment* (2nd ed.). San Diego, CA: Delmar Cengage Learning.

Andrews, M. L. (2000). Voice disorders. In E. P. Dodge (Ed.), *The survival guide for school-based speech-language pathologists.* San Diego, CA: Delmar Cengage Learning.

Andrews, M. L., & Champley, E. H. (1993). The elicitation of vocal responses from preschool children. *Language, Speech and Hearing Services in Schools,* 24(3), 156–167.

Andrews, M. L., & Shank, K. H. (1983). Some observations concerning the cheering behavior of school-girl cheerleaders. *Language, Speech, and Hearing Services in Schools, 14,* 150–156.

Andrews, M. L., & Summers, A. C. (1988). *Voice therapy for adolescents.* San Diego, CA: Singular Publishing Group.

Andrews, M. L., & Summers, A. C. (1991). The awareness phase of voice therapy: Providing a knowledge base for the adolescent. *Language, Speech and Hearing Services in Schools,* 22(3), 118–162.

Andrews, M. L., & Summers, A. C. (1993). A voice stimulation program for preschoolers: Theory and practice. *Language, Speech and Hearing Services in Schools,* 24(3), 140–145.

Andrews, M. L., Shrivastav, R., & Yamaguchi, H. (2000). The role of cognitive cueing in eliciting vocal variability. *Journal of Voice, 14*(4), 494–501.

Andrews, M. L., Tardy, S. J., & Pasternak, L. G. (1984). The modification of hypernasality in young children: A programming approach. *Language, Speech and Hearing Services in Schools, 15*, 37–39.

Arnold, G. E. (1963). Vocal nodules. In J. F. Daly (Moderator), Voice problems and laryngeal pathology. *N.Y. State Journal of Medicine, 63*, 3096–3110.

Aronson, A. E. (1973). *Psychogenic voice disorders: An interdisciplinary approach to detection, diagnosis and therapy: Audio seminars in speech pathology*. Philadelphia: Saunders.

Aronson, A. E. (1980). *Clinical voice disorders: An interdisciplinary approach*. New York: Brian C. Decker.

Arvedson, J., & Lefton-Greif, M. A. (1998). *Pediatric videofluoroscopic swallow studies: A professional manual with caregiver guidelines*. San Antonio, TX: Communication Skill Builders.

Arvedson, J., Crary, M., Groher, M., Mann, G., Miller, R., & Rosenbeck, J. (2000, June). The Second Annual Florida Dysphagia Institute, Orlando, FL.

Aslin, R. N., Pisoni, D. B., & Jusczek, P. W. (1983). Auditory development and speech perception in infancy. In P. Mussen (Ed.), *Carmichael's manual of child psychology* (4th ed.). *Vol. II: Infancy and the Biology of Development* (M. M. Haith & J. J. Campos, Eds., pp. 573–687). New York: Wiley.

Atoynatan, T. H. (1986). Elective mutism: Involvement of the mother in the treatment of the child. *Child Psychiatry and Human Development, 17*, 15–27.

Baken, R. J. (1977). Estimation of lung volume change form torso hemi-circumferences. *Journal of Speech and Hearing Research, 20*, 808–812.

Baken, R. J. (1979, June). Respiratory mechanisms: Introduction and overview. *Transcripts of the Eighth Symposium: Care of the Professional Voice, 2*, 9–13.

Baken, R. J. (1987). *Clinical measurement of speech and voice*. San Diego, CA: College-Hill Press.

Baken, R. J., Cavallo, S. A., & Weissman, K. J. L. (1979). Chest wall movements prior to phonation. *Journal of Speech and Hearing Research, 22*, 862–872.

Bales, D. W., & Sera, M. D. (1995). Preschoolers' understanding of stable and changeable characteristics. *Cognitive Development, 10*, 69–107.

Baltaxe, A., & Simmonds, J. O., III. (1995). Speech and language disorders in children and adolescents with schizophrenia. *Schizophrenia Bulletin, 21*, 677–692.

Baltaxe, C. A. M. (1994, November). *Communication issues in selective mutism*. Paper presented at the American Speech-Language-Hearing Association Convention, New Orleans, LA.

Baranak, C., Potsic, W. P., Miller-Bauer, L., & Marsh, R. R. (1983, December). *Changes in sleep patterns with adenotonsillectomy*. Paper presented at the annual meeting of SENTAC, San Diego, CA.

Bastian, R. W., Keidar, A. K., & Verdolini-Marston, K. (1990). Simple vocal tasks for detecting vocal fold swelling. *Journal of Voice, 4*, 172–183.

Battle, D. W., & Van Hattum, R. J. (1982). Scheduling. In R. J. Van Hattum (Ed.), *Speech-language programming in the schools* (2nd ed., pp. 448–509). Springfield, IL: Thomas.

Baynes, R. A. (1967). Voice therapy with children—a global approach. *Journal of the Michigan Speech and Hearing Association, 3*, 11–14.

Begley, S. (2000, May 8). A world of their own. *Newsweek*, 53–56.

Bell, R. (1980). *Changing bodies, changing lives (A book for teens on sex and relationships)*. New York: Random House.

Bennett, S. (1983). A three-year longitudinal study of school-aged children's fundamental frequencies. *Journal of Speech and Hearing Research, 26*, 137–141.

Benson, H. (1975). *The relaxation response*. New York: Morrow.

Bent, J. P., & Porubsky, E. S. (1998). Acute laryngeal trauma in the pediatric population. *Annals of Otology, Rhinolology, and Laryngology, 107*, 104–106.

Berryman, J. D. (1986). Clinical techniques and materials. In W. R. Neal (Ed.), *Speech-language pathology services in secondary schools* (pp. 99–122). Austin, TX: Pro-Ed.

Bittleman, D. B., Smith, R. J. H., & Weiler, J. M. (1994). Abnormal movement of the arytenoids region during exercise presenting as exercise-induced asthma in an adolescent athlete. *Chest, 106*, 615–616.

Black, B., & Uhde, T. (1995). Psychiatric characteristics of children with selective mutism: A pilot study. *Journal of the American Academy of Child and Adolescent Psychiatry, 34*, 847–856.

Blager, F., Brugman, S., Howell, G., Mahler, G., & Rosenberg, D. (1998, June). *Predictive factors in adolescents with vocal fold dysfunction*. Paper presented at the 27th Symposium of the Voice Foundation: Care of the Professional Voice, Philadelphia.

Blahova, O., & Brezovsky, P. (1981). Stenozing processes due to endotracheal intubation and tracheostomy in children. *International Journal of Pediatric Otorhinolaryngology, 3*, 191–203.

Bless, D. M., & Abbs, J. H. (1983). *Vocal fold physiology: Contemporary research and clinical issues*. San Diego, CA: College-Hill Press.

Blonigen, J. A. (1978). Management of vocal hoarseness caused by abuse: An approach. *Language, Speech and Hearing Services in Schools, 9*, 142–150.

Bloom, B. S. (Ed.). (1956). *Taxonomy of educational objectives: Cognitive domain*. New York: David McKay.

Blos, P. (1962). *On adolescence*. New York: The Free Press.

Blyth, D. A., Thiel, K. S., Mitsch, D., & Simmons, R. G. (1980). Another look at school crime: Student as victim. *Youth and Society, 11*, 369–388.

Böhme, G. & Stuchlik, G. (1995). Voice profiles and standard voice profile of untrained children. *Journal of Voice, 9*, 304–307.

Boliek, C., Hixon, T. J., Watson, P. J., & Morgan, W. J. (1996). Vocalization and breathing during the first year of life. *Journal of Voice, 10*, 1–22.

Boliek, C., Hixon, T. J., Watson, P. J., & Morgan, W. J. (1997). Vocalization and breathing during the second and third years of life. *Journal of Voice, 11*, 373–390.

Boltezar, I. H., Burger, Z. R., & Zargi, M. (1997). Instability of voice in adolescence: Pathologic condition or normal developmental variation? *Journal of Pediatrics, 130*, 185–190.

Boone, D. R. (1974). Dismissal criteria in voice therapy. *Journal of Speech and Hearing Disorders, 39*, 133–139.

Boone, D. R. (1977). *The voice and voice therapy*. Englewood Cliffs, NJ: Prentice Hall.

Boone, D. R. (1983). *The voice and voice therapy* (2nd ed.). Englewood Cliffs, NJ: Prentice Hall.

Bordo, S. (1998). Sexual harassment is about bullying, not sex. *Chronicle of Higher Education, 44*(34), B6.

Bordo, S. (1999). Gay men's revenge. *Journal of Aesthetics & Art Criticism, 57*, 21–26.

Bradford, M. A., Hosea, K. L., & Neal, W. R., Jr. (1977, November). *National survey of speech pathology services in the secondary schools*. Paper presented at the annual convention of the American Speech-Language-Hearing Association, Chicago.

Brammer, L. M. (1973). *The helping relationship process and skills*. Englewood Cliffs, NJ: Prentice Hall.

Bramson, R., & Bramson, S. (1985). *The stressless home*. Garden City, NY: Anchor-Doubleday.

Broad, D. J. (1973). Phonation. In F. Minifie, T. Hixon, & F. Williams (Eds.), *Normal aspects of speech, hearing and language*. Englewood Cliffs, NJ: Prentice Hall.

Brodnitz, F. S. (1963). Goals, results and limitations of vocal rehabilitation. *Archives of Otolaryngology, 77*, 148–156.

Brodnitz, F. S. (1971). *Vocal rehabilitation*. Rochester, MN: American Academy of Ophthamology and Otolaryngology.

Brugman, S., & Newman, K. (1993). Vocal cord dysfunction. *Medical Scientific Update*, National Jewish Center for Immunology and Respiratory Medicine, *111*(5), 1–5.

Brumberg, J. J. (1997). Silicone Valley. *Nation, 265*(22), 38–41.

Budoff, P. W. (1981). *No more menstrual cramps and other good news*. New York: Penguin Books.

Bzoch, K. R. (Ed.). (1972). *Communicative disorders related to cleft lip and palate*. Boston: Little, Brown.

Calvert, D. R., & Silverman, S. R. (1975). *Speech and deafness*. Washington, DC: Alexander Graham Bell Association for the Deaf.

Carkhuff, R. R. (1969). *Helping and human relations* (Vol. 2). New York: Holt, Rinehart & Winston.

Carr, M. M., Nguyen, A., Nagy, M., Pizzuto, C., Poje, C., & Brodsky, L. (1999). *Utility of symptoms in identifying children with gastroesophageal reflux disease (GERD).* Paper presented at the annual meeting of the Society for Ear, Nose, and Throat Advances in Children, Williamsburg, VA.

Carrow, E. A. (1974). A test using elicited imitations in assessing grammatical structure in children. *Journal of Speech and Hearing Disorders, 39,* 437–444.

Case, J. L. (1991). *Clinical management of voice disorders* (2nd ed.). Austin, TX: Pro-Ed.

Cavo, J. W., Jr. (1985). True vocal cord paralysis following intubation. *Laryngoscope, 95,* 1352–1359.

Chait, D. H., & Lotz, W. K. (1991). Successful pediatric examination using nasoendoscopy. *Laryngoscope, 101,* 1016–1018.

Champley, E. (1977). *A comparison of four methods of eliciting vocal responses from preschool children.* Unpublished master's thesis, Indiana University, Bloomington.

Chandler, M. J. (1973). Egocentrism and antisocial behavior: The assessment and training of social perspective-taking skills. *Developmental Psychology, 9,* 326–333.

Cherry, J., & Margulies, S. I. (1968). Contact ulcer of the larynx. *Laryngoscope, 73,* 1937–1940.

Chethik, M. (1973). Amy: The intensive treatment of an elective mute. *Journal of the American Academy of Child Psychiatry, 12,* 482–498.

Clark, H. H. (1969a). Linguistic processes in deductive reasoning. *Psychological Review, 76,* 387–404.

Clark, H. H. (1969b). The influence of language in solving three-term series problems. *Journal of Experimental Psychology, 82,* 205–215.

Clary, R. A., Pengilly, A., Bailey, M., Jones, N., Albert, D., Comins, J., & Appleton, J. (1996). Analysis of voice outcomes in pediatric patients following surgical procedures for Laryngotrocheal stenosis. *Archives of Otolaryngology–Head and Neck Surgery, 122,* 1189–1194.

Cline, T., & Baldwin, S. (1994). *Selective mutism in children.* San Diego, CA: Singular Publishing Group.

Cohn, J. R., Sataloff, R. T., Spiegel, J. R., & Cohn, J. B. (1997). Airway reactivity induced reversible voice dysfunction in singers. *Allergy-Asthma-Proceedings, 18,* 1–5.

Cole, J. D., Dodge, K. A., & Coppotelli, H. (1982). Dimensions and types of social status: A cross age perspective. *Developmental Psychology, 18,* 557–570.

Cole, R. B., & Mackay, A. D. (1990). *Essentials of respiratory disease* (3rd ed.). Edinburgh, UK: Churchill Livingstone.

Colton, R. H., & Casper, J. K. (1990). *Understanding voice problems: A physiological perspective for diagnoses and treatment.* Baltimore, MD: Williams & Wilkins.

Conger, J. J. (1973). *Adolescence and youth.* New York: Harper & Row.

Contencin, P., Maurage, C., Ployet, M. J., Seid, A. B., & Sinaasappel, M. (1995). Gastroensophageal reflux and ENT disorders in childhood. *International Journal of Pediatric Otorhinolaryngology, 32*(Suppl.), S135–S144.

Cook, J. V., Palaski, D. J., & Hanson, W. R. (1979). A vocal hygiene program for school age children. *Language, Speech and Hearing Services in Schools, 10,* 21–26.

Cooksey, J. M. (1977). The development of a contemporary eclectic theory for the training and cultivation of the junior high school male changing voice: Part I. Existing theories. *The Choral Journal, 18*(2), 5–14.

Cooper, I., & Kuersteiner, K. O. (1970). *Teaching junior high school music* (2nd ed.). Boston: Allyn & Bacon.

Cooper, M. (1973). *Modern techniques of vocal rehabilitation.* Springfield, IL: Thomas.

Cooper, M. (1977). Direct vocal rehabilitation. In M. Cooper & M. H. Cooper (Eds.), *Approaches to vocal rehabilitation* (pp. 22–42). Springfield, IL: Thomas.

Cooper, M. (1984). *Change your voice, change your life.* New York: Noble Books.

Coopersmith, S. (1967). *The antecedents of self-esteem.* San Francisco: W. H. Freeman.

Cotton, R. T. (1990). Management and treatment of subglottic stenosis in infants and children. In C. Bluestone & S. S. Stool (Eds.), *Pediatric otolaryngology* (pp. 1194–1204). Philadelphia: W. B. Saunders.

Covey, S. R. (1989). *The seven habits of highly effective people.* New York: A Fireside Book.

Crystal, D. (1981). *Clinical linguistics.* New York: Springer-Verlag.

Curry, E. (1940). The pitch characteristics of the adolescent male voice. *Speech Monographs, 7,* 48–62.

Curry, E. (1949). Hoarseness and voice change in male adolescents. *Journal of Speech and Hearing Disorders, 16,* 23–24.

Dalton, K. (1977). *Premenstrual syndrome and progesterone therapy.* Chicago: Year Book.

Dalton, K. (1979). *Once a month.* Pomona, CA: Hunter House.

Daniels, A. C. (2000). *Bringing out the best in people: How to apply the astonishing power of positive reinforcement.* New York: McGraw-Hill.

Darley, F. L. (1965). *Diagnosis and appraisal of communication disorders.* Englewood Cliffs, NJ: Prentice Hall.

Darwin, C. (1872). *The expression of emotions in man and animals.* London: Murray.

Davitz, J. R. (Ed.). (1964). *The communication of emotional meaning.* New York: McGraw-Hill.

Deal, R. E., McClain, B., & Sudderth, J. F. (1976). Identification, evaluation therapy and follow-up for children with vocal nodules in a public school setting. *Journal of Speech and Hearing Disorders, 41,* 390–397.

Dejonckere, P. H. (1999). Voice problems in children: Pathogenesis and diagnosis. *International Journal of Pediatric Oto-Rhino-Laryngology, 32* (Suppl. 1), 5311–5314.

DeVito, J. A. (1980). *The interpersonal communication book* (2nd ed.). New York: Harper & Row.

DeWeese, D. D., & Saunders, W. H. (1973). *Textbook of otolaryngology* (4th ed.). St. Louis, MO: C. V. Mosby.

Diehl, C. F., & Stinnett, C. D. (1959). Efficiency of teacher referrals in a school speech testing program. *Journal of Speech and Hearing Disorders, 24,* 34–36.

Dobres, R., Lee, L., Stemple, J. C., Kummer, A. W., & Kretschmer, L. W. (1990). Description of laryngeal pathologies in children evaluated by otolaryngologists. *Language, Speech and Hearing Services in Schools, 27,* 282–291.

Dobson, J. (1984). *Preparing for adolescence.* New York: Bantam.

Dodge, K. A. (1981, April). *Attributional bias in aggressive children.* Paper presented at the biennial meeting of the Society for Research in Child Development, Boston.

Dodge, K. A., Coie, J. D., & Brakke, N. P. (1982). Behavior patterns of socially rejected and neglected preadolescents: The roles of social approach and aggression. *Journal of Abnormal Child Psychology, 10,* 389–409.

Dodge, K. A., Schlundt, D. G., Delagach, J. S., & Schocken, I. (1982, November). *Multivariate information theory analysis of children's peer group entry behavior.* Paper delivered at the annual meeting of the Association for the Advancement of Behavior Therapy, Los Angeles.

Douvan, E., & Adelson, J. (1966). *The adolescent experience.* New York: Wiley.

Dow, S. P., Sonies, B. C., Scheib, D., Moss, S. E., & Leonard, H. L. (1995). Practical guidelines for the assessment and treatment of selective mutism. *Journal of the American Academy of Child and Adolescent Psychiatry, 34,* 836–846.

Drudge, M. K., & Phillips, B. J. (1976). Shaping behavior in voice therapy. *Journal of Speech and Hearing Disorders, 41,* 398–411.

Duffy, R. (1970). Fundamental frequency characteristics of adolescent females. *Language and Speech, 13,* 14–24.

Eckel, F., & Boone, D. (1981). The s/z ratio as an indication of laryngeal pathology. *Journal of Speech and Hearing Disorders, 46,* 147–149.

Edelman, N. H. (1997). *The American Lung Association's family guide to asthma and allergies.* Boston: Little, Brown.

Eguchi, S., & Hirsh, U. (1969). Development of speech sounds in children. *Acta Otolaryngologica, 257*(Suppl.), 543.

Eklund, S. J. (1967). A comparison of behavior modification and traditional evocative therapies. *Peabody Papers in Human Development, 5*(2).

Ekman, P., & Oster, H. (1979). Facial expression of emotion. *Annual Review of Psychology, 30,* 527–554.

Ekstrom, R. C. (1959). *Comparison of the male voice before, during and after mutation.* Unpublished doctoral dissertation, University of Southern California, Los Angeles.

Engleman, S. G., & Turnage-Carrier, C. (1997). Tolerance of the Passy-Muir speaking valve in infants and children less than 2 years of age. *Pediatric Nursing, 23,* 571–575.

Espenschade, A. I., & Eckert, H. (1967). *Motor development.* Columbus, OH: Merrill.

Fairbanks, G., Herbert, E., & Hammond, J. (1949). An acoustical study of vocal pitch in seven- and eight-year-old girls. *Child Development, 20,* 71–78.

Fairbanks, G., Wiley, J., & Lassman, F. (1949). An acoustical study of vocal pitch in seven- and eight-year-old boys. *Child Development, 20,* 63–69.

Fay, J., & Flerchinger, B. J. (1982). *Top secret.* Renton, WA: King County Rape Relief.

Fellows, J. D. (1976). The speech pathologist in the high school setting. *Language, Speech and Hearing Services in Schools, 7,* 61–63.

Ferrand, C. T. (2000). Harmonics-to-noise ratios in normally speaking prepubescent girls and boys. *Journal of Voice, 14,* 17–21.

Fisher, H. B. (1975). *Improving voice and articulation* (2nd ed.). Boston: Houghton Mifflin.

Fixsen, D., Phillips, E. L., Baron, R., Coughlin, D., Daly, D., & Daly, P. (1978). The Boys Town revolution. *Human Nature, 1*(11), 54–61.

Flach, M., Schwickardi, H., & Simon, R. (1969). What influence do menstruation and pregnancy have on the trained singing voice? *Folia Phoniatrica, 21,* 199–205.

Flynn, P. (1978). Effective clinical interviewing. *Language, Speech and Hearing Services in Schools, 9,* 265–271.

Flynn, P. T. (1983). Speech-language pathologists and primary prevention: From ideas to action. *Language, Speech and Hearing Services in Schools, 2,* 99–104.

Flynn, P., Andrews, M. L., & Cabot, B. (1990). *Using your voice wisely and well.* Tucson, AZ: Communication Skill Builders.

Fonagy, I. (1981). Emotions, voice and music. In *Research aspects on singing.* Published by the Royal Swedish Academy of Music, No. 33.

Forner, L. L., & Hixon, T. J. (1977). Respiratory kinematics in profoundly hearing-impaired speakers. *Journal of Speech and Hearing Research, 20,* 373–408.

Fox, D. R. (1978). Evaluation of voice problems. In S. Singh & J. Lynch (Eds.), *Diagnostic procedures in hearing, language and speech* (pp. 485–527). Baltimore: University Park Press.

Frable, M. S. (1972). Hoarseness, a symptom of premenstrual tension. *Archives of Otolaryngology, 75,* 66–67.

Frances, S. J. (1979). Sex-differences in nonverbal behavior. *Sex Roles, 5,* 519–535.

Frassinelli, L., Superior, K., & Meyers, J. (1983). A consultation model for speech and language intervention. *ASHA, 25,* 25–30.

Frazier, C. A. (1978). *Parent's guide to allergy in children.* New York: Grossett and Dunlap.

Freeman, S. R., & Garstecki, D. C. (1973). Child directed therapy for a nonorganic voice disorder: A case study. *Language, Speech and Hearing Services in Schools, 4,* 8–12.

Froy, M. (1978). *The prolongation of /s/ and /z/ by preschool children.* Unpublished master's thesis, Indiana University, Bloomington.

Friesen, J. H. (1972). *Vocal mutation in the adolescent male: Its chronology and a comparison with fluctuations in musical interest.* Unpublished doctoral dissertation, University of Oregon.

Frisch, R. E. (1972). Weight at menarche: Similarity for well-nourished and under-nourished girls at differing ages, and evidence for historical constancy. *Pediatrics, 50,* 445–450.

Frisch, R. E. (1978). Critical weights, a critical body composition, menarche and the maintenance of menstrual cycles. In *Biosocial interrelation in population adaptation.* The Hague, Netherlands: Mouton.

Frisch, R. E., & Revelle, R. (1970). Height and weight at menarche and a hypothesis of critical body weights and adolescent events. *Science, 169,* 397–399.

Frisch, R. E., & Revelle, R. (1971a). Height and weight of girls and boys at the time of initiation of the adolescent growth spurt in height and weight and the relationship to menarche. *Human Biology, 43,* 140–159.

Frisch, R. E., & Revelle, R. (1971b). Height and weight at menarche and a hypothesis of menarche. *Archives of Disease in Children, 46,* 695–701.

Frisch, R. E., Revelle, R., & Cook, S. (1973). Components of the critical weight at menarche and at initiation of the adolescent growth spurt: Estimated total water, lean body mass and fat. *Human Biology, 45,* 469–483.

Fuller, C. W. (1970). Differential diagnosis. In F. S. Berg & S. G. Fletcher (Eds.), *The hard of hearing child: Clinical and educational management* (pp. 203–215). New York: Grune & Stratton.

Gay, T., Hirose, H., Strome, M., & Sawashima, M. (1972). Electromyography of the intrinsic laryngeal muscles during phonation. *Annals of Otology, Rhinology and Laryngology, 81,* 401–409.

Geist, R., & Tallett, S. E. (1990). Diagnosis and management of psychogenic stridor caused by a conversion disorder. *Pediatrics, 86,* 315–317.

Gentile, R. D., Miller, R. H., & Woodson, G. E. (1986). Vocal cord paralysis in children one year of age and younger. *Annals of Otology, Rhinology and Laryngology, 95*, 622–625.

Giddan, J. J. (1991a). Communication issues in attention deficit hyperactivity disorder. *Child Psychiatry and Human Development, 22*, 45–51.

Giddan, J. J. (1991b). School children with emotional problems and communication deficits: Implications for speech-language pathologists. *Language, Speech and Hearing Services in Schools, 22*, 291–295.

Giddan, J. J., Bade, K. M., Rickenberg, D., & Ryley, A. T. (1995). Teaching the language of feelings to students with severe emotional and behavioral handicaps. *Language, Speech and Hearing Services in Schools, 26*, 3–10.

Giddan, J. J., Ross, G. J., Sechler, L. L., & Becker, B. R. (1997). Selective mutism in elementary school: Multidisciplinary interventions. *Language, Speech and Hearing Services in Schools, 28*, 127–133.

Giddan, J. J., Trautman, R. C., & Hurst, J. B. (1989). The role of speech and language clinician on a multidisciplinary team. *Child Psychiatry and Human Development, 19*, 190–195.

Glaze, L. (1996). Treatment of voice hyperfunction in the pre-adolescent. *Language, Speech and Hearing Services in Schools, 27*, 244–250.

Glaze, L. E., Bless, D. M., Milenkovic, P., & Sasser, R. D. (1988). Acoustic characteristics of children's voices. *Journal of Voice, 2*, 312–319.

Goda, S., (1970). *Articulation therapy and consonant drillbook.* New York: Grune & Stratton.

Gold, S. M., Gerber, M. E., Shott, S. R., III, & Myer, C. M. (1997). Blunt laryngotrauma in children. *Archives of Otolaryngology–Head and Neck Surgery, 123*, 83–87.

Goldfarb, W. (1961). *Childhood schizophrenia.* Cambridge, MA: Harvard University Press.

Goldfarb, W., Braunstein, P., & Lorge, I. (1976). A study of speech patterns in a group of schizophrenic children. *American Journal of Orthopsychiatry, 56*, 544–555.

Goldstein, M. N., & Abramson, A. L. (1983, December). *Airway obstruction in the lung due to allergy: Uncommon pediatric problem.* Paper presented at the annual meeting of SENTAC, San Diego, CA.

Goleman, D. (1995). *Emotional intelligence.* New York: Bantam Books.

Goleman, D. (1997). *Working with emotional intelligience.* New York: Bantam Books.

Gracco, C., Jones-Bryant, N., Fahey, J., DeStephens, R., & Naito, W. (1995, June). *Videoendoscopic and cardiopulmonary measures of exercise induced upper airway dysfunction.* Paper presented at the 25th Symposium of the Voice Foundation: Care of the Professional Voice, Philadelphia.

Gray, S. D., Hammond, E., & Hanson, D. F. (1995). Benign pathologic responses of the larynx. *Annals of Otology, Rhinology and Laryngology, 104*, 13–18.

Gray, S. D., & Smith, M. E. (1996). Voice disorders in children. *NCVS Status and Progress Report, 10*, 133–150.

Gray, S., Smith, M., & Schneider, H. (1996). Voice disorders in children. *Pediatric Otolaryngology, Pediatric Clinics of North America, 43*, 1357–1384.

Green, G. (1989). Psycho-behavioral characteristics of children with vocal nodules: WPBIC ratings. *Journal of Speech and Hearing Disorders, 54*, 306–312.

Greenberg, J. H. (1966). *Language universals.* The Hague, Netherlands: Mouton.

Greene, M. C. L. (1972). *The voice and its disorders.* (3rd ed.). New York: Pitman.

Gregory, H. H. (1986). The clinician's attitudes. In *Counseling Stutterers* (No. 18, pp. 9–17). Memphis, TN: Speech Foundation of America.

Grey, P. (1973). Microlaryngostroboscopy and "singer's nodes." *Journal of the Otolaryngology Society of Australia, 3*, 525–527.

Grinder, R. E. (1973). *Adolescence.* New York: Wiley.

Groden, J. (1989). *High anxiety: The need for focusing on stress and anxiety in people with developmental disabilities.* Paper presented at the convention of the Association for Persons with Severe Handicaps, San Francisco, CA.

Gumpert, L., Kalach, N., Dupont, C., & Contencin, R. (1998). Hoarseness and gastroesophageal reflux in children. *Journal of Laryngology and Otolaryngology, 112*(1), 49–54.

Gurian, M. (1999). The moral reader. *Christian Science Monitor, 91*(222), 14.

Hacki, T., & Heitmuller, S. (1999). Development of the child's voice: Premutation, mutation. *International Journal of Pediatric Otorhinolaryngology, 49*(Suppl. 1), S141–S144.

Hamachek, D. E. (1978). *Encounters with the self* (2nd ed.). New York: Holt, Rinehart & Winston.

Handler, S. D., & Wetmore, R. (1982). Otolaryngologic injuries. *Clinical Sports Medicine, 1*, 431–447.

Hanley, T. D., & Thurman, W. L. (1970). *Developing vocal skills* (2nd ed.). New York: Holt, Rinehart & Winston.

Harris, P. L., Olthof, T., & Terwogt, M. (1981). Children's knowledge of emotion. *Child Psychology and Psychiatry, 33*, 247–261.

Harrison, H. (1983). *The premature baby book.* New York: St. Martin's Press.

Harrison, M. (1982). *Self-help for premenstrual syndrome.* Cambridge, MA: Matrix Press.

Harvey, G. L. (1996). Treatment of voice disorders in medically complex children. *Language, Speech and Hearing Services in Schools, 27*, 282–291.

Harvey, P. L. (1979). The young adult patient. *Journal of Voice, 11*, 144–152.

Hasek, C., Singh, S., & Murry, T. (1980). Acoustic attributes of preadolescent voices. *Journal of the Acoustical Society of America, 68*, 1262–1265.

Haskell, J. A. (1987). Vocal self-perception: The other side of the equation. *Journal of Voice, 1*, 172–179.

Hately, B. W., Evison, G., & Samuel, E. (1965). The pattern of ossification in the laryneal cartilages: A radiological study. *British Journal of Radiology, 38*, 585–591.

Hayden, T. L. (1980). Classification of elective mutism. *Journal of the American Academy of Child Psychiatry, 19*, 118–133.

Helmi, A. M., El-Ghazzawi, I. F., Mandour, M., & Shehata, M. A. (1975). The effect of estrogen on the nasal respiratory mucosa. *Journal of Laryngology and Otology, 89*, 1229–1241.

Henry, D. P., Pashley, N. R. T., & Fan, L. (1983, December). *Anticipation of laryngeal injury incurred by an endotracheal tube in children.* Paper presented at the annual meeting of SENTAC, San Diego, CA.

Herman-Giddens, M. E., Slora, E. J., Wasserman, R. C., Bourdony, C. J., Bhapkar, M. V., Koch, G. G., & Hasemeier, C. M. (1997). Secondary sexual characteristics and menses in young girls seen in office practice: A study from the Pediatric Research in Office Settings Network. *Pediatrics, 98*, 505–512.

Hershenson, M. (1992). The respiratory muscles and chest wall. In R. Beckermann, R. Brouillette, & C. Hunt (Eds.), *Respiratory control in infants and children* (pp. 28–46), Baltimore: Williams & Wilkins.

Herzel, H., & Reuter, R. (1997). Whistle register and biphonation in a child's voice. *Folia Phoniatrica, 49*, 216–224.

Hesselman, S. (1983). Elective mutism in children 1977–1981. A literary summary. *Acta Paedopsychiatrica, 49*, 297–310.

Heymans, H. S. A. (1996). Current recommendations for the management of gastro-esphageal reflux in children. In G. Pons & C. Dupont (Eds.), *Les medicaments du RGO et de l'infection à helicokacter pylori chez l'enfant* (pp. 75–85). Paris: Springer-Verlag.

Hirano, M. (1974). Morphological structure of the vocal cord as a vibrator and its variations. *Folia Phoniatrica, 26*, 89–94.

Hirano, M. (1981). Structure of the vocal fold in normal and disease states: Anatomical and physical studies. In C. L. Ludlow & M. O. C. Hart (Eds.), *Proceedings of the Conference on the Assessment of Vocal Pathology: Report II.* Rockville, MD: American Speech and Hearing Association.

Hirano, M., Kurita, S., & Nasashima, T. (1981). The structure of the vocal folds. In *Vocal fold physiology* (pp. 33–44). Tokyo: University of Tokyo Press.

Hlastala, M. P., & Berger, A. J. (1996). *Physiology of respiration.* New York: Oxford University Press.

Holinger, P. H., & Brown, W. T. (1967). Congenital webs, cysts, laryngoceles and other anomalies of the larynx. *Annals of Otolaryngology, Rhinology and Laryngology, 76*, 1967.

Hollien, H., & Malcik, E. (1962, March). Adolescent voice changes in southern Negro males. *Speech Monographs, 29*, 53–58.

Hollien, H., & Malcik, E. (1967). Evaluation of cross-sectional studies of adolescent voice change in males. *Speech Monographs, 32*, 87–90.

Hollien, H., Malcik, E., & Hollien, B. (1965). Adolescent voice changes in southern White males. *Speech Monographs, 32*, 87–90.

Homer, E. M. (2000). Scheduling and collaborative planning. In E. P. Dodge (Ed.), *The survival guide for school-based speech-language pathologists.* San Diego, CA: Delmar Cengage Learning.

Hood, L., & Bloom, L. (1979). What, when and how about why: A longitudinal study of early expressions of causality. *Monographs of the Society for Research in Child Development, 44* (6, Serial No. 181).

Hu, F. Z., Preston, R. A., Post, J. C., White, G. J., Kikuchi, L. W., Wang, X., Leal, S. M., Levenstien, M. A., Oh, J., Self, T. W., Allen, G., Stiffler, R. S., McGraw, C., Pulsifer-Anderson, E. A., & Ehrlich, G. D. (2000). Mapping of a gene for severe pediatric gastroesophageal reflux to chromosome 13q14., *JAMA, 284*(3), 325–334.

Huang, S. W., & Kimbrough, J. W. (1997). Mold allergy is a risk factor for persistent cold-like symptoms in children. *Clinical Pediatrics, 36,* 695–699.

Inhelder, B., & Piaget, J. (1964). *Early growth of logic in the child: Classification and seriation.* New York: Harper & Row.

Isshiki, H. (1964). Regulatory mechanism of voice intensity variation. *Journal of Speech and Hearing Research, 7,* 17–29.

Itoh, M., Horii, Y., Daniloff, R. G., & Binnie, C. A. (1982). Selected aerodynamic characteristics of deaf individuals during various speech and nonspeech tasks. *Folia Phoniatrica, 34,* 191–209.

Jeffrey, W. E. (1958). Variables in early discrimination learning: 11. Mode of response and stimulus difference in the discrimination of tonal frequencies, *Child Development, 29,* 531–538.

Jensen, P. (1964). Hoarseness in cheerleaders, *ASHA, 6,* 406.

Jerome, J. (1980). *The sweet spot in time* (pp. 242–264). New York: Summit Books.

Jones, D., Austin, C., MacLean, D., & Warkomski, R. (1973). Task force report on traditional scheduling procedures in schools. *Language, Speech and Hearing Services in Schools, 4,* 100–109.

Jones, M. C. (1958). A study of socialization patterns at the high school level. *Journal of Genetic Psychology, 93,* 87–111.

Jones, M. C. (1965). Psychological correlates of somatic development. *Child Development, 36,* 899–911.

Jones, M. C., & Bayley, N. (1950). Physical maturing among boys as related to behavior. *Journal of Educational Psychology, 41,* 129–148.

Jones, M. C., & Mussen, P. H. (1958). Self-conceptions, motivations, and interpersonal attitudes of early and late maturing girls. *Child Development, 29,* 491–501.

Jones, M. M. (1983, August). Premenstrual syndrome: Part 1. *British Journal of Sexual Medicine, 10,* 9–11.

Joseph, L., & Mills, A. (1983). *A doctor discusses allergy: Fact and fiction.* Chicago: Budlong.

Joseph, W. (1963). Vocal growth in the human adolescent and the total growth process. *Journal of Music Education, 13,* 135.

Josselyn, I. M. (1962). *The adolescent and his world.* New York: Family Service Association of America.

Judson, L. S. V., & Weaver, A. T. (1965). *Voice science* (2nd ed.). New York: Appleton-Century-Crofts.

Kagan, J. (1971). A conception of early adolescence. *Daedalus, 100,* 997–1012.

Kahane, J. C. (1975). *The developmental anatomy of the human prepubertal and pubertal larynx.* Unpublished doctoral dissertation, University of Pittsburgh.

Kahane, J. C. (1978). A morphological study of the human prepubertal and pubertal larynx. *American Journal of Anatomy, 151,* 11–20.

Kahane, J. C. (1980). Age related histological changes in the human male and female laryngeal cartilages: Biological and functional implications. In V. Lawrence (Ed.), *Transcripts of the Ninth Symposium: Care of the Professional Voice, Part I* (pp. 11–20). New York: Voice Foundation.

Kahane, J. C. (1982). Growth and development of the human prepubertal and pubertal larynx. *Journal of Speech and Hearing Research, 25,* 446–455.

Kahane, J. C. (1983). Age related changes in the elastic fibres of the adult male vocal ligament. In V. Lawrence (Ed.), *Transcripts of the Eleventh Symposium: Care of the Professional Voice.* New York: The Voice Foundation.

Kahane, J. C. (1983). Postnatal development and aging of the human larynx. *Seminars in Speech and Language, 4,* 189–203.

Kahane, J. C. (1996). Life span changes in the larynx: An anatomical perspective. In W. S. Brown, B. P. Vinson, & M. A. Crary (Eds.), *Organic voice disorders: Assessment and treatment* (pp. 89–106). San Diego, CA: Singular Publishing Group.

Kahane, J. C., & Mayo, R. (1989). The need for aggressive pursuit of healthy childhood voices.

Language, Speech and Hearing Services in Schools, 20, 102–107.

Kalb, C. (2000, May 8). Unhealthy habits. *Newsweek*, 66–68.

Kamel, P. L., Hanson, D., & Kahrilas, P. J. (1994). Prospective trial of omeprazole in the treatment of posterior laryngitis. *American Journal of Medicine, 96*, 321–326.

Kantner, R. M. (1983). *The change masters*. London: Counterpoint, Unwin Paperbacks.

Karnell, M. P., Scherer, R. S., & Fischer, L. B. (1991). Comparison of acoustic voice perturbation measures among three independent voice laboratories. *Journal of Speech and Hearing Research, 34*, 781–90.

Kaslon, K. W., & Stein, R. E. (1985). Chronic pediatric tracheostomy: Assessment and implications for habilitation of voice, speech and language in young children. *International Journal of Pediatric Otorhinolaryngology, 76*, 744–752.

Katz, S., McDonald, J. L., & Stuckey, G. K. (1972). *Preventive dentistry in action*. Upper Montclair, NJ: D. C. P. Publishing.

Kelly, H. D. B., & Craik, J. E. (1952). Laryngeal nodes and the so-called amyloid tumour of the cords. *Journal of Laryngology and Otolaryngology, 66*, 339–358.

Kent, R. (1976). Anatomic and neuromuscular maturation of the speech mechanism: Evidence from acoustic studies. *Journal of Speech and Hearing Research, 19*, 421–447.

Kereiakes, T. J. (1996). Clinical evaluation and treatment of vocal disorders. *Language, Speech and Hearing Services in Schools, 27*, 240–243.

Kero, P., Puhakka, H., Erkinjuntti, M., Iisalo, E., & Vilkki, P. (1983). Foreign body in the airways of children. *International Journal of Pediatric Otorhinolaryngology 6*, 51–59.

Kiell, N. (1964). *The universal experience of adolescence*. Boston: Beacon Press.

Klingholz, F., & Martin, F. (1985). Quantitative spectral evaluation of jitter and shimmer. *Journal of Speech and Hearing Research, 28*, 169–74.

Klock, L. E., Jr. (1968). *The growth and development of the human larynx from birth to adolescence*. Unpublished master's thesis, University of Washington School of Medicine, Seattle.

Knorr, D., Bidlingmaier, O., Butenandt, H. F., & Ehrt-Wehle, R. (1974). Plasma testosterone in male puberty. *Acta Endocrinologia, 75*, 181–194.

Kohlberg, L. (1975). Moral development in the schools: A developmental view. In R. E. Grinder (Ed.), *Studies in adolescence* (3rd ed.). New York: Macmillan.

Kolbenschlag, M. (1981). *Kiss Sleeping Beauty goodbye*. New York: Bantam.

Kolvin, I., & Fundudis, T. (1981). Elective mute children: Psychological development and background factors. *Journal of Child Psychology and Psychiatry, 22*, 219–232.

Koufman, J. A. (1991). The otolaryngologic manifestations of gastroesophageal reflux disease (GERD). *Laryngoscope, 101*(Suppl. 53), 1–78.

Koufman, J. A. (1995). Gastroesophageal reflux and voice disorders. In J. S. Rubin, R. T. Sataloff, G. S. Korovin, & W. G. Gould (Eds.), *Diagnosis and treatment of voice disorders* (pp. 161–175). New York: Igaku-Shoin.

Kreiman, J., & Gerratt, B. R. (1996). The perceptual structure of pathologic voice quality. *Journal of the Acoustical Society of America, 100*, 1787–1795.

Krohn, D. D., Weckstein, S. M., & Wright, H. L. (1992). A study of the effectiveness of a specific treatment for elective mutism. *Journal of the American Academy of Child and Adolescent Psychiatry, 31*, 711–718.

Kronberg, J., Tyano, S., Apter, A., & Wijsenbeck, H. (1981). Treatment of transsexualism in adolescence. *Journal of Adolescence, 4*, 177–185.

Kruttschnitt, C., McLeod, J., & Dornfeld, M. (1994). The economic environment of child abuse. *Social Problems, 41*, 299–315.

Kubler-Ross, E. (1969). *On death and dying*. New York: Macmillan.

Kulin, H. E., Grumbach, M. M., & Kaplan, S. L. (1972). Gonadal-hypothalamic interaction in prepubertal and pubertal man: Effect of clomisphene citrate on urinary follicle-stimulating hormone and luteinizing hormone and plasma testosterone. *Pediatric Research, 6*, 162–171.

Kummer, A. W., & Lee, L. (1996). Evaluation and treatment of resonance disorders. *Language, Speech and Hearing Services in Schools, 27*, 271–281.

Kuppersmith, R., Rosen, D. S., & Wiatrak, B. J. (1993). Functional stridor in adolescents. *Journal of Adolescent Health, 14*, 166–171.

Kussmaul, A. (1877). *Die Stoerungen der Sprache* [Disturbances in linguistic function] (p. 21). Basel, Switzerland: Benno Schwabe.

Labbe, E. E., & Williamson, D. A. (1984). Behavioral treatment of elective mutism: A review of the literature. *Clinical Psychology Review, 4,* 273–292.

Large, J., & Patton, R. (1979). The effects of weight training and aerobic exercise on singers. *Transcripts of the Eighth Symposium: Care of the Professional Voice* (Vol. 1, pp. 29–35). New York: The Voice Foundation.

Laughlin, H. P. (1970). *The ego and its defences.* New York: Appleton-Century-Crofts.

Launer, P. G. (1971). *Maximum phonation time in children.* Unpublished master's thesis, State University of New York at Buffalo.

Laupus, W. E., & Pastore, P. N. (1967). The larynx. In E. L. Kendig, Jr. (Ed.), *Disorders of the respiratory tract in children* (pp. 204–212). Philadelphia: W. B. Saunders.

Laver, J. (1980). *The phonetic description of voice quality.* New York: Cambridge University Press.

Lazarus, R. S. (1968). Emotions and adaptation: Conceptual and empirical relations. In W. J. Arnold (Ed.), *Nebraska symposium on motivation.* Lincoln: University of Nebraska.

Lazarus, R. S. (1975). The self-regulation of emotions. In L. Levi (Ed.), *Emotions—their parameters and measurement.* New York: Raven Press.

Lebrun, Y. (1990). *Mutism.* London: Whurr.

Leff, A. R., & Schumacker, P. T. (1993). *Respiratory physiology: Basics and applications.* Philadelphia: W. B. Saunders.

Lehiste, I. (1976). Suprasegmental features of speech. In N. J. Lass (Ed.), *Contemporary issues in experimental phonetics.* New York: Academic Press.

Leinonen, L., & Poppius, H. (1997). Voice reactions to histamine inhalation in asthma. *Allergy, 52,* 27–31.

Leonard, H. L., & Topol, D. A. (1993). Elective mutism. In H. L. Leonard (Ed.), *Child and adolescent psychiatric clinics of North America: Anxiety disorders* (pp. 695–708). Philadelphia: W. B. Saunders.

Lerman, J. W., & Damste, P. H. (1969). Voice pitch of homosexuals. *Folia Phoniatrica, 21,* 340–346.

Lesser-Katz, M. (1986). Stranger reaction and elective mutism in young children. *American Journal of Orthopsychiatry, 56,* 458–469.

Lewis, J. R., Andreassen, M. L., Leeper, H. A., Macrae, D. L., & Thomas, J. (1993). Vocal characteristics of children with cleft lip/palate and associated velopharyngeal incompetence. *Journal of Otolaryngology, 22,* 113–117.

Lieberman, P. (1975). *Intonation, perception and language.* (Research Monograph No. 38, 3rd ed.). Cambridge, MA: MIT Press.

Ling, D. (1975). Amplification for speech. In D. R. Calvert & S. R. Silverman (Eds.), *Speech and deafness* (pp. 64–88). Washington, DC: Alexander Graham Bell Association for the Deaf.

Ling, D. (1976). *Speech and the hearing-impaired child: Theory and practice.* Washington, DC: Alexander Graham Bell Association for the Deaf.

Logemann, J. A., & O'Toole, T. J. (2000). Identification and management of dysphagia in the public schools: Prologue to LSHSS clinical forum. *Language, Speech and Hearing Services in Schools, 31,* 26.

Luchsinger, R., & Arnold, G. E. (1965). *Voice-speech-language. Clinical communicology: Its physiology and pathology.* (G. E. Arnold & E. R. Finkbeiner, Trans.). Belmont, CA: Wadsworth.

Lundy, D. S., Casiano, R. R., Shatz, D., Reisberg, M., & Xue, J. W. (1998). Laryngeal injuries after short- versus long-term intubation. *Journal of Voice, 12,* 360–365.

Lyons, J. (1963). *Structural semantics.* Oxford, England: Blackwell.

MacArthur, C. J., & Healy, G. B. (1995). Acquired voice disorders in the pediatric population. In J. S. Rubin, R. T. Sataloff, G. S. Korovin, & W. J. Gould (Eds.), *Diagnosis and treatment of voice disorders.* New York: Igaku-Shoin.

Maccoby, E., & Jacklin, C. N. (1974). *The psychology of sex differences.* Stanford, CA: Stanford University Press.

Mallick, S. K., & McCandless, B. R. (1966). A study of catharsis aggression. *Journal of Personality and Social Psychology, 4,* 591–596.

Marshall, W. A., & Tanner, J. M. (1969). Variations in the pattern of pubertal changes in girls. *Archives of Disease in Children, 45,* 291–303.

Marshall, W. A., & Tanner, J. M. (1970). Variations in the pattern of pubertal changes in boys. *Archives of Disease in Childhood, 45,* 13–23.

Martin, R. J., Blager, F. B., Gay, M. L., & Wood, R. P. (1987). Paradoxic vocal cord motion in presumed asthmatics. *Seminars in Respiratory Medicine, 8,* 332–337.

Mason, M., Jerome-Ebel, A., & Romey, P. (1994). *Voicing! Communication approaches for tracheostomized and ventilator dependent patients.* Newport Beach, CA: Voicing! Inc.

Masuda, T., Ikeda, Y., Manako, H., & Komiyama, S. (1993). Analysis of vocal abuse: Fluctuations in phonation time and intensity in 4 groups of speakers. *Acta Otolaryngologica, 113,* 547–552.

McAllister, A., Sederholm, E., Sundberg, J., & Gramming, P. (1994). Relations between voice range profiles and physiological and perceptual voice characteristics in ten-year-old children. *Journal of Voice, 8,* 230–239.

McAllister, A., Sederholm, E., Ternstrom, S., & Sundberg, J. (1996). Perturbaton and hoarseness: A pilot study of six children's voices. *Journal of Voice, 10,* 252–261.

McCandless, B. R., & Coop, R. H. (1979). *Adolescents: Behavior and development* (2nd ed.). New York: Holt, Rinehart & Winston.

McDonald, T., & Chance, B. (1964). *Cerebral palsy.* Englewood Cliffs, NJ: Prentice Hall.

McFall, R. M., & Dodge, K. A. (1982). Self-management and interpersonal skills learning. In P. Karoly & F. H. Kanfer (Eds.), *Self-management and behavior change.* Elmsford, NY: Pergamon.

McGlone, R. E., & Hollien, H. (1963). Vocal pitch characteristics of aged women. *Journal of Speech and Hearing Research, 6,* 164–167.

McKenzie, D. (1956). *Training the boy's changing voice.* New Brunswick, NJ: Rutgers University Press.

McKinley, N. L., & Lord-Larsen, V. (1985). Neglected language-disordered adolescent: A delivery model. *Language, Speech and Hearing Services in Schools, 16,* 2–15.

McLeod, J. D., & Shanahan, M. J. (1996). Trajectories of poverty and children's mental health. *Journal of Health and Social Behavior, 37,* 207–220.

McMahon, O. (1961, May). Exploring music with children. *Australian Pre-school Quarterly, 1,* 10–15.

McNamara, A. P., & Perry, C. K. (1994). Vocal abuse prevention practices: A national survey of school-based speech language pathologists. *Language, Speech and Hearing Services in Schools, 25,* 105–111.

Merritt, R., Bent, J., & Porubsky, E. (1998). Acute laryngeal trauma in the pediatric patient. *Annals of Otology, Rhinology and Laryngology, 107,* 104–107.

Michel, J. F., & Tait, N. (1977, November). *Maximum duration of sustained /s/ and /z/.* Paper presented at annual convention of the American Speech and Hearing Association, Chicago, IL.

Miller, D. (1974). *Adolescence: Psychology, psychopathology and psycho-therapy.* New York: Jason Aronson.

Miller, G. A., Galanter, E., & Pribram, K. H. (1960). *Plans and the structure of behavior.* New York: Holt, Rinehart & Winston.

Mischel, W. (1970). Sex-typing and socialization. In P. H. Mussen (Ed.), *Carmichael's manual of child psychology* (Vol. 2, 3rd ed., pp. 3–72). New York: John Wiley.

Moncur, J. P., & Brackett, I. P. (1974). *Modifying vocal behavior.* New York: Harper & Row.

Money, J., & Clopper, R. R., Jr. (1974). Psychosocial and psychosexual aspects of errors of prepubertal onset and development. *Human Biology, 46,* 173–181.

Montague, J. C., & Hollien, H. (1973). Perceived voice quality disorders in Down's syndrome children. *Journal of Communication Disorders, 6,* 76–87.

Moore, G. P. (1971a). *Organic voice disorders.* Englewood Cliffs, NJ: Prentice Hall.

Moore, G. P. (1971b). Voice disorders organically based. In L. E. Travis (Ed.), *Handbook of speech pathology and audiology* (pp. 535–570). New York: Appleton-Century-Crofts.

Morris, H. L., Spriesterbach, D. C., & Darley, F. L. (1961). An articulation test for assessing competency of velopharyngeal closure. *Journal of Speech and Hearing Research, 4,* 48–55.

Morris, R. J. (1997). Speaking fundamental frequency characteristics of 8- through 10-year-old White and African-American boys. *Journal of Communication Disorders, 30,* 101–116.

Morris, S., & Dunn Klein, M. (1987). *Prefeeding skills.* Tucson, AZ: Therapy Skill Builders.

Mowrer, D. (1978). Speech problems: What you should and shouldn't do. *Learning, 6,* 34–37.

Murray, D. M., & Lawler, P. G. (1998). Case report: All that wheezes is not asthma: Paradoxical vocal cord movement presenting as severe acute asthma requiring ventilatory support. *Anaesthesia, 53,* 1006–1111.

Mussen, P. H., & Jones, M. C. (1957). Self-conceptions, motivations and interpersonal attitudes of late- and early-maturing boys. *Child Development, 28,* 243–256.

Muuss, R. E. (1975). *Theories of adolescence* (3rd ed.). New York: Random House.

Myer, C. M., Orobello, P., Cotton, R. T., & Bratcher, G. O. (1987). Blunt laryngeal trauma in children. *Laryngoscope, 97,* 1043–1048.

Mysak, E. D. (1971). Cerebral palsy speech syndromes. In L. E. Travis (Ed.), *Handbook of speech pathology and audiology* (pp. 673–695). New York: Appleton-Century-Crofts.

Mysak, E. D. (1980). *Neurospeech therapy for the cerebral palsied: A neuroevolutional approach* (3rd ed.). New York: Teachers College Press.

Naidr, J., Zbořil, M., & Ševšik, K. (1965). Die pubertalen veränderungen der stimme bie junger im verlauf von 5 jahren. *Folia Phoniatrica, 17,* 1–18.

Neal, W. R., Jr. (1976). Speech pathology services in secondary schools. *Language, Speech and Hearing Services in Schools, 7,* 6–16.

Neal, W. R., Jr. (1986). *Speech-language pathology services in secondary schools.* Austin, TX: Pro-Ed.

Neidecker, R. A. (1980). *School progress in speech-language: Organization and management.* Englewood Cliffs, NJ: Prentice Hall.

Neubauer, P. (Ed.). (1965). *Concepts of development in early childhood education.* Springfield, IL: Charles C. Thomas.

Nilson, H., & Schneiderman, C. R. (1983). Classroom program for the prevention of vocal abuse and hoarseness in elementary school children. *Language, Speech and Hearing Services in Schools, 14,* 121–127.

Novak, A. (1972). The voice of children with Down's syndrome. *Folia Phoniatrica, 24,* 182–194.

Nowicki, S., & Duke, M. P. (1992). *Helping the child who doesn't fit in.* Atlanta, GA: Peachtree Publishers, Ltd.

Noyce, P. W. (1983, December). *The shape of the infant sub-glottis.* Paper presented at the annual meeting of SENTAC, San Diego, CA.

O'Toole, T. J., & Zaslow, E. L. (1969). Public school speech and hearing programs: Things are changing. *ASHA, 11,* 499–501.

Osterrieth, P. A. (1969). Adolescence: Some psychological aspects. In G. Caplan & S. Lebovici (Eds.), *Adolescence: Psychosocial perspectives* (pp. 11–21). New York: Basic Books.

Pabon, J. H. P. (1991). Objective acoustic voice-quality parameters in the computer phonetogram. *Journal of Voice, 5,* 203–216.

Pannbacker, M. (1984). Classification systems of voice disorders: A review of the literature. *Language, Speech and Hearing Services in Schools, 15,* 169–174.

Papousek, M. (1989). Determinants of responsiveness to infant vocal expression of emotional state. *Infant Behavior and Development, 12,* 507–524.

Parisier, S. C., & Henneford, G. E. (1969). Surgical correction of acquired vocal cord webs. *Archives of Otolaryngology,* 90, 103–107.

Parker, E. B., Olsen, T. F., & Throckmorton, M. C. (1960). Social casework with elementary school children who do not talk in school. *Social Work, 5,* 64–70.

Pasquariello, P. S., Potsic, W. P., Miller, L., & Corso, C. (1983, December). *Nutrition in adenotonsillar hyperplasis.* Paper presented at the annual meeting of SENTAC, San Diego, CA.

Pedry, C. P. (1945). A study of voice change in boys between the ages of eleven and sixteen. *Speech Monographs, 12,* 30–36.

Pellegrini, A. D. (1982). Applying a self-regulating private speech model to classroom settings. *Language, Speech and Hearing Services in Schools, 13,* 129–133.

Peppard, R. C. (1996). Management of functional voice disorders in adolescents. *Language, Speech and Hearing Services in Schools, 27,* 257–270.

Perkins, W. H. (1977). *Speech pathology: An applied behavioral science* (2nd ed.). St. Louis, MO: C. V. Mosby.

Peters, T., & Guitar (1991). *Stuttering: An integrated approach to its nature and treatment.* Baltimore: Williams and Wilkins.

Peters-Johnson, C. (1992). Why voice problems should be considered an educational disability. *Language, Speech and Hearing Services in Schools, 23,* 189–190.

Phillips, E. L., Shenker, S., & Revitz, P. (1951). The assimilation of the new child into the group. *Psychiatry, 14,* 319–325.

Piaget, J. (1926). *Judgment and reasoning in the child.* New York: Harcourt Brace Jovanovich.

Piaget, J. (1929). *The child's conception of the world.* New York: Harcourt Brace Jovanovich.

Piaget, J. (1930). *The child's conception of physical causality.* London: Kegan Paul.

Piaget, J. (1974). Adolescence: Thought and its operation: The affectivity of the personality in the social world of adults. In Z. M. Cantwell & P. N. Svajian (Eds.), *Adolescence: Studies in development* (pp. 34–56). Itasco, IL: Peacock.

Piliavin, J. A., & Martin, R. R. (1978). Effects of sex composition in groups on style and social interaction. *Sex Roles, 4*, 281–296.

Pope, S., & Whiteside, L. (1993). Low-birth-weight infants born to adolescent mothers. *Journal of the American Medical Association, 269*, 1396–1401.

Pope, H. G., Jr., Gruber, A. J., Choi, P., Olivardia, R., & Phillips, K. A. (1997). Muscle dysmorphia: An underrecognized form of body dysmorphic disorder. *Psychosomatics, 38*, 548–557.

Powell, M., Filter, M., & Williams, B. (1989). A longitudinal study of the prevalence of voice disorders in children from a rural school division. *Journal of Communication Disorders, 22*, 375–382.

Prange, A. (1974). *The thyroid axis, drugs and behavior*. New York: Raven Press.

Prater, R. J., & Swift, R. W. (1984). *Manual of voice therapy*. Boston: Little, Brown.

Proctor, A. (1989). Stages of normal non-cry vocal development in infancy: A protocol for assessment. *Topics in Language Disorders, 10*, 26–42.

Prutting, C. A., & Connolly, J. E. (1976). Imitation: A closer look. *Journal of Speech and Hearing Disorders, 41*, 412–422.

Ptacek, P. H., & Sander, E. K. (1963). Maximum duration of phonation. *Journal of Speech and Hearing Disorders, 28*, 171.

Punt, N. A. (1967). *The singer's and actor's throat* (2nd ed.). Oxford, England: Alden Press.

Punt, N. A. (1979). *Singer's and actor's throat* (3rd ed.). New York: Drama Book Specialists.

Punt, N. A. (1983). Laryngology applied to singers and actors. *Journal of Laryngology and Otology, 97*(Suppl. 6), 1–24.

Putallaz, M., & Gottman, J. M. (1981a). Social skills and group acceptance. In S. R. Asher & J. M. Gottman (Eds.), *The development of children's friendships: Description and intervention*. New York: Cambridge University Press.

Putallaz, M., & Gottman, J. M. (1981b). An interactional model of children's entry into peer groups. *Child Development, 52*, 986–994.

Putnam, P. E., & Orenstein, S. R. (1992). Hoarseness in a child with gastroesophageal reflux. *Acta Paediatrica, 81*, 635–636.

Randolph, T., & Moss, R. (1981). *An alternative approach to allergies*. New York: Lippincott & Crowell.

Rastatter, M. P., & Hyman, M. (1984, January). Effects of selected rhinologic disorders on the perception of nasal resonance in children. *Language, Speech and Hearing Services in Schools, 15*, 44–50.

Ratto, A., Diaco, P., & Perillo, L. (1990). Epidemiological survey of dysphonia in school children. *Archives of Stomatology, 31*, 85–91.

Reed, V. A., McLeod, K., & McAllister, L. (1999). Importance of selected communication skills for talking with peers and teachers: Adolescents' opinions. *Language, Speech and Hearing Services in Schools, 30*, 32–49.

Reese, H. W. (1970). Imagery in children's learning: A symposium. *Psychological Bulletin, 73*, 404–414.

Reich, A., McHenry, M., & Keaton, A. (1986). A survey of dysphonic episodes in high school cheerleaders. *Language, Speech and Hearing Services in Schools, 17*, 63–71.

Reiter, E. O. (1981). Delayed puberty in boys. *Medical Aspects of Human Sexuality, 15*, 79–80.

Richard, B. A., & Dodge, K. A. (1982a). *Children's competence at persuasion: The relation between cognitive skills and behavioral performance*. Paper presented at the annual meeting of the Association for the Advancement of Behavior Therapy, Los Angeles.

Richard, B. A., & Dodge, K. A. (1982b). Social maladjustment and problem solving in school-aged children. *Journal of Consulting and Clinical Psychology, 50*, 226–233.

Robb, M., & Saxman, J. (1985). Developmental trends in vocal fundamental frequency of young children. *Journal of Speech and Hearing Research, 28*, 421–427.

Rogers, C. R., (1961). *On becoming a person*. Boston: Houghton-Mifflin.

Rosin, D. F., Handler, S. D., Potsic, W. P., Wetmore, R. F., & Tom, L. W. C. (1990). Vocal cord paralysis in children. *Laryngoscope, 100*, 1174–1179.

Sacks, O. (1995). *An anthropologist on Mars*. New York: Alfred A. Knopf.

Sadewitz, V. L., & Shprintzen, R. J. (1985, December). *Changes in velopharyngeal closure with age*. Paper presented at the annual meeting of SENTAC, Dallas, TX.

Sander, E. (1989). Arguments against the aggressive pursuit of voice therapy for children.

Language, Speech and Hearing Services in Schools, 20, 94–101.

Sapienza, C., & Stathopoulos, E. T. (1994). Respiratory and laryngeal measures of children and women with bilateral vocal fold nodules. *Journal of Speech and Hearing Research, 37*, 1229–1234.

Sapir, E. (1944). Grading: A study in semantics. *Philosophy of Science, 11*, 93–116.

Sataloff, R. T. (1981, August). Professional singers: The science and art of clinical care. *American Journal of Otolaryngology, 2*, 251–266.

Sataloff, R.T. (1991). *Professional voice: The science and art of clinical care.* New York: Raven Press.

Sataloff, R. T. (1995). Rational thought: The impact of voice science upon voice care. *Journal of Voice, 9*, 215–230.

Sataloff, R. T., Hawkshaw, M., Hoover, C. A., & Spiegel, J. R. (1998). Vocal fold nodule and cyst. *Ear, Nose, & Throat Journal, 77*, 728.

Satter, E. (2000). *Child of mine: Feeding with love and good sense.* Palo Alto, CA: Bull Publishing.

Schachter, S. (1975). Cognition and peripheralist—centralist controversies in motivation and emotion. In M. S. Gassaniga & C. Blakemore (Eds.), *Handbook of psychobiology*. New York: Academic Press.

Scherer, N. J. (1999). The speech and language status of toddlers with cleft lip and/or palate following early vocabulary intervention. *American Journal of Speech, Language, and Pathology, 8*, 81–93.

Schiffman, H. R. (1976). *Sensation and perception.* New York: Wiley.

Schoen, P., Gill, G., & Wallace, K. (1983, December) *Tracheostomized school children.* Paper presented at the annual meeting of SENTAC, San Diego, CA.

Sederholm, E., McAllister, A., Dolkvist, J., & Sundberg, J. (1995). Aetiologic factors associated with hoarseness in ten-year-old children. *Folia Phoniatrica et Logopedia, 47*, 262–278.

Senior, B.A., Radowski, D., & MacArthur, C.J., Sprecher, R. C., Jones, D. (1994). Changing patterns in pediatric supraglottis: A multi-institutional review, 1980 to 1992. *Laryngoscope, 104*, 1314–1322.

Senturia, B. H., & Wilson, F. B. (1968). Otorhinolaryngic findings in children with voice deviations *Annals of Otology, Rhinology and Laryngology, 77*, 1027–1042.

Shao, W., Chung, T., Berdon, W. E., Mellins, R. B., Griscom, N. T., Ruzal-Shapiro, C., & Schneider, P. (1995). Fluoroscopic diagnosis of laryngeal asthma (paradoxical vocal cord motion). *American Journal of Radiology, 165*, 1229–1231.

Shipp, T., & McGlone, R. E. (1971). Laryngeal dynamics associated with voice frequency change. *Journal of Speech and Hearing Research, 14*, 761–768.

Shrivastav, R. (1997). *Transformation of speech of the hearing impaired.* Unpublished master's thesis, University of Mysore, India.

Shrivastav, R., Yamaguchi, Y., & Andrews, M. (2000). The effects of stimulation techniques on vocal responses: Implications for assessment and treatment. *Journal of Voice. 14*(3), 322–330.

Silverman, E. M., & Zimmer, C. H. (1975). Incidence of chronic hoarseness among school-aged children. *Journal of Speech and Hearing Disorders, 40*, 211–215.

Silverman, E. M., & Zimmer, C. (1978). Effect of the menstrual cycle on voice quality. *Archives of Otolaryngology, 104*, 7–10.

Simon, B. M., Fowler, S. M., & Handler, S. D. (1983). Communication development in young children with long-term tracheostomies: Preliminary report. *International Journal of Pediatric Oto-Rhino-Laryngology, 6*, 37–50.

Simon, B., & Handler, S. D. (1981). The speech pathologist and management of children with tracheostomies. *Journal of Otolaryngology, 10*, 440–448.

Skinner, B. F. (1971). *Beyond freedom and dignity.* New York: Knopf.

Sluckin, S. (1977). Children who do not talk at school. *Child: Care, Health and Development, 3*, 69–79.

Sluzki, C. E. (1983). The sounds of silence: Two cases of elective mutism in bilingual families. *Family Therapy Collections, 6*, 68–77.

Smith-Frable, M. A. (1961). Hoarseness, a symptom of premenstrual tension. *Archives of Otolaryngology, 75*, 66–68.

Sorenson, D. N. (1989). A fundamental frequency investigation of children ages 6–10 years. *Journal of Communication Disorders, 22*, 115–123.

Specter, P., Subtelny, J. D., Whitehead, R. L., & Wirz, S. L. (1979). Description and evaluation of a training program designed to reduce vocal tension in adult deaf speakers. *Volta Review, 81*, 81–90.

Spiegel, J. R., Sataloff, R. T., & Emerich, K. A. (1997). The young adult voice. *Journal of Voice, 11*, 138–143.

Spivack, G., & Shure, M. B. (1974). *Social adjustment of young children: A cognitive approach to solving real-life problems*. Washington, DC: Jossey-Bass.

Stathopoulos, E. T. (1986). Relationship between intraoral air pressure and vocal intensity in children and adults. *Journal of Speech and Hearing Research, 29*, 71–74.

Stathopoulos, E. T. (1995). Variability revisited: An acoustic, aerodynamic and respiratory kinematic comparison of children and adults during speech. *Journal of Phonetics, 23*, 375–385.

Stathopoulos, E. T., & Sapienza, C. M. (1993). Respiratory and laryngeal measures of children during vocal intensity variation. *Journal of the Acoustical Society of America, 94*, 2531–2543.

Stathopoulos, E. T., & Weismer, G. (1985). Oral air flow and intraoral air pressure: A comparative study of children, youths and adults. *Folia Phoniatrica, 37*, 152–159.

Statistical Abstract of the United States. (1999). *Table 140*. Washington, DC: U.S. Census Bureau.

Staub, E. (1975). *The development of prosocial behavior in children*. Morristown, NJ: General Learning Press.

Steinsapir, C. D., Forner, L. L., & Stemple, J. C. (1986). *Voice characteristics among black and white children: Do differences exist?* Paper presented at the American Speech and Hearing Association Convention, Detroit, MI.

Stemple, J., Lee, L., D'Amico, B., & Pickup, B. (1994). Efficacy of vocal function exercises as a method of improving voice production. *Journal of Voice, 8*, 271–278.

Strik, H., & Boves, L. (1992). On the relation between voice source parameters and prosodic features in connected speech. *Speech Communication, 11*, 167–174.

Strodtbeck, F. L., & Mann, R. D. (1956). Sex role differentiation in jury deliberation. *Sociometry, 19*, 3–11.

Swanson, F. J. (1960). Music teaching in the junior high and school music. *Music Education Journal, 46*, 50.

Tait, N. A., Michel, J. P., & Carpenter, M. A. (1980). Maximum duration of sustained /s/ and /z/ in children. *Journal of Speech and Hearing Disorders, 45*, 239.

Tanner, J. M. (1969). Growth and endocrinology of the adolescent. In L. Gardner (Ed.), *Endocrine and genetic diseases for childhood*. Philadelphia: W. B. Saunders.

Tanner, J. M. (1971). Sequence, tempo, and individual variation in the growth and development of boys and girls aged twelve to sixteen. *Daedalus, 100*, 907–930.

Taranger, J., Engstrom, I., Lichtenstein, H., & Svennkerg-Redegren, I. (1976). The somatic development of children in a Swedish urban community. A prospective longitudinal study. *Acta Paediatrica Scandinavica, 258*(Suppl.), 121–135.

Tavris, C. (1982). *Anger, the misunderstood emotion*. New York: Simon & Schuster.

Thomas, J. T. (1973). Adolescent endocrinology for counselors of adolescents. *Adolescence, 8*, 395–406.

Titze, I. R. (1976). On the mechanics of vocal-fold vibration. *Journal of the Acoustical Society of America, 60*, 1366–1380.

Titze, I. R. (1980). Comments on the myoelastic-aerodynamic theory of phonation. *Journal of Speech and Hearing Research, 23*, 495–510.

Titze, I. R. (1981). Biomechanics and distributed-mass models of vocal fold vibration. In M. Hirano & K. N. Stevens (Eds.), *Vocal fold physiology*. Tokyo: University of Tokyo Press.

Todd, T. (1983, August). The steroid predicament. *Sports Illustrated, 59*, 62–72.

Toppozada, H., Michaels, L., Toppozada, M., El Ghazzawi, E., Talaat, A., & Elwany, S. (1981). The human nasal mucosa in the menstrual cycle. *Journal of Laryngology and Otology, 95*, 1237–1247.

Tosi, O., Postan, D., & Bianculli, C. (1976). Longitudinal study of children's voices at puberty. In E. Lorbell (Ed.), *Proceedings of the XVIth International Congress on Logopedics and Phoniatrics* (pp. 486–490). Basel, Switzerland: Karger.

Trautman, R. C., Giddan, J. J., & Jurs, S. (1990). Language risk factors in emotionally disturbed children within a school and day treatment program. *Journal of Childhood Communication Disorders, 13*, 123–133.

Travis, L. E. (Ed.). *Handbook of speech pathology and audiology* (pp. 673–695). New York: Appleton-Century-Crofts.

Treole K., & Trudeau, M. D. (1997). Changes in sustained production tasks among women with bilateral vocal nodules before and after voice therapy. *Journal of Voice, 11*, 462–469.

Truax, C. B., & Carkhuff, R. R. (1967). *Toward effective counseling and psychotherapy.* Chicago: Aldine.

Trudeau, M. D. (1998, April). Paradoxical vocal cord dysfunction among juveniles. *SIDS, Voice and Voice Disorders Newsletter,* 11–13.

Tucker, H. M. (1993). *The larynx: Neurological disorders* (2nd ed.). New York: Thieme Medical Publishers.

Van Gelder, L. (1974). Psychosomatic aspects of endocrine disorders of the voice. *Journal of Communication Disorders, 7,* 263–267.

Van Hattum, R. (1969). Program scheduling. In R. J. Van Hattum (Ed.), *Clinical speech in schools: Organization and management* (pp. 163–195). Springfield, IL: Thomas.

Vandell, D. L., & George, L. B. (1981). Social interaction in hearing and deaf preschoolers: Successes and failures in initiations. *Child Development, 51,* 627–635.

Van Riper, C. (1972). *Speech correction: Principles and methods* (5th ed.). Englewood Cliffs, NJ: Prentice Hall.

Van Riper, C., & Irwin, J. V. (1958). *Voice and articulation.* Englewood Cliffs, NJ: Prentice Hall.

Vendler, Z. (1968). *Adjectives and nominalizations.* The Hague, Netherlands: Mouton.

Volin, R. (1991). Microcomputer-based systems providing biofeedback of voice and speech production. *Topics in Language Disorders, 11,* 65–79.

Von Leyden, H. (1985). Vocal cord modules in children. *ENT Journal, 64,* 473–480.

Vuorenkoski, V., Lenko, H., Tjernlund, P., Vuorenkoski, L., & Perheentupa, J. (1978). Fundamental voice frequency during normal and abnormal growth and after androgen treatment. *Archives of Disease in Childhood, 53,* 201–209.

Wagner, J. (1992). *Pulmonary function testing: A practical approach.* Baltimore: Williams & Wilkins.

Walton, J., & Orlikoff, R. C. (1994). Speaker race identification from acoustic cues in the vocal signal. *Journal of Speech and Hearing Research, 37,* 738–745.

Warr-Leeper, Y. A., McShea, R. S., & Leeper, H. A. (1979). The incidence of voice and speech deviations in a middle school population. *Language, Speech and Hearing Services in Schools, 10,* 14–20.

Wegscheider-Gruse, S. (1983). *Choice making for co-dependents, adult children and spirituality seekers.* Pompano Beach, FL: Health Communications.

Weinberg, B., & Zlatin, M. (1970). Speaking fundamental frequency characteristics of five- and six-year-old children with mongolism. *Journal of Speech and Hearing Research, 13,* 418–425.

Weinberger, S. E. (1992). *Principles of pulmonary medicine.* Philadelphia, PA: W. B. Saunders.

Weiss, D. A. (1950). The pubertal change of the human voice. *Folia Phoniatrica, 2,* 30–32.

Welsh, R. C., & Harvin, V. R. (1976). Strategies for developing concepts in elementary school mathematics. *Viewpoints* [Bulletin School of Education, Indiana University], *5,* 13–26.

Wergeland, H. (1979). Elective mutism. *Acta Psychiatrica Scandinavica, 59,* 218–228.

Werner, H., & Kaplan, B. (1963). *Symbol formation: An organismic-developmental approach to language and the expression of thought.* New York: Wiley.

Westlake, H., & Rutherford, D. (1961). *Speech therapy for the cerebral palsied.* Chicago, IL: National Society for Crippled Children and Adults.

White, P. (1999). Formant frequency analysis of children's spoken and sung vowels using sweeping fundamental frequency production. *Journal of Voice, 13,* 570–582.

Wilson, D. K. (1972). *Voice problems of children.* Baltimore: Williams & Wilkins.

Wilson, D. K. (1979). *Voice problems of children* (2nd ed.). Baltimore: Williams & Wilkins.

Wilson, D. K. (1987). *Voice problems of children* (3rd ed.). Baltimore: Williams & Wilkins.

Winder, A. E. (1974). Normal adolescence: Psychological factors. In A. E. Winder (Ed.), *Adolescence: Contemporary studies* (2nd ed.). New York: Van Nostrand.

Wolf, L., & Glass, R. (1992). *Feeding and swallowing disorders in infancy: Assessment and management.* Tucson, AZ: Therapy Skill Builders.

Wright, H. H., Miller, M. D., Cook, M. A., & Littmann, J. R. (1985). Early identification and intervention with children who refuse to speak. *Journal of the American Academy of Child Psychiatry, 24,* 739–746.

Zajac, D. J., Farkas, Z., Dindzans, L. J., & Stool, S. E. (1993). Aerodynamic and laryngographic assessment of pediatric vocal function. *Pediatric Pulmonology, 15,* 44–51.

Zalzal, G. H., Loomis, S. R., & Fischer, M. (1993). Laryngeal reconstruction in children: Assessment of vocal quality. *Archives of Otolaryngology–Head and Neck Surgery, 119*, 504–507.

Zehr, A. (1983). *Beating the blues. Potentials in human development* (pp. 1–4). Bloomington, IN: South Central Community Mental Health Center.

Zemlin, W. R. (1968). *Speech and hearing science: Anatomy and physiology.* Englewood Cliffs, NJ: Prentice Hall.

Zemlin, W. R. (1981). *Speech and hearing science* (2nd ed.). Englewood Cliffs, NJ: Prentice Hall.

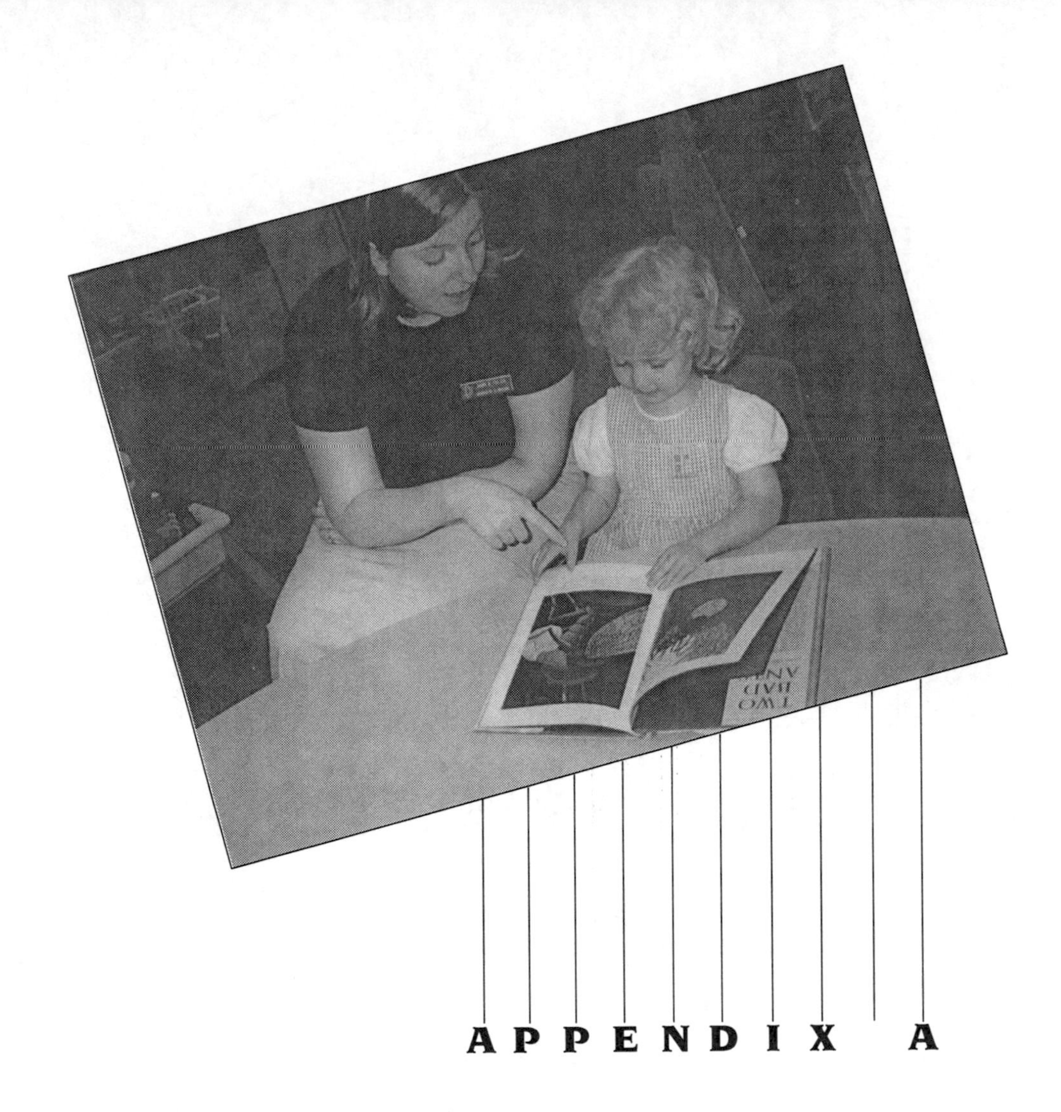

APPENDIX A

Practice Materials and Worksheets for Voice Therapy for Preschool Children

In the following appendices, specific examples of practice materials for awareness, facilitating production, easy vocal production, and complex vocal production are presented. These activities can be used with a variety of voice disorders.

Contents

Voice Assessment for Preschoolers: A Sample Protocol to Elicit Vocal Responses

Today's date: ________________

Child's name: ______________________ Birthdate: ________________

Gender: _____ Location of Testing: ______________ Referred by: ________________

Materials needed: picture of a playground, glass, water, straw, small motorcycle, small garage (or box), big brown bear, small toy snake, small box for cave, picture of a birthday cake, small baby doll picture, 2 small toy chickens, picture of steps, small toy fire truck, 2 puppets (large and small)

General instructions: Today we are going to play some games. I will tell you what to do. You must listen carefully and do exactly what I tell you to do. Are you ready to play?

Activities

Task instructions	Scoring
1. Spontaneous sample	
When I play outside, I like to swing and slide. (Present picture.) What do you like to do?	Total number of words ________________ Description of voice during spontaneous speech ________________ Comments ________________
2. Inhalation and exhalation	
Make bubbles for as long as you can. Examiner models a deep breath and blows bubbles in a plastic glass of water, through a straw. Multiple trials as needed for best responses.	Type of inhalation ________________ Length of best exhalation __________ seconds Comments ________________ ________________

3. Prolongation of /z/

The motorcycle goes /z/. Keep going until it gets to the garage. Examiner models 10-second production of /z/ and moves motorcycle. Multiple trials as needed for best response.	Number of seconds ________
	Continuous voicing ____ yes ____ no
	Understood task ____ yes ____ no
	Comments ________
	________

4. Prolongation of /s/

Sammy snake goes /s/. Keep going until it gets to the cave. Examiner models 10-second production of /s/ and moves snake. Multiple trials as needed for best response.	Number of seconds ________
	Continuous voicing ____ yes ____ no
	Understood task ____ yes ____ no
	Comments ________
	________

5. Prolongation of /a/

Here is the big brown bear. He says /a/ for a long time. You be the big brown bear and say /a/ for as long as you can. Examiner models 10-second production of /a/. Multiple trials as needed.	Number of seconds ________
	Continuous voicing ____ yes ____ no
	Voice breaks ____ yes ____ no
	Quality ________
	Comments ________
	________

6. Pitch pattern (singing)

Let's pretend we're at a birthday party!	Number of lines completed ________
Sing "Happy Birthday" to the teacher.	Pitch variability ________
Present cake with candle. Examiner sings	Quality ________
"Happy Birthday."	Recognizable tune ______ yes ______ no
	Recognizable rhythm ______ yes ______ no

7. Relaxed phonation

(Present baby doll.) Look at baby. She is tired.	Imitates yawn ______ yes ______ no
Pretend you are yawning and say /ha/.	Prolongs relaxed /ha/ ______ yes ______ no
(Examiner models.) Do it again for a long time.	Length prolonged ________ seconds

8. Imitation of high pitches

Mrs. Chicken says /a/. She goes up the	Pitch variation ______ yes ______ no
steps. Examiner moves Mrs. Chicken up	Number of discernible notes ________
steps, accompanied by vocal scale.	Understood task ______ yes ______ no
Multiple trials as needed.	Pitch changed quality ______ yes ______ no
	Comments ________
	________

9. Imitation of low pitches

Make Mr. Chicken go down the steps. Mr. Chicken says /a/. He goes down the steps, accompanied by vocal scale. Make Mr. Chicken go down the steps.	Pitch variation ________ yes ________ no Number of discernible notes ________ Understood task ________ yes ________ no Pitch changed quality ________ yes ________ no Comments ________________ ________________

---

10. Identification of high and low /i/

Mrs. Chicken talks in a high voice. (Place Mrs. Chicken at top of steps.) She says /i/. (Model high /i/.) Mr. Chicken talks in a low voice (Place Mr. Chicken at the bottom of the steps.) He says /i/. (Model low /i/.) Show me who says this. Is this Mrs. Chicken or Mr. Chicken? Point to the one who is talking. (Multiple trials randomized.)	Trials (score + or –) High ________ 1 ________ 2 ________ 3 Low ________ 1 ________ 2 ________ 3

---

11. Imitation of loudness variation

This is a fire truck. It goes "whoo." It is getting louder. The fire engine is going home. It is getting softer. Pretend you are the fire truck. Start at home. Put	Loudness variation ______ yes ______ no Understood task ______ yes ______ no Effects of loudness changes on quality? ________ yes ________ no

the fire out and go back home. Remember the fire truck goes "whoo." Examiner models target behavior.	Comments ____________

12. Identification of loud and soft

This is a big puppet and his voice sounds loud. (Present big puppet.) He says /u/. Model loud /u/.	Trials (score + or –) Loud 1 ______ 2 ______ 3 ______
This puppet's voice sounds soft. (Present little puppet.) He says /u/. (Model soft /u/.) Show me who says this. Point to the one who is talking. (Multiple trials randomized.)	Soft 1 ______ 2 ______ 3 ______

13. Verbal analogies to listen for voice resonance

Listen to what I say, then finish what I say. (Examiner presents entire analogy once, repeats analogy deleting last word, but presents picture.)

1. I hit a baseball with a (<u>bat</u>). ________ normal balance

2. Mother is a woman. Daddy is a (<u>man</u>). ________ hyponasal

3. Summer is hot. Winter is (<u>cold</u>). ________ hypernasal

4. Bow-wow goes the dog. Meow goes the (<u>cat</u>).

5. On my feet I wear shoes. On my head I wear a (<u>hat</u>).

Total number of tasks presented: ______________________________

Total number of tasks completed appropriately: ______________________

Total number of tasks with no response: __________________________

Comments on understanding of tasks: ____________________________

Comments on stimulability (which cues helped): ____________________

Speech–language pathologist's impressions of receptive and expressive voice skills relative to age:

Relevant reports from other caregivers:

Hearing test results:

Recommendations and referrals:

Reference:

Andrews, M. L., and Champley, E. H. (1993). The elicitation of vocal responses from preschool children. *Language, Speech and Hearing Services in Schools,* 24(3): 156–167.

Worksheet: Character Rhymes

Goal: Do the actions as you say the rhymes. Try to keep the rhythm for both the actions and the words.

I am a soldier
Tall as can be
March, march, march
For everyone to see

I am a pony
Trotting down the street
Trot, trot, trot
On four little feet

I am a carpenter
Making things with wood
Hammer, hammer, hammer
My work is very good

I am a barber
Cutting people's hair
Snip, snip, snip
Sit in my chair

I am a race driver
Steering round the track
Vroom, vroom, vroom
My race car is black

I am a fisherman
I pull fish from the sea
Heave ho, heave ho
Nets with fish for me

I am a floppy doll
Relaxed as you can see
Jiggle, jiggle, jiggle
Loose as can be

I am a scarecrow
Made of stiff sticks
Jerky, jerky, jerky
Arms doing tricks

I am a dancer
Light on my feet
Pretty, pretty, pretty
Moving dainty feet

Worksheet: Action Rhymes

Goal: To speak with rhythm while performing the appropriate actions. Keep the beat.

1. Run run run
   To catch the sun

2. Prance prance prance
   All around France

3. Sway sway sway
   All of the day

4. Skip skip skip
   Do not trip

5. Walk walk walk
   Do not talk

6. Creep creep creep
   Do not sleep

7. Jump jump jump
   Over a bump

8. Wriggle wriggle wriggle
   And don't giggle

9. Shiver shiver shiver
   Try to quiver

10. Stoop stoop stoop
    Bend and droop

Worksheet: Ocean Rhyme for Preschoolers

Goal: Say the words "wiggle, wiggle, wiggle" as you wiggle your hips during each refrain

There are many awesome creatures
In the deep blue sea
Lots of creatures wiggle there
Smoothly as can be

Pretend you are a slippery eel
In the deep blue sea
Wiggle wiggle wiggle
Smoothly as can be

Pretend you are a great big whale
In the deep blue sea
Wiggle wiggle wiggle
Smoothly as can be

Pretend you are a little shrimp
In the deep blue sea
Wiggle wiggle wiggle
Smoothly as can be

Pretend you are a dark gray shark
In the deep blue sea
Wiggle wiggle wiggle
Smoothly as can be

Pretend you are a colored fish
In the deep blue sea
Wiggle wiggle wiggle
Smoothly as can be

Pretend you are a tough old crab
In the deep blue sea
Wiggle wiggle wiggle
Smoothly as can be

1. Draw some pictures of humpback whales who are known for their songs.
2. Did you know that dolphins and porpoises are small whales?
3. Blue whales are the largest of all whales.
4. There are some fun books about whales. Maybe there are some in your library.

Suggested reading about whales:

Davis, M. S. A. (1993). *Garden of Whales.* Columbia, SC: Camden House.

Sheldon, D. (1991). *The Whale's Song.* New York: Dial.

Wells, R. E. (1993). *Is a Blue Whale the Biggest Thing There Is?* Morton Grove, IL: Albert Whitman.

Worksheet: Hats for Young Children

Goal: To breathe out plenty of air on the word "hat" and on the other "h" words. Sing using a light "head" voice.

Activities

1. Provide children with paper plates that have had the center removed. Provide them with scrap materials and tissue paper and glue to decorate their hats. As they model their hats, the children describe them.

2. Play "Simon Says" using the words, "Harry Hatter says" instead.

3. Play "Hit the Hat" (see below) by throwing pennies into a hat. At each turn, the child says, "I hit the hat" or "I didn't hit the hat."

4. Sing "A Hip Hap Song" and perform the actions while singing (see next page).

5. Practice saying these sentences. Feel the breath on your hands.

   Harry Hatter has a hat.
   Hold the hats here.
   Hard hats for hard heads.

6. Hats can tell about the people who wear them. Think about and describe the hats worn by:

   A firefighter
   A police officer
   A sailor
   A pilot
   A chef
   A coal miner

7. People wear hats for protection as well as for decoration. Helmets are like hats. They protect cyclists and football players. Headgear can also show a person's rank. Think about what kings and queens wear on their heads.

A Hip Hat Song

(Sung to the tune of "If you're happy and you know it, clap your hands.")

Put your hat on your head, clap your hands (clap twice)
Put your hat on your head, clap your hands (clap twice)
Put your hat on your head, put your hat on your head,
Put your hat on your head, clap your hands (clap twice).

Put your hands on your hips, clap your hands (clap twice)
Put your hands on your hips, clap your hands (clap twice)
Put your hat on your neighbor, your hat on your neighbor,
Put your hands on your hips, clap your hands (clap twice).

Put your hat on your hoof, clap your hands (clap twice),
Put your hand on your hoof, clap your hands (clap twice),
Put your hat on your head, take your hat off your head,
Put your hat on your head, clap your hands (clap twice).

Worksheet: Bears' Picture Hunt

Goal: The teacher puts pictures of different bears in hiding places in the room. The child marches around the room in time to the verse and describes each bear he finds in a clear, easy voice.

Bear Picture Safari

Teacher: Let's go on a bear hunt
March along with me
When you find a picture
Tell me what you see

Child: I found a big black bear

Repeat until all of the bears are found.

Other types of bears:

- Yogi Bear
- Smoky Bear
- panda bear
- koala bear
- teddy bear
- polar bear

Talk about books you have read that have bears in them. Remember Goldilocks?

Suggested reading about bears:

Newman, N. (1994). *There's a Bear in the Bath.* New York: Harcourt.
Rosen, M. (1989). *We're Going on a Bear Hunt.* New York: Macmillan.

Worksheet: Slow Tommy and Fast Roger

Goal: To demonstrate the difference between slow and fast rate and duration while participating in story telling about a tortoise and a rabbit.

One night Caitlin and Robbie asked their mom to tell them a story. She told them a story about Tommy the Tortoise. All tortoises move very slowly and can't go fast at all. Tommy was a very old tortoise, which made him go even slower because his legs were stiff and creaky. Tommy made a humming sound as he crept through the grass. Each time he moved an inch, he hummed with pleasure "Hmm." Then he would stop for a while before he moved again. He made very slow progress, and he sounded like this. Hums with long pauses between them.

Hmm (pause) Hmm (pause) Hmm (pause) Hmm

Tommy had a friend, Roger Rabbit. He was a quirky and lively young rabbit who liked to scamper around his neighborhood. He also liked to hum. He made a lot of quick humming sounds as he scampered through the grass very fast. He never paused at all so his hums sounded like this:

Hmm Hmm Hmm Hmm Hmm Hmm Hmm

Roger did a lot of hums. He was a fast hummer.

Caitlin and Robbie's mom asked them to guess who was humming, Tommy or Roger. Caitlin and Robbie found it easy to guess because Tommy's hums were slow with pauses between. Roger's hums were fast with no pauses between them. Listen and tell me if I am humming fast like Roger or slowly like Tommy.

Now let's continue the story and you provide the sound effects. Remember if it's Roger, hum fast. If it's Tommy, hum slowly with pauses.

Tommy was thirsty, so he set out to the pond. He crept along slowly and sounded like this . . . Soon he was passed by Roger, who was scampering by and humming fast like this . . . Tommy crept on past a big old tree, but he kept humming in his slow way like this . . . Roger came to a patch of flowers, but he didn't have time to smell them as he rushed on humming like this . . . Soon Roger passed by a big brown cow, but he kept on moving fast and humming like this . . . He had no time to talk to cows. Tommy crept along on his creaky legs and slowly moved toward the pond, but it took him a very long time. On his way, he hummingly said "Hello" to Toscia Tortoise, who was coming by on her way back from the pond. Tommy liked Toscia very much, so he hummed especially slowly and sweetly like this . . . He also saw Harry Horse, who was so busy eating grass that he almost stepped on Tommy. Tommy had to hum loudly, but still in his slow way, so Harry would know it was him and be careful. When Harry heard Tommy hum like this . . . , he quickly moved away and said "Oops, sorry Tommy,

I didn't see you there in the grass. Take care now." Tommy hummed a slow hum to thank Harry, like this . . . and kept on creeping. Soon he reached the pond and had a long drink of nice cool water. He hummed slowly, with great satisfaction, like this . . . His long slow trip had been worth it. Sometimes it takes a long time to get where you need to be.

Receptive Voice Story: Friends of Frona Frog

Goal: To listen to and discuss a story about distinctive voices.

Once upon a time there was a green frog named Frona. Frona Frog lived in a pool in a meadow. Lots of creatures lived in the meadow, and although Frona wasn't exactly best friends with all of her neighbors she felt she knew them all quite well because she always recognized their voices. They all came to drink water from her pool, so she heard the noises they made. All of them had quite different voices. She especially liked to hear the birds when they played in her pool. They fluttered and splashed and bathed in the water each day. Some of them sang lovely songs that made Frona's heart melt with longing to sound like they did. The mourning doves had gentle smooth coos that caressed Frona's ears and soothed and calmed her. She loved the mourning doves. They weren't bright like the dashing red male cardinals; in fact they were a drab grey color. Frona thought her own green color was much prettier, but she really loved those doves' voices. Their voices made her want to have them stay near the pool forever, as they were so pleasant to have around. One creature who she certainly did not like to have to listen to for long was Crikey Crow. He was a big black bird with the harshest voice she had ever heard. "Caw, caw, caw" screeched Crikey Crow every time he came for a drink. "Caw, caw, caw" over and over, and it really grated on Frona's ears and made her feel agitated and nervous until he flew off.

The cows who came to drink at the pool stirred up the mud a lot because the earth was soft around the edge of the pool. Frona didn't like that. She liked their low-pitched mooing though. She liked the cow's moos a lot. They sort of vibrated as they came out of their big mouths, which they opened so wide. Frona could almost feel the "moo" sounds vibrating on those big teeth they had and making the sound richer. It was funny the way those big animals could make such loud sounds in such an easy relaxed way. Long, smooth, rich-sounding moos that made Frona think of the rich, creamy milk they gave to the farmer who kept them. The cows had such satisfying voices. It seemed right for such big, solid, gentle animals to have big, solid, gentle voices. Although their moos could be very loud, they never sounded scary or angry, just easy and smooth to Frona's listening ears.

Frona also liked to hear Harriet Horse and her newborn foal, Flasher, when they came to the pool. They snorted and nickered and whinnied to each other after they had drunk the water. Harriet would toss her head and give a long, low whinny and Flasher would answer in his high voice. His high-pitched whinnies always sounded happy and excited, and he made the sound go on for a long, long time. Flasher has a lot of air in his lungs to be able to make such long whinnies in one breath, thought Frona. Her own sounds were so much shorter, but then she was smaller than a horse, even a tiny baby horse, like Flasher. She tried to prolong her "glup" sounds but couldn't. All she could do was repeat the short "glup" over and over again. After awhile she gave up trying to make her "glup" sound like Flasher's long whinny. She thought to herself that horses whinny, cows moo, crows caw, doves coo, and frogs croak and that's just the way it is. Of course, since she was such a small frog, her croaks were soft glups that were a lot easier to listen to than the croaks that Brody Bullfrog made.

Frona thought about all the voices of creatures she knew and how she could always recognize who it was making the different sounds. In fact, she could often learn lots of things just from the sound of their voices. She knew that Flasher was a baby horse and Harriet was older than him, just from their whinnies. Flasher's whinny was high and Harriet's was low. She could also tell that birds were small and cows were big, just from their voices. Moos were certainly louder than the doves' coos. Also, it was interesting the way the different voices made her feel. The doves made her feel relaxed and so did the cows. Flasher made her feel happy and carefree, and Harriet Horse's voice had a pleased motherly sound when she whinnied in answer to Flasher. Mothers often sound loving when they talk to their children, Frona thought. Though sometimes Flasher misbehaved and Harriet's whinny would have a warning sound in it at those times.

How lucky I am to live in a pool where other creatures come to get their water, Frona said to herself. How lucky I am to be able to hear all these interesting and different voices. Voices tell us so much about creatures: who they are, how they feel, and even how old they are. When I listen carefully I can learn a lot about all of my neighbors and how different we all are. Wouldn't it be boring if we all had exactly the same voices? Frona hopped up on a rock to sun herself and looked across the meadow. "Glup" she said. If any of her neighbors were listening they would have known, for sure, that Frona was feeling that she was a very, very lucky frog.

Activities

1. Talk about the different voices in your world. Think about age (grandparents, babies, etc.)
2. See if you can match the sound the creature makes to the name of the creature.

dogs ________	cats ________	pigs ________
lambs ________	snakes ________	bees ________
lions ________	frogs ________	cows ________
horses ________	doves ________	chickens ________
roosters ________	elephants ________	monkeys________

3. Here are some fun rhymes to say:

    a) Elephants trumpet
    Monkeys chatter
    Voices tell us
    Things that matter

    b) Horses whinny
    and nicker too
    Crows caw
    They really do

    c) Ducks quack
    And snakes hiss
    (and bite too)
    It's not a kiss!

    d) Cows moo
    Frogs croak
    Turkeys gobble
    It's not a joke!

4. Now we'll play another game. I'll say the sound, you say the name. Example "If it barks, it's a ______.

Talking About Voice With Preschool and School-Age Children

I. Voice is the basic component of oral communication, and all children can benefit from understanding more about the effects of vocal behaviors.
  A. Awareness of Voice Use
    1. I can describe why voices are important
      a. Animals, birds, people all have special voices
    2. I can describe why voice is important to me
      a. I recognize people by their voices
      b. Voices tell me important information
        i. age
        ii. gender
        iii. health
        iv. wakefulness/tiredness
        v. feelings
        vi. meanings
      c. I can describe how people respond to different voices
        i. familiar/unfamiliar
        ii. pleasant/unpleasant
        iii. natural/phony
        iv. calm/stressed
      d. I can describe how voice is important to me in my daily life
        i. It is the "me" others hear
        ii. It can help me feel confident/anxious
        iii. It can draw others to me/turn others from me
        iv. It can help me/stop me from getting what I want
  B. Exploration of Voice Use
    1. I can show my feelings with my voice.
      a. "I'm scared, my voice is shaking."
    2. I can make friends.
      a. "I'm Lauren, what's your name?"
    3. I can ask for what I want.
      a. "Mom, can I have a cookie, please?"
    4. I can get information.
      a. "Is there a soda machine here?"
    5. I can keep in touch.
      a. "Hi Grandma, Happy Birthday!"
    6. I can make music with my voice.
      a. Making the beat
      b. Making the best (actions and movements)
      c. Making patterns (beads on a string)
      d. Singing songs, showing feelings
II. Behaviors to Emphasize
    1. Breathing
      a. Lower chest movement
      b. Extended exhalation phase
      c. Frequent replenishing breaths

2. Relaxed, easy talking
   a. Body alignment/posture (not like a turtle)
   b. Downward movement of jaw-mouth opening
   c. Use plenty of air–feel on hand
3. Easy onsets of vowel initial words
   a. Blending words smoothly (legato not staccato)
   b. Inserting semi vowels
   c. Lengthening vowels
   d. Breathing out the vowel (with /h/ first)
4. Oral and nasal resonance
   a. Prolonging voiced continuants (facial buzz)
   b. Humming
   c. Finishing words (voicing final consonants)
   d. The vowel is the heart of the word (e.g., "worm")
5. Loud talking without strain
   a. Use lips to help throw the words
   b. Use "head voice" (like singing)
   c. Practice the Australian bush call (e.g., "coo-ee")
   d. Increase articulatory movements/mouth opening

III. Basic Concepts

1. Relaxation
   a. Tense/relaxed; smooth/jerky; loose/tight; uptight/laid back
2. Prolongation/duration
   a. Stop/go/keep going; long/short
3. Speech breathing
   a. Breathe in/breathe out; sniff/blow; chest/tummy; pull in/push out; air/voice; hiss/buzz
4. Resonance
   a. Nose sounds/mouth sounds, trapdoor open/closed
5. Pitch
   a. Up/down; high/low; happy tune/sad tune
6. Loudness
   a. Loud/soft; getting louder/getting softer; outside voice/inside voice; turn the volume up/down (soft, medium, loud)
   b. Feeling cues

soft	*loud*
calm	uptight
kind	angry
scared	bragging

   c. Meaning cues

soft	*loud*
tiptoe	thump
tapping	banging
tinkling	crashing
a tiny bunny	a big bear

d. Situational cues
   Voice in a library, hospital, playground, church
e. Listener cues
   mom has a headache
   friend scores a homerun
   elderly grandparent

IV. Information
1. Anatomy and physiology
2. Hydration
3. Abusive practices/alternatives
4. Interpersonal dynamics
5. Characteristics of effective speakers
6. Variability for getting and holding attention

V. Dissemination of information about voice
1. Provide classroom materials for science, health, and speech lessons
2. Consult with music teachers, teachers, aides, coaches, caregivers of preschoolers; parents
3. Arrange for in-services; posters; conflict resolution activities; cheerleaders sessions
4. Put materials in physician's offices (coloring sheets)
5. Include voice goals in preschool languages programs
6. Talk about the link between children's ability to identify voice (and other paralinguistic) cues and their interpersonal skills.
7. Give stories that illustrate the link between voice and listeners' reactions to teachers of young children.
8. Measure children's knowledge about voice (e.g., quizzes, pretests/post-tests) to document progress in treatment and to be considered part of dismissal criteria.

Guess Who Is Breathing the Best Way?

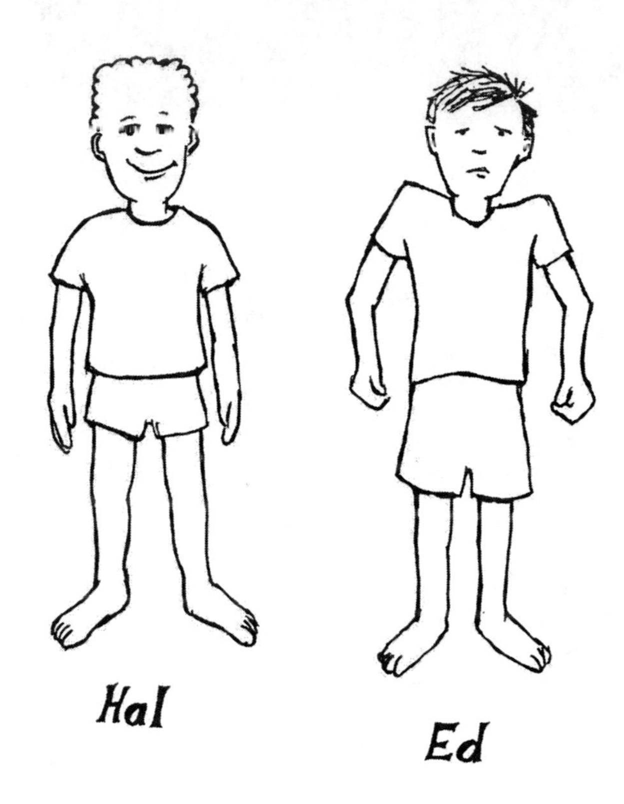

Handout for Parents: Providing Positive Oral and Facial Experiences for Children With Tracheostomy and/or Feeding Tubes

1. Distract infants during suctioning times. Eliminate oral or facial stimulation also during suctioning. This will reduce association of negative behaviors with oral and facial stimulation.
2. Encourage staff to complete suctioning and changing of tracheostomy and NG tubes as carefully as possible.
3. Encourage oral stimulation through sucking on a pacifier, finger, or toys.
4. Encourage sucking activities during feeding times to create associations between satiation and oral motor movements.
5. Tastes of breast milk and formula can be introduced on the tip of a pacifier or gloved finger. This can be completed when the child is able to tolerate non-nutritive stimulation and the speech–language pathologist feels the child is ready for further stimulation.

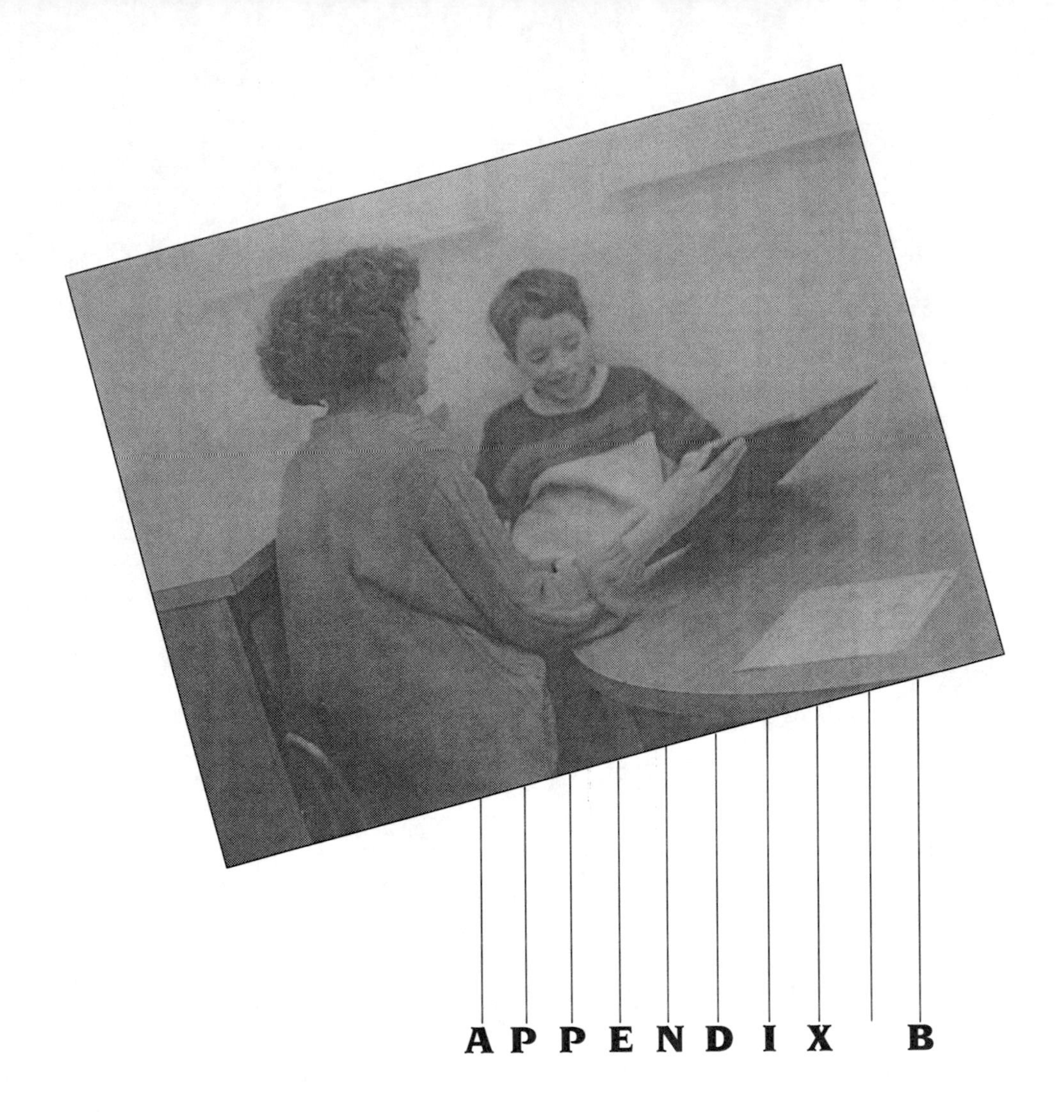

APPENDIX B

Practice Materials and Worksheets for Voice Therapy With School-Age Children

Contents

Worksheet: Voice Pictures (Pitch Changes)

Goal: To learn about and practice pitch variation.

1. We can make word pictures by making our voice sound like a picture in our minds. We can make a word sound high or low. A squeak is high, and a grunt is __________. Color the high words red and the low words blue, and then read the words aloud.

roof	deep	father	thunder	sky
basement	twinkle	baby	piglet	dark
tunnel	tweet	mice	kite	moose
air	moo	elephants	anchor	pin

2. Sometimes we slide our voices up or down. Pretend you are sliding down a slide. Move your finger down the picture of the slide as your voice goes down on "ah." Slide your voice as you say these words:

fell down ⤵

climbed up ⤴

kites fly up ⤴

arrows shoot up ⤴

leaves fall down ⤵

elevators go up ⤴ and down ⤵

helicopters lift off ⤴ and land ⤵

dive down ⤵ and pop up ⤴

3. When we ask a question, the end of the sentence goes up. Let's make questions from these words and sentences.

Who?	Me?	You?
Now?	Today?	He can play?
Are you coming?	Whose is it?	

Let's take turns saying the same words. You say it like a question, and I'll say it like an answer. Then we'll switch.

Yours?	Yours!	Tomorrow?	Tomorrow!
Chocolate?	Chocolate!	Um?	Um!
OK?	OK!	No?	No!
Maybe?	Maybe!	Bedtime?	Bedtime!

4. When we are feeling good, our voices show it. Our voices can smile and make happy voice pictures, or our voices can frown.

   Draw a happy face or a frowning face beside the words as I say them. Then you read the words to me. (Did you match your voice to the face you drew?)

No way	recess	swimming
I won't do it	Christmas	angry
It's my birthday	It's broken	scared
He's a bully	ice cream	movies

5. Find some words and phrases in your reading book that make good voice pictures. Write them on this sheet and then practice saying them either high or low.

Worksheet: Voice Pictures (Loudness Changes)

Goal: To talk about and practice loudness variation.

1. One way to make words interesting is to make pictures of the words with our voices. This makes an important word sound different from the others near it. Sometimes we make a word loud so that people will really notice it. Underline words you think should be said louder than the other words in these sentences.

   The gun went bang.

   She hit the water with a splash.

   The boy yelled at me.

   The plane crashed.

   "Stop," he said.

2. Most people know about making words loud, but that is not the only way to make people take notice of a special word. Sometimes, if a word is soft, it gets noticed even more.
   Think about the words that are underlined and how a soft voice might make the best pictures.

   The story made me <u>shiver</u>.

   It was <u>dead</u> as could be.

   I <u>hate</u> it.

   It's <u>delicious</u>.

   <u>Warm</u> cocoa.

   The dog's ears are <u>silky</u>.

   I know a <u>secret</u>.

   A <u>gentle</u> animal.

   A <u>slimy</u> snake.

   A <u>ghost</u> lives here.

3. Feelings show through our voices. The way we use our voices affects how other people feel when they hear us, too. Finish the sentences below.

   a. When people yell loudly at me, I feel ____________________.

   b. My mom makes me feel good when she talks to me in a ____________________ voice.

   c. When people are tense, their voices sound ____________________.

   d. Some people get a headache if the voices around them are ____________________.

   e. If I want to frighten someone, I sometimes use a ____________________.

   f. If I want to comfort or calm someone, I try to use a ____________________ voice.

4. A voice that is always loud or a voice that is always soft is boring to listen to. We need to vary our voices if we want people to listen to what we are saying. Practice saying the sentences that follow in different ways. At least two words in each sentence are picture words. Circle them first and then think how you'll say them.

a. It was quiet, and then came the thunder.

b. The scream made him scared.

c. The ship exploded and sank.

d. The dog crouched, then attacked.

e. The siren got louder and louder.

f. The door banged, and the tap dripped.

g. It was eerie before the tornado hit.

h. I lay still but my heart was pounding.

i. There was a drumroll, a pause, then applause.

j. Ladies and gentleman, the next President of the United States . . . .

k. The coach tapped his shoulder and said "Go, get in there and get a goal!"

l. I like dainty little earrings, not clunky stuff.

m. He loves the quiet of the mountains away from the noise of cities.

n. After the teacher asked who was making the noise, the whole room was totally still.

Worksheet: Voice Pictures (Duration Changes)

Goal: To learn about and practice timing variation

1. When we talk slowly or quickly all the time, our words all sound the same. We can make different word pictures if we have a change of pace. Read this sentence in six different ways.

   The man went down the road. (He was walking fast. He was on crutches. He stopped after every second step. He was running. He walked jerkily. He drove smoothly in a big car.)

2. Sometimes it is fun to make pictures by changing the rate of different groups of words. Some words can be made long, and others can be made short to make special pictures. What words in the paragraph below would you make long or short? Say them aloud and then fill in the columns.

   The Indian trod carefully through the forest. A twig snapped. He quickened his pace and began running. He ran faster and faster and then stopped. A slow smile crossed his face.

Long	Short
carefully	quickened

   Now read the passage aloud, varying the rate of each sentence.

3. When we stop talking, we give our listeners time to think about what we have said. We use pauses to make our meaning clear and to take in air. Periods and commas tell us to stop, but we have to choose other places to pause, too. In the following paragraph, mark places where you would pause. Then read it aloud.

   The boy who was wearing a red shirt and blue pants was walking faster than the girl who was trailing behind him. He suddenly came to a halt and turned to her and called "Come on or we'll miss the bus."

4. Sometimes we stop before or after important words so that they stand out from the others. In the following sentence, try to think of as many different places to pause as you can. Then discuss how pausing alters the meaning. For example,

   I . . . . hate you.

   I *hate* . . . . you.

   I hate *you* . . . .

   a. Give it to the most deserving person.
   b. Peanut butter sticks to the roof of your mouth.
   c. Cigarettes have been proven to cause lung cancer.
   d. Give me time to answer the question please.

e. I thought I knew what her answer would be.
f. You don't know her at all do you?

5. Some sentences have a main idea and then extra additional information is added between commas. Thus, the phrase between the commas is adding to the main idea but is not a critical part of that idea.

   For example: My mother, a very clever woman, never went to college. It is as if the phrase "a very clever woman" is an aside, or bracketed in parentheses. Thus, sentences like those are called parenthetical sentences. The parenthetical phrase, between the commas, must be set off by pauses and also said at a different rate or in a different voice. This indicates to the listener that it is not part of the main idea.

   Use timing changes when you read the following parenthetical sentences.

   a. My favorite television programs, which I watch on Saturday mornings, are cartoons.
   b. My favorite ice cream flavor, which I eat every day, is mint chocolate chip.
   c. My dog, a Jack Russell Terrier, got loose in the park.
   d. I went to the Hard Rock Cafe, the one in New York City, when I was on vacation.
   e. Chandra, she is my favorite cousin, is coming to visit me this summer.
   f. Mrs. Novotny, she lives in my neighborhood, gives me cookies.

Worksheet: Evaluation of Anticipatory and Retroactive Nasality

Goal: To practice appropriate velopharyngeal closure.

1. Listed below are a list of syllables and a list of words using the syllables. Practice saying these words and syllables into a tape recorder and then listen to how you sound.

Syllables		Words	
nar	arng	mar	arm
nor	orng	nor	horn
noo	oong	new	tune
ner	erng	nerve	burn
nee	eeng	meat	teen

2. Now make up some sentences using these words and syllables. Write them down and then say them into the tape recorder.

____

____

____

____

____

____

I can tell when I open the door

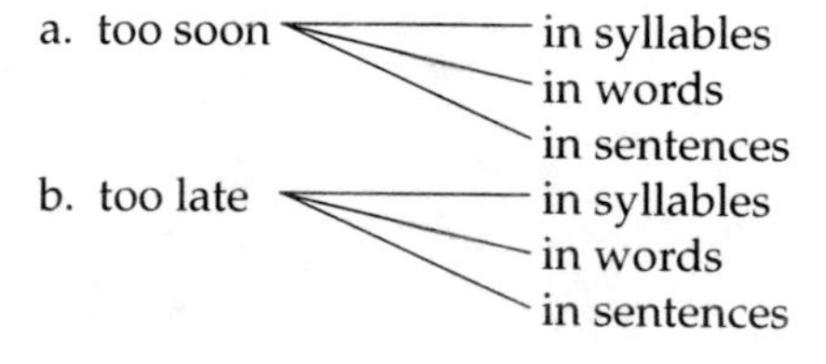

Worksheet: Evaluation of Production

Goal: To learn self-monitoring of oral resonance.

I made the mouth sounds well because

______ **1.** I opened my mouth wide.
______ **2.** I talked slowly.
______ **3.** I lengthened the vowels.
______ **4.** I thought about closing the door.
______ **5.** I marked the hard words on the page before I started to read.
______ **6.** I kept my tongue down/relaxed.
______ **7.** I used my lips well.
______ **8.** I used a low pitch.
______ **9.** I dropped my jaw.
______ **10.** I took a deep breath.
______ **11.** I said it loudly.

I can make the mouth sounds well in

______ **1.** Syllables
______ **2.** Words
______ **3.** Carrier phrases
______ **4.** Reading sentences
______ **5.** Sentence completions
______ **6.** Conversation

Sentences to practice:

a. Where will the wedding be?
b. Is it a house, a church or a hall?
c. I like red, blue, or black shirts.
d. I go upstairs to bed at eight o'clock.
e. She chews with her back teeth clenched.
f. He grabbed the collar of Jonah's jacket.
g. Dad said I was silly to worry about it.

Worksheet: Timing of the Evaluation

Goal: To practice avoidance of nasality on vowels.

Fill in the blanks below by inserting words that rhyme with **clown.** Think about the vowel sound. See if you can prevent opening the trap door too soon. Then listen to the tape recording of the sentences as we play them back, and judge them!

a. Smile, don't ________________.

b. My shoes are ________________.

c. Another name for a city is a ________________.

d. A naming word is a ________________.

e. A dress can be called a ________________.

f. Not up, but ________________.

I knew it was correct–incorrect
______ a. after I said it.
______ b. while I was saying it.
______ c. when I was getting ready to say it.

Sentences to practice:

a. Andy and Mandy like sugar candy.
b. Anna Banana played the piano.
c. Gran made a banner for a spanish dancer.
d. Ninety-nine men were sent to France.
e. Nail those green signs up, Joanna.
f. Nathan knows not to frown.
g. Moaning and groaning never ends.
h. Noreen whines and whines every day.
i. You'll never be alone if you smile.
j. May means it will soon be summer.

Worksheet: Resonance Self-Evaluation Checklist

Goal: To practice self-monitoring of resonance patterns.

______ **1.** I can identify mouth and nose sounds.
______ **2.** I can tell when the door is open or closed.
______ **3.** I can say all vowels with the door closed.
______ **4.** I can tell when a vowel sound comes out of my nose, and I can change it.
______ **5.** I can describe all of the rules.
______ **6.** I can say words with all mouth sounds.
______ **7.** I can say sentences with all mouth sounds.
______ **8.** I can say both mouth and nose sounds in one word.
______ **9.** I can say sentences containing both nose and mouth sounds.
______ **10.** I know when I make a mistake with nose and mouth sounds in words.
______ **11.** I can think of a "trick" to correct any mistake I've made.
______ **12.** I can use a "trick" to prevent making mistakes.

Sentences to practice:

a. I like oranges best.
b. Mother loves me a lot.
c. Dad gave us candy at Easter.
d. Clowns travel with the circus.
e. Katie lives down by the river.
f. Mr. Chan is a gifted teacher.
g. Maddy has red hair.
h. The moon shines brightly.
i. Do you know your spelling words?
j. She asked the girls their names.

Worksheet: Maximizing Resonance (Sound Carriers)

Goal: To practice improved resonance to increase the carrying power of the voice.

1. In the following word list circle all the "sound-carrying" consonants. Some are short sounds that are exploded and are over quickly. Some continue longer, and we can hang on to the vibrations.

ham	find	zip	bell	Vi
melt	zonk	lemon	than	melon

Now list all the voiced plosives and all the voiced continuants.

Voiced Plosives (short sounds)		**Voiced Continuants (long sounds)**	
1. ______	4. ______	1. ______	4. ______
2. ______	5. ______	2. ______	5. ______
3. ______	6. ______	3. ______	6. ______

2. Vowels are good "sound carriers" too. Write down all the different vowels in the words above.

1. ____________________	6. ____________________
2. ____________________	7. ____________________
3. ____________________	8. ____________________
4. ____________________	9. ____________________
5. ____________________	10. ____________________

3. Listen to some vowels and consonants together in small words. When I say the words, put a check beside the ones where I make the most of the "sound-carrying" consonants.

am	zee	no	ill	my	Ev
I'm	vee	all	owl	lie	in

4. Some people say the vowel too fast and don't give it time to vibrate well. Remember that the vowel is the heart of the word—if I say the vowel too quickly, the word is "scrunched up" and has no heart. Draw a heart over the words where I "open up" and vibrate the vowel sound well. Draw an "X" through the ones I don't say well.

hat	boy	down	moon	sell
fail	go	ways	trees	pies

5. Some hints for making our voices carry are these:
a. Open the mouth well.
b. Make sure the vowel vibrates on the bones of the face.
c. "Vibrate" the sound-carrying consonants on the front of the face.
d. "Hang on to" the consonants that can be continued.
e. Use lips and tongue well to explode the consonants that are short.
f. Linger on the vowel: it is the heart or center of the word.

6. While I say these words, you tell me what I can do to improve them:

me	oil	Lyn	need
bees	nob	I've	them

7. Now *you* say the words, and I'll tell you which of the hints you remembered and which you forgot. Before you begin, tell me again what the hints are. I'll put an "X" beside each hint every time you forget it.

Hints	Trials
Mouth opening	
Vibrations on face	
Use of lips and tongue	
"Hang on to" the continuants	

8. Some people like gym a lot because you exercise your whole body. When we "work out" on words, using the muscles of our lips and tongue and throwing vibrations to the front of our face, it is sometimes called "mouth gym." Do some "mouth gym" on the following words. After each try, mark the columns. Say each word three times or until it is as good as you can do it.

Words practiced	Felt like a good workout	Could be better	Lots of vibrations	Could be more vibrations
1. maybe				
2. yellow				
3. Mommy				
4. Zambia				
5. Miami				
6. navy				
7. thieves				
8. Lulu				
9. weary				
10. neon				

9. Here are some rhymes to practice focusing your voice on the front of your face.

a. Rooms for rent
Inquire within
You move out
And I'll move in.

b. Red white and blue
Stars shine on you
Red white and pink
What do you think?

c. Polly Molly talks like this
Dolly Dimple throws a kiss
Jenny Penny went to France
To teach children how to dance.

d. Put a penny in the dish
Make just a tiny wish
Put a dollar in a pan
Make any wish you can.

e. I like butter on my bread
I like hats upon my head
I like movies and T.V.
I like you and I like me.

f. Sheep in the meadow
Cows in the corn
I am very glad
That I was born.

Worksheet: Maximizing Resonance (Projected Speech)

Goal: To practice voice projection.

1. Write down as many suggestions as you can think of to help people improve the way their voices carry.

2. Imagine you are playing outdoors and you want someone to hear you. Show me how you would throw your voice across the distance as you say the following:

"I'm coming."

"No, I don't want any."

"The ball wasn't in."

"Throw it to me."

3. Put slashes to show where to pause in the following passage if you were practicing it to speak in a large hall at a school.

> Ladies and gentlemen. You all know that our principal is leaving our school. On behalf of all of the children I would like to present him with this gift.

Now stand up and pretend you are speaking the words in the large, noisy hall.

4. Record the following sentences or fragments using the best tone focus and richest voice you can. Then listen while they are replayed and mark the sentences with a + or a − to show the ones you think need more practice.

______ **1.** Rising and soaring, the birds flew away.
______ **2.** Boys and girls running to school
______ **3.** No one knows the trouble I've seen.
______ **4.** I'm never able to buy pies and peas.
______ **5.** These plains belonged to the Indians.
______ **6.** I've got spurs that jingle and jangle.
______ **7.** *Fee, fi, fo, fum,* I smell an Englishman.
______ **8.** Yo, ho, ho and a barrel of rum
______ **9.** The pirates of Penzance sang of their treasure with pleasure.

5. Prepare five questions that you would ask me in an interview on television. Write them down for homework. Practice them aloud. When you ask me the questions, pretend you are a professional speaker in front of a large studio audience.

6. Review the paragraphs below, planning where to pause and underlining important words to emphasize. Then practice reading aloud as if you were giving a speech in a large hall. Remember to open your mouth well and project your voice by using forward tone focus.

   a. In 600 B.C., soap was invented by the Phoenicians when they mixed goat's tallow and wood ashes together. Still, in many parts of the world, the laundry is done in the nearest river without soap at all. Clothes are just pounded on rocks and then spread out in the sun to bleach and dry.
   b. In America, the early colonists found washing clothes to be such a hard job that they only did it about four times a year. There was a barrel in which clothes were pounded in water with a long pole to move them around. Later, washboards were made of wood and the wet clothes were rubbed against the ridges on the board. Then they were draped over bushes to dry. Later, clothes lines were invented and the wash was pinned on the lines to dry using clothespins.
   c. Before the washing machine was invented, clothes were boiled in water in copper boilers over wood fires outdoors. In the early part of the nineteen century, washing moved indoors as machines were invented. By 1939, many different brands of washing machines were available, though they were not as efficient as those we have today.

Worksheet: Describing Angry Feelings

Goal: To learn about expressing anger.

1. Circle the things that you believe make most people feel angry with others:

being called names

being put down

being treated unfairly

not being given an equal share (treats, time, attention, etc.)

being physically hurt

having others touch their property

having others take their property

having others destroy their property

feeling they are not respected (liked, loved, believed, listened to)

2. Add any other things (or situations) that you can think of.

3. Circle the things that you believe make most people angry with themselves:

when they do something dumb

when they break something

when they don't do as well as they'd hoped (in school, in sports, in handling a tough situation, etc.)

when they lie or cheat

when they don't do something to correct an unfair situation

when they lose control

when they feel bad inside

4. Add any other things (or situations) that you can think of.

5. Everyone gets angry. Some people get more angry at some things than at others. Can you think of some examples? For example, what is something your mom gets angry about that you don't (e.g., mud on the kitchen floor)? Your teacher (e.g., too much noise in the room)? Why do you think people react differently?

6. Anger can be expressed in many different ways. We often *choose* the way we want to express it. How we choose to express it depends on

   a. the situation. What if your sister makes a face at you in church?
   b. the person we are angry with. Compare your reaction to someone spilling your soft drink—an infant, your worst enemy, and so forth.
   c. what we know (or suspect) about a person's intentions. Think about someone who "forgets" to give you an important message.
   d. the possible penalty. If you are angry with your teacher or your brother would you express it the same way?
   e. how badly you feel.

7. Getting angry is OK as long as we do not let our anger keep spoiling our chances of getting what we want. Think of all of the different ways anger can be expressed. We make different choices at different times. Some ways we can choose to express our anger follow:

   a. using our voice (list some ways)
   b. using our body
   c. confronting the cause head-on
   d. redirecting or transforming the feelings
   e. putting off expressing the feelings until later

8. List some situations in which you saw other people get angry. Describe the choices they made in expressing their anger.

9. Complete these sentences:

   a. When my mom is angry, her voice sounds ____________________.

   b. I know my teacher is angry when ____________________.

c. If I want to make my friend angry, I ____________________.

d. When I'm a parent, I'll get angry if my kids ____________________.

e. When people get angry, they should ____________________.

10. It is important to use your voice to assert your rights calmly and not rudely or with violence. The way you ask for what you want affects your chances of success. Practice saying these sentences firmly but politely. Try not to sound defiant or whiny.

a. Excuse me sir, but I need to get by.
b. Could I please use the phone to telephone my Mom?
c. Miss, I don't think you gave me the correct change.
d. Jason, would you check to be sure that you didn't pick up my jacket by mistake.
e. Bill, excuse me but I was ahead of you.

Worksheet: Handling Our Angry Feelings

Goal: To practice appropriate expression of anger.

1. List some things that always make you angry.

2. Describe the last time you were really angry at someone.

3. Describe the last time you were really angry at yourself.

4. How did you handle your anger? Did your choice work well for you? What benefits or penalties did you receive?

5. Describe the things you do most often when you are angry:

   a. with your voice
   b. with your body
   c. to make yourself feel better
   d. what do you think you most want to achieve when you express your anger?

6. What are some ways you know to express your feelings of anger without hurting yourself (your own feelings, your own body, etc.); without hurting others (their feelings, their body, their things); without hurting your voice; without damaging your relationships?

7. Here are some situations to talk about and to role play.

a. Aaron is drinking at the water fountain. Daniel is running in the hall and accidentally runs into Aaron. Aaron immediately thinks Daniel has done it on purpose. He turns, grabs Daniel, and punches him. The teacher sees them fighting, breaks it up, and sends them both to the principal's office. Aaron screams defiantly at the teacher, "It's not my fault! He started the fight on purpose."

Questions:

a. Why did Aaron punch Daniel? What could he have done instead? How would you deal with this problem if you were Aaron, Daniel, or the principal.
b. Jordan wants to join a group of boys playing with action figures on the playground. He rushes over, grabs some figures and yells "I've got better ones at home." The others angrily push him aside and say "Get away from our stuff. We don't want you around here."
c. Cassie went to look for her lunch box and couldn't find it. She started crying and screaming, soon her face was all red and her throat hurt. She sobbed hysterically and the teacher on duty asked her what was wrong. "Someone stole my lunch" Cassie yelled rudely to the teacher.

Worksheet: Describing Anxious Feelings

Goal: To learn about anxious feelings.

1. Underline the things that you believe make most people anxious:

When the doctor wants to give a shot.

When someone wants a fight.

When someone is mad with them.

When they are alone in the dark.

When they don't feel cared for (loved, understood).

When something is their fault.

When they've told a lie.

When they are in a strange place.

When they don't have any friends.

When they don't know what to expect.

When they think they'll fail or be punished.

Can you think of some other things?

2. Everyone feels scared and anxious sometimes. List some situations that you know cause some of your friends to be anxious or worried.

3. What are some signs that a person is anxious or worried?

   a. in their voice?

   b. in their body?

   c. in things they do?

4. Think about some of the ways different people try to deal with their feelings of anxiety.

a. Admitting that they are anxious sometimes helps.
b. Identifying the cause of the problem may be useful.
c. Talking about it sometimes makes them feel better.
d. Asking questions about what is happening can help, too.
e. Yelling and screaming sometimes makes people feel worse.
f. Strained, tense talking is hard on their throat if they do it too much.
g. Trying to relax can sometimes ease pain.
h. Some people talk too loudly or too much when they are frightened.

5. Complete these sentences:

a. It's hard for me to ______________________________.

b. I feel silly when ______________________________.

c. Sometimes I'm afraid of ______________________________.

d. I hate it when ______________________________.

e. I am afraid to ______________________________.

f. I would hate to lose my ______________________________.

g. I was really scared once when ______________________________.

h. When I am scared, my voice sounds ______________________________.

i. When I am frightened, I cover it up by ______________________________.

j. After I cry, I ______________________________.

6. Taking deep breaths sometimes makes a person feel calmer. Take some deep breaths before reading each of the sentences below.

a. Count to ten before you yell at your brother.
b. I try to breathe deeply when I am scared.
c. I go to my mother for a hug when I'm worried.
d. Reading a book sometimes takes my mind off bad things.

Worksheet: Handling Our Anxious Feelings

Goal: To use self-talk to calm anxious feelings.

1. List some things that always make you anxious.

2. Describe the last time you were really anxious about something.

3. How did you handle your anxiety? Did you feel better because of what you did to deal with your feelings?

4. Suggest some ways you could deal with your anxiety (without straining your voice) in the following situations:

   a. when someone is mean or teases you

   b. when you want to act as if you are not scared

   c. when someone blames you for something you didn't do

   d. when someone tries to pick a fight with you

5. Sometimes, the way we talk to ourselves (inside our heads) helps us to feel better when we are frightened or anxious. Check the things you sometimes say to yourself:

   ______ It will be over soon.
   ______ It's not that bad, really.
   ______ Just pretend you feel fine.
   ______ Please, God, help me through this.
   ______ I can do it.
   ______ Even grown-ups feel scared sometimes.

   What are some other things you say to yourself?

6. Here is a story about how one girl dealt with anxiety about a missing jacket. Read the story aloud.

   > Missy left her new jacket on the school bus. She knew her mother would ask her where it was and Missy was anxious because she knew her mother would say she was careless. So when she got home she made up a story about how two big boys had stolen her jacket and run away with it. Her mother said she'd call the school and report the thieves. Missy screamed "The teacher will just think you're stupid if you do that."

   Think about how Missy could have dealt with her problem without telling a lie and without letting her fears make her mean to her mom.

7. Retell the story with a better ending.

Worksheet: Words to Practice Easy Onset of Phonation

Goal: To practice easy onset on vowel–initial words.

and	extra	ashen
add	amateur	Ellen
ouch	amiable	Eleanor
all	Edgar	American
ant	elephant	oozing
art	eggplant	underground
eat	animosity	uncle
ate	expert	unaware
old	appetite	ostrich
ache	anxious	onion
Andy	alternate	office
Alfie	eccentric	oddity
ill	excruciating	autumn
Eve	outsize	evenings
our	outhouse	ancient
every	instinct	undecided
own	Asia	ostentatious
each	Africa	unrolled
ice	Australia	awesome
out	Iceland	oatmeal
I'd	outer	ocean
eyes	igloo	Oxford
is	inland	Ottawa
easy	irrigate	oxygen
able	Easter Islands	outpost

Projected speaking

1. "It's out of bounds" called the umpire.
2. "Anyone eager to eat?" called the mom to her children across the park.
3. "Oh, Amy, stop that" called the big sister.

Worksheet: Action Words

Goal: To make up action words (verbs) and to make the voice show the action.

Instructions: Make up some words and write them in a list. The trick is that each word must start with the last letter of the word that comes before it on your list. Start with the word "zigzag."

Examples:

Words	Expand into a Sentence
zigzag	zigzag along the path
gasp	gasp in surprise
pant	pant like a dog
tiptoe	tiptoe up the stairs
exercise	exercise with energy
empty	empty out all the water
yell	yell for help
Leah	Leah, push the car up the hill
hiss	hiss like a snake
slurp	slurp the milk shake
pick	pick up your boys now!
kiss	kiss the baby gently
sob	sob, whimper and wail
burp	burp and cover your mouth

Worksheet: Allergy Facts to Read Aloud[1]

Goal: To read the following sentences aloud without tension in the throat.

1. Boys under age 10 are twice as likely as girls of the same age to experience symptoms of hay fever
2. Americans spend more than $2 billion each year on allergy treatments.
3. Ragweed is responsible for 75% of hay fever in the eastern and midwestern United States.
4. Pollen can travel up to 500 miles on dry, windy days.
5. Particles expelled by sneezing can travel up to 103.6 miles per hour.
6. One in eleven visits to the doctor are allergy related.
7. Nasal congestion is the symptom that most allergy sufferers complain of most.
8. People with allergies lose three million days of work and two million days of school every year in the United States.
9. Sneezing, coughing, and sore throats are frequent symptoms for allergy sufferers.
10. On January 13, 1981, a young girl in Great Britain began sneezing and continued to sneeze for 977 consecutive days. She sneezed an estimated one million times in the first 365 days alone.

[1]Adapted from "Allergy Problems Abound" by Alyssa Emory, *Indiana Daily Student,* May 13, 1999.

Worksheet: Anagrams

Goal: To discuss what an anagram is and to read some examples using an easy voice. An anagram is a word or phrase made by rearranging the letters of another word or phrase.

	Given Words	**Rearranged Words**
1.	straw	warts
2.	no	on
3.	mug	gum
4.	sleep	peels
5.	ton	not
6.	lee	eel
7.	part	tarp
8.	gem	meg
9.	violet	to live
10.	dormitory	dirty room
11.	desperation	a rope ends it
12.	astronomer	moon starer
13.	a decimal point	I'm a dot in place.
14.	the Morse code	Here come dots.
15.	snooze alarms	alas! no more Zs
16.	eleven plus two	twelve plus one
17.	The public art galleries	Large picture halls, I bet.
18.	Alec Guiness	genuine class
19.	animosity	is no amity
20.	contradiction	accord not in it

Find some words of your own that can become other words when spelled backward. Also, you could rearrange the letters in words you find in the newspaper. For example:

A suggestion	A guest is on
year two thousand	a year to shut down

Anagrams in sentences

Here are some sentences made with words that are anagrams on your list. Read them aloud. Can you find the two words in each sentence?

a. Violet Brown went to live in Malaysia.
b. Peels of bells woke him from a deep sleep.
c. It is not good for a ton of bricks to fall.
d. The math teacher said 13 can be made up of eleven plus two or twelve plus one.
e. Alec Guiness is an actor with genuine class.

f. No actor is on the stage now.
g. Snooze alarms signal that alas, no more Zs are possible this morning.
h. Amity means kindliness and animosity is no amity or kindliness, but rather quite bad feelings.
i. Meg was given gem earrings on her birthday.
j Part of the tarp was torn so everything it was covering got wet when the rain came down heavily.

Worksheet: Body Parts

Goal: To find the body parts in the words listed below and to say the words in an easy voice.

Instructions: Circle the body parts in the words listed below:

1. legume
2. hearty
3. mottoes
4. worship
5. charming
6. keyed
7. caliper
8. browsing
9. snail
10. disjointed
11. redskin
12. behead
13. chintz
14. slashing
15. deliver

Now make up some sentences describing where the body parts are, what they do, and why we need them.

Examples:
1. A leg is one of a pair that we have, and we need legs to walk.
2. We have nails on our fingers and toes to protect them.
3. Our skin is like a coat over our whole body that keeps germs out.

Worksheet: Buzz the Buzzy Sounds

Goal: To say the words buzzing your voice on the front of your face.

Instructions: All of the words on this page have "z" sounds in them. When you say the words, make your teeth buzz and feel your voice on the front of your face.

A.

Beginning	**Middle**	**End**
zoo	cousin	buzz
zulu	raisin	whiz
zelda	razor	does

B. Now find eight or more words by drawing lines connecting the circled letters below. Each word has a "z" sound. You must go straight but may go in any direction. Letters can be used in more than one word

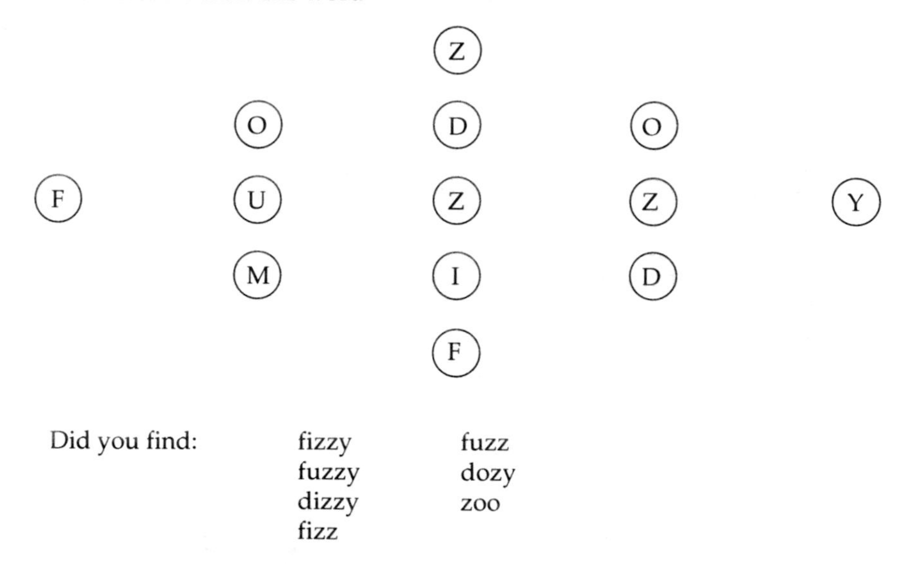

Did you find:

fizzy
fuzzy
dizzy
fizz
fuzz
dozy
zoo

Worksheet: Using Sentences for Cognitive Cueing

Cognitive cueing is a method to stimulate children to vary their voices. No model is provided, just questions to simulate their thinking about the ideas and images. Listed below are sentences with sample cues.

Goal: To practice voice variation using cues.

1. The meowing came from outside the door. Brian opened the door and saw a scruffy little kitten staring at him. The kitten was wet and shivering as the icy wind roared in the dark and shook the house.

   - What do you think Brian felt when he saw the kitten?
   - How old is Brian? What does he look like? Does he like cats?
   - Is a kitten's meow loud or soft?
   - What color is the kitten? Why do you think he's outside the door?
   - How could you say "scruffy" to show what it means?
   - How can your voice make us see how "little" it is?
   - Think about a picture in your mind as you say "staring." Is a stare something that takes a long or short time?
   - Feel the feelings as you say "shivering" and "icy," "dark" and "shook." Is "dark" a word that sounds best in a low or high voice? What about "icy"?
   - Can you make your voice "roar" like the wind? Is the "roaring" loud or soft?
   - What do you think Brian will do? Why?
   - Read each part two or three times until it sounds right to you.
   - Now try the whole passage. Listen while we play it back. Which parts sounded too overdone? Which parts sounded the way you wanted them to? Why?

2. **Other Sentences**

   - There was a quick ping as an arrow whizzed by (high pitch and rate).
   - It rained for days and days, the ground was black and muddy, and my feet squished when I walked to get the bus (low pitch and rate).
   - The door slammed after him, suddenly the house was perfectly still, and his mother sighed (loudness changes and pauses).
   - The fish leapt out of the water, jiggling on the end of the line, the sun glinting on its scales (pitch and duration).
   - After the crashing thunder, there was a moment of quiet, and then the rain came beating down on the roof (loudness and rate).
   - She whined and whined, and it was so very tiresome (pitch, loudness, and rate).
   - The classroom was in an uproar; girls squealed, boys threw books that thudded against the walls, and then the principal came in and it was quiet as a tomb (loudness, pitch, pauses, rate).
   - The TV blared, the dog barked, and Ashley crouched in a corner with her hands over her ears, sobbing as if her heart would break (loudness, rate, pitch, pauses).

- They rolled on the floor laughing hysterically until they got so tired that they fell asleep (loudness, rate).
- "No one understands me" the girl sobbed, and then her mother's cool hand on her forehead calmed her and she was still (loudness and rate).
- The surfers in wet suits are out today and the huge waves are hurtling them through the crashing waves (loudness and rate).
- The wailing sirens came closer and closer to the school until the firetruck stopped in front of the building, and the firemen rushed into the smoke (pitch, loudness, rate).

Worksheet: Sentences for Cognitive Cueing

Goal: To imagine the ideas and feelings and express them in the voice during reading.

1. Sirens shriek, wheels squeal, and the ambulance races through the night with lights flashing wildly until the hospital is reached, and it comes to a halt. Help is at hand.

2. There was not much breeze—just a little movement of the leaves on the big solid oak standing sentinel in the bottom of the garden. Nothing else moved, the air felt heavy with humidity, and the heat seemed to rise from the ground in sickening waves that made the frail old woman feel as if she would faint. It was too much to bear as she trudged toward the door of the house, her head bent and her back humped; she looked as if she would fall. Bill raced up the path and took her arm and steadied her. "There," he said gently, "you're almost home now."

Instructions

1. Think about who could be in the ambulance and what the problem might be. Describe the scene inside and outside the ambulance. How far do they have to go? What will happen when they get to the hospital? What feelings do the sound and lights evoke in people who see and hear the ambulance go by?

2. Who do you think this woman is? What is she wearing? What does she look like? Why is she out when it's so hot? Who is Bill? What is inside the house? Describe how she and Bill feel and why you think he ran to help her.

Worksheet: Homonyms, Rhyming Pairs, and Homographs

Goal: Read the words clearly and talk about the differences between pairs of words that are homonyms, homographs, and pairs that rhyme.

a. Homonyms are word pairs where both words have the same sounds but different meanings. Rhyming words usually have the same vowel sounds, and the end of the words sound similar, but they have different beginning sounds and different meanings.

Homonym Pairs

1.	pair	pear
2.	guest	guessed
3.	road	rowed
4.	build	billed
5.	stair	stare
6.	real	reel
7.	steal	steel
8.	knight	night
9.	sale	sail
10.	male	mail
11.	cue	queue
12.	loot	lute

Rhyming Pairs

1.	sad	lad
2.	light	bite
3.	quite	right
4.	never	ever
5.	quiet	riot
6.	double	trouble
7.	cool	pool
8.	far	star
9.	funny	money
10.	slight	fright
11.	night	flight
12.	sane	shane

b. See if you can identify the rhyming words in the list above from the following descriptions:

1. unhappy young man (sad lad)
2. perfectly correct
3. a gleam in the distant sky
4. a refreshing body of water
5. an evening airplane ride
6. a small snack
7. counterfeit notes and coins
8. a mild scare
9. a noncrazy man
10. not at any time

c. Homographs are words that are spelled exactly alike and yet have different meanings. Some change their vowel sounds, change the sound of the letter /s/, or shift the stress to different syllables. Read the lists below. Then make up sentences using the words.

permit	per′mit
present	pres′ent
progress	prog′ress
project	proj′ect
rebel	re′bel

tear = rip and eye moisture

wind = a stiff breeze and a motion

row = a fight and propel a boat

does = female deer and past tense of "do"

sow = female pig and scatter seeds

refuse	ref'use	abuse = verb and noun
reject	rej'ect	close = shut and intimate
resume	resume'	drawer = artist and part of cabinet
separate	separ'ate	house = verb and noun
subject	sub'ject	
suspect	sus'pect	
transport	trans'port	

Worksheet: Interchangeable Sentences

Goal: To choose words to complete the sentences below so that they sound sensible when read aloud. Use your best voice to create word pictures.

Words

1. squeezed	He grabbed my hand and 1, 3, 6, 9, 10.
2. whistled	When I heard her voice, I, 2, 4, 8, 9, 7.
3. danced	I was sorry that I, 7, 8, 9, 10.
4. flipped	The boy was punished after he 2, 7, 8, 9, 10.
5. smacked	It isn't fun to be 1, 4, 5, 6, 7.
6. jerked	She was so happy that she 2, 3, 9, 10.
7. interrupted	When he 7, the girl 9, 10, 8, 4.
8. exploded	When he 1, 9, 2, the girl 10, 8, 3.
9. laughed	She 8 angrily when he 1, 7, 2.
10. giggled	George 3 and 4 and 2 and 9.

Now think of names that start with the first letter of each word on the list above.

1. Susie squeezed
2. Wanda whistled
3. Daisy danced
4.
5.
6.
7.
8.
9.
10.

Worksheet: Jokes and Riddles

Goal: To vary the voice appropriately so as to make the listener enjoy the jokes and riddles. Use a different pitch for each speaker.

1. Cinema attendant: That's the sixth ticket you've bought!
   Customer: Yes, I know. There's a girl in there who keeps tearing them up.
2. Question: What do you get when you cross a chicken with a cement mixer?
   Answer: A brick layer.
3. Question: Why did the little girl tiptoe past the medicine cabinet?
   Answer: She didn't want to wake the sleeping pills.
4. Patient: "Doctor, doctor, I keep thinking I'm a goat!"
   Doctor: "How long have you had this feeling?"
   Patient: "Since I was a kid."
5. John King went to the dentist. The receptionist wrote—
   Name: King, John
   Complaint: Crown came off.
6. Teacher: Why are you late?
   Student: Because of the sign!
   Teacher: What sign?
   Student: The one that says: "School ahead. Go slow."
7. Child: Dad, can you write in the dark?
   Father: I think so. What do you want me to write?
   Child: Your name on this report card.
8. Teacher: In this box, I have a 10-foot snake.
   Child: You can't fool me. Snakes don't have feet.
9. Teacher: George, go to the map and find Australia.
   George: Here it is.
   Teacher: Now class, who discovered Australia?
   Class: George!
10. Teacher: Tommy, why do you always get so dirty?
    Tommy: Well, I'm a lot closer to the ground than you are.
11. Teacher: Willy, name one important thing we have today that we didn't have 10 years ago.
    Willy: Me.
12. Teacher: How old were you on your last birthday?
    Child: Seven.
    Teacher: How old will you be on your next birthday?
    Child: Nine.
    Teacher: That's impossible!
    Child: No it isn't. I'm eight today.
13. Patient: Doctor, doctor, will you help me out?
    Patient: Certainly, which way did you come in?
14. Doctor: Did you drink your orange juice after your bath?
    Patient: After drinking the bath, I had no room for the juice.

15. Customer: Waiter, waiter, there's a button in my salad!
    Waiter: It must have fallen in while the salad was dressing.
16. Question: What did the dirt say to the rain?
    Answer: If this keeps up, my name will be mud.
17. Question: When do words hurt most?
    Answer: When someone throws a dictionary at you.
18. Question: What do monsters do when they lose a hand?
    Answer: They go to a second-hand store.
19. Question: What did the river say when the elephant sat in it?
    Answer: Well, I'll be damned!
20. Question: Who invented the 5-day workweek?
    Answer: Robinson Crusoe. He had all his work done by Friday.
21. Question: What did the barman say when the ghost wanted a drink?
    Answer: We don't serve spirits.
22. Question: Why couldn't the elephants go swimming together?
    Answer: They only had one pair of trunks between them.
23. Doctor: You need glasses!
    Patient: How do you know?
    Doctor: I could tell as soon as you walked through the window.
24. Doctor: Mr. Beazley, that pain in your leg is simply due to old age.
    Mr. Beazley: Well my other leg is just as old, and it doesn't hurt.
25. First tonsil: What you are getting dressed up for?
    Second tonsil: Oh, the doctor is taking me out tonight.
26. Man: Ouch! A crab just bit my toe!
    Doctor: Which one?
    Man: I don't know! All crabs look alike to me.
27. Question: What do they call Dracula?
    Answer: A pain in the neck.
28. Question: Who invented fire?
    Answer: Oh! Some bright spark!
29. Question: What part of a fish weighs the most?
    Answer: The scales.
30. Teacher: How can you prevent diseases caused by biting insects?
    Child: Don't bite any!
31. Teacher: Give me a sentence beginning with "I."
    Child: "I is."
    Teacher: No dear, always say, "I am."
    Child: All right! I am the ninth letter of the alphabet.
32. Teacher: If I had seven oranges in one hand and eight oranges in the other hand, what would I have?
    Child: Big hands!
33. Question: What is an "ig"?
    Answer: An Eskimo house without a "loo."
34. Questions: What does one invisible man say to another invisible man?
    Answer: It's nice not to see you again.

Worksheet: Names, Real or Imagined

Goal: To write down names to match the initials that are provided. Then read the names aloud in a voice that carries well. Linger on the voiced sounds.

Initials	Names
MM	Mickey Mouse
LR	Lone Ranger
KL	Kathy Lee
BC	Bill Clinton
BP	Brad Pitt
AA	
LN	
OR	
WE	
QE	
PD	
BH	
BG	
PL	
IT	
ZR	
RL	
VW	
PS	
NK	

Worksheet: Oronyms

Goal: To talk about how running sounds from one word onto another word changes the meaning of phrases.

An oronym is a phrase or sentence that has the same sounds in it but can be changed by connecting those sounds differently. If we slur certain sounds and change the word boundaries, we can dramatically change the meaning. An example is "a name/an aim."

a. Read the following examples:

1. A notion; an ocean
2. A nice man; an ice man
3. Great ape; grey tape
4. I scream; ice cream
5. Plum pie; plump eye
6. Tulips; two lips
7. Grade A; grey day
8. May cough; make off
9. Night rate; nitrate
10. A near ring; an earring

b. Now guess which phrase on the above list is meant by the following description:

1. A cold person
2. A cold food
3. Spring flowers
4. Fruit-filled dessert
5. A large animal
6. A fat thing to see with
7. A chemical
8. A piece of jewelry
9. I do it when I'm frightened.
10. An idea or the Atlantic

Worksheet: Oxymorons

Goal: To learn what an oxymoron is and to say them in sentences using an easy voice.

An oxymoron is a saying that seems to be contradictory. For example, two words that have seemingly quite the opposite meaning such as, "good grief." Now "grief" is usually *not* good is it? Yet "good grief" has become a common saying in our everyday language. Despite the individual meanings of the two words being so different, when they are said together everyone realizes what is meant by the phrase.

Jon Agee is a writer who has written a book about these peculiar kinds of word combinations that have become commonplace in our language. In his illustrated book, *Who Ordered the Jumbo Shrimp? And Other Oxymorons* (published by Michael di Capua/Harper Collins), he discusses these nonsensical phrases. Some of his examples are listed below, and it is fun to think of others you have heard:

pretty ugly

almost perfect

calculated risk

minor catastrophe

open secret

near miss

instant classic

hot water heater

bitter sweet

sweet sorrow

thunderous silence

dry ice

evil angel

Sentences to practice:

a. The evil angel is pretty ugly.
b. The movie was an instant classic.
c. Don't worry about a near miss or minor catastrophe.

Worksheet: Planning a Party

Goal: Practice short, spontaneous utterances in your best voice.

Instructions: Fill in the blanks with words you find on the lists and to say those words in your best voice.

a.

Something green	Crunchy food	Liquids
lettuce	chips	root beer
lime sherbet	pretzels	olive oil

1. For our party, we will have some funny refreshments. ______________ (something green) dip and ______________ (crunchy food). We will drink ______________ (liquid) punch with ______________ (liquid).

Plural nouns	Part of a room	Room of house
tooth brushes	ceiling	bathroom
sneakers	floor	kitchen

2. For the decorations, ______________ (plural noun) will be hung from the ______________ (part of a room) in the ______________ (room of a house).

Living things	Furniture	Party favors
eels	pianos	paper hats
cocker spaniels	sofas	whistles

3. Guests will include ______________ (living things), who will be provided with ______________ (furniture) and ______________ (party favors).

   It will be a wonderful occasion.

b. Now complete the sentences below with words from the previous lists.

1. At parties I love to eat ______________ and ______________.
2. At parties I love to drink ______________ and ______________.
3. At parties I love to decorate with ______________.

c. Now make up any words you like to insert in the blanks in the following paragraph.

On the fourth of July I always have a party for ______________. I get fireworks of many kinds and especially like the ones that look like ______________. I invite ______________ and ______________ to attend and give them party favors such as ______________ and ______________. The refreshments include ______________, ______________, and ______________. The games I like to play are ______________ and ______________. Songs we sing include ______________ and ______________ and ______________. I tell everyone to wear ______________ clothes. When guests arrive at my party I greet them by saying ______________. When they leave I tell each one ______________.

Worksheet: Poetry to Practice Picture Words

Goal: To read the poems in a clear voice highlighting the picture words. Keep the rhythm and breathe in appropriate places.

1. I planted seeds in my garden
   I watered them with such care
   Lettuce, tomatoes and onions
   Were growing everywhere

   I watched the plants all growing
   And imagined the salads I'd taste,
   But some deer sneaked in one evening
   Oh! What a terrible waste!

2. As long as earth lasts,
   seedtime and harvest, cold and heat,
   summer and winter, day and night,
   they will never cease.

   Genesis 8:22

3. The words you say
   May come back to you
   So think of how they sound
   To the ears of those
   They travel to . . .
   Bad feelings stick around!

4. Something purely you
   Is the sound of your voice
   You surely make the choice
   To whine or sound blue
   Or to laugh and rejoice.

5. It's not what you do with a million,
   if riches should e'er be your lot,
   but what are you doing at present
   with the dollar and quarter you've got?

   Unknown

6. This is the song of the bee,
   Buzz, buzz, buzz
   A jolly good fellow is he.
   Buzz, buzz, buzz
   In days that are sunny
   He's making his honey
   Buzz, buzz, buzz

Unknown

7. Three little rabbits
   Were eating their lunch,
   Their heads were down
   And how they did munch
   They nibbled and nibbled
   and nibbled some more
   Crunch, crunch, crunch!

Unknown

Worksheet: Portmanteau Words

Goal: To talk about words in the English language made by combining two other words and to make sentences out of some of those words.

Instructions: Portmanteau words are the result of combining two words into a new word. Usually two ideas are combined also. For example, "motel" is a combination of "motor" and "hotel" because it is a hotel you drive to. Read the list of other words like this and discuss the ideas that were combined in the portmanteau words. Remember to use your best voice.

Note: A portmanteau is a case or bag used to carry things. In some countries "ports" are the same as "suitcases." The word "portmanteau" is French and derived from "porter" (to carry) plus "manteau" which is a clock. The plural is "portmanteaux."

1. flame + glare = flare
2. breakfast + lunch = brunch
3. squirm + wiggle = squiggle
4. chuckle + snort = chortle
5. smoke + fog = smog
6. gleam + shimmer = glimmer
7. glamour + Ritz = glitz
8. fantastic + fabulous = fantabulous

Sentences to practice:

1. If you chuckle and snort you chortle.
2. If there's smoke and fog together it is smog.
3. If you miss breakfast, just have brunch.

Worksheet: Proverbs

Goal: To discuss the meaning of each proverb and then to read them so the meaning is reflected in your voice.

1. A friend is one to whom we may pour out the contents of our hearts, chaff, and grain together, knowing that the gentlest of hands will sift it, keep what is worth keeping, and with a breath of kindness, blow the rest away *(Arabian proverb)*
2. It takes a year to make a friend, but you can lose one in an hour. *(Chinese proverb)*
3. He who gives, teaches me to give. *(Danish proverb)*
4. A friend in need is a friend indeed. *(English proverb)*
5. The man who thinks he can live without others is mistaken; the one who thinks others can't live without him is even more deluded. *(Hasidic proverb)*
6. A cheerful heart is a good medicine, but a downcast spirit dries up the bones. *(Proverbs 17:22)*
7. Shared joy is double joy, and shared sorrow is half sorrow. *(Swedish proverb)*
8. A kind word warms for three winters. *(Japanese proverb)*
9. He who does kind deeds becomes rich. *(Hindu proverb)*
10. Sympathy is a little medicine to soothe the ache in another's heart. *(Jewish proverb)*
11. I have learned silence from the talkative; tolerance from the intolerant; and kindness from the unkind. *(Kahil Gibran)*
12. One can pay back the loan of gold, but one dies forever in debt to those who are kind. *(Malayan proverb)*
13. With a sweet tongue and kindness, you can drag an elephant by a hair. *(Persian proverb)*
14. Your own soul is nourished when you are kind; it is destroyed when you are cruel. *(Proverbs 11:17)*
15. He who is narrow of vision cannot be big of heart. *(Chinese proverb)*
16. Where the heart is willing, it will find a thousand ways, but where it is unwilling, it will find a thousand excuses. *(Dayak proverb)*

17. The heart sees better than the eye. *(Jewish proverb)*

18. He who has lost his freedom has nothing else to lose. *(German proverb)*

19. A willing helper does not wait until he is asked. *(Danish proverb)*

20. Help thy brother's boat across, and lo! thine own has reached the shore. *(Hindu proverb)*

21. Fear less, hope more; eat less, chew more; whine less, breathe more; talk less, say more; hate less, love more; and all good things are yours. *(Swedish proverb)*

22. A bit of fragrance always clings to the hand that gives you roses. *(Chinese proverb)*

23. It is better to light one small candle than to curse the darkness. *(Confucius, 551–479 B.C.)*

24. I will charge you nothing but the promise that thee will help the next person thee finds in trouble. *(Mennonite proverb)*

25. Charity begins at home but should not end there. *(Scottish proverb)*

26. By always taking out and never putting in, the bottom is soon reached. *(Spanish proverb)*

27. Tell me, I'll forget. Show me, I may remember. But involve me, and I'll understand. *(Chinese proverb)*

28. One mother achieves more than a hundred other teachers. *(Jewish proverb)*

29. One joy shatters a hundred griefs. *(Chinese proverb)*

Talk about proverbs and how the same ideas are stated in proverbs of many different cultures. What is your favorite proverb? Why?

Can you tell me some proverbs you have known from your past? Do you know one about "sticks and stones" or "people in glass houses?"

Explain what is meant by the following:

1. A rolling stone gathers no moss.
2. Buy low sell high.
3. Do unto others as you would have them do unto you.
4. Birds of a feather flock together.
5. You cannot shake hands with a clenched first.
   Indira Ghandi
6. A stitch in time saves nine.

Worksheet: Quotations

Goal: To read the quotations in a voice that shows the meaning is understood. Talk about the meanings, too.

1. The World is so full of a number of things, I'm sure we should all be happy as kings.
   (Robert Louis Stevenson)

2. Animals are such agreeable friends. They ask you no questions. They pass no criticisms.
   (George Eliot)

3. Write it on your heart that every day is the best day of the year.
   (Ralph Waldo Emerson)

4. If there's anything half so much fun as being alive, I'd like to know what it is.
   (Frederick Buechner)

5. Give me your tired, your poor, your huddled masses yearning to breathe free, the wretched refuse of your teeming shore. Send these, the homeless, the tempest-tossed to me. I lift my lamp beside the golden door. *(Emma Lazarus)*

6. Live and work to make a difference, to make things better, even the smallest things. Give full consideration to the rights and interests of others. No business is successful, even if it flourishes, in a society that does not care for or about its people. *(Eugene C. Dorsey)*

7. If a man does not make new friends as he passes through life, he may find himself alone.
   (Samuel Johnson)

8. What is charity? It is silence when your words would hurt. It is patience when your neighbor is hurt. It is deafness when a scandal flows. It is thoughtfulness for others' woes. It is promptness when duty calls. It is courage when misfortune falls.
   (Unknown)

9. The Spirit of Christmas is always near; it shines like a beacon throughout the year. Don't look in a store or high on a shelf, for sharing and giving are found in yourself.
   (Unknown)

10. Iron rusts from disuse, stagnant water loses its purity, and in cold weather becomes frozen; even so does inaction sap the vigors of the mind. *(Leonardo da Vinci)*

11. The best of all things is to learn. Money can be stolen, health and strength may fail, but what you have committed to your mind is yours forever. *(Louis L'Amour)*

12. A school is a building that has four walls and tomorrow inside. *(Unknown)*

13. None of us has gotten where we are solely by pulling ourselves up by our own bootstraps. We got here because somebody bent down and helped us up.
(Thurgood Marshall)

14. There is not another country in the world that can come close to matching the generosity of America. *(Jerold Panas)*

15. Some people think that they are generous because they give away free advice.
(Unknown)

16. Give to all generations by saving the earth. *(Christina R. Newman)*

17. Reflect upon your present blessings of which everyone has many; not upon your past misfortunes of which all have some. *(Charles Dickens)*

18. Remember that happiness doesn't depend upon who you are or what you have. It depends solely upon what you think. *(Dale Carnegie)*

19. He who plants a tree provides a kindness for many generations. *(Henry Van Dyke)*

20. Sympathy sees, and says, "I'm sorry." Compassion feels, and whispers, "I'll help."
(Unknown)

21. I expect to pass through life but once. If, therefore, there be any kindness I can show, or any good thing I can do to any fellow being, let me do it now, and not defer or neglect it, as I shall not pass this way again. *(William Penn)*

22. Success is going from failure to failure without loss of enthusiasm.
(Winston Churchill)

Worksheet: Removable Letters

Goal: To practice reading words with a common trait while remembering to use the best voice you have available.

Here are some words that share a common trait. You can remove letters from the front of them and still have a recognizable word left. For example "space pace ace." Now find as many different words as you can in the list below.

1. alone
2. braid
3. chair
4. crash
5. crate
6. grant
7. ozone
8. phone
9. stone
10. place
11. plaid
12. plate
13. price
14. scare
15. scold
16. score
17. shall
18. snail
19. spear
20. spill
21. spray
22. stale
23. start
24. skill
25. please

Sentences using words above:

1. I braid my hair while I sit on my chair.
2. Phone home if you feel alone.
3. A snail moves more slowly than any other creature.
4. Score a goal if you can.
5. Grant me the patience to study for the test.
6. The firefighters will spray water on the flames.

Worksheet: Rhymes to Say Rhythmically

Goal: Say the rhymes rhythmically but with meaning and feeling. Don't forget the picture words!

1.

Aunt Isabella has a very long nose
Nobody knows
Why it grows
So long and so thin and as red as a rose

Uncle Marcus has very big ears
Does nobody know
Why they grow
So lumpy and hairy, oh why, such ears?

Cousin Mabel has very big feet
Does nobody know
Why feet grow
So long and fat, like plates of meat?

Nephew Billy has quite knobbly knees
And nobody knew
Why they grew
So lumpy and crooked like knots on trees.

Sister Sally has a wobbly chin
And nobody knew
Why it grew
So floppy and wide and not more thin.

Those are my relatives mentioned above
All can see
Even me
That what's inside is what I love!

2.

I love the sound of raindrops
Gentle dripping rain
Sprinkling in a pattern
On the windowpane.

I love the sound of thunder
Banging all around
Booming, cracking, crashing
Reverberating sound.

I love the sound of music
Sweet notes in a refrain
Bringing so much pleasure
Time and time again.

I love the sound of traffic
Passing in the street
Cars and buses whooshing
And people's clacking feet.

I love the sound of water
It pours and drips and flows
Splashes, cools and nurtures
Everything that grows.

I love the sound of horses
Canter, gallop, trot
The rhythm of their hoof beats
The snorting when they're hot.

I love the sound of children
As they run and play
Enjoying summer weather
Free from school all day.

I love my family's voices
And wherever I may roam
Those precious voices call me
Reminding me of home.

3.

Birds twitter
Dogs bark
Babies cry
In the dark.

Grandmas laugh
Leaves rustle
Dads say
"Let's hustle."

Mothers soothe
Sisters whine
Brothers tease
Especially mine!

Worksheet: A Scary Halloween Story

Goal: Read the story filling in the blanks with the words listed in the columns. Make your voice reflect the meanings and feelings as you read.

Story

Sometimes I get scared at Halloween. I ____________ (verb) in my ____________ (noun) and imagine ____________ (noun + s) in my ____________ (noun) making my skin crawl and my heart ____________ (verb). It is dark, and there is no moon at all shining through the window. I think I see a cat's ____________ (noun) in the dark. I hear the wind ____________ (verb + ing) outside the window and ____________ (noun + s) move around me. I'm scared to ____________ (verb) and lie as still as can be hardly ____________ (verb + ing) at all. My ____________ (noun) thuds in my chest. I want my mom to turn on the ____________ (noun) and ____________ (verb) ____________ (verb + ing) ____________ (noun + s) to keep me from ____________ (verb + ing) that ____________ (noun + s) are ____________ (verb + ing) to frighten her ____________.

Verbs	Nouns	Nouns + s (Plural Nouns)	Verb + ing
lie	bed	witches	gleaming
shriek	pyjamas	houses	glowing
snuggle	sleeping bag	ghosts	whistling
beat	hair	shadows	whining
say	room	words	breathing
stop	eyes	footsteps	comforting
move	heart	boys	feeling
breathe	light	girls	coming
thump	daughter	eyes	blowing
sleep	son	whiskers	moving

Which words make the scariest voice pictures? Here are some to say in a soft voice.

ghosts

shadows

whiskers

blowing

breathing

Here are some to say in a low voice.

thump

beat

comforting

witches

snuggle

Here are some to say in a high voice.

shriek

whistling

light

gleaming

Worksheet: Verses

Goal: To speak the lines rhythmically but with meaning and feeling, without breaking the flow.

1. Sheep Shut Eye

Sheep shouldn't sleep in a shack.
Sheep should sleep in a shed.
Sheep shouldn't sleep on their back
and certainly not in a bed.

Talk about where and how sheep sleep. Count how many "sh" sounds there are in this tongue twister.

2. Owlish not Scowlish

He's as wise as an owl,
And, as he gives me a pat,
He says "Don't ever scowl
as no one likes that!

Talk about who this person might be. A grandfather perhaps? Why would he give this advice?

3. Envy (by Edgar Guest)

I wonder if the poppy shows
the slightest envy of the rose?
Or if the pansy wastes its time
regretting that it cannot climb?
Do blossoms of a yellow hue
complain because they are not blue?
I cannot say, but fancy not.
Each seems contented with his lot.
Tis only man who thinks that he
some other man would rather be.

Talk about things you have felt envious about. Also talk about how "man" is used in the poem to mean "all mankind" including, of course, girls and women.

Worksheet: Vocal Expressiveness

Goal: To practice varying the voice on target words to suggest the meaning.

1. As **solid** as a brick
   (Substitute other words, e.g., hard, rough, heavy)
2. As **treacherous** as quicksand
   (Substitute other words, e.g., shifting, unsafe, scary)
3. As **deep** as the ocean
   (Substitute other words, e.g., blue, wide, calm)
4. As **sleek** as a panther
   (Substitute other words, e.g., dangerous, deadly, powerful)
5. As **delicious** as chocolate
   (Substitute other words, e.g., dark, smooth, creamy)
6. As **sweet** as sugar
   (Substitute other words, e.g., white, fine, crunchy)
7. As **cuddly** as a kitten
   (Substitute other words, e.g., wriggly, soft, adorable)
8. As **sour** as a lemon
   (Substitute other words, e.g., bitter, yucky, juicy)
9. As **golden** as the sun
   (Substitute other words, e.g., bright, warm, glowing)
10. As **pretty** as a picture
    (Substitute other words, e.g., colorful, beautiful, gorgeous)

Worksheet: All Voiced Sounds

Goal: To read the words making sure no sounds are devoiced.

Word List

melons	elbows	legs
lavender	oval	ivy
wild	noses	meadow
Indiana	nine	windows
Iowa	mauve	granola
Alabama	ear	bananas

Choose appropriate words from the lists above to fill in the blanks.

1. A ______________ animal lives in ______________.
2. ______________ is where we grow these ______________.
3. Imagine ______________ arms, ______________, and ______________ on one unusual man.
4. Ron's ______________ wears a gold earring.
5. Marilyn wore an old ______________ and ______________ gown.
6. Mary's nails are ______________ and long.
7. Melvin's ______________ and arms are brown.
8. Mom grew ______________ and roses in the garden.
9. I'll have ______________ and ______________ for my meal on Monday evening.
10. The view from the ______________ is of a lovely green ______________.

Worksheet: Weather Sayings

Instructions: Read the sayings written below in your most authoritative voice, but don't strain or tense your throat. Use your lips and tongue to say the words clearly and with authority.

1. If fleecy white clouds cover the heavenly way,
   no rain should mar your plans that day.

2. Frost or dew in the morning light
   shows no rain before the night.

3. If the woolly bear caterpillar
   has a narrow band,
   colder winter weather
   will freeze your hand.

4. Rain before seven
   clear by eleven.

5. A ring around the moon
   means it will rain soon.
   The larger the ring
   the more rain birds sing.

6. Short notice, soon to pass
   long notice, long will last.
   (Clouds that form quickly bring short rain;
   cloudy for a long time and rain will remain.)

Worksheet: What Happened Next?

Goal: To make up sentences that follow each other and to practice your best voice.

Instructions: Read the beginning sentences in a clear voice. Then continue the story starting each new sentence with the last letter in the previous sentence. Use your imagination, and don't forget about your voice!

When I came out of the school building, I went to get my bike. "Eek!" I screamed, "My bike isn't here where I left it." "Tell the teacher," said my best friend. "Did you really ride your bike today?" said my brother, Rollo. "Of course, I did, you know I did," I wailed. "Don't cry" said my brother, "I will use my cell phone to call home." "Mom will be upset if I have lost my new bike" I said. "Don't you think you should notify the police too?" said my friend Holly. "Yes, of course," said my brother, "I will call them on my cell phone too." "Oh," I wailed, "I am so upset and rattled by all this."

Worksheet: Word Square

Goal: To find as many words as you can in the square and to say those words in your best voice.

Instructions: Start with any letter and move one square at a time in any direction, even diagonally, to spell a word. See how many words you can make.

S	T	A	N
O	H	E	D
N	G	A	R
K	I	W	B

Examples:

ward

dean

heat

ghost

kin

bard

When you have found all the words you can in this square, perhaps you can make up a new square of letters yourself.

Worksheet: Word Stress

Goal: To vary the stress of bisyllabic words while producing them in an easy voice.

Sometimes the meaning of a word changes depending on the part of the word that is stressed (or has the strong beat). There are even some words in English where we know whether the word is a noun (naming word) or a verb (doing word) by the stressed syllable. The rule is that the second syllable is stressed if the word is a verb, and the first syllable is stressed if it is being used as a noun. Read the lists below and then try making up sentences using the words.

Verbs	Nouns
exploit	exploit
convert	convert
excuse	excuse
project	project
entrance	entrance
convict	convict
import	import
console	console
conduct	conduct
insult	insult
rebel	rebel
compress	compress
contract	contract
compact	compact
reject	reject
commune	commune
contest	contest
escort	escort
combat	combat
content	content

Here are some where the stress stays the same:

reward	reward
respect	respect
refill	refill

Can you think of any others?

Sentences with two versions of the same word:

1. She was a learned woman and he learned a lot from her.
2. We are blessed by this birth of a child, which is a truly blessed event.
3. I was interrupted when typing my resumé and had to resume doing it later.
4. Separate the separate elements of the puzzle.
5. A moderate politician was chosen to moderate the event.
6. I will intimate to the viewers that my cousin is not an intimate friend of the contestant on the quiz show.
7. I will lead you to the house with the dangerous lead paint.
8. In a minute I will show you the minute particles of gold.
9. I live near a studio where live television shows are produced.
10. The invalid went in her wheelchair to vote, but her vote was invalid.

Worksheet: A Story About Quiet Breathing: George the Giraffe

George the Giraffe was walking through the zoo eating lunch. His long neck came in very handy for eating the leaves off the top of the trees. The only problem with his long neck was that when he had a cold and his throat was sore, the whole long thing was sore. *OUCH!* Having such a long neck, George had to breathe very carefully and deeply to get the air all the way into his lungs. The air had a long way to go (trace George's neck with your finger to see how far the air had to go). Even though his air had so far to go, you could never hear him breathing. It was amazing how quiet he could be.

One day George the Giraffe was stopped by his friend Leo the Lion. "George, how can it be that with such a long neck, you are such a quiet breather?" "That's easy," said George, "I know a secret." Well, Leo loved secrets, and he wanted to know this one. "George, please tell me. I'd like to breathe a lot more quietly so I can sneak up on people." "Well," said George, "All you need to do to breathe quietly is to breathe deeply, relax your shoulders **(Jiggle)**, relax your neck **(Roll it)**, and relax your jaw **(Wiggle)**." "Just stay relaxed and you won't make any sound while breathing." "Thanks," said Leo, "I think I'll go practice."

Continuing on his walk, George met Benny Bear. "Oh dear, oh dear," said Benny. "What's wrong?" asked George. "Hunting season is coming, and I am scared of the hunters." Now most bears are mean and frighten folks. But not Benny; he was afraid of his own shadow. "I am scared that some hunter will hear my noisy breathing and trap me. I wish I had quiet, easy breathing like you, George," said Benny. "That's easy," said George, "let me teach you." So George explained, what you need to do is to breathe deeply, relax your shoulders **(Jiggle)**, relax your neck **(Roll it)**, and relax your jaw **(Wiggle)**." When you stay relaxed, you won't make any sound." Benny was very nervous that a hunter would hear him, and when he tried what George told him to do, he tensed up. By tensing up, he sounded like this: HH HH HH (loud breathing). "Don't worry Benny, just relax, practice, and you'll be fine. I didn't learn how to breathe this quietly in one day," George said. "I'll keep trying," replied Benny.

As George continued walking he saw Zippy Zebra crying by a tree. "Zippy," George asked, "what's wrong?" "Oh George, I have such noisy breathing, and I am afraid that people will make fun of me. Listen." Zippy began breathing, and it was louder than George thought it would be. George noticed that Zippy was tensing his neck, his shoulders, and his jaw, and his throat was so tight that it was no wonder his breathing was so loud. George told Zippy that he knew a secret that would help him to breathe quietly and easily. "Zippy," George said, "all you need to do is to breathe deeply, relax your shoulders **(Jiggle)**, relax your neck **(Roll it)**, and relax your jaw **(Wiggle)**." If you remember to keep yourself relaxed, than your breathing will be quiet in no time."

As George walked away from Zippy, he felt very happy. For many different reasons, quiet, easy breathing was important to his friends. He had always been told what a quiet breather he was, and now his breathing secrets could help some of his friends. George the Giraffe stood by himself relaxing his shoulders **(Jiggle)**, relaxing his neck **(Roll it)**, and relaxing his jaw **(Wiggle)** and breathing deeply and as quietly as he possibly could. He felt so relaxed that he fell asleep—standing up of course!! Good night George.

Written by Jodi K. Bloom

Worksheet: Waltzing Matilda*

Goal: To speak or sing the words with the voice reflecting changes in meaning.

Instructions: Act out this popular Australian song by singing or speaking the words as the characters would do it.

Once a jolly swagman
Camped by a billabong
Under the shade
Of a coolibah tree
And he sang as he watched
And waited till his billy boiled
You'll come a-waltzing Matilda with me.

<u>*Refrain*</u>

Waltzing Matilda, Waltzing Matilda
You'll come a-waltzing Matilda with me
And he sang as he watched
And waited till his billy boiled
You'll come a-waltzing Matilda with me.

Up came a jumbuck
To drink at the billabong
Up jumped the swagman
And grabbed him with glee
And he sang as he stuffed
That Jumbuck in his tucker bag
You'll come a-waltzing Matilda with me.

<u>*Refrain*</u>

Waltzing Matilda, Waltzing Matilda
You'll come a-waltzing Matilda with me
And he sang as he stuffed
That Jumbuck in his tucker bag
You'll come a-waltzing Matilda with me.

Up rode the squatter
Mounted on his thoroughbred
Up came the troopers
One two three
"Where's that jolly jumbuck
You've got in your tucker bag
You'll come a-waltzing Matilda with me" } sternly

<u>*Refrain*</u>

Waltzing Matilda, Waltzing Matilda
You'll come a-waltzing Matilda with me
"Where's that jolly jumbuck
You've got in your tucker bag
You'll come a-waltzing Matilda with me."

Up jumped the swagman
And sprang into the billabong
"You'll never catch me alive" said he
And his ghost may be heard
As you pass by that billabong
You'll come a-waltzing Matilda with me. } softly

<u>*Refrain*</u>

Waltzing Matilda, Waltzing Matilda
You'll come a-waltzing Matilda with me
And his ghost may be heard
As you pass by that billabong
You'll come a-waltzing Matilda with me. } softly

Glossary:

- Waltzing Matilda refers to the movement of the swag as a swagman (hobo) walks.
- A coolibah tree is a eucalyptus or gum tree.
- A billabong is a water-hole or pond.
- A billy is a tin in which tea is made over an open fire.
- A jumbuck is a sheep.

Note: If this is a group activity, children can be trees as well as the jumbuck and the other characters mentioned. A blue cloth on the floor can be the billabong.

Worksheet: Changing Pitch to Show Meaning

Goal: To contrast pitch on key words and phrases.

chirp	tuba	up the stairs
squeak	bass	down the stairs
whistle	foghorn	at dusk
flute	basement	in the mist
sing	stomped	warm rich bass

Instructions A
Underline the words in the lists above, and talk about how to say them, before you read the sentences below.

1. She stomped down the stairs to the basement.
2. Some birds sing and others chirp.
3. At dusk, in the mist, the foghorn scares us.
4. She started at the bottom and climbed up the stairs.
5. My favorite is the flute, but he likes the tuba.
6. He can sing beautifully in a warm rich bass.
7. She'll whistle a happy tune for you.

Instructions B
See which words fit best in the blanks in the sentences below. Then read them aloud.

1. If I were a bird I would ______________.
2. When I walk downstairs I ______________.
3. To come from the basement I ______________ ______________ ______________.
4. The tuba makes a deeper sound than the ______________.
5. Ships need the ______________ to warn them of danger.
6. If I were a mouse you'd hear me ______________.
7. Mom sings soprano but Dad sings ______________.
8. I went ______________ ______________ ______________ to the attic.
9. Foghorns blast, birds ______________ and children ______________.
10. Mom calls me indoors ______________ ______________.

Worksheet: Cognitive Cueing of Sentences

Goal: Practice how your voice reflects meanings and feelings. Try these sentences. Read the sentences silently. Picture it in your mind as you read it and then say it aloud.

Reinforcements provided include prompts such as:
  a. "Yes, I could really see that in my mind as you said it."
  b. "I could really feel it!"

The sentences and the associated cues:

1. The submarine sank to the bottom of the sea.
   a. Let me hear how the sailors felt as the submarine sank.
   b. Think about the surface of the water. Start your voice there and show me how the submarine goes down.
2. The red wagon maneuvered the curve.
   a. Think about what kind the wagon is? Maybe a Mercedes? Make your voice show how smoothly it took the curve!
   b. Let me feel that smooth ride!
3. The bomber dived way down in the ocean.
   a. Diving is quick and perhaps the bomber disintegrated. Make your voice show me the effect on the ocean.
   b. Let me feel the shock!
4. Roseanne ran away in May.
   a. Why do you think Roseanne ran away?
   b. How did she feel?
5. Those wars are all over now.
   a. Contrast the impact of wars with the peace that followed.
   b. Make me feel the relief.
6. There were eleven oily wheels.
   a. What kind of wheels were they? Make your voice "oily" and the wheels move as you wonder why there were eleven.
   b. Make me feel the rhythm of the wheels going around.
7. I'll remember my money.
   a. Did something happen to your money before? Think why it is important to you to have the money with you and let me hear you remembering.
   b. Feel the importance of money to you.
8. Whose arms are these?
   a. You have discovered a part of a body. Let me hear how you feel as you think whose they might be.
   b. Feel the horror of it.

Pretest and Posttest Items

Respiration

Length of Exhalation

Blows through a straw in water to make bubbles . . . . . ________ secs

Prolongs s. . . . . ________ secs

Inspiratory Patterns

Observable tension. . . . . ☐ yes ☐ no
Lower chest expansion . . . . ☐ yes ☐ no
Raises shoulders . . . . ☐ yes ☐ no

Replenishing Breaths

Replenishes before supply is exhausted . . . . ☐ yes ☐ no
Voice fades at ends of breath groups . . . . ☐ yes ☐ no
Voice sounds "pressed" for air . . . . ☐ yes ☐ no

Phonation

Prolongations

Prolongs voiced and unvoiced cognates *s/z* . . . . ________ secs /s/

. . . . ________ secs /z/

Prolongs vowel *a* . . . . ________ secs

Quality during prolongation of *a* (Circle items that apply.)

voice breaks   hoarse
tense   clear
continuous   harsh
breathy   diplophonic

Loudness

Adjusts loudness levels . . . . ☐ yes ☐ no (when cued)
☐ yes ☐ no (spontaneously)
Sustains soft phonation . . . . ☐ yes ☐ no (prolonged sounds)
☐ yes ☐ no (phrases)

Vocal abuse (Circle items that apply.) . . . . ☐ yes ☐ no

hard attacks   tension
habituated loudness   other practices

Pitch

Adjusts pitch levels . . . . ☐ yes ☐ no (when cued)
☐ yes ☐ no (spontaneously)
Uses pitch variability . . . . ☐ yes ☐ no (contrastive words)
☐ yes ☐ no (reading)
☐ yes ☐ no (speaking)

Sings "Happy Birthday" . . . .☐ yes ☐ no (melodic accuracy)
☐ yes ☐ no (monotone)
☐ yes ☐ no (some pitch variations)

Duration/Rate/Rhythm

Sings "Happy Birthday" . . . .☐ yes ☐ no (correct timing and beat)
Phrases appropriately . . . .☐ yes ☐ no (spontaneous speech)
☐ yes ☐ no (reading)
Uses variation for meaning . . . .☐ yes ☐ no (spontaneously)
☐ yes ☐ no (when cued)

Number of syllables produced in one breath . . . . .______________ syllables

Rate during speech sample . . . . .______________ words per minute

Resonance

Adequacy of velopharyngeal mechanism . . . .☐ yes ☐ no
(note medical documentation)

Nasal emission on oral productions
(Circle items that apply.) . . . .☐ yes ☐ no

plosives	fricatives
affricatives	vowels
words	phrases

Voice quality during connected speech (Circle items that apply.)

hypernasal	appropriate balance
hyponasal	inadequate resonance

Maximizes resonance . . . .☐ yes ☐ no (vowels)
☐ yes ☐ no (voiced continuants)
☐ yes ☐ no (projected speech)
☐ yes ☐ no (conversational speech)
Assimilated nasality (regionalisms) . . . .☐ yes ☐ no

Psychosocial Aspects

Adjusts vocal behavior . . . .☐ yes ☐ no (effect on listeners)
☐ yes ☐ no (context)
☐ yes ☐ no (when cued)
Discusses vocal options . . . .☐ yes ☐ no
Lists rules for vocal hygiene . . . .☐ yes ☐ no
Balances talking/listening time . . . .☐ yes ☐ no
Demonstrates conversational skills . . . .☐ yes ☐ no (turn-taking)
☐ yes ☐ no (question asking)
☐ yes ☐ no (topic maintenance)

Significant factors related to voice use (Circle items that apply.)

abusive habits	mouth opening	loudness level
role in family	amount of talking	posture
attitude	relationships	self-esteem

Note: This sample Pretest/Posttest may be used either in part or as a whole to check children's behaviors that are relevant to voice production. (For a more detailed assessment protocol and directions for implementation, see Moya L. Andrews, *Manual of Voice Treatment: Pediatrics Through Geriatrics.* San Diego, CA: Singular Publication Group.)

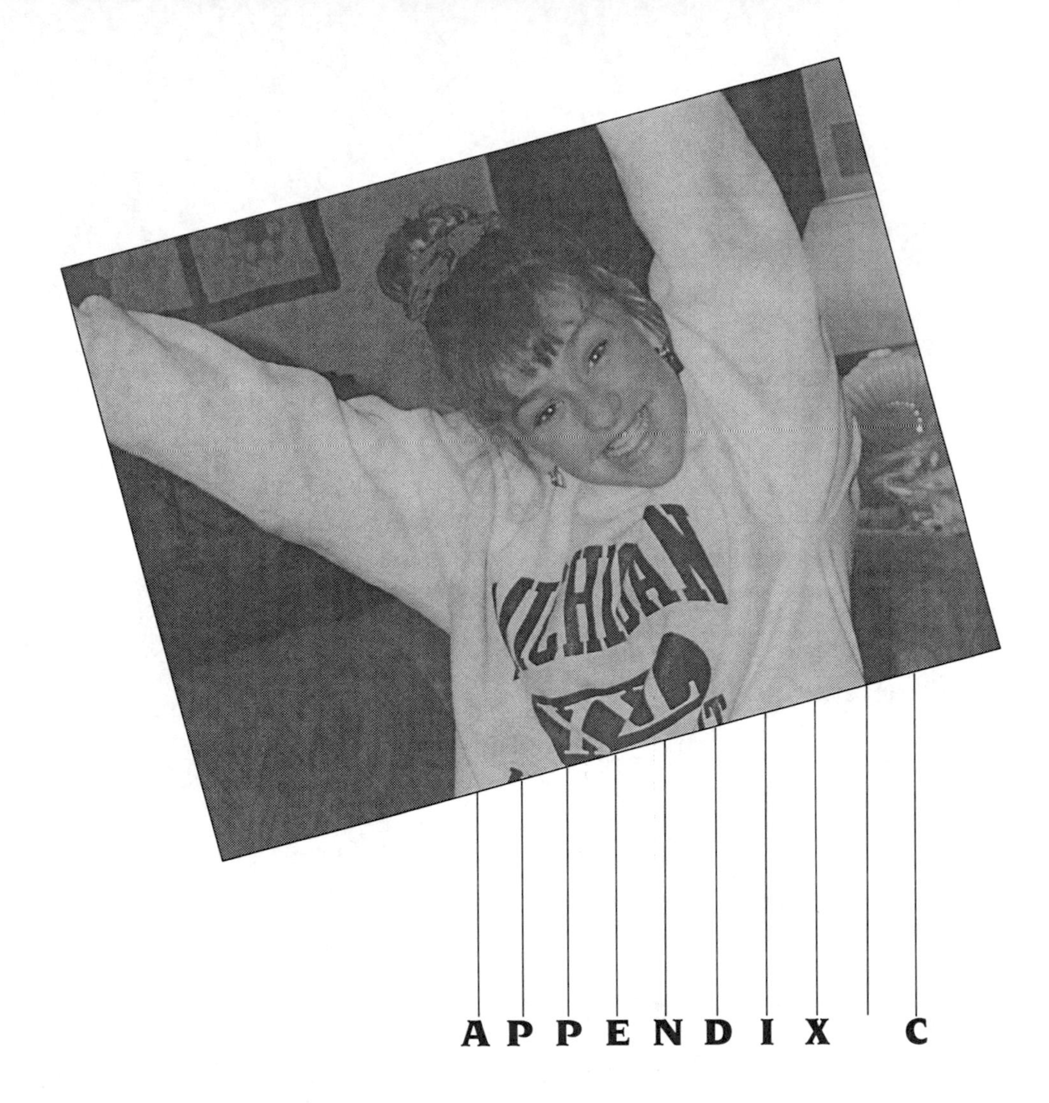

APPENDIX C

Practice Materials for Voice Therapy for Adolescents

Contents

Facilitators

Facilitators are used to stimulate an appropriate phonational pattern and are cues that are eliminated as the desired behavior stabilizes.

To Increase Laryngeal Tension

(Useful when vocal fold closure needs strengthening)

1. Push/press while phonating
   a. push against a wall with two hands
   b. push a chair across the room
   c. push clasped hands together
   d. push hands down on seat of chair (while seated)
   e. push feet firmly against floor
   f. push clasped hands together behind body (this keeps shoulders back and enhances breathing)
   g. push hands against a table edge while seated
2. Pull while phonating
   a. pull on own fingers
   b. pull on a cord held by clinician
   c. pull on a lock of hair
   d. pull on a ledge or table edge
3. Sudden body movements while phonating
   a. thrust arm (with clenched fist) forward from chest position to full extension in front of chest
   b. kick leg forward (as in a chorus line kick)
   c. quick deep knee bends
   d. quick side bends (arm moves down outer leg)
   e. partial sit-ups
   f. "reach for the sky"
4. Visualization while phonating
   a. squeezed or constricted images (e.g., necktie too tight)
   b. frightening situations (e.g., standing on the edge of a cliff and loosing balance)
   c. strong emotional states (e.g., shrieks, cries, closed vowels, clenched jaw)

To Decrease Laryngeal Tension

(Useful when folds are adducted with too much tension)

1. Vegetative movements while phonating
   a. chewing
   b. sighing
   c. yawning
   d. panting
   e. whistling
2. Body movements while phonating
   a. head rolls
   b. shoulder shrugs and rolls (can be done in unison and alternately)
   c. flop over at waist (Raggedy Ann style)
   d. lie flat on floor or table
   e. relaxed deep breathing
   f. twist back and forth from the torso
3. Speech movements
   a. drop jaw (to release tension in suprahyoids)
   b. blow out on voiceless continuants in a relaxed manner
   c. blow out on "whoo"
   d. hum to relaxing music
   e. intersperse "hums" with "h" in a relaxed sequence
   f. let voice flow through an open throat as "flow" is prolonged
   g. contrast very tense "i" with an open relaxed "a"
4. Images/visualization while phonating
   a. float on water while saying "hmm"
   b. feel "fat cheeks" like chipmunk while saying "aah"
   c. sink onto a soft feather bed while saying "oh"
   d. recapture own most relaxed situation or image
   e. drop word "blop" into a deep well (gradually increase number of "blops")
   f. think of honey or velvet (or other substance) and say "soothing"
   g. pretend to be quieting an agitated child/animal and murmur "There, there"
   h. visualize and adopt a relaxed posture; align head and torso and stand tall

To Increase Forward Placement of Voice

(Useful to improve oral resonance)

1. Body position while phonating
   a. bend over from waist and feel voice falling forward toward floor
   b. place chin on folded arms on a table (while seated) and feel facial bones vibrating
   c. place hands on face and feel vibration
   d. push hands against sternum with an upward movement
   e. cup hands on either side of mouth, feel mouth opening, and project
2. Tactile cues while phonating
   a. hum and make the lips tickle
   b. practice frontal voiced plosives with vowels and "throw" the voice past the plosive (CVs)
   c. sing a song to "la," emphasizing tongue movement and mouth opening
   d. use the lips to push the voice forward
   e. "bite off" each word with precise articulation
   f. feel as if mouth opening and lip and tongue movements are exaggerated; watch in a mirror to check perceptions
3. Visualization while phonating
   a. pull an imaginary string of voice from the mouth
   b. "throw" the voice to a distant surface, listener, object
   c. pretend to have a hinged jaw and open it wide like a ventriloquist's dummy
   d. pretend to be an authority figure and speak with a declamatory vocal style
   e. pretend to be angry and "hit" the listener with each firmly articulated word

Practice Materials Without Nasal Sounds

Words With Voiced Continuant Consonants

These words are suitable for improving oral resonance. Initially, words can be read in a "chanting" style, prolonging the vowels and voiced consonants. When appropriate oral resonance has been achieved, the words should be read in a conversational style, maximizing the consonants as "sound carriers." Care should be taken to avoid devoicing continuant consonants in final positions.

Monosyllabic		Multisyllabic	
rye	woe	rely	arouse
wave	woo	visa	rally
there	raise	Zulu	lazy
ooze	eyes	yellow	viral
live	ray	vowel	viva
rail	loaves	valley	volley
wise	raves	value	layers
use	zoo	vary	ravel
views	eve	very	losers
lull	wool	lathers	always
these	lathes	lazily	razor
owes	rouge	treasure	levers
veil	will	weasel	rather
vial	lose	lilly	lovely
zeal	veal	rosy	easily
czar	valve	revel	Lizzie
awes	low	Loyola	every
laws	zee	zero	early
Liz	zoe	rosary	leveler
rose	ewes	revise	livelier
whiz	lies	Eloise	easel
the	owes	they'll	zither
thou	wheeze	although	Louisa
thy	wise	leather	whereas
writhes	they	weather	realize
lair	though	worthy	they've
Lou	loathe	Larry	either
ale	wreathes	worthily	whithers
oil	Lear	Laura	worrier
raw	liar	Leah	larvae
row	eel	leeway	lava
rouse	zeal	really	layer
wave	real	olive	leery
wall	reels	oily	leisure
weave	rise	velour	resolve
all	rolls	evolve	valves
weigh	rules	revolve	elves

Words Without Nasal Consonants

The plosive and fricatives should be produced with emphasis on mouth opening and articulatory precision. These words are useful for students who need to experience "orality" and concentrate on continuity of velopharyngeal closure to generate appropriate oral pressure. Sentences to practice production of pressure consonants may also be used, such as, "These chillies are cheaper, but these chips of Charlie's are best" and "Space visitors are cheapskate shoppers who are churlish to shopkeepers."

Monosyllabic		Multisyllabic	
take	weld	police	broccoli
clock	scold	bracelet	jeweled
beach	gauze	luggage	outrigger
coat	bat	breakfast	tablecloth
dart	cut	attractive	spaghetti
sport	dot	delicious	factory
book	feet	parachute	distributor
glue	hut	vegetable	duplicator
hook	put	selective	hospital
five	pit	shapeless	operator
puff	tot	tadpole	diversity
tip	let	helicopter	favorable
dead	rat	freaky	behavior
hit	root	disbelief	fertilizer
pill	spit	relative	vaporizer
cave	bite	variety	pleasure
kite	bath	perspire	precipice
fuzz	door	powerful	precocious
wag	deer	isolated	rebellious
bug	house	reflective	ridiculous
shout	row	celebrate	phosphorus
touch	food	bicycle	addressed
tell	hook	practical	righteous
light	bait	jealous	accessory
brow	good	pretzel	asphalt
cold	cash	shoelace	scoreboard
fruit	couch	cockroach	stethoscope
street	race	witchcraft	wastebasket
chop	sail	sauerkraut	escalator
rush	shake	chapter	discouraged
huge	chair	acrobatics	exposure
bulge	chill	chocolate	exchequer
golf	verb	irradiate	luxurious
fresh	loaf	refrigerate	paperbacks
tweed	haul	jubilee	preserved
froze	yield	valuable	biweekly
doubt	child	exclusive	backlash
drool	vase	exclude	heckler

Sentences Without Nasal Consonants

1. I will purchase the vegetables for supper.
2. Bagels are Phillip's favorite food.
3. You are requested to stay here, Patricia.
4. Steve works at a very large store.
5. The subway fire caused great fright.
6. Jack always washes his face with soap.
7. Where do you wish to go?
8. He shouted loudly to the lady across the street.
9. The holidays passed altogether too quickly.
10. The picture of you is absolutely beautiful.
11. Who will give us the gist of this topic?
12. What vegetables would you like to have at the party?
13. She had to go back to school.
14. How do you like your eggs cooked?
15. I saw her go out to greet Peter.
16. Yesterday she wore a bright red suit with white shoes.
17. The celebrity was happy to receive the key to the city.
18. The girl was a popular Ohio State cheerleader.
19. The letter gave her a severe shock.
20. Food is so costly these days that it costs us $60 for a week's groceries.
21. He will be grateful to you for it.
22. There was too little variety of topics listed.
23. I had the watch repaired at the local jewelers.
24. The crawl stroke is easy to do.
25. This toothpaste is available at all reputable drug stores.
26. Tell her to be sure to address the parcels correctly.
27. The effects of alcohol are quite disastrous for drivers.
28. The college is situated here.
29. There will be a large art display at the state gallery this week.
30. The sailors had good weather throughout their voyage.
31. We have to stay at the library to study effectively.
32. Is she very seriously hurt?
33. I'd like a table for two over by the fireplace.
34. The subdued lights threw weird shadows about the hall.
35. I would like to travel overseas this year.
36. Basketball develops athletic skill.
37. The gatekeeper told the picketers to go away.
38. Will you give this boy a piece of paper?
39. I walked up the stairway before he did.
40. At sea the air is oppressively sultry.
41. We took the videotape to the class party.
42. Read your words aloud to the class.
43. Look before you leap or you'll fall up the stairs.
44. Good posture is a requisite to good speech.
45. The political party usually forgets its earlier pledges.
46. The library clerk is very polite.
47. Yes, I shall wait here for you.

Paragraphs Without Nasal Sounds

Our resort offers exotic local food that tastes as good as it looks. Beautiful, fresh, delicious appetizers to desserts are offered here. Fruits, vegetables, cakes, plus pies are all available for you. There are lots of places to go. These trips take you everywhere. Places such as Europe, Israel plus Florida. There is lots to do at these resorts. Your are able to sail, water ski, scuba dive, horseback ride, or sit at the pool. You will see lots of people at the resort; the guests plus workers will help you feel relaxed as well as happy.

Everybody loves to eat pizza. There are several foods that are good to top pizza. Cheese is the best, but I also like sausage. Chili peppers are delicious, too. Olives are also OK. If I go to the pizzeria, I also order garlic bread. Plus, I'll get a salad. Rarely do I order all three together, though. I'd be obese if I did. As it is I eat a lot of pizza, so I usually have to watch what I eat. If I eat pizza everyday, I'll look like a hippo.

Just outside of Chicago, there's a little old village called Libertyville. It is a beautiful area filled with history. A circle of large rosebushes that flatters the aged village hall borders the village square. Daily visitors cheerfully gaze at the colorful roses. The village square is a place for local artists or actors. People love to watch or participate with these activities while the sky is bright above. After the dark sky has appeared, refreshed visitors stroll by the lake that glows like a colorful glass. Few people realize Libertyville has this delightful character.

Charles just switched jobs. Because his wife, Debbie, works, too, they have extra cash to pay for a house. They hope to locate a big yellow house with a large yard that's close to the busy city. They chose the colors for the various places—lots of blues or reds. They have already picked out the chairs, tables, pillows plus little objects with which to decorate. They're really excited to look for a house especially because they expect their first baby after a short while.

There are very few areas of life that allow us to regard this world without disgust, but there is a beauty that people create out of the chaos: the pictures they produce, the lyrics they create, the books they write, plus the lives they lead. Of all these, the richest beauty is a life well lived. That is the perfect work of art.

Koala bears look like large, gray teddy bears. They are 2 to 3 feet tall with thick woolly fur. Trees serve as the chief habitat for koalas, especially eucalyptus trees. The foliage of the eucalyptus, as well as a few other trees, provides food for the creatures. Koalas occupy various parts of Australia. There is a risk that the species will disappear as eucalyptus trees are destroyed. To forestall this, koalas are protected by law.

Here are a few tips for the racquetball player. First, buy a good quality glove. Good sturdy plastic glasses are also a good idea to protect your eyes. You will also have to buy two racquetballs. After you have bought all the prerequisite articles, you are ready to play. Always be sure to keep the face of the racquet parallel to the wall you wish to hit. Last, try to hit the ball as close to the floor as possible.

Oral–Nasal Contrast Words

/m/	/b/	/m/	/b/
me	be	bomb	Bob
mail	bail	boom	boob
mar	bar	bum	bub
mass	bass	came	Cabe
mess	Bess	come	cub
my	bye	cram	crab
mill	Bill	dam	dab
mole	bowl	dim	dib
moss	boss	dumb	dub
muff	buff	limb	lib
mug	bug	loam	lobe
male	bail	game	Gabe
moan	bone	gram	grab
mow	bow	rim	rib
mile	bile	Jim	jib

/n/	/d/	/n/	/d/
gnome	dome	an	add
knave	Dave	ban	bad
knead	deed	been	bead
new	dew	Ben	bed
knock	dock	bin	bid
know	dough	bone	bode
Nan	Dan	bun	Budd
near	dear	clan	clad
neck	deck	clown	cloud
nice	dice	cone	code
Nile	dial	crown	crowd
nip	dip	dune	dude
nun	done	green	greed
nor	door	hen	head
nose	doze	Jane	jade
knot	dot	June	Jude
noun	down	lane	laid
numb	dumb	lean	lead
neigh	day	moon	mood
Newell	dual	prune	prude
name	dame	gone	God
note	dote	brawn	broad

(continued)

Oral–Nasal Contrast Words *(continued)*

/ŋ/	/g/	/ŋ/	/g/
bang	bag	lung	lug
bing	big	ping	pig
bong	bog	rang	rag
bring	brig	ring	rig
ding	dig	rung	rug
dong	dog	sang	sag
dung	dug	slang	slag
fang	fag	spring	sprig
gang	gag	swing	swig
hang	hag	tongue	tug
hung	hug	wing	wig
long	log	tang	tag

Practice Materials With Nasal Sounds

Words With Nasal Consonants

Monosyllabic (Vowels and voiced continuants only)		**Monosyllabic** (Other consonants)	
name	male	mange	march
ming	mall	mink	mask
mane	nine	mound	mat
man	ring	monk	mace
mean	knees	mind	mash
numb	nouns	mumps	math
moan	mourn	manned	mass
moon	gnarl	mount	month
none	noun	malt	ninth
mine	gnaw	map	nip
gnome	known	nod	nix
noon	men	north	nook
norm	maim	not	neat
mine	ma'am	nest	next
mum	nun	knife	gnats
maize	noise	gnash	nights

Multisyllabic (Vowels and voiced continuants only)		**Multisyllabic** (Other consonants)	
aiming	mammogram	neutron	Cincinnati
morning	aluminum	amend	snakeskin
meaning	neon	nomad	centennial
Maureen	immune	mandate	monkey
family room	mammal	maintain	humdrum
linoleum	numbing	member	income
neoplasm	minimum	mental	nimble
enamel	membrane	milky	mushroom
mingle	hangman	minstrel	phantom
newsmen	Miami	mountain	springtime
ringing	normal	madam	symptom
anagram	animal	moonbeam	addendum
dining room	noisy	phoneme	pantomime
nasals	Norman	random	chrysanthemum
northern	neither	sternum	almond
naval	nylon	tandem	compendium

(*continued*)

Words With Nasal Consonants *(continued)*

Multisyllabic (Vowels and voiced continuants only)	Multisyllabic (Other consonants)	
pneumonia	anteroom	Hinduism
nominee	antonym	cannibalism
nouveau	Christendom	crematorium
lunar	maximum	abnormal
manner	synonym	informal
money	journalism	monument
owner	mongolism	ornament
inner	Anglicanism	number
airliner	condominium	magnificent
another	subnormal	coming
honors	almanac	England
lanolin	Monday	metholatum
lawn mower	lenient	international
maneuver	November	Pan-American
Manila	nonentity	nuisance
vanilla	ping pong	semifinal
mariner	gangplank	newborn
manually	Michigan	symposium
minerals	moment	nutmeg

Names With Nasal Consonants

Ways to use name lists include (a) reading all names of people you know, (b) reading all names containing more than one nasal sound, (c) reading all names that can be either a first or last name, (d) making up surnames containing nasal sounds to go with the first names, (e) making up nicknames for as many of the names on the list as possible.

Mame	Mable	Moya	Murray
Maureen	Maurice	Mickie	Myrna
Marc	Marcus	Millie	Myron
May	Marie	Milton	Myrtle
Marvin	Marshall	Mandy	McArthur
Michael	Marsha	Mitchell	McIntosh
Matthew	Martin	Molly	Madeline
Myles	Mary	Morris	Madonna
Manuel	Mercedes	Meredith	Miranda
Amy	Emma	Jimmy	Jamie
Mimi	Omar	Remus	Sammy
Simon	Tammy	Timothy	Tommy
Kenneth	Edmond	Clementine	Pamela
Kimberly	Naomi	Adam	Christine
Alma	Elmer	Wilma	Thelma
Selma	Selina	Andrew	Edna
Nancy	Erma	Norma	Charmaine
Angela	Nanette	Smith	Neil
Nell	Nicholas	Nelson	Noel
Nina	Natalie	Napoleon	Anna
Annette	Lena	Benjamin	Bonny
Daniel	Dennis	Frances	Gina
Janet	Jeanette	Lana	Penelope
Venus	Robin	Mona	Blaine
Glenn	Donald	Dean	Jean
John	Joan	Lynn	Ronald
Stan	Shawn	Shane	Elaine
Eugene	Gordon	Helen	Herman
Irene	Karen	Susan	Colleen
Clinton	Aileen	Lyndon	Loraine
Sharon	Sanford	Sheldon	Sylvan
Allison	Sandra	Geraldine	Josephine
Shirleen	Magdalene	Vernon	Janice
Brandy	Cynthia	Indira	Blondie
Roland	Mary Ann	Ingrid	Bernard
Arnold	Ernest	Lorna	Lillian
Lorne	Spencer	Penny	Garland

Sentences With Nasal Consonants

1. No one knows Norman's nickname.
2. The Indians camped around the mountain.
3. Ken wants to go to Sweden next autumn.
4. The annoying random humming seemed too much for him to handle.
5. The garden smelled fragrant in summer.
6. Jane went to Norway last winter.
7. The baron came from Munich.
8. Never make a mean man mad.
9. Neal needs some lumber to build extensions.
10. Nancy knows that Mike might marry me.
11. Newton's comprehension of science knew no boundaries.
12. Mervin made a mess of the musical number.
13. Not under any circumstances can he be included as a member.
14. Nixon never ran again.
15. Mr. Morris met my neighbor Madeline in March.
16. Millie made lemon and lime marmalade.
17. Many men named Ned as a nominee.
18. Marsha and Mallory went to Macy's in New York.
19. That singing telegram made me angry.
20. A nasty note was sent to my neighbor anonymously.
21. Norman never sings in the morning or even at night.
22. Novocain numbs my mouth and tongue.
23. Diamonds make nice engagement rings.
24. *Mademoiselle* printed a column on anorexia nervosa.
25. Mike needed money to take Nancy on a romantic honeymoon in Miami.
26. Many men or women never learn knitting or needlework.
27. The man smiled with contentment when his team won the Indianapolis 500.
28. Don't smoke in the newly painted dining room.
29. Many men and women work in amusement parks such as Disneyland and Disneyworld.
30. My most memorable moment came when I sang with the Minneapolis Symphony.
31. Muriel will live in Merrillville near Adrienne Nowell's.
32. Can Nancy remember Noreen's phone number?
33. Bananas and melons grow in warm climates.
34. My new neighbors are Norwegian immigrants.
35. Natchez is an historic town in Mississippi.

Paragraphs With Nasal Consonants

Most men and women make many decisions, and one's friends may often be influential. Decisions made now may have major implications for many moons to come! Smart decisions are not made on impulse. Much information, not only emotion, is mandatory.

Marshall McLuhan maintained that the medium is the message. Many mass media managers market television time emphasizing the subliminal impact of commercial messages on teenagers.

Humor has significant benefits. One man experienced pain in his joints and wondered, "If negative emotions bring negative chemical changes, might humor contribute to my treatment?" He programmed himself for optimum benefits, and noted increased pain-free time minus tension following sessions of merriment.

Muriel Montgomery married a minerologist named Emmanuel Glenn in Manila and moved around many times during her marriage to him. On one occasion, when residing in Arizona, Muriel became enamored of Indian customs and handicrafts. The museum in Phoenix presented a marvelous opportunity for Muriel to become immersed in many interesting readings and programs on Navajo Indians.

Rhonda Simonson came from an unfortunate family situation. It seemed that her parents never had time to spend at home and were always running around town with friends. Consequently, dinner was never a family occasion and mostly consisted of weiners and canned or frozen entrees. Rhonda resented having to mind the small children and assume her parents' responsibilities. Her teenage years were miserable until she became determined to compensate for the emptiness in the home environment. She began to prepare nutritious meals for the family, related to the children more warmly, and encouraged open communication during dinner times.

A psychologist in Alabama, Dolf Zillmann, has studied the anatomy of rage. He found that a universal trigger for anger is the feeling of being endangered. It may be a physical or symbolic threat to self-esteem or dignity. It may be a feeling of being unjustly treated or feeling insulted or demeaned. It may even be frustration, if one is blocked in achieving an objective. Anger from earlier frustrating circumstances may cause someone to become enraged later on when some minor event triggers what seems like an overreaction. Thus the man who kicks the poor dog in the evening following a frustrating day at the office.

Words With Voiced Continuant Consonants
(Suitable for improving oral-nasal resonance)

Words should be said slowly so that voicing may be prolonged throughout the entire word.

Monosyllabic		Multisyllabic	
new	rhyme	neon	loving
vine	loan	moving	movies
zoom	Mel	mellow	Molly
maze	loom	miser	muzzle
zing	mauve	mainly	zoning
thine	knees	nuzzling	venial
moan	zone	lion	leaning
kneels	noise	lonely	longing
mom	rain	morning	vision
man	ring	rolling	raisin
nose	worm	lemon	ozone
run	mine	million	alone
name	muse	immune	only
mine	aim	oozing	evening
hum	nose	numeral	manly
wing	wrong	Milan	mural
long	lung	muslin	minor
limb	maize	maneuver	manual
lamb	lime	mariner	menial
room	lame	Miami	millionaire
whim	vim	malaria	millinery
yam	whom	memorial	memorize
realm	elm	among	Amen
I've	knell	Emma	amuse
gnome	knoll	layman	mammal
known	nerve	Mimi	numbing
news	Nile	omen	Omar
noon	nor	rumor	amnesia
noun	none	amusing	alum
knave	Anne	memorize	annual
line	Verne	emery	vermilion
rhine	then	anomaly	alimony
than	vein	realism	living room
wane	whine	linoleum	aluminum
yawn	ram	Wilma	enamel
lean	lawn	naive	amazing

Practice Materials for Frontal Tone Focus

Words Containing Front Vowels and Tongue-Tip Consonants

To improve forward tone focus emphasizing tongue and lip movement. Useful for clients exhibiting cul-de-sac resonance, laryngeal hyperfunction, and limited mouth opening.

Monosyllabic			Multisyllabic		
neat	tip	net	lethal	chamois	shifty
knit	pat	nail	tipsy	shampoo	tennis
tab	tape	tea	patent	sheba	able
tail	deep	team	mitten	shiny	lady
tap	teal	knee	talent	babyish	Pepsi
teeth	lap	peat	bitten	demolish	tiptoe
thin	babe	bade	little	finish	taboo
tight	bad	bail	table	relish	tasty
cheat	bait	ban	tattoo	Danish	relish
chip	bat	bay	Lizzy	blemish	debate
laugh	bead	been	lowly	initial	tedious
tint	beet	bent	Lynette	beneficial	tally
tithe	bet	bib	pity	leadership	teddy
gnats	bill	bite	patter	tinsel	litter
feet	den	dam	batter	fiddle	teepee
sheath	date	dead	eighteen	chisel	petite
ship	deal	debt	belittle	chili	Betty
thieves	deed	deep	termite	achieve	Lilly
she'll	did	dip	petty	feature	tissue
shell	type	laid	battle	inches	British
shaft	lamb	lamp	city	moocher	fitted
shall	lane	lap	attention	peaches	latin
till	late	lead	Terrence	ditches	nineteen
fish	leap	tide	ballerina	chitchat	satan
leash	Lent	let	tablets	bleachers	title
flip	lid	light	nimble	busy	vital
fill	pad	line	peppers	fizzy	timidity
fifth	lip	lit	brittle	befit	lettuce
fib	paid	pail	bitters	Philippines	Teddy
chill	paint	peat	visited	fashion	aviation
tight	peal	peep	altimeter	differ	apple
teach	pep	pet	diameter	efface	tipped
tiff	pill	pipe	perimeter	jiffy	dainty
beach	pip	tape	nevertheless	infinity	thimble
cheese	cheap	sheen	lazily	pencil	athlete

Sentences Containing Front Vowels and Tongue-Tip Consonants

1. "Tiptoe through the tulips," trilled Tiny Tim in falsetto.
2. We drank a pint of bitters and ate tasty tortillas, but Ted was a teetotaler.
3. Billy stuck ten tiny pins and needles in my voodoo doll.
4. Lynn and Liz raced to the sea to take a dip.
5. Write the letter on this white tablet.
6. Read the list of names to them at bedtime.
7. Their feet tapped the tiles as they danced to the band that night.
8. Sit in the seat at the left end of the little theater.
9. People vanish every day from city streets.
10. Terrence touched his front teeth lightly.
11. Lizards eat many little flies and gnats.
12. Linda prepares a tasty Bibb lettuce salad every day.
13. Penny needs an advance in salary to pay her bills.
14. Tea and sympathy help mend many ills.
15. Even if tired, Ted never buys tablets to help revive him.
16. Embarrassed people rarely interview easily anytime.
17. Betty made a beer batter bread with raisins in it and iced it with lemon essence.
18. Steve's dentist feels peanut brittle is sweeter than he needs and increases his cavities.
19. The stars in the Little Dipper light the heavens at night.
20. The Apache Indians stitched the skins into a nice teepee.
21. Neal appreciates that people feel differently in stressful situations.
22. Pop the top of the cereal box, but don't tear it.
23. The Smithsonian is a museum in Washington, D.C.
24. The baby-sitter hid the Ninja Turtles.
25. September is my favorite time of the year.
26. The L. L. Bean catalog is free.
27. They sell everything you need for the season.
28. Don't miss out on the free gift certificates.
29. Visit our Web site that has 88 hits a day.
30. Infants are high-maintenance roommates.

Sentences Containing Voiced Continuant Consonants

1. The razor is always so noisy.
2. We run early Monday morning.
3. We'll all stroll home the long way.
4. He's as wise as an owl.
5. No one loves misery.
6. The royal family is rarely alone.
7. Mel loathes liver with onions.
8. No man or woman is an island.
9. The lonely woman raises those roses.
10. I envision a long, lazy summer.
11. The man oiled the machinery every morning.
12. Will the sling harm my arm?
13. We will have more lemons than ever this year.
14. The sun shines warmly in summer.
15. Summer in London is lovely.
16. Mollie's new mother has a lovely home.
17. When he is lonely, we run over there in the morning.
18. The falling rain ran in waves along the railing.
19. Many luxurious yellow pillows were seen in their home.
20. Cinnamon was in misery when wearing his muzzle.
21. Lemon jam is yummy on melon.
22. I mainly remember rain in November.
23. Levi was a miner in rural Virginia.
24. Jean always irons Myron's jerseys.
25. Wally examines the enzymes in oil.
26. Money is never evil when owners are wise.
27. Angel loves wearing ruby earrings.
28. Ease along the railing avoiding the wires.
29. Joy is realizing all will be well.
30. The lion and the unicorn were images.

Activities to Practice Forward Projection

The clinician sits on the far side of the room and asks a group member a question. The group member turns to the next person and says the answer at a conversational level. The group member then turns to the clinician and says the answer again using forward projection techniques (e.g., increased mouth opening, increased lip/tongue movement, and forward tone focus). This exercise contrasts conversational projection and distance projection strategies.

The student hums the tune of a favorite song then hums a stanza alternating humming and saying the words of the song. The student makes sure the reverberation felt during humming is carried over into the words. Finally, the student hums first as a cue then says all of the words of the song. If the tone focus is lost at any time, cue with a "hum" to regain it.

The student makes strings of /m/ words by changing one letter at a time. For example: mind, mild, mold, mole, mile, mill. The words are produced maximizing reverberation of the /m/ sounds.

The student thinks of favorite memories and uses appropriate projection, resonance, and the carrier phrase, "I mainly remember ____________________." Voiced continuants are emphasized.

Students in a group choose a country (e.g., France), and each group member, in turn, uses the carrier phrase, "I'm reminded of _______________." A variation of this activity is for each person to choose a word in alphabetical order. For example:

"I'm reminded of Antoinne."

"I'm reminded of Bordeau."

"I'm reminded of croissants."

Voiced continuants and vowel sounds are emphasized.

The student relives a favorite moment, experience, or day and describes it. If projection is lost, other group members hiss softly to prompt the student who is speaking. It usually helps if the speaker stands across the room from the rest of the group.

The student imagines receiving $50,000 from a benefactor and discusses ways the money could be spent on the school. Appropriate tone focus must be maintained during the discussion. At the end of the discussion, the student summarizes the plans for use of the money, demonstrating projected speech techniques.

The student writes letters to famous people and reads them aloud, using appropriate tone focus during the reading.

The student counts aloud by tens from 7 to 77, prolonging the voiced continuant /v/ sounds in each repetition of "seven," and maximizing frontal tone focus.

Practice Materials to Eliminate Hard Glottal Attacks

Vowels in Initial Position in Words

Monosyllabic		Multisyllabic (First syllable stressed)	
arm	eat	oilskin	Oscar
own	ache	apple	angry
aunt	off	enter	over
act	old	exit	entrance
ice	oil	instant	enemy
ink	ox	operator	oodles
on	elk	open	eastern
oops	east	outward	ample
end	ear	outside	uncle
ax	of	obvious	anyone
each	out	everyone	unaware
itch	ease	utter	ugly
age	inch	ulcer	ultra
egg	ours	oboe	engine
odd	eight	oval	accident
edge	ash	ankle	angel
off	aisle	alcohol	alimony
ape	ale	altitude	igloo
aim	aid	olive	under
eel	up	edible	aardvark
oat	oak	alligator	afternoon
owl	ouch	artichoke	office
us	is	osteopath	amateur
in	eve	earthworm	outskirt
ooze	earn	afterthought	earthquake
and	oh	orchestra	orthodox
earth	oink	editor	oversight
oil	eye	auctioneer	optional
I've	ill	ice pick	ordinance
are	as	ape-man	islander
asp	ounce	icicle	oxygen
air	ache	Asian	oxidize
arch	add	eggshells	ex officio
oaf	I'll	opposite	officer
elf	aft	odious	emphasis
I'm	all	asking	embassy

Additional Practice Activities

The student identifies as many differences between hard and easy onsets as possible.

occur mainly on vowels

occur on stressed syllables

occur when there is too much effort or tension

neck feels tight

sounds like a grunt or click

feels jerky

The speech–language pathologist reads a word list, and the student checks the words on which hard attacks occurred.

The student practices the transition from air flow to voicing in slow motion, prolonging a breathed sound and gradually adding smooth voicing.

/s/ – /z/

/θ/ – /ð/

/f/ – /v/

/ʃ/ – /ʒ/

The student makes a list of vowel sounds, practices producing the vowels preceded by an /h/, then produces the vowel sounds "thinking" the /h/ but not actually producing it.

The student practices word pairs:

whose	ooze	hit	it
hate	ate	heel	eel
he's	ease	hive	I've
hill	ill	his	is
ha	ah	how	ow
has	as	hoops	oops
heat	eat	hotter	otter
ham	am	high	eye
hay	eh	hail	ale
hi	eye	heave	Eve
howl	owl	hash	ash

The speech–language pathologist questions and the student responds with the same answer each time, but varying vocal expressiveness. This activity involves practice of conversational timing and vocal and facial expressiveness, while the target response remains short. For example:

"oh" "uh uh"

"always"

"I will/I won't"

"I do/I don't"

The student counts from 8 to 98 by tens (8, 18, 28 . . .). This is tape-recorded and then self-evaluated.

The students say names of people, states, cities, foods, or substances that start with vowel sounds. In a group situation, group members take turns and monitor each other's production.

The speech–language pathologist begins a sentence, such as, "I went to Alaska and I ate. . . ." and students repeat the carrier phrase and add items until each member has had a turn. The students repeat the entire sentence each turn. For example, "I went to Alaska and I ate avocados, eggs, oranges, artichokes, apples, and asparagus." Other progressive sentences such as, "At Oxford I acquired . . ." and "In Iceland Eskimos argue over . . ." may be used.

Students share tricks used to facilitate easy onset. For example: elongating the vowel, linking the preceding consonant (e.g., "his answer"), "thinking" an /h/ before the word, saying the word softly, and breathing out on the word. After a discussion of various tricks, students read word lists and listeners try to guess the trick they were using.

The student has 5 minutes to construct practice sentences of words beginning with vowels and then read them aloud. Examples follow:

An ounce of ore equals an ounce of iron.

I am to exercise expertly all October in Ohio.

Our annual auction is always an exciting affair and attracts onlookers.

Ancient automobiles always act up in August.

Ann's Aunt Ursula exercises every evening in April.

Ellie asks for everyone's ideas and answers Anthea angrily afterward.

Evelyn Ellis is always excited in autumn.

The student uses a dictionary to make paragraphs containing as many words as possible beginning with "ex."

The student thinks of words beginning with vowels as the speech–language pathologist reads the following list and writes the student's responses in blank spaces in a story. The student then reads the story aloud.

a plural noun ______________________

an adjective ______________________

a number ______________________

a verb (past tense) ______________________

a plural noun ______________________

an adjective ______________________

a verb (past tense) ______________________

a noun ______________________

a proper noun ______________________

Almost everyone is excited about art. Art is sometimes hung in ______________ (plural noun) and sometimes in ______________ (adjective) people's homes. On occasions at art auctions, bids of ______________ (number) million dollars, or even in excess of that amount, are offered. Once upon a time in ancient civilizations, art treasures were ______________ (verb, past tense) in the tombs of kings and queens. Our ancestors painted on the walls of ______________ (plural noun). Many ______________ (adjective) carvings were made by our ancestors. The value of art is often in the ______________ (noun) of the beholder. No two individuals always agree on everything and art is not an exception. Although angels are ______________ (verb, past tense) on the ______________ (noun) of the Sistine Chapel, not everyone adores Michaelangelo or even ______________ (proper noun).

Additional Sentences to Practice Easy Onset

1. Aaron asked for Amy's address.
2. In Alaska I observed interesting and unusual animals.
3. Emily is eating unflavored ice cream.
4. Andrew annihilated the annoying insect.
5. Aaron arranged exciting outings.
6. Obsequious people overpraise others.
7. Actually I am older than anyone else around.
8. The airplane en route to Israel arrived in Afghanistan at 8:00 in the evening.
9. Isabelle underestimates her own abilities.
10. Is anyone interested in investigating the accident?
11. Adam attends an auction every August.
12. Is anyone interested in another opinion?
13. Across the aisle Eddie ignored Annette.
14. Amy and Andrea are engaged in an angry argument.
15. Anthropologists are always interviewing Apache Indians.
16. Approximately 80 artists arrived early at the Australian Opera.
17. Understandably, Anna was appreciative of all your efforts.
18. The opposite of in is out.
19. Anne, Elizabeth, and Alice all entered the arena at 8 o'clock.
20. Everyone exhibited opposing ideas.
21. Isn't everyone educated enough in arithmetic?
22. I am interested in elementary education.
23. Imagination expresses an organism's inner ideas.
24. I am eating an apple an hour.
25. Eight egotistical egotists eagerly echoed their egotistical ecstasy.
26. Are any of you eating at Ellen's apartment?
27. Ask an instructor of economics about Eastern affairs.
28. Our annual auction is always an exciting affair.
29. Athletic activities are important elements on everyone's agenda.
30. In August I am attending a university orientation event.
31. Ordering oranges in an afternoon is an edible arrangement.
32. An ounce of ore equals an ounce of iron.
33. Ann's Aunt Ursula exercises everyday at an old exercise emporium.
34. All instructors of education are allotted an enormous amount of empathy.
35. Alice owes Ed about $80 and offered an IOU instead.
36. Alice observed Andrea eating apples, oatmeal, eggs, and onions all at once.
37. Elizabeth's errors outweigh Eric's.
38. Evidently Ann's accounts are unbalanced.
39. Emily's anger over Adrienne's evil attitudes and actions is apparent in her eyes.
40. Albert's expectations are unreasonable.
41. Elliot's arithmetic is unsatisfactory.
42. Indians of Indiana are always undergoing every aid.
43. I always ask if all evidence is orderly.

44. Every iceberg acts icy.
45. If Agnew aches at apples, Edward eeks at eggs.
46. Edward entertains ingenues every evening at eight o'clock.
47. Any analysis of an active agent is utterly ostentatious.
48. An idiot accepts almost anything, even if it is incredibly unbelievable.
49. All irate adults insist upon alligators ingesting investigators of electrifying events.
50. An ardent admirer of Elizabeth admittedly inspected her assets.

Paragraphs to Practice Easy Onset

The amount of energy I am able to expend at any instance increases and decreases according to the environment around me. If, for instance, I am in a group of individuals with whom I am acquainted, the amount of available energy is enormous, and I laugh and talk incessantly. If, in another instance, I am talking with an extremely close acquaintance alone, I am under no obligation to be extremely outgoing but am allowed to "undo myself," so to speak, and do as I please. The in-between amount of energy I expend is in a place where I sit quietly, as in class or when watching a television program. Then I am attentively alert, yet I talk more infrequently to others.

Almost 80 years ago, at age 18, my Uncle Ed traveled alone across the Atlantic Ocean and arrived in America. While on this excursion, he became engaged to my Aunt Edith, another immigrant from England. Their early years of marriage were not easy. Against Edith's intuition, Uncle Ed invested in the oil industry. Unfortunately, he lost his entire estate. They were forced to auction off all of their assets and start all over again. At this time, Uncle Ed announced that he intended to enlist in the army. Because of his ethnic origin, he was assigned as a special envoy to England. Edith accompanied him. They eventually returned to America in 1948 and ended up in Evanston, Illinois. In their older age, Edith enjoyed attending many social activities. Uncle Ed, still agile and active, spent every afternoon ambling about in the park, dressed in an overcoat and toting an umbrella.

Every afternoon at about 1:18, I experience an empty ache in my abdomen. I get anxious to eat an apple or an orange. In order to accomplish anything in the afternoon, I must acquire only an apple or only an orange. Other appetizers I enjoy include apricots, artichokes, avocados, etc., but they do not appease the empty ache in the afternoon.

Edward Anderson accepted an invitation to accompany the ambassador of Afghanistan across the ocean to Eastern Asia. An extremely independent envoy, Edward embarked on an exciting adventure in India. After his arrival at the airport, he elected to amble around an unpopulated area. He approached an enormous amphitheater and exclaimed, "This is absolutely awesome!" Afterward, he enthusiastically accompanied the ambassador to the Afghanistan embassy where he was introduced to an assembly of Indian actresses and their escorts.

Amy Oliver, anchorwoman of the eight o'clock news, is only 18 years old. It all started in Arkansas when she was asked by Allen Osborn, owner of ABC News, to announce the entertainers involved in an Arthritis Telethon. Everyone expressed awe at Amy's ability. Ike Underwood was immediately attracted to Amy's emerald eyes. In a whisper, Ike asked Amy out, and Amy, of course was elated. You will be amazed to know that Ike has emerald eyes and was only 18 years old, too. Amy and Ike have remained together since that exciting evening. In fact, Amy Oliver will become Amy Underwood on August 18! They are both ecstatic!

On October 8, in the autumn, Ann Engle arrived in Oxford, Ohio, from Anchorage, Alaska. She entered into aerobic and acrobatic activities immediately. Unfortunately, she injured her ankle, and it ached unbearably. She asked an orthopedic specialist for advice. He allayed her anxiety after examining her ankle. His expert opinion was for her to exert no effort for eight days before resuming exercise.

Paragraphs to Practice Replenishing Breaths

"I desire so to conduct the affairs of this administration that if at the end, when I come to lay down the reins of power, I have lost every other friend on earth, I shall at least have one friend left, and that friend shall be down inside of me." (Abraham Lincoln)

When I graduated from high school, located in Chestnut Hill, Massachusetts, I decided to take a summer off before I started college in the fall. My roommate, Tracy Donaldson, a very wonderful and close friend, asked me if I would like to spend the summer with her and her family in Lebanon, New Hampshire. Knowing how wonderful her family was and also, more importantly, how close Boston was to Lebanon, I decided to live with the Donaldson family. Why did I care about the proximity of Boston, you may ask? Well, I had a close group of friends, about 20 of us altogether, at high school, and since none of them were going on to college, they all decided to look for jobs in Boston. I, however, had decided to go to college in, of all places, Bloomington, Indiana, which is at least 1,500 miles away from Boston and all my friends. Knowing how much I was going to miss all of my friends in the years to come, I wanted to spend as much time with them as I possibly could, and the best way to do that was to live in Lebanon during the week and drive down to Boston every weekend, a short $2\frac{1}{2}$ hour drive. Well, that is exactly what I did, and now that I am far away from all my friends, whenever I start to miss them, I just think of the wonderful times we shared while still in school, and also the times we shared during that wonderful summer in Lebanon, New Hampshire, and Boston, Massachusetts.

Allan and Bert May have owned the Apache Daycamp, located at 1600 Winding Brook Road, Hartford, Illinois, for approximately 17 years. The camp is actually composed of two divisions, one for children 3 to 5 years old, and one for children 5 to 14 years old. Approximately 200 to 300 children attend both divisions of the daycamp during the months of June through August each year. During the spring, both Allan and Bert May travel around high schools and colleges in the state of Illinois and interview male and female students who have applied to work as counselors at the Apache Daycamp during the summer. Most counselors are paid from $40 to $75 per week, plus room and board, and many enjoy the experience so much that they return for additional summers at the camp. Allan and Bert May supply transportation, which is usually in the form of a minibus, a large bus, or a van, and these vehicles are driven by the counselors who are 21 years old or older.

My little neighbor, Billy, the one with the red hair who always chases my dog around the block, has this annoying habit of collecting "treasures" from everyone's garbage cans and storing them in the bushes in my backyard. He is such a pest, and you wouldn't believe what he found on his last expedition and stashed amongst my rose bushes (the expensive ones I try so hard to maintain). He had been scrounging through the neighborhood, going from garbage can to garbage can, trash heap to trash heap, looking for something wonderful and valuable. Well, he found something, and it was something I did not want stored in my backyard, since I work very hard to keep my yard in good condition. I was looking out of my window, the large picture window in my living room, when I saw that little terror carrying something carefully tucked under his arm. It was black and furry and for a moment I thought it was a stray kitten, but I was horrified to see that it was my old fur hat, which I had thrown out when it hadn't sold in my garage sale last week!

Since time began, people have been fascinated by beautiful and visually exciting gemstones used for jewelry and adornment. In former centuries, precious stones were reserved for the ruling classes only, but nowadays, if one includes costume or fashion jewelry, gemstones are so numerous that it is hardly possible for the layperson to judge what is available. There is much to be learned about the formation, properties, deposits, manufacture, synthesis, and imitations of gemstones that it would take a lifetime of study to become expert in their categorization and description. The beauty of the stones and the appeal of brilliance and color do not always correlate exactly with monetary value. Individual's taste and preference vary, although knowledgeable collectors usually look for clarity and purity in gemstones as well as consider such factors as rarity, size, and cut. Some believe that as people age and feel the loss of their own beauty, they are increasingly drawn to collecting and wearing gemstones for adornment.

Some of the traditional symbols still seen today on dishes, furniture, tools, and barns were created by talented colonists who came from the Rhineland during the 1700s. The Pennsylvania Dutch colonists represented many religious groups. They developed a new way of life and a different style of art. Their folk-art motifs depicted flowers and birds and traditional symbols from their homeland. Their paintings, carvings, and textiles reflected their religious beliefs, their joy in their homes, and their pride in their craftsmanship. Pennsylvania Dutch homes were sturdy structures made of wood and stone and were extremely well kept, while the barns were built in the European tradition with oak beams and rafters. The women were wonderful cooks and contributed many recipes that have been incorporated into the culinary heritage of our country, the United States of America.

American colonial music was especially important to the early settlers, who did not have television as we do today, and the banjo was introduced to America by the slaves who brought their musical tradition from Africa. Many of the early colonists were religious people to whom hymn singing was an important part of their daily life, and wealthy families were influenced by European music and harpsicords, spinets, and violins were played by their children. New songs were created by the colonists as time passed, and the folk music of early America reflects the struggles of the new nation to describe the experiences of the colonists as they moved toward independence. As we listen to early American music, we are stirred by the tunes to which soldiers marched, that farmers hummed as they went about their daily work, and that women and children sang in the nursery, kitchen, and parlor. It helps us feel the everyday struggles in the new land, the happy optimistic spirit of the colonists, and the transformation of 13 young colonies into the United States of America, when we listen to the variety of music that characterized the emergence of the American spirit as we know it today.

Early explorers who thought they had found a western route to India named our Native Americans "Indians." Early settlers from Europe, who were inexperienced in understanding how to use materials at hand, learned much from the Native Americans, who understood how to maintain the balance of nature, and colonists learned from them, for example, how to get sap from maple trees and how to plant pumpkins and squash. The colonists saw corn growing in the villages of the first Americans, and soon this crop became one of the most important to their survival in the new vast land. Corn could be eaten fresh or ground into meal, the husks could be braided into ropes and made into brooms and mattress stuffing, and in addition, dolls and ornaments could be made from corn husks. The early colonial families owed a great deal to the willingness of the Native Americans to share their knowledge of how to make the best use of the materials available in their natural surroundings in the new land.

Isaac Newton was a man who by the age of 43 had already invented calculus, broken white light into its component colors, and built a telescope whose design is so good it is still in use today. Eight years after he arrived as a student at Cambridge, the university appointed him in 1669, at age 26, as Lucasian Professor of Mathematics, which is still one of the most prestigious positions in the scientific world. However, most of us remember Newton mainly because of the story of the apple, which by hitting him on the head, although it probably didn't actually hit him at all, gave him the idea about gravity.

Practice Materials for Vocal Variety in Pitch, Loudness, and Duration

Words to Stimulate Pitch Changes Through Meaning
Onomatopoeic Words

Defintion: Onomatopoeic words—the naming of a thing or action by a vocal imitation of the sound associated with it. (Webster's Dictionary, 7th edition)

High Pitch	Low Pitch	Low Pitch
squeak	dungeon	boomed
creak	cave	sunk
teeny	deep	dump
peak	low	under
hiss	buzz	bummer
squealed	submerge	tomb
shrill	mellow	below
cheep	fruity	groan
yipped	thunder	moan
peep	doom	plunged
screech	thump	depths
tingle	thud	grave
rippling	murmur	humming
whistling	stroked	snore
snicker	plummeted	snarl
eek	tumbled	dreaming
tinkle	growled	sadly
surprise	grumbled	buried
chirp	shudder	gurgled
piercing	guzzled	slurp
twitter	gruff	burp
jingle	filthy	gloomy
trill	cascaded	dreary
soprano	dive	musty
piccolo	sank	rut
flitter	dud	fell
crest	delved	dropping

Contrastive Pairs			
ping	pong	ceiling	floor
ding	dong	up	down
light	dark	smooth	rough
treble	bass	jump	hesitate
high	low	hissed	buzzed

Contrastive Pairs			
hill	valley	fun	work
comedy	tragedy	minutes	hours
happy	sad	air	earth
delight	remorse	tinkled	crashed
flute	drum	top	bottom
sniff	snarl	bip	bop
piccolo	tuba	light	heavy
chatter	drawl	fly	elephant

Loud		Soft	
bang	howling	velvet	hush
roar	smash	feathery	muffled
crash	dash	mellow	peaceful
thunder	bash	tender	mist
slam	mash	silky	slumber
ouch	clash	tiptoe	coo
fire	bellowed	silent	delicate
clang	Stop!	soft	rustled
shattered	raucous	cloud	billowy
rumbled	shout	gentle	shushed
boom	explode	cuddly	swished
blast	noisy	fluffy	pastel
boisterous	brash	gauzy	furry
resounding	strident	quiet	souffle
blaring	deafening	soothe	whisper

Duration			
Fast		**Slow**	
tick/tock	halt	slithered	pull
blitz	galloped	pulled	blend
fleet	tap	strolling	molasses
flip	clap	stretch	creep
slam	shoot	linger	casually
pop	gushed	elongate	inched
flashed	swoop	trickled	leisurely
zip	snatch	oozed	snarl
zoom	wiggled	boring	sneer
whip	hurriedly	slowly	drawl
snort	knocked	slumber	languished
sniff	ran	murmur	waddled
sneeze	bounced	sustain	lazily
chatter	launched	wandering	sluggish
jabber	rushing	long	drizzle
lightning	gingerly	winding	dawdling
energetic	plucked	sleepily	doddery
plopped	grab	hesitate	marathon
suddenly	snap	prolonged	trudge
flitter/flutter	flicker	measured	dragged
accelerate	cracked	suffered	squeeze
bubbled	twitter	tardy	linger
babbled	catapult	waited	lulled
jump	splat	straining	languidly
immediately	hasty	poky	eternity
brisk	swift	plodding	lagging

Sentences to Facilitate Use of a Higher Pitch

1. The cook made a light, fluffy souffle that was airy and high.
2. He sang when he felt happy.
3. When we found out the news, we were so thrilled!
4. She floated out onto the dance floor.
5. The pretty bird chirped and flitted about.
6. The effervescent champagne sparkled in the light.
7. Peter's eyes crinkled when he laughed.
8. In the high wind, the rafters creaked and squeaked.
9. Look at the star right up there.
10. We can see the balloon float right into the blue sky.
11. Did you see her climb to the very top of the ladder?
12. Did Jack and Jill climb the high hill?
13. His eyes twinkled and he said, "You're happy, too, aren't you?"
14. His parachute opened and jerked him upward.
15. Did you really think I'd do that?
16. On the night of the prom, Kitty was very excited.
17. As they looked up, the sky seemed filled with millions of stars, all twinkling.
18. She was at the pinnacle of happiness.
19. The politician's popularity rating shot up.
20. She climbed onward and upward, striving for the top.
21. The plane soared high above the clouds.
22. Is anyone interested in another opinion?
23. The tennis ball bounced over the net, then high into the air.
24. There was a tinkling sound from the wind chimes.
25. I always have sweet dreams when I sleep with music.

Sentences to Facilitate Use of Lower Pitch

1. The submarine sank slowly to the bottom of the sea.
2. The miner went down to the depths of the earth.
3. The man crawled down into the deep, dark hole.
4. The mountaineer lost his footing and plummeted down to the valley.
5. I felt myself sinking down into a deep, deep sleep.
6. The parachutist jumped from the plane and floated slowly down to earth.
7. I sank deep into the plush velvet chair.
8. Grandfather spoke in a deep, gruff voice.
9. The prisoner was flung into a dank, dark hole in the dungeon.
10. I've been working and working all day and I'm so tired.
11. As we dug for gold, the hole got deeper and deeper.
12. The movie was interesting, but very sad at the end.
13. No one could have foreseen the terrible tragedy.
14. The *Titanic* sank to the bottom of the ocean.
15. The shark swam slowly in the murky depths.
16. Most people suffer from some depression.
17. The sun sank on the western horizon.
18. We delved into his deep, dark, and sordid background.
19. They toiled under the blazing sun.
20. The drums rolled mournfully following his death.
21. The mole tunneled away in the dark earth.
22. She stopped dead in her tracks when she spotted her old boyfriend.
23. My heart sank in despair.
24. We crawled along the bottom of the cavern.
25. We sat in awe as the soothsayer spoke.

Sentences Contrasting High and Low Pitch

1. The hang glider soared and then plunged into a down draft.
2. You take the low road and I'll take the high way.
3. Are you going to finish this, or do I have to?
4. She lifted her eyes upward to the sky, then down to the sleeping child in her arms
5. The athletes stretched their arms upward, then bent down to touch their toes.
6. That woman sings soprano, but her husband sings bass.
7. As the men pulled down the rope, the boy was lifted into the air.
8. The kite soared up into the air, then landed with a thud.
9. After a long, hard climb, they suddenly reached the peak.
10. The party was great, but the morning after was a downer.
11. He scored a goal, but it was disallowed.
12. The low, dull drum roll accompanied the high-pitched, squeaky flute.
13. The fat, blobby snake slithered all the way up the tree to the very tip-top.
14. They enjoyed the picnic, but felt violently ill afterward.
15. "To be, or not to be. That is the question." (Shakespeare)
16. "If life is a bowl of cherries, how come I'm left with the pits?" (Erma Bombeck)
17. After a long, cold winter, tiny green leaves appeared on the trees.
18. I'm sorry, but can you repeat the question, please?
19. The young woman was happy and carefree until she received word of her father's accident.
20. Can you reach the top? I'm too short.
21. Don't get into a rut. Experience life! Live a little!
22. Will you help me please? I can't find it.
23. The boys swung higher and higher, but the rope broke and they fell to the ground.
24. The talented actress, at the peak of her career, became despondent and withdrawn.
25. He aimed for the last goal, but time had run out.
26. Those who reach for the stars never get bogged down in mediocrity.
27. Laugh and the world laughs with you, cry and you cry alone.
28. Tip your hat to spring, and wave goodbye to winter.
29. The trail climbs through the hills where the temperature is 40 degrees below zero.
30. The road twists upward and then plunges straight down.

Activities for Pitch Variation

Students ask questions of each other. The response is limited to "um hmm" but must be inflected in a variety of ways to reflect different meanings.

The days of the week are repeated with a different pitch level on each syllable. For example:

high pitch:	Mon		Tues	
low pitch:		day		day

A variation of this activity is to require the student to generate multisyllabic words and speak each syllable on different pitches.

The student makes a statement and then adds a tag to convert the statement to a question. For example:

He's really crazy

He's really crazy, isn't he?

A variation of this activity is for the student to be given a list of different tags and then frame questions using those tags.

The student says a telephone number, using ascending or descending pitch levels in sequence. A variation of this exercise is to repeat the number, choosing various digits for inflectional emphasis. Students can also try to find as many different pitch inflections for their telephone numbers as possible.

The student generates as many pairs of "opposites" as possible and repeats the word pairs, contrasting the pitches. For example:

up	down
tall	short
over	under
overhead	underground

The student makes up sentences that have parenthetical clauses. The parenthetical clauses are information that is not central to the main idea and are spoken at a different pitch level. For example:

Bill, *he's my brother,* is a very good football player.
England, *where my relatives live,* has a lot of historic landmarks.

The student reads a passage aloud, beginning every second sentence on a lower (or higher) pitch.

The student reads a sentence aloud, stressing (with pitch variation) a different word on each successive reading. The student discusses how the meaning is changed and generates additional sentences. For example:

That woman insulted her boss after dinner.

Students think of a list of verbs that suggest motion and use them in sentences, varying pitch to suggest the motion. For example:

Eagles soar in the air
Leaves fall from the trees
The wind howled all night
The athlete jumped the barrier
The train lurched to a halt

The clinician presents a list of sentences to the group, and each student reads a sentence aloud. Then the student chooses an adjective to add to the sentence. On the second reading, the adjective is highlighted with an appropriate pitch change. Example: "The Christmas decorations were in all the shop windows." (Insert "sparkling")

Each student prepares a 1-minute speech and presents it to the group. The goal is to use pitch variation to suggest meaning and feeling appropriately. A variation is to use pitch changes inappropriately and to discuss the incongruity, thus reviewing general rules for pitch usage. Example: "My most exciting day" and "Demons that visit me in the night."

"Feeling states" are written on slips of paper. Each student chooses one and then reads a short paragraph, reflecting the "feeling" in his or her voice. Other students identify the "feeling" from the vocal behaviors the student who is reading exhibited (e.g., envy, greed, malice, compassion, affection, sarcasm, bewilderment, excitement).

Students discuss vocal behaviors associated with a variety of characters. They then practice simple sentences, attempting to create the appropriate vocal behavior (e.g., a distraught teenager, an irritable parent, an injured athlete, a mean teacher, and a jubilant lottery winner).

Students discuss vocal behaviors associated with a variety of roles and ages. They then practice simple sentences, attempting to create the appropriate vocal behavior (e.g., authority figures of different ages and professions, such as a young police cadet and an elderly police officer).

Students practice the following phrases and sentences. They say each one three times to reflect feelings of anger, surprise, and puzzlement.

That is not yours.
My test results were mailed.
My brother did that.
No way, no way.
I am going to the party.
That check is made out to me.
You don't even know her name.
Mr. Gillespie didn't call me.
My cell phone isn't working.

Sentences Contrasting Loud and Soft Volume

1. The music swelled to fill the room and then faded away to a solitary note.
2. The small, frail whimper grew into an anguished roar.
3. The children sat quietly in their seats until the school bell brought shouts of laughter.
4. The screams and cries of alarm sent everyone running, but the deaf old woman heard nothing.
5. The brothers argued in loud voices, but no one said a word when their mother walked in.
6. After the clamor and noise of the battle, there was an eerie silence in the field.
7. The bomb exploded, there was a moment's silence, and then the sirens began to wail.
8. The thunder rumbled and the lightning flashed violently; suddenly it was quiet and a rainbow appeared.
9. The girls were whispering across the room when the teacher suddenly slammed his book down on the desk.
10. The party was in full swing and the music was blaring; then John heard his parents' car in the driveway.
11. Take a piece of meat, pound the heck out of it, and fry it till it sizzles.
12. When I say I got up, I mean I GOT UP. About three feet, covers and all.
13. With snarls and barks and squeals the fight erupted, while I watched in terror, rooted to the spot.
14. He launched into a chorus of "Jingle Bells" at full lung power, followed by a soft-voiced reverential singing of "Silent Night."
15. He stood silently at first, then grabbed the bars of the cage and rattled them so loudly that the zookeeper came running.

Sentences Contrasting Fast and Slow Rates

1. The hunter crept along quietly, aiming carefully, yet the sharp gunshot was unexpected.
2. She had waited patiently for hours, but the abrupt tap on her shoulder frightened her.
3. The voice on the phone droned on, but the click of the receiver brought sudden silence.
4. The thief crawled stealthily out the window, then took off down the street.
5. The runner slowly kept pace until the last lap, sprinted feverishly to the finish line, then collapsed from sheer exhaustion.
6. The leopard crept quietly through the grass, paused, then pounced on his prey.
7. My head was sinking into the pillow when suddenly I awoke, but soon I drifted back to sleep.
8. We stretched and pulled the taffy, then quickly snipped it into little pieces.
9. The stranger slowly stalked the scene of the crime and then ran with amazing speed when the police chased him.
10. The race driver's car sped by the crowd and around the curve until it blew a tire and slid slower and slower to a halt.
11. I yawned, opened one eye cautiously, and then jumped up and took off.
12. Uplifted, exalted, excited, overwhelmed by the music, with my earphones on, I gradually drifted off to sleep.
13. I was jumping and twisting to the beat, and the floor was vibrating, until the neighbors downstairs called the police.
14. There are people who encourage us, cheer us on, give us a quick push toward our goal, and yet somehow we never seem to manage to do it.
15. The rapping on the door was sharp, urgent, and insistent, a foreboding of a crisis, and I froze, listening and waiting.

Sentences Combining Pitch, Loudness, and Rate Changes

1. Each day is a grand adventure that ends with quiet sleep.
2. As your body races, keep your concentration still.
3. Love suffereth long and is kind.
4. Time can hang heavily, even as the minutes tick fast.
5. The rain felt soft but cold on her skin.
6. Sometimes anxiety can cause feelings of paralysis.
7. Whispering sweet nothings today, he would be hurling accusations tomorrow.
8. Some people who ride on an emotional roller coaster come to a grinding halt.
9. Tension and drama are sometimes used as substitutes for real intimacy.
10. An ardent Romeo wooed an impetuous Juliet.
11. She was exhausted by his restless energy.
12. Over the din of battle they could not even hear themselves speak.
13. Some laughed uproariously at the movie while others just waited it out.
14. Sometimes I fantasize about Europe while I do the dishes.
15. He wanted status and she wanted privacy.
16. The marriage of friends may be the funeral of friendship.
17. Violin strings can make beautiful music, but if drawn too tight, they snap.
18. My father had a quick temper, but he also had extraordinary courage.
19. The sun sank, showering the sand with a golden glow and sending a chill through the air.
20. As I stood in the sunset, I heard my grandmother's voice telling me stories I thought I had forgotten.
21. Susan saw him sizing her up and then smiling confidently at her.
22. In Alaska, chopping ice and hauling water is hard work.
23. Berries can be eaten on cereal or enjoyed one-by-one.
24. "To every thing there is a season, and a time to every purpose under the heaven: A time to be born, and a time to die; a time to plant, and a time to pluck up that which is planted." (Ecclesiastes 3:1–2)
25. Potatoes are nutritious and low in calories, but be careful about adding rich toppings.
26. Sleep through the night and you'll wake up refreshed.
27. The television news blared as he picked at his frozen dinner.
28. A quick question should be given serious consideration at this time.
29. Building walls to protect yourself won't prevent you from getting hurt.
30. He was just passing through life, while she was enjoying every minute.
31. When someone says you have bats in the belfry, they imply you are crazy or weird.
32. "Life is mostly froth and bubble, but two things stand like stone: kindness in another's trouble and courage in your own." (Anonymous)
33. Pop it in the microwave and then savor it at leisure.

Paragraphs Combining Pitch, Loudness, and Rate Changes

He hit the ball and it flew high, arching against the blue sky. The spectators looked up and squinted as they were dazzled by the bright sun. Then they gasped and groaned as the ball suddenly fell to the ground, out of bounds. The excitement, so intense a minute before, evaporated. The game was over and done. Victory had been snatched from the home team.

Sam was zipping along the freeway at 90 miles an hour and weaving in and out of the traffic. The top of his convertible was down and he felt the air whiz by his face and blow his hair. Then, ahead, he caught sight of a police car. He squeezed his foot down hard on the brakes and watched as the speedometer needle dropped back—80—70—60—50. . . . It seemed now as if he was merely crawling along the ribbon of road under the hot California sun. There was no exhilarating breeze to cool his face and body, and he felt as if he was hardly moving.

A mighty herd of elephants was ponderously grazing under the hot sun on that open plain. They lumbered slowly in the intense noonday heat, a slow mountainous group of flesh on padded feet. A bull raised his head and listened. A shiver raced through the herd and suddenly they were off, thundering faster and faster across the open plain, stirring a huge storm of dust in their wake, until they were a blur on the horizon. Then all was quiet on the plain again.

The assassin, dressed in black, slipped through the doorway into the dark night. He moved stealthily and made no sound at all. Everyone in the command post slept peacefully. High in the watchtower, a beam of light raced across the night sky. Suddenly a fuse was lit. There was a hiss as it ignited, and then a red line snaked through the blackness. A shriek penetrated the night, a high piercing wail of terror. Then the crack of an explosion as fire and smoke spewed into the air, and the building blew asunder with a deafening roar.

The band played jaunty tunes as the members marched across the green grass. Balloons danced in the air overhead, and a few white wisps of cloud dotted the blue sky. Spectators lounged on the side of the field, a few babies wailed in their strollers, and the hot dog vendors did a lot of business. The mayor mopped his brow, huffing and puffing with importance as he ascended the platform, and cleared his throat to begin his opening remarks.

Jayne was home late. She quietly turned her key in the door, gently opened it, and tiptoed up the stairs, her heart in her mouth. There was no light under her parents' bedroom door. She prayed the stairs would not creak. She could hear the dull thudding of her heart in the stillness. Then something brushed against her leg, and she gasped in fright—but it was just the cat. She was almost to the top of the stairs when she heard her father's voice, "Is that you, Jayne?"

Practice Materials Using Short, Easy Utterances

Redundant Phrases

This activity is useful in a group when the length of the target utterance is to be limited to two words but where spontaneous production is desirable. A list of nouns is presented to the student, who is asked to make an adjective from each noun and then to repeat the adjective and noun as a phrase. Phrase production is evaluated.

Example: slime—"slimy slime"; ghoul—"ghoulish ghoul"; actor—"acting actor."

Anagrams

One student suggests a multisyllable word and the other students break it down into as many small words as possible. At the end of 3 minutes, the students read their lists using appropriate vocal production.

Example: Photography—pot, path, pray, hot, hag, hop toy, trophy, toga.

Alliteration

The students think of sentences in which each word begins with the same sound. Each group member adds words to the sentence. For example: "Zany Zelda xeroxed Zion's Zebras."

Associations

The students choose a general topic (e.g., music) and find suitable word associations related to it. A variation of this (at the sentence level) is to name as many musical titles as possible. Each group member can take turns and other members can evaluate appropriate vocal production. To increase the cognitive complexity of this activity, the associations can be alphabetized.

Another association activity is to ask a student to think of something that:

is over 50 years old.

juice is derived from.

has angles.

comes in a pump dispenser.

is made from synthetic material.

originates in Asia.

is a trademark.

is an amphibian.

The student responds, "An example is ______________________________."

Cumulative Sentence

One group member begins a sentence. The other members progressively add information. For example:

The teacher

The teacher said

The teacher said no one

The teacher said no one passed

The teacher said no one passed the exam.

Chain Sentences

One student says a sentence. The next student must continue by beginning a new sentence with the last letter of the last word of the preceding statement. The sentences must contain a logical progression of ideas. The group effort is tape-recorded and replayed for evaluation of vocal behaviors.

Count Your Blessings

Each student is asked to enumerate 12 blessings, one associated with each month of the year. A variation of this activity is to enumerate "pet peeves."

Famous People

Each student names famous people whose first and last names begin with the same letter (e.g., Alan Alda).

Each student names as many rock groups as possible and then pretends to be a disc jockey introducing each group in turn.

Opposing Proverbs

The clinician asks the student to state a proverb with an opposite meaning from the one the clinician quotes. For example, the clinician says, "Look before you leap" and the student volunteers, "He who hesitates is lost."

This activity may be used as a homework assignment or as a spontaneous group activity. It is hardest when students must think up the proverbs on their own. An easier version can be used by providing the students with a set of proverbs from which to choose. In this latter task, the activity becomes one of reading sentences.

An example of another activity involving proverbs is "scrambled sayings." For example:

Moss a stone gathers rolling no.

Nine a saves stitch in time.

Is saved a penny penny a earned.

Nose to your off spite your cut don't face.

Bush a bird the in the in worth hand is two.

Message on Answering Machine

The speech–language pathologist writes situations on index cards. Students select an index card from a container and respond in 20 seconds or less with a message to leave on an answering machine. The message must be spoken in accordance with the student's vocal objectives. Situations might include the following:

Call your parents' office(s) and explain why you'll be late returning home from school.

Call the vet to make an appointment for your cat.

Call a friend to arrange driving plans for the ball game.

Call your date and explain why you have to change your plans.

Students must be sure to state their names, the date and time of the call, and a succinct message.

Imaginary Auction

Give each student $20,000 in imaginary money. Inform the students that once their money is spent they cannot bid any longer. Bidding opens on each item at $200 and increments are $100 or multiples. The speech–language pathologist is the auctioneer. Even though bidding may become spirited, appropriate voice rules must be maintained throughout or bids will not be acknowledged. Items to be "auctioned" might be selected from the following list, or students could be encouraged to make their own lists.

Having the wardrobe of your choice for life

Having a lot of money

Having good health all through life

Being attractive to the opposite sex

Getting the very best education possible

Being famous

Postcard Inscriptions

The student is given a situation and asked to think about what to say on a postcard to friends.

on a beach at spring break
on a school trip to Washington, D.C.
on a visit to grandparents
at a family reunion
at the Grand Canyon
at the Hard Rock Cafe in L.A.

Practice Materials Using Long, Complex Utterances

Ten Years From Now . . .

Students prepare the sentence completion activity below as a homework assignment. At the group meeting, each student pretends to give an extemporaneous speech at a class reunion and presents a summary of what has occurred during the ten years since high school graduation. The other students monitor vocal behavior and provide written feedback.

In 10 years my age will be ______________.

I'll be living in ______________.

I'll be the kind of friend who ______________.

One of my strengths that others admire will be ______________.

My future goals will be ______________.

My responsibilities will include ______________.

My most important personal possessions will be ______________.

The highlights of the last 10 years will be ______________.

Rhyming Activity

This activity is useful for students who are working on vocal production at the sentence level. Increased complexity of processing is introduced while the length of utterance remains reasonably short.

A student thinks of two words that rhyme and announces one of the words by saying, "I'm thinking of a word that rhymes with foal." Other players ask questions by framing definitions. For example: "Is it a receptacle in which fruit is kept?" The student must guess the correct word from the definition (e.g., bowl) and answer in sentence form. The game continues until the correct word emerges. For example:

Statement: I'm thinking of a word that rhymes with foal.

Question: Is it a type of fuel?

Response: No, it is not coal.

Question: Is it a dark blemish on the skin?

Response: No, it is not a mole.

Question: Is it the spirit inside a person's body?

Response: Yes, it is soul.

"Ear Aches"

The name of this activity can be varied depending on the goal for the target response. For example, for students working to decrease hard glottal attacks, the target response "ear aches" can be used.

A student thinks of a word (preferably a common noun) and keeps it a secret from the other players, who ask simple questions to determine the secret word. In formulating each answer, the student must frame a response that includes the secret word, but substitutes "ear aches" for the secret word, with emphasis on the easy onset of phonation. Questioning continues until the players guess the secret word.

Example: (secret word = daffodil)

Question: What is the weather like today?

Answer: It is the kind of weather when there are ear aches.

Question: What did you do yesterday?

Answer: I gathered ear aches.

Question: Where do you live?

Answer: In a house with ear aches in the back garden.

Coffee Pots

This activity involves the choice of pairs of homophonic words. It is an effective group activity that can be used when students are practicing vocal targets in sentences with conversational timing and considerable cognitive complexity.

A student thinks of a pair of words that sound alike but are spelled differently but does not reveal them to the group. Group members question the student, and the student must use answers that include one of the secret words. Instead of saying the secret word, however, the words "coffee pots" are substituted and inflected. The activity continues until the word pair is guessed correctly.

Example: (stare/stair)

Question: What is your favorite sport?

Answer: I like coffee potting at people walking along the street.

Question: What did you do in school today?

Answer: I walked up a lot of coffee pots.

Question: When is your birthday?

Answer: Don't coffee pot at me when I tell you that it is tomorrow.

Question: Where do you live?

Answer: In a house with lots of coffee pots.

One-Minute Spontaneous Speeches

Students each choose a piece of paper on which a topic is written. Each student prepares an extemporaneous one-minute speech and presents it to the rest of the group. Sample topics follow:

Describe a character from a soap opera

Basketball greats

My dream wardrobe

My fantasy vacation

CDs I couldn't live without

A nightmare day

Decisions

The speech–language pathologist presents students with a list of ways in which decisions can be dealt with:

Allowing others to decide

Putting off the decision

Drawing straws to decide alternatives

Not deciding at all

Impulsive, arbitrary choosing

Making a list of pros and cons

Evaluating and researching a number of alternative solutions

Students are then asked to generate examples of situations to illustrate the various approaches. They discuss the advantages, disadvantages, and possible consequences of each method.

The speech–language pathologist introduces the idea that "mistakes" are often the result of inappropriate decision-making strategies. Students are asked to consider the task of buying a car and discuss how the outcome is influenced by the following:

Personal values

Time available

Money (e.g., initial outlay, maintenance costs, insurance, cost per mile to run)

Significant others involved

Consideration of all options (e.g., new, used)

Empathy

Empathy is not agreement with another's point of view but understanding and appreciation of another's experience. Empathy is expressed with both vocal and nonvocal cues. The students are asked to convey the following ideas to a listener, phrasing them in their own words using empathetic cues.

Example: Someone's father treats him unfairly "You're very angry with your father because he's treating you so unfairly."

A girl needs help with a drug problem.

Someone's pet dies.

A girl is not selected for a team.

A boy flunks an exam.

A girl isn't asked to the prom.

Topics for Spontaneous Speech Tasks of at Least Three Minutes' Duration

1. You can get good jobs without finishing high school.
2. A person who decides not to have children is selfish.
3. Girls should help pay on dates.
4. Fathers should feed, diaper, and bathe babies.

5. Life is a game of chance, so why plan.
6. Having a baby is a good way to get attention.
7. Men can make good nurses, flight attendants, and secretaries.
8. Life was much better before the Women's Liberation Movement.
9. There are some jobs that should be left to men.
10. It's a man's duty to provide financially for the family.
11. It's wrong to have sex if you are not married.
12. "A woman's place is in the home."
13. If you haven't had sex by your senior year, you're weird.
14. It's okay for a man to cry.

Formulating Solutions to Dilemmas

Students are given pieces of paper on which the speech–language pathologist has written short paragraphs describing certain problem situations. Students take turns presenting a dilemma to the group. The presenter is responsible for guiding discussion and reviewing alternatives.

Sample Dilemmas

Maria, in the 11th grade, has a chance to get a job working for her uncle. She could have the job immediately and have her own money. The job is replacing the receptionist in her uncle's office for 6 months while the present receptionist is on maternity leave. She would have to drop out of school. What should she do?

Carol, age 15, is really attracted to Mario, who is on the football team. Mario has never paid her any attention, and her friend says that she should ask him for a date. What should she do?

Ron is always being teased by his friends because of his squeaky voice. He avoids talking because of his embarrassment. The English teacher gives bonus points for oral reports in class. These are optional, but Ron badly needs to improve his grade by the end of the semester. Nonetheless, he is afraid of making a fool of himself. What should he do?

Sean's girlfriend calls him a chicken because he won't smoke grass. Sean has poor eyesight and his optometrist told him drugs can affect people's eyes. He is afraid that his girlfriend will dump him if he continues to be a spoil sport at her friends' parties, however. What should he do?

Jeff has vocal nodules and has been told not to abuse his voice by yelling loudly. His father has a hearing problem and always gets irritated with Jeff and complains when he talks softly. Jeff hates fighting with his father but wants to get rid of the nodules. What should he do?

Diane talks a lot and is always amusing her friends with her impersonations and anecdotes. She is often hoarse because of the strain she puts on her voice. Although she knows she should be careful with her voice, she is afraid to give up her role as "life of the party." She thinks her friends will think she's dull and mousy if she isn't talkative. What should she do?

John's father is dying of cancer, but John doesn't want anyone at his school to know about it. He doesn't want people talking about his family or pitying him. Yesterday he got into a terrible fight with some of his best friends and acted very aggressively toward them. Now he feels bad and his friends aren't speaking to him. What should he do?

Megan finished a hard test and went to meet some friends at a fast food restaurant. She bought a shake and some french fries, and just as she was about to start eating, her two friends arrived. Neither ordered anything, but both proceeded to eat her fries. What should she do?

Standing Up for Yourself

The speech–language pathologist discusses the differences between assertiveness and aggressiveness. Students are asked to think of situations in which they find it difficult to stand up for themselves with family and friends. The speech–language pathologist then writes a list of strategies on a chart and asks students to apply them to the situations they've identified. Role playing may be used. Strategies might include:

Express feelings honestly.

Offer solutions rather than complain.

Respect others' rights.

Criticize behavior, not people.

Take responsibility for own feelings.

Verbally disagree without physical or verbal abuse.

Gather facts before jumping to conclusions.

Say "no" without feeling guilty.

Rock Art

Have students select their favorite rock song, draw a picture to illustrate the song's lyrics, and then discuss the finished artwork.

Worksheet: Reading Passage on Clouds

A cloud is made up of minute particles of dust, very tiny minerals, water, and sometimes ice. There are water clouds and ice clouds, and clouds are grouped into four basic categories. Cirrus clouds are high clouds that occur at altitudes ranging from 20,000 to 40,000 feet. Alto describes middle clouds, ranging from 6,500 to 20,000 feet. Cumulus is the name given to clouds that look packed or heaped so that the clouds appear like heaps of fluffy cotton. When clouds appear to be layered instead of heaped together, they are named stratus clouds. The four names (cirrus, alto, cumulus, and stratus) are all Latin names that describe cloud characteristics. For example, cirrus clouds have a delicate appearance and are seen as tufts or lines across a clear sky. People have called them names such as "mares' tails," "hen feathers," and "spider webs." They are composed of ice particles.

Stratus clouds are light to dark gray and are usually uniform in appearance, but they may have ragged pieces. The precipitation from these clouds is usually drizzle, light rain, or snow. Sometimes sun shines through them, and at sunset they can look spectacular. Cumulus clouds can also look striking. Cirrocumulus clouds are ice clouds in sheets like ripples in sand or like fish scales. Sometimes they are said to look like a "mackerel sky." This usually signals that strong winds are coming. Altocumulus are usually white clouds and may look like waves or rolls and only the upper parts have ice particles. Altocumulus are darker though the shapes are similar to cirrocumulus clouds. Stratocumulus are water clouds and can bring either rain or snow. They often appear to be lighted from behind, and the precipitation they bring is fairly light although it may last a while. When the word *nimbus* is added to the other cloud names, as in nimbostratus, it means the cloud is gray and dense and will bring rain. A sure sign of approaching rain is a changing progression of cloud formations from cirrus, cumulus, and stratus to nimbus. Winds usher in the changes. Fair weather usually comes with northwest, west, and southwest winds. Winds from the northeast, east, and south bring unsettled weather. For example, if the sky is cloudy and the wind shifts from southwest to southeast or from northwest to northeast, then a squall can be expected. A morning sky of Indian-red altocumulus clouds usually brings rain, winds, and summer thunderstorms. Thus, the old saying "red sky at night, sailor's delight; red sky in the morning, sailors take warning" is true.

Worksheet: Reading Passage on Time

In 1759, John Harrison constructed the first clock, the first timepiece able to keep reliably precise time at sea. British sailors therefore were able to measure longitude accurately even when they were away from land. This changed the course of history and had long-lasting effects on world trade, exploration, and opportunities for war.

Before Harrison, many people had tried to find ways to measure time. Cavemen carved grooves in bones to represent changes in the sun, moon, and the seasons. One of the first actual devices seems to have been the sundial. By 3500 B.C., the Egyptians had constructed elaborate obelisks whose moving shadows broke the day into two parts, divided by noon. It took 2000 years for the obelisk to evolve into the smaller sundial, or shadow clock. For millennia, it was the most advanced device for dividing days into hours, but of course it only worked if the sun was shining. Because water flowed both day and night, a water clock was then invented. Time was kept by measuring water as it dripped into a hole in the bottom of a bowl. A series of lines in the bowl marked the passage of time.

With refinements in glass making in 18th century Europe, the hourglass filled with sand was used to measure short periods of time. By 1300, mechanical clocks struck a bell every hour, but they had no hands or faces. It was not until the mid 1400s that European craftsmen discovered that they could use coiled springs to move the hands on a timepiece. The development of the pendulum in 1656 by a Dutch astronomer was based on Galileo's discovery that a pendulum swings at a constant rate. The longer the pendulum, the greater the accuracy—and so the "longcase," or grandfather clock with a glass door to show the pendulum, became popular. But even the best 18th century, pendulum clocks were worthless at sea as the motion of the ship interfered with the accuracy. To calculate longitude, sailors had to have accurate time measurements; so in 1714 the British Parliament offered a prize equal to several million dollars today to anyone who could solve the problem.

John Harrison was a carpenter's son, and he worked for 6 years on his first attempt to win that prize. His 3-foot-high clock, now called the H_1, took a test run on a round-trip sea journey to Lisbon. Harrison was so sick that he never went to sea again after that 5-week voyage. His H_1 was good but not accurate enough to win the prize. Finally, his fourth version, H_4 was a small watch-type timepiece only 3 pounds in weight. On a second $6\frac{1}{2}$ week voyage from Britain to Jamaica (1761–1762), H_4 lost only 5 seconds. Harrison's son went on this trip in his place. In 1772, the son pleaded with King George III to give his father the prize and recognition he deserved. It had taken 45 years, but John Harrison was finally recognized for his efforts.

Other clock makers made refinements on the H_4, and by the 19th century, chronometers, as they are now known, were standard equipment on all ships. Navigation was much more precise and sailors more safe because John Harrison had solved a technological problem that had baffled scientists for centuries. He contributed mightily to the growth of trade that built the British Empire.

Reading Passages: Native American Customs

Goal: To read the passages in an easy voice. Phrase carefully to take plenty of replenishing breaths during long sentences.

1. The Hopi were monogamous, and weddings were very ritualized events. The ritual began with an exchange of food between the two families as a pledge of marriage, then the subsequent wedding rites extended over 4 days. On the first night, the bride's relatives brought her to the house of her prospective husband, where she remained in seclusion for 3 days, occupying herself grinding the meal that her bridegroom's female relatives would cook during the fourth night. The next morning was devoted to the wedding feast, and the final act was the washing of the bride's head by her mother-in-law. The couple then remained at the husband's family home until his relatives had completed the bride's wedding garments, and then they went to live with the bride's people.

2. The Cheyenne Indians ate like other Plains Indians, chiefly relying on the buffalo for most of their food supply. They supplemented this with the flesh of other animals, however, deer and antelope mainly, as well as gathering native fruits and vegetables, roots, and berries.

3. The most noteworthy industry practiced by the Indians of the north Pacific coast was working with wood. They felled giant yellow cedars, which they burned and hewed to make seaworthy canoes using implements that were utterly primitive in both design and material. They made canoes of various sizes and design from the tiny, blunt-nosed river crafts capable of carrying, somewhat precariously, two passengers, to the great seaworthy vessels accommodating 20 to 30 people besides a considerable cargo of household utensils and food.

4. The Sioux were a seminomadic people. Throughout the summer months they moved their camps to follow the buffalo herds, and day after day, their hunting parties went out to the killing. Great stores of meat were cut into thin strips, dried, and pounded for use during the winter months when they could not hunt or kill. When autumn came and the cold northern winds began to sweep across the plains, the hunting parties, large and small, sought out a valley by a stream, and settled into the protection of a wooded area to remain until spring came. Furs were accumulated for winter clothing and bedding and were heaped into the tipis. The women gathered stores of roots and berries to supplement the dried meat the men had provided to last the people through the cold winter months. Thus, the seasons provided a rhythm that dictated the movement and the settling periods in the life of the Sioux communities.

5. The Apache made maternity belts from the skins of mountain lions, the black-tailed deer, the white-tailed deer, and the antelope because all of these animals were known to give birth to their young easily and with no complications. Medicine men were called in to pray to the spirits of these animals when a woman approached confinement and put on a maternity belt to be worn constantly during the critical period of labor and delivery, never removed until after the child was born. Prayers were said, first by the mother and father for their daughter, then by the medicine man, and finally by the mother-to-be; the prayers were directed to the gods and to the animals whose images were depicted on the belt.

Practice Materials Using Vocal Function Exercises

Goal: To understand the rationale and to practice vocal function exercises.

Joseph Stemple has popularized some exercises to modify laryngeal function. They are like "physical therapy" for the vocal folds and are useful for patients with problems of the laryngeal musculature (Stemple et al., 1994).

Selected Exercises

1. Warm-up: Sustain the sound "E" for as long as possible on the musical note "F." The goal is to increase the number of seconds the note can be held.
2. Stretching: Glide from lowest to highest note on the sound "O." The goal is to do is with no voice breaks.
3. Contracting: Glide from high to low on the vowel "O." The goal is to glide without any voice breaks.
4. Power: Sustain the musical notes "C, D, E, F, G" for as long as possible on the sound "O." The goal is to increase the number of seconds the notes can be sustained.

Do the exercises twice per day as softly as possible. Use easy onset and frontal tone focus. Voice breaks, wavering, and breathiness will gradually disappear as the vocal folds strengthen with practice.

Challenge Voice Practice

Goal: To practice reading using a well projected voice. Take plenty of air and use your lips and tongue well to focus the voice at the front of your mouth. Don't push from the throat.

1. You're joking about making fun of that poor devil, but you can't really expect any sane person to think that cruelty is funny.
2. I've heard you say you'll do more exercise a thousand times. Words are nothing, it's action that counts. So get off your butt and move those muscles.
3. It's good to have a feeling of strength and resolve. You know it's not going to be easy, but it's great to have decided to start to become the person you want to be.
4. I'm the teacher and if one more of you smart-alecky kids gives me any more lip, I will give you all detention. You are supposed to develop self control but I've yet to see any evidence of it in this classroom. Now, get on with the assignment. You only have 20 more minutes.
5. Speak aloud the words of "America, the Beautiful."

Confidential Voice Practice

Goal: To practice reading using a voice that is relaxed and easy. Imagine you are confiding in a friend, using reduced vocal power but using your lips and tongue so that the words are clear to the listener.

1. The last time something like this happened, I told myself that next time I would just keep my mouth shut and mind my own business. How did I get into this mess again?
2. I got into another fight with Jody in the lunchroom. I didn't mean to but I did anyway because she always bugs me with her smug condescending attitude. She thinks she's better than all the rest of us put together. I got sent to the Principal's office and he said he'd deal with me tomorrow. I'm scared that I could get into a lot of trouble over this as it's not the first time.
3. You'll never guess who asked me for a date. It was just now at the lockers when he came up to me. I nearly died of shock, he's so cool. Asked me to go to the game this Saturday.
4. The coach grabbed Damon by the neck and yelled at him like crazy. That man is a demon about discipline as he calls it. I call it harassment.

Note: The terms *challenge* and *confidential* voice are attributed to Dr. Janina Casper.

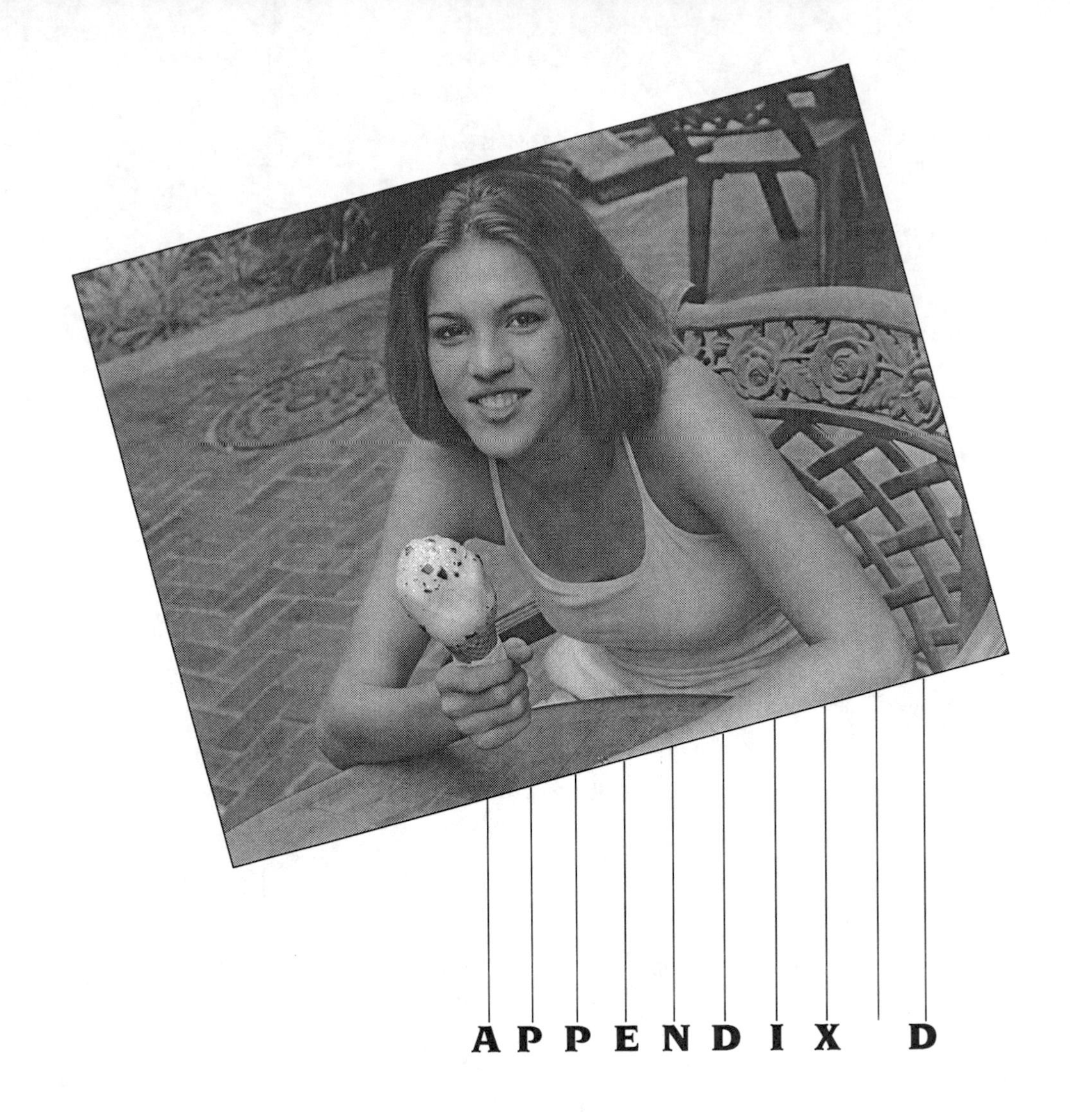

APPENDIX D

Practice Materials and Worksheets for Personal Growth and Awareness for Adolescent Students

Contents

Personal High-Risk Inventory

This inventory can help a student identify the many factors relevant to a vocal pattern. It can also be used as a format for students to interview peers in a voice group and may be followed by a discussion. A variation, where the student interviews the speech–language pathologist, allows the clinician to model responses and discuss individual differences in reactions to triggers.

Name: ____

Address: ____

Telephone: ____

Check the following factors that you feel may affect your vocal condition:

Environmental Factors

Smoking ____
Alcohol ____
Noise level ____
Dust in the air ____
Pollen ____
Recreational demands ____
Other (specify) ____

Health Factors

Eating disorders ____
Postnasal drip ____
Throat clearing ____
General fatigue ____
Sore throat ____
Illness ____
Frequent upper respiratory infections ____
Use of antihistamines and decongestants ____
Inadequate energy release ____

PMS ____
Allergies ____
Coughing ____
General tension ____
Aspirin ____

Other ________________

Excessive mucus or dryness (specify) ________________________

Vocal Habits

Specific neck tension _____
Number of replenishing breaths _____
Shortened exhalations _____
Shallow breathing pattern _____
Specific laryngeal fatigue _____
Hard glottal attacks _____
Inappropriate pitch _____
Strained vocalizations _____
Excessive singing _____
Excessive shouting, talking, cheering _____
Limited vocal variety _____

Other ____

Personality

Afraid of silence _____
"On" all the time _____
Excitable _____
Nervous _____
Volatile _____
Depressed _____
Shy _____

Other ____

Comments:

Worksheet: Managing Stress

Goal: To talk about do's and don'ts for handling stress.

DO'S

1. Physical exercise.
2. Take time to relax.
3. Eat regularly and well.
4. Try to sleep for 8 hours each night.
5. Express your feelings before they build up to stressful levels.
6. Make time to regenerate your emotional energy.
7. Temporarily remove yourself from a stressful scene.
8. Control what you can and accept what you must.
9. Devise a plan to work through a problem.
10. Prioritize tasks and break them into small steps.
11. Establish some order in the way you keep your belongings (not necessarily the same as neatness).
12. Give away (to charitable organizations) those excess belongings that overwhelm your space.
13. Take one thing at a time.
14. Establish goals for the future.
15. Adapt positive attitudes and perspectives.
16. Reframe expectations and perspectives in a positive way.

DON'TS

1. Avoid sweets, fats, caffeine, alcohol, tobacco, and drugs.
2. Avoid people, places, and situations that cause stress.
3. Don't procrastinate.
4. Don't obsess about a problem.
5. Don't focus on the problem but learn from it.
6. Don't feel sorry for yourself or imagine the worst.
7. Don't have unrealistic expectations for yourself or others.
8. Don't take yourself too seriously.
9. Don't pretend nothing is wrong by denial.
10. Don't use food to console yourself.
11. Don't have a judgmental attitude or seek revenge.
12. Don't be stubborn and demanding and inflexible.

What other advice could you think of to help manage stress?

Lifestyle Worksheet

The amount of time spent in vocally challenging activities may affect an adolescent's motivation to change vocal behaviors. This worksheet focuses attention on the importance of time allotted to quiet versus vocally strenuous activities and can provide the basis for further discussion.

Instructions: Rank order areas of your life in terms of importance to you as an individual and amount of time spent (weekly).

Activities	Importance	Amount of Time
Television		
Sports (spectator)		
Sports (participant)		
Reading		
Religion/Church		
Family		
Clubs (specify)		
Paid work		
School		
Music		
Friends		
Movies		
Service to community		
Quiet time alone		

Comic Collage

Comic books often illustrate vocally abusive behaviors. In this activity, students identify examples of abuse and list ways to avoid them. Alternate strategies can further be explored through discussion and role playing.

Examples of Vocal Abuse Cut From Comic Books	Ways to Avoid These Types of Abuse

Interviews About My Voice

Through interviews, students can learn to discuss more openly the positive and negative effects of their vocal behavior on others and gain insight into the overall pattern of how they use their voices.

Myself	Brother or Sister
Positive: Negative:	Positive: Negative:
Teacher	**Friend**
Positive: Negative:	Positive: Negative:

Voice Image

This activity stimulates insight and motivation. By providing practice in discussing their voices with the speech–language pathologist, students can define feelings about their vocal behavior and identify aspects of others' voices that they admire and could emulate.

Things I like about my voice: ______________________________

____

Things I don't like about my voice: ______________________________

____

Things about my personality that can be identified from listening to my voice: ______________________________

____

People who have voices I admire: ______________________________

____

Pleasing aspects of admired voices: ______________________________

____

Which of these aspects do I possess? ______________________________

____

Which pleasing aspects could I acquire? ______________________________

____

Gestures and Expressions: Alternatives to Talking

Through discussion and role playing, students explore nonverbal expression as an adjunct and alternative to oral communication.

The speech–language pathologist writes the following words on index cards (one word per card):

rejection	nervousness	exhaustion
anger	fear	eagerness
disappointment	shyness	joy
surprise	determination	disgust

Students "draw" one of the cards and act out, through gesture and expression, the word on the card until other group members guess the word. Students discuss what additional gestures and expressions can be used and in what situations these gestures and expressions can serve as alternatives to voice use. Then students role play, using both words and nonverbal communication, to convey the meaning.

Revising Accusatory Statements

Sentence structure as well as vocal delivery can convey a negative message to the listener. By learning to revise accusatory statements, students become aware of how to constructively say what they mean.

The speech–language pathologist provides a box containing slips of paper, each of which has an accusatory sentence written on it. For example:

You never call me.

Your room is a mess.

You won't have time, but I need help with my homework.

You're never going to take me to the game.

Don't yell at me.

That's a stupid idea.

You shouldn't do that.

Nobody here cares about me.

You always ignore what I say.

I just know you're going to stop dating me.

You're always lying.

You make me feel bad.

Each student must select a slip of paper, read the message aloud in an accusatory style, and then reword it. The revision must be worded to reflect the student's needs, feelings, or reactions. Beginning the statements with "I feel," "I need," or "I like" should be encouraged. Tone of voice and wording should reflect a positive, constructive attitude rather than an accusatory one. The group should be encouraged to discuss and evaluate the effects of the revisions. Characteristics such as loudness level, facial expression, and inflection should be noted.

Family "Messages" About Communication

All families and social groups have individual styles of communication. In this exercise, students analyze the direct and indirect messages inherent in communications between family members.

On index cards, the speech language pathologist writes, "What does your family tell you, either in words or by actions, gestures, or facial expressions about . . . ?"

Tone of voice

Yelling through the house

Loudness level of CDs

Loudness level of television

Dinner table conversation

Verbally sharing daily experiences

Cards are placed in a container and randomly drawn out for students to answer verbally or in written form. Sometimes there may be competing messages (i.e., say one thing but behave in another way). Discuss these differences.

Listening Responses

Whether listening responses are verbal or nonverbal, they convey important information. In this activity, the speech–language pathologist discusses the nature of communication as a two-way interaction. Students then list as many different kinds of listening responses as they can.

For example:

Telling an anecdote that tops the last one

Offering advice

Saying, "uh uh"

Frowning

Changing the subject

Being offended

Refusing to answer

Letting eyes wander

Asking questions for clarification

Interrupting before the speaker is finished

Talking to a friend while someone else is talking

Making a snide comment

Giggling

Complimenting the speaker

Saying, "I understand how you feel"

Saying, "It's stupid to feel that way"

Paraphrasing the meaning

Students pair off, and one tells a story while the other uses a particular listening response. At the end of 1 minute, they discuss the effect the listener has on the speaker, then switch roles. At the end of 10 minutes, all students form a large group and evaluate and discuss the strategies used.

Rank the Value of Interpersonal Communication Strategies

By analyzing their own reactions to interpersonal communication strategies, students become more aware of the effectiveness of their own strategies. The speech–language pathologist can help facilitate emerging insights through questions or examples provided in the discussion. A student discussion leader can be appointed to prepare examples in advance of the session.

The clinician lists communication strategies (e.g., turn taking, question asking, active listening, affirming statements, advice giving, sarcasm, giggling, lying) and asks students to rank in order the strategies in terms of importance to them as listeners.

Discuss:

Which has the most important or least important value?

Which strategies have you not thought about before?

Does the value of certain strategies change in different situations?

Is complete honesty always possible? How can a speaker be honest and kind at the same time?

Can tone of voice help to make a negative statement more palatable to a listener? How?

How can a speaker's tone of voice devalue the effect of their words on their listeners?

Which communication strategies communicate respect for an individual who is being addressed? Does this increase their value? If so, how?

Predicting the Outcome

Every communication has some effect on others and on oneself. For example, control of one's behavior helps to make one feel good about oneself. This activity explores the outcomes of various strategies.

Have students predict possible outcomes of the following actions by writing the answers on a piece of paper.

Discuss:

You scream and yell all the time.

You speak calmly even when upset.

Your eyes wander when you are talking to a person.

You maintain eye contact with your conversational partner.

You interrupt when you have something to say.

You allow others to finish speaking before talking yourself.

You usually do most of the talking.

You usually do most of the listening.

Sentence Completion

When students are practicing short, spontaneous utterances, sentence completions provide a helpful structure. The sentences may be tape-recorded and then played back and evaluated. The initial portion of each sentence is read, and the ending is spoken extemporaneously. The student may be encouraged to compare the vocal production during the sections involving both reading and speaking. For example, was the target vocal behavior maintained even during the part that was uttered spontaneously?

By next semester, I hope to have enough money to ________________________________

____.

One thing I'd like to accomplish in school is to ________________________________

____.

An evening of fun includes ________________________________

____.

Something I'd like to try this semester is ________________________________

____.

One habit I'd like to change now is ________________________________

____.

When I have children, something I'd like to do is ________________________________

____.

After school, the job I'd like to have is ________________________________

____.

Some things I'd like to have accomplished in two years include ________________________________

____.

My highest priorities in life are ________________________________

____.

Worksheet: Learning Styles

Goal: To understand and apply information through discussion of the reading.

People learn in different ways. When we understand how we learn best, it is easier for us. We can develop strategies that are effective for us. This kind of self-awareness also is useful in helping us overcome problems that arise when a teacher's teaching style is a mismatch with our own type of learning style. We can compensate by organizing the class material in a way that helps us learn it more easily when we study. This is a skill we need to develop to succeed in school, both today and later in college. It is also an important step in understanding more about our own uniqueness and how we can adapt to what happens in our world. Some writers call this dawning self-awareness "learning to be the author of our own lives." It is almost as if we can see ourselves living our life each day, in class as well as outside of it, and can determine ways to tell ourselves how to do it more efficiently.

Learning, in school as well as in life, is a process of becoming who we are meant to be. So the more we know about ourselves and the ways we learn new things, the easier it is for us to solve the problems we come up against. If we learn to do this well, we will have more energy, and we will also perform better, which usually makes us feel better about ourselves, too.

Think about your preferred method of learning. Do you think you rely more on hearing or seeing? Do you recall the way you remember things on a page? What do you know about emotional intelligence?

References

Covey, S. R. (1989). *The seven habits of highly effective people.* New York: A Fireside Book.

Daniels, A. C. (2000). *Bringing out the best in people: How to apply the astonishing power of positive reinforcement.* New York: McGraw-Hill, Inc.

Goleman, D. (1995). *Emotional intelligence: Why it can matter more than I.Q.* New York: Bantam Books.

Goleman, D. (1997). *Working with emotional intelligence.* New York: Bantam Books.

Worksheet: Short Rhythmic Readings

Goal: Read the following items maintaining the rhythm as well as an easy clear voice.

1. Money can buy a house, but not a home
   Money can buy medicine, but not health
   Money can buy fun, but not happiness
   Money can buy sex, but not love
   Money can buy a church, but not heaven.
2. I like to spend time out of doors
   admiring the meadows and trees
   but my allergies cause me a problem
   and I sneeze and sneeze and sneeze.
3. What is wealth
   But the rich means to gratify desire?
   What is empire?
   The privilege to punish and enjoy;
   To feel our power in making others fear it;
   To taste of pleasure's cup till we grow giddy,
   And think ourselves immortal!
   Hannah More (1790)

Worksheet: Career Paths

Goal: To talk about career paths and think of specific occupations.

Instructions: Use your best voice to talk about various occupations and what path they follow.

Business, Management, and Technology

(Business Path)

- People who like to work with numbers and be organized
- Specific careers
  Accountant
  Salesperson
  Computer programmer
  What occupations can you think of?

Arts and Communications and Entertainment

(Creative Path)

- People who like to draw, write, or perform
- Specific careers
  Artist
  Athlete
  Photographer
  Musician
  Journalist
  Actor
  Florist

Natural Resources and Agriculture

(Nature Path)

- People who like to work outside with plants or animals
- Specific careers
  Groundskeeper
  Agricultural engineer
  Naturalist
  Veterinarian
  Dog groomer
  Farmer

Industrial and Engineering Technology

(Fixing and Building Path)

- People who like to figure out how things work and build things
- Specific careers
  Architect
  Engineer
  Carpenter
  Plumber
  Scientist
  Electrician

Human Service and Social and Personal Services

(Helping Path)

- People who like to work with people to help make things better for others
- Specific careers
  Minister
  President of the United States
  Teacher
  Swimming instructor
  Coach
  Personal trainer
  Camp counselor
  Police officer

Health Services

(Health Path)

- People who like to take care of animals and people
- Specific careers
  Speech pathologist
  Pharmacist
  Doctor
  Dental hygienist
  Dentist
  Emergency medical technician

Career Skills Identification

Many careers require a wide range of vocal skills. By tying vocal behavior to career objectives, the speech–language pathologist can encourage greater motivation in some students. By first identifying those skills already possessed, the student may feel less overwhelmed by the effort involved in changing other aspects of his or her vocal behavior.

Identify students' vocation or career objectives on index cards (one career per card).

List vocal requirements of each vocation or career on individual index cards.

Identify those requirements the student currently possesses.

List those skills the student must acquire to be successful in each vocation or career.

Worksheet: Short Practice Utterances

Goal: Say the following sentences in a clear voice.

1. The winner asks, "May I help?"
   The loser asks, "Do you expect me to do that?
2. "It is a nuisance that knowledge can only be acquired by hard work."
   Somerset Maugham
3. Your future depends on many things, but mostly on you.
4. "Don't write merely to be understood. Write so that you cannot possibly be misunderstood."
   Robert Louis Stevenson
5. "Opportunity is missed by most people because it is dressed in overalls and looks like work."
   Thomas Edison
6. "Character is defined by what you're willing to do when the spotlight has been turned off, when the applause has died down, and no one is around to give you credit."
   Anonymous
7. "The reason most people fail, instead of succeeding, is because they trade what they want most for what they want at the moment."
   Anonymous
8. "One of the most time-consuming things is to have an enemy."
   E. B. White
9. "The average person puts only 25% of his [or her] energy and ability into work. The world takes off its hat to those who put in more than 50% of their capacity and stands on its head for those few-and-far between souls who devote 100%."
   Andrew Carnegie
10. "The reason why worry kills more people than work is that more people worry than work."
    Robert Frost

Worksheet: Short Reading Passages

Goal: To read the passages using your best voice and using vocal variation.

1. Imagine a bank that credits your account each morning with $1,440. It carries over no balance from the previous day. Every evening it deletes whatever part of the balance you failed to use during the day. What would you do? Draw out every dollar of course. Each of us has such a bank. Its name is "time." Every morning it credits you with 1,440 minutes. Every night it writes off as lost, whatever of this you have failed to invest to good purpose. It carries over no balance, and it allows no overdraft. Every day it opens a new account for you. Every night it burns the remains of the day. If you fail to use the day's deposits, the loss is yours. There is no going back. There is no drawing against tomorrow. You must live on today's deposit. Invest it so you will get from it the utmost in health, happiness, and success. The clock is running. Make the most of today.

2. To realize the value of 1 year, ask a person who has been sick in bed for a year. To realize the value of 1 month, ask a student who had her leg in a cast. To realize the value of 1 week, ask the editor of a weekly newspaper. To realize the value of 1 hour, ask the lovers who are waiting to meet. To realize the value of 1 minute, ask a person who missed the train. To realize the value of 1 second, ask the person who just avoided an accident. To realize the value of 1 millisecond, ask the person who won a silver medal at the Olympics. Treasure every moment that you have.

3. Treasure every moment you share with someone special who is special enough to spend your time with. Remember that time waits for no one. Yesterday is history. Tomorrow is a mystery. Today is a gift. That is why it is called the present.

4. We could learn a lot from crayons: Some are sharp, some are pretty, some are dull, some have weird names, and all are different colors . . . but they all have to learn to live in the same box.

5. Oh give me your pity, I'm on a committee
Which means that from morning to night
We attend and amend and contend and defend
Without a conclusion in sight.
We confer and concur, defer and demur
And reiterate all of our thoughts.
We reverse the agenda with frequent addenda
And consider a load of reports.
We compose and propose, we suppose and oppose
And the points of procedure are fun!
But though various notions are brought up as motions
There's terribly little gets done.
We resolve and absolve, but never dissolve
Since it's out of the question for us
Where else could we make such a fuss?

6. **The Hippopotamus**
I had a hippopotamus, I kept him in a shed
I fed him upon vitamins, vegetables and bread
I made him my companion on many cheery walks
And had his portrait done, by a celebrity, in chalks.

His charming eccentricities were known on every side
The creature's popularity was wonderfully wide.
He frolicked with the rector in a dozen friendly tussles
Who could not but remark about his hippopotomuscles.

If he should be afflicted by depression or the dumps
The hippopotomeasles or the hippopotomumps
I never knew a particle of peace till it was plain
That he was hippopotomasticating properly again.

I had a hippopotamus, I loved him as a friend
But beautiful relationships are bound to have an end
Life takes alas, our joys from us and robs us of our blisses
My hippopotamus turned out to be a hippopotomissus.

My housekeeper regarded him with jaundice in her eye
She did not want a colony of hippopotami
She borrowed a machine gun from her soldier nephew Percy
And showed my hippopotamus no hippopotomercy.

My house now lacks the glamor that the charming creature gave
The garage where I kept him is as silent as the grave
No joy that life can give me will be strong enough to smother
My sorrow, for what might have been, a hippopotomother.

7. **The Bath**
Broad is the gate and wide the path
That leads one to one's daily bath
But ere you spend that shining hour
With sponge and spray and sluice and shower
Remember! Where so ere you be
To lock the door and turn the key

I had a friend, my friend no more
Who failed to lock the bathroom door.
A maiden aunt of his, one day
Walked in, as half submerged he lay.
She did not notice nephew John
And turned the boiling water on!

He had no time, or even scope
To camouflage himself with soap.
But gave a cry and flung aside
The sponge neath which he sought to hide.
It fell to earth, I know not where
He beat his breast in his despair.
And rising, naked from the foam
Sprang into view and made for home.

His aunt fell fainting to the ground
Alas! they never brought her round.
She died, intestate, in her prime
The victim of another's crime
And John can never quite forget
How, by a breach of etiquette
He lost at one fell swoop, or plunge
His aunt, his honor, and his sponge!

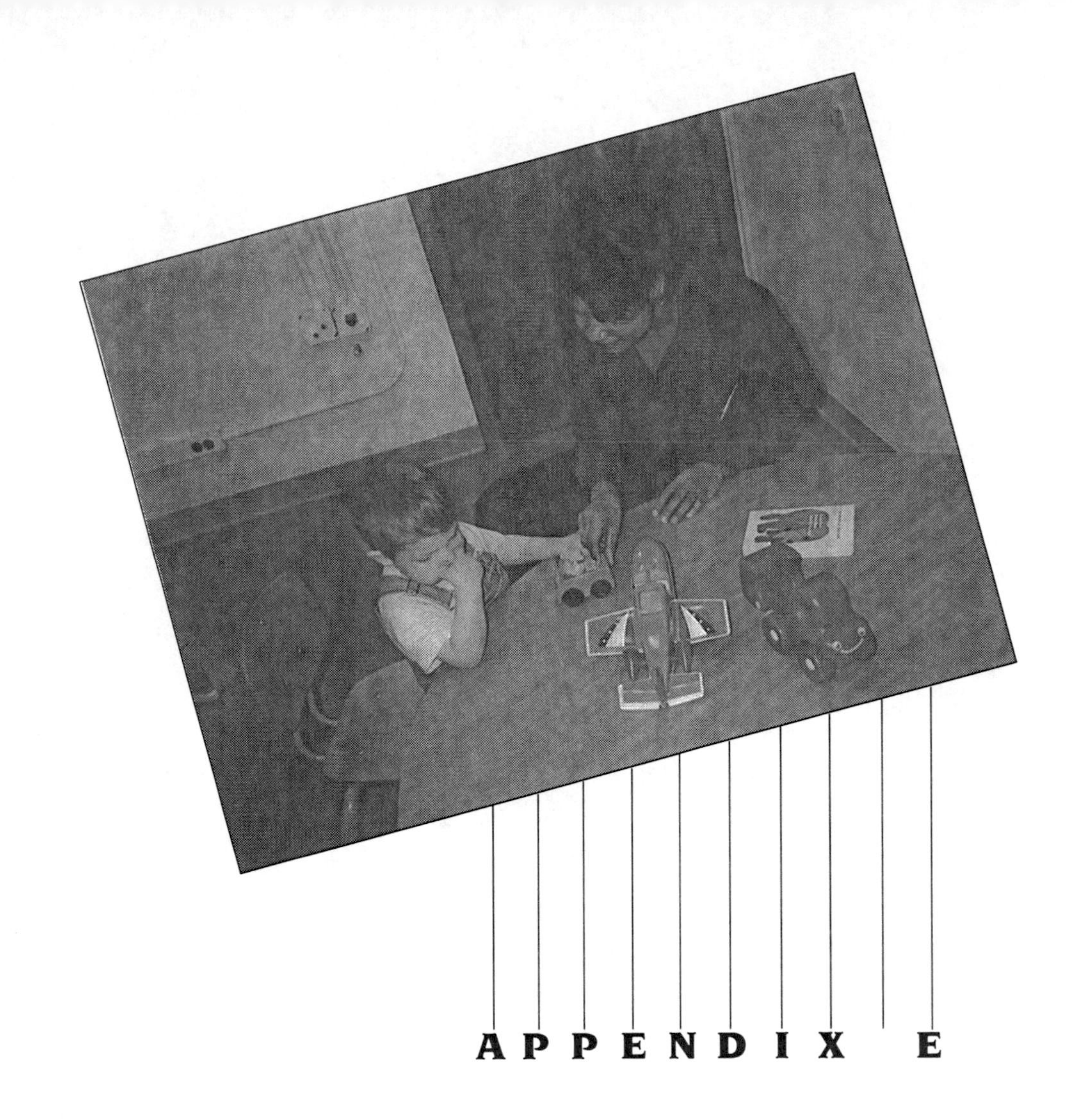

APPENDIX E

Clinician's Information

Contents

A Handout for Parents: Acknowledging Children's Feelings

Even young children need adults to acknowledge their feelings. Even bad feelings need to be acknowledged to be diffused and also to help the child to explore the feelings and find constructive ways to deal with them. For example, when a child is angrily acting out, it is best to remind him to use words instead of actions.

Example: If a child tries to knock over another child's toys, say, "Use words to tell her how you feel instead."

Consider the following interaction:

Melanie: I hate my brother.

Mom: You sound very mad at him.

Melanie: I am.

Mom: What did he do to upset you?

Melanie: He went into my closet and messed up my stuff.

Mom: No wonder you're so angry.

Melanie: He shouldn't go into my closet.

Mom: So you want your brother to know he should leave your things alone?

Melanie: I sure do, and I'm going to tell him right now.

Melanie's mom helped her to express her anger and understand just why she felt the way she did. By thinking through the situation, Melanie knew what she needed to say to her brother, and her anger was diminished.

Allergies: Information for Parents and Caregivers

Goal: To review information about allergies.

Identify whether your child's symptoms are seasonal or occur consistently all year. Talk this over with your physician.

- Mold, animal dander, and food allergens result in year-round symptoms.
- Pollen from trees, grass, and weeds is seasonal.
- Keep a diary of your child's symptoms to ascertain a pattern of cause and effect.

Examples

- Tree pollens: symptoms begin February to March and are finished by May.
- Grass pollens: symptoms usually subside in late July.
- Weed allergies begin in August and continue through fall. Ragweed continues until frost.

Medications

Allergy seasons vary by geographic area, so monitoring the local conditions is important because it impacts medication schedules. To be most effective, many medications must be taken 2 or 3 weeks before the exposure to the allergen occurs.

Treatments can be tailored to individual symptoms, and drugs can be combined by physicians who take into account factors such as patient's age, health status, lifestyle, and allergy history.

Antihistamines are the first class of drugs to treat allergic rhinitis (inflammation or infection of the membranes of the nose). They work by blocking the effects of histamine, the chemical responsible for many allergy symptoms. Now there are antihistamines available that do not make children drowsy.

Decongestants are sometimes used to treat symptoms like a stuffy nose. They may be combined with antihistamines in some products.

Corticosteroid nasal sprays are inhalers used to alleviate allergic rhinitis. Children as young as 6 years old can use them.

Cromolyn nasal sprays also relieve nasal inflammation and are frequently used for mild to moderate allergic rhinitis.

Allergy shots work like a vaccination. Patients receive small injections of the substances to which they are allergic. As the doses increase over time, the body builds up immunity. Anaphylaxis is a life-threatening reaction to an allergen that causes airways to constrict. It occurs suddenly, and patients need immediate medical attention. Bee stings and food allergies cause this reaction, and a shot of epinephrine must be administered quickly. There is a remote possibility that patients taking shots for desensitization may have such a reaction. For this reason, physicians ask patients to wait in the office for at least 20 minutes following a shot to see if a reaction develops.

Pitch Characteristics of 8- to 10-Year-Old White and African-American Boys

Morris (1997) studied the speaking fundamental frequencies (SFF) and the standard deviations of the SFF (pitch sigmas) of 90 boys aged 8 to 10 years when they read and when they described a picture; 45 of the boys were African American, and 45 were White. He found no significant differences for modal SFF between the two groups. The comparison of pitch sigma between groups, however, revealed that the 9- and 10-year-old African-American boys had significantly greater variability. Also, the 10-year-old African-American boys exhibited greater variability than the younger African-American boys. No significant differences in modal SFF were found to be related to age differences in either of the racial groups.

Modal Speaking Fundamental

Age	SFF *Range*	*Subjects*
8–10 years	233–215	African American
8–10 years	232–220	White

From Morris (1997); N = 90.

Puberty

Studies have shown that the onset of puberty varies considerably with respect to age and that factors such as race and ethnicity, nutrition, and environment affect it. In 1997, Dr. Marcia Herman-Giddens reported on a study of 17,077 girls ages 3–12 years examined by pediatricians all over the United States. About 90% were White, and 10% were African American. Results showed that by age 8, 15% of the White girls and 48% of the African-American girls had some breast development, pubic hair growth, or both. Additionally, 7% of the White girls and 27% of the African-American girls had begun puberty by age 7.

Joan Jacobs Brumberg (1997) wrote about the way girls today focus on physical characteristics and that the lean, taut female body ideal, combined with the idea that bodies are perfectible, heightens pressure on adolescents. Although girls have always been self-conscious about their looks, she noted a marked contrast in New Year resolutions of young women in the 1890s versus young women today. The ideal in the 1890s was to be of good character, to be self-restrained and dignified, and to think of others rather than self. In the 1990s, the ideal was to lose weight or to obtain various items to improve one's appearance: contact lenses, a good haircut, makeup, clothes, and accessories.

The obsession with physical appearance is also a problem experienced by male adolescents in our culture. Some experts view body image as something young men think about all the time and some male adolescents suffer from extreme body image disorders. Pope (1993) discussed "muscle dysmorphia," which involves an excessive preoccupation with muscularity. This syndrome could be called "reverse anorexia nervosa" because sufferers think they are too small, skinny, and weak to the point that their obsession with bodybuilding interferes with work and relationships.

Starting in middle school, other boys taunt the fat, the skinny, the short, and even if the boys eventually outgrow the body image that oppressed them as adolescents, the memories linger through adult life. Writing about both men and women, Susan Bordo (1999) noted that the standards for achieving physical acceptance in modern society are more stringent and rigorous than before. The feminist complaint has been that women internalize being treated as objects, and this damages their self-esteem; now men are judged not by who they are, but by how they look, especially without a shirt.

Michael Gurian (1999) drew on biology, anthropology, literature, and his own experience to explain why young men in our society are often impulsive at best and violent at worst. He believes boys need an extended family with male relationships and role models so that elders can train young men and boys. He believes that at adolescence male role models can help teenagers control and cope with inherent urges and drives. He said that every time you raise a loving, wise, and responsible man, you help create a better world for women.

References

Brumberg, J. J. (1997). *The body project: An intimate history of American girls.* New York: Random House.

Gilbert, S. (1997, April 9). "Early puberty onset seems prevalent." *New York Times.*

Gurian, M. (1999). *The good son: Shaping the moral development of our boys and young men.* New York: Putnam.

Hall, S. S. (1999, August 22). "The bully in the mirror." *The New York Times Magazine.*

Herman-Giddens, M. E., Slora, E. J., Wasserman, R. C., Bourdony, C. J., Bhapkar, M. V., Koch, G. G., & Hasemeier, C. M. (1997). Secondary sex characteristics and menses in young girls seen in office practice: A study from the Pediatric Research in Office Settings Network. *Pediatrics, 98,* 505–512.

Pope, H. G., Jr., Gruber, A. J., Choi, P., Olivardia, R., & Phillips, K. A. (1997). Muscle dysmorphia: An underrecognized form of body dysmorphic disorder. *Psychosomatics, 38,* 548–557.

Paradoxical Vocal Cord Dysfunction

Paradoxical vocal cord dysfunction (PVCD) is characterized by shortness of breath and stridor; it is diagnosed by laryngoscopy, pulmonary function tests, or both. During attacks the vocal folds adduct on either inspiration or expiration. It has also been referred to in the literature as paradoxical vocal fold motion, Munchausen's stridor, factitious asthma, psychogenic asthma, and laryngospasm. Dr. Florence Blager (Martin, Blager, Gay, & Wood, 1987) was the speech pathologist who published extensively on therapy protocols used at the National Jewish Medical and Research Center (1400 Jackson St., Denver, Colorado 80206 [www.njc.org]). Michael Trudeau (1998) of Department of Speech and Hearing Sciences, The Ohio State University, has studied juveniles with PVCD referred by pulmonologists and otolaryngologists. He found more female than male subjects in his sample, although the youngest children he saw were boys. He also did not find a significant history of abuse, although he recommended that clinicians "should remain cautiously observant for signs of abuse" in this population. He did find typical stressors as a possible trigger for PVCD but believed that it is possible that it is multiple stressors that trigger PVCD in nonadult clients. He noted divorce, deaths of family members or friends, crowded schedules (especially seen in athletes), and conflict with authority figures (most commonly coaches). Sensitive interviewing of both the students and their parents allows the clinician to make appropriate recommendations and discover links between possible stressors and their effects on the individual. Trudeau found evidence of gastroesphageal reflux on videoendoscopy in some subjects in his study, causing edema and erythema of the posterior larynx. A few children also demonstrated laryngeal tremor during phonation.

Treatment

1. Referrals to other professionals, for example, to mental health professionals for stress and to a physician for gastroesphageal reflux (esophageal manometry or Ph monitoring tests) to maximize the benefits of a team approach.
2. Information to families and students to clarify anatomy and physiology, the role and effect of stressors, the reason for any medications or treatment strategies, and the need for lifestyle changes. Handouts summarizing key points are useful, and the establishment of a trusting and supportive relationship is essential
3. Reprogramming cognitively, emotionally, and physiologically to establish the individual's sense of control over the condition generally, and over the laryngeal spasm specifically.

    - Verbalization of anxieties concerning the symptoms and the learning of more direct ways to express emotion and deal with the problem
    - Focus of attention away from the larynx and the inspiratory phase of breathing
    - Relaxation of the oropharyngeal, neck, shoulder, and chest muscles and concentration on deep, relaxed abdominal breathing
    - Teach the child to use abdominal breathing at the first sign of tightness in the throat or stridor
    - Use cognitive images of openness in the laryngeal-pharyngeal area: "open hose or tube" versus "tight or kinked hose or tube" or "a wide tunnel for the air to flow through"

- Focus on exhalation to break the pattern of fighting to get air in. It stops attempts to hold the breath and efforts to gasp for air. The child may count silently as the air is expelled. Audible exhalation (e.g., /s/) can be practiced but not to maximum duration
- Stress the natural easy rhythm of breathing and the helpfulness of breathing frequently so that there is always plenty of air flowing in and out; increase self-awareness of the "easy" versus "tight" breathing
- Optimize hydration by drinking plenty of water and eliminate drying agents such as decongestants, aspirin, caffeine
- Teach the following ways to establish relaxed patterns of breathing lip pursing, nasal inspiration, and sniffing, which maximally adduct the folds; exhaling available air so that the next inhalation occurs spontaneously; and exhalation of breathed sounds such as /s/ /sh/
- Devise rituals to deal with night chokes and difficulties experienced during physical exertion

Differential Diagnosis

Other causes of upper airway obstruction can produce symptoms similar to PVCD and must be ruled out. These include:

- neoplasma
- granulomatous diseases
- aspiration of foreign bodies
- stenotic lesions from trauma
- hypertrophic tonsils
- external airway compression

Reference

Brugman, S. M., & Newman, K. (1993). Vocal cord dysfunction. *Medical/Scientific Update, National Jewish Center for Immunology and Respiratory Medicine, 111* (5), 1–5.

Rules for Voice Class

(If you do not know a person in the group, be sure to tell him or her your name and ask the person to tell you his or her name.)

1. Say kind things
2. Don't interrupt
3. No fighting
4. Don't yell at someone
5. Talk slowly
6. Talk so that they can understand you
7. Don't tell people what to say
8. Don't talk too much
9. Don't play with things or throw things at people
10. Take turns talking
11. No showing off or distracting others
12. No talking or giggling while others are talking
13. No making fun of others
14. Don't be rude
15. Greet people
16. Wait for answers

Good "Friend Talking" Sample Form

Week of:	3/23	3/30	4/20	5/4	
Sharing talking time:	+	+	+		
Ask questions:	–	+			
Eye contact:	+	+	+		
Acknowledge good ideas:	–				
Avoid interruptions:		+	+		
Avoid putdowns:					
Say kind things:					
Greet people:	+		+		
Wait for answers:					
Avoid showing off or distracting:					
No name calling:					
Posture/breaths:	– posture				
Transitions (links):					

Good "Friend Talking" Form

Week of:					
Sharing talking time:					
Ask questions:					
Eye contact:					
Acknowledge good ideas:					
Avoid interruptions:					
Avoid putdowns:					
Say kind things:					
Greet people:					
Wait for answers:					
Avoid showing off or distracting:					
No name calling:					

Topics to Discuss in Voice Class

What Do You Think About?

Privacy

Allowance

Sick pet

Hairstyles

Fighting in the car

Visiting Grandma

Rules about watching television

Dad's new friend

Respecting property

Homework habits

Sharing space

Loud music

Drugs

Alcohol

Name calling

Group reports

Holiday pageants

Gossip

Bullies

Forging a note

Being ignored

Copying a report

Stolen bicycle

Choosing a team

Too many animals

Rating as a friend

Friendly gestures

Cheating on a test

Incorrect grade

Forbidden friend

Movie restrictions

Defending a friend

Shoplifting

Voice Goals for Individualized Educational Programs

Proficiency 1: Awareness and Discrimination of Factors Related to Voice Problems

Objectives

- Increase motivation for self-improvement
- Awareness of non-speech sounds the body can make (e.g., lip smacking, tongue clicks, kissing, sniffling, coughing, etc.)
- Awareness of speech-related sounds (e.g., Boo!, Sh!, hissing, slurping, panting, etc.)
- Awareness of the relationship between your voice and reactions by other people
- Awareness of the relationship between sounds and feelings
- Awareness of parts of the face, mouth, and body that are used in speech and voice
- Awareness of the way the voice works
- Awareness of the causes of voice problems and how they affect the vocal folds
- Identify physical behaviors that contribute to inappropriate voice (e.g., posture, breathing, muscular tension, etc.)
- Identify health factors that might contribute to inappropriate voice (e.g., allergies, colds, reflux, hydration, hearing loss, etc.)
- Identify lifestyle factors that contribute to inappropriate voice (e.g., noisy environment, sleeping or eating habits, air pollution, etc.)
- Identify vocally abusive practices that contribute to inappropriate voice (e.g., throat clearing, coughing, smoking, cheering, etc.)
- Identify interpersonal behaviors that contribute to inappropriate voice (e.g., talking too much, ignoring feedback, competing for attention, etc.)
- Awareness of high/low, loud/soft, fast/slow qualities of sound
- Discriminate high/low, loud/soft, fast/slow qualities of sound
- Identify high/low, loud/soft, fast/slow qualities of voice
- Identify target pitch, loudness, or rate range
- Discriminate target/error pitch, loudness, or rate
- Awareness of respiratory conditions that affect breathing efficiency (e.g., allergies, smoking, infections)
- Understand how to compensate for respiratory conditions that affect breathing efficiency
- Awareness of physical conditions that affect voice quality (e.g., medications, mouth breathing, hormones)
- Understand how to compensate for physical conditions that affect voice quality
- Awareness of lifestyle and environmental conditions that affect voice quality (e.g., cheering, sports, air pollution, noisy environment)
- Understand how to compensate for lifestyle and environmental conditions that affect voice quality

Proficiency 2: Use Appropriate Respiration and Phrasing Patterns in Spontaneous Speech

Objectives

- Understand the concept of inhalation
- Understand the concept of exhalation
- Increase amount of air on inhalation phase
- Increase amount of air on exhalation phase
- Understand concept of abdominal versus upper chest breathing
- Use abdominal breathing for deep inhalation
- Increase control of exhalation phase (stopping and starting airflow)
- Increase efficiency of air use on exhalation phase
- Identify phrasing which is inappropriate to meaning of sentence
- Identify inappropriate replenishing breath patterns
- Identify appropriate places for replenishing breaths
- Increase rhythmical flow of inhalation, exhalation, and replenishing segments in spontaneous speech
- Identify limited variety of phrasing, pitch, loudness, or rate in speech patterns
- Identify appropriate inflectional patterns to meaning by changing pitch, loudness, rate, or pause patterns (e.g., question, statement, command)

Proficiency 3: Apply Relaxation Strategies for Optimal Use of Vocal Mechanism

Objectives

- Understand concepts of tension and relaxation
- Increase awareness of tense and relaxed states in the body
- Discriminate tense and relaxed states
- Increase awareness of tension sites in the upper chest, neck, and jaw
- Identify various relaxation strategies (e.g., deep breathing, physical, visual, and mental exercises)
- Voluntarily relax the laryngeal and upper chest areas
- Use relaxation techniques in structured speech situations
- Use relaxation strategies during everyday and stressful activities

Proficiency 4: Use Appropriate Voice Quality in Everyday Speaking Situations

Objectives

- The student's voice quality will be monitored by the speech–language pathologist
- Compare own voice sound to normal voice sound
- Identify appropriate voice quality characteristics
- Identify inappropriate voice quality characteristics
- Produce target voice quality varying length of utterance
- Monitor and self-correct voice quality target with accuracy
- Use target voice quality in everyday speaking situations

Proficiency 5: Understand and Use the Oral Mechanism Appropriately

Objectives

- Increase fluid intake to 6–8 glasses of water a day
- Raise head of bed 4–6 inches
- Use humidifier in bedroom
- Reduce smoke in environment
- Know parts of the face and body used in speech production
- Learn exercises for lips, tongue, jaw, and cheeks
- Increase lip and tongue movement
- Increase mouth opening by lowering jaw during speech
- Direct air stream through the mouth
- Understand the difference between frontal and back tone focus in the mouth
- Use frontal tone focus on sounds, words, and sentences
- Use facilitators to increase laryngeal tension (e.g., push/pull)
- Use facilitators to decrease laryngeal tension (e.g., jaw drop, head roll, visualization)
- Use facilitators to improve frontal tone focus (resonance; e.g., lip tickle, voice "throw")

Proficiency 6: Use Appropriate Non-Verbal Body Actions in Everyday Speaking Situations

Objectives

- Be aware of the relationship between posture and voice quality
- Discriminate posture positions
- Imitate good posture
- Use good posture in voice class
- Use good posture in everyday life

- Understand how non-verbal factors can convey information (e.g., gestures, facial expressions, body movements, eye contact)
- Describe what feelings are sent by different gestures, facial expressions, body language, and eye contact
- Role-play different feelings with gestures, facial expressions, body language, and eye contact
- Use appropriate gestures, facial expressions, body language, and eye contact in everyday life

Proficiency 7: Use Appropriate Resonance in Everyday Speaking Situations

Objectives

- Understand concepts of tone focus: frontal, back, nasal
- Direct air stream through the lips and through the nares (nose)
- Sustain nasal resonance on a hum
- Increase adequacy of velopharyngeal closure
- Increase mouth opening and lip and tongue movement to decrease nasality
- Prolong vowels without nasal emission
- Produce appropriate oral/nasal balance on words, phrases, and sentences
- Produce appropriate oral/nasal balance during conversation

Proficiency 8: Use Appropriate Onset of Voice in Everyday Speaking Situations

Objectives

- Initiate phonation on vowel
- Prolong phonation
- Start-stop-start phonation
- Understand the concept of hard glottal attacks
- Identify words that start with vowel sounds and words that start with consonant sounds
- Identify hard glottal attack and easy onsets when hearing words that begin with vowels
- Produce easy onset vowels
- Identify hard glottal attack and easy onsets when producing words that begin with vowels
- Avoid hard glottal attacks in reading sentences and paragraphs
- Avoid hard glottal attacks in conversation with the speech pathologist present
- Avoid hard glottal attacks in everyday speaking situations

Proficiency 9: Use Appropriate Pitch, Loudness, and Rate in Everyday Speaking Situations

Objectives

- Awareness of how pitch, loudness, and rate can vary
- Discriminate high/low pitch, loud/soft loudness, fast/slow rate
- Imitate high/low, loud/soft, fast/slow aspects of voice
- Produce pitch, loudness, and rate variations in isolated vowels and series of vowels
- Vary pitch, loudness, and rate in words
- Vary pitch, loudness, and rate in sentences
- Vary pitch, loudness, and rate in structured speech situations
- Vary pitch, loudness, and rate in everyday speech situations
- Describe pitch, loudness, and rate variations in phrases and sentences to alter the meaning of the phrases and sentences
- Use pitch, loudness, and rate variations appropriate to sentence meaning
- Use pitch and rate changes rather than loudness to get and hold attention

Proficiency 10: Use Nonabusive Vocal Practices in Everyday Speaking Situations

Objectives

- Identify characteristics of atypical voices (e.g., breathy, harsh, low, aphonic episodes, pitch breaks, etc.)
- Identify and describe how a voice should sound
- Understand the vocal mechanism and how voice is produced
- Understand abuse of the vocal mechanism and how the vocal folds become damaged
- Identify behaviors that cause voice problems
- Identify ways to improve posture, breathing and relaxation skills
- Identify ways to alter lifestyle to decrease vocal abuse
- Identify ways to decrease irritation to vocal folds caused by health factors
- Avoid repeated throat clearing and non-productive coughing
- State alternative behaviors for behaviors that cause voice problems
- Identify alternative non-verbal behaviors to vocally abusive practices
- Role play alternative behaviors to vocally abusive practices
- Reduce vocal abuse in specific adverse situations
- Use alternative behaviors to yelling and screaming in everyday situations

Proficiency 11: Use Interpersonal Skills to Decrease Vocal Stress in Everyday Speaking Situations

Objectives

- Awareness of tension sites (jaw, neck, upper chest)
- Awareness of interpersonal behaviors that adversely affect voice quality (e.g., incessant talking, competing for attention, aggressive behavior)
- Identify interpersonal behaviors that increase vocal effectiveness
- Use pleasant tone of voice instead of whining and screaming
- Be a good questioner and encourage others to talk
- Avoid asking the same question over and over
- Use polite methods of interrupting a conversation
- Reduce the distance between yourself and the listener to lessen the tendency to shout
- Use nonverbal attention-getters (e.g., clapping, waving, etc.) whenever possible
- Maintain good posture while relaxing neck, jaw, and shoulders
- Avoid talking during periods of upper respiratory problems or when in the presence of loud noises
- Increase the ratio of listening versus talking time
- Identify positive strategies for managing stress (e.g., exercise, seek alternatives, prioritize, talk-it-out)
- Use positive self-talk
- Analyze perspectives of others
- Learn conflict resolution skills
- Read self-help articles

Special Interest Division of ASHA (Division 3) Voice and Voice Disorders Listserv

If the following instructions do not adequately guide you through the process of joining sid3voice contact the listserv manager.

sid3voice

This listserv is sponsored by the American Speech-Language Hearing Association's Special Interest Division for Voice and Voice Disorders and the University of Iowa Department of Otolaryngology–Head and Neck Surgery. Its purpose is to promote discussion among health care professionals, scientists, and professional voice users regarding clinical and scientific issues relating to the normal and disordered human voice.

sid3voice Subscribe Instructions

To subscribe to sid3voice, you may access the sid3voice webpage at:

http://list.medicine.uiowa.edu/scripts/lyris.pl?enter=sid3voice&text_mode=0&lang=english

click on the button "Join sid3voice"

Alternatively, you may subscribe by email as follows:

1. Address an e-mail message to lyris@list.medicine.uiowa.edu
2. In the body of the message type:

   subscribe sid3voice firstname lastname
   quit

3. Send the message

You will receive an automated confirmation message that you've been added to the Sid3voice mailing list. SAVE THE CONFIRMATION MESSAGE! It has important instructions, including how to sign off the listserv.

After you have subscribed, address messages to the listserv as follows:
sid3voice@list.medicine.uiowa.edu

If you have any problems, contact:
michael-karnell@uiowa.edu
Michael Karnell, Ph.D.
sid3voice Listserv Manager

Individuals With Disabilities Education Act (IDEA)

Voice Problems Are an Educational Disability

Students with voice disorders may fail to receive speech services because it is thought that their disability does not adversely affect academic performance (a criterion used by many special educators when citing IDEA regulations for determining if a student qualifies for special education or related services). *In a letter of interpretation, the Office of Special Education Programs (OSEP) clarified the term educational performance,* as used in IDEA, *to include effect upon academic and nonacademic areas. Furthermore, if the presence of a speech-language impairment has been established by a SLP through appropriate appraisal procedures, the receipt of services is not conditional upon academic performance. A child who is achieving at grade level can still qualify as having a speech–language disability.*

Vocal disability includes disorders of misperception of one's own voice, vocal misperception by others, and difficulties with vocal production. Students with voice disorders can face many difficulties that affect academic and related educational, as well as social-emotional aspects of life. Oral communication is basic to all classroom learning and is the major vehicle of instructional interaction between teachers and children. Children with unusual or strained voices, attention-getting compensations, restricted vocal options for seeking and holding attention, and inadequate understanding of the vocal correlates of meaning generally require intervention to offset educational deficits.

Impact of Voice Disorders on Education

Children with voice disorders can be negatively affected in a variety of ways:

1. Attempts to conceal atypical vocal production, or feelings of inferiority about their voices may seriously limit their classroom participation, giving them fewer opportunities to practice and receive feedback. Furthermore, their preoccupation with concealing deviant vocal behaviors may interfere with concentration during academic activities.
2. Social-emotional implications of a voice disorder are many. Children may become withdrawn and reticent, or vocally aggressive and defiant in attempting to compensate for their disability. These problems can become worse without early intervention and seriously impact learning.
3. Children with a limited number of vocal strategies for solving interpersonal problems (e.g., whining, using a baby voice, talking loudly and incessantly) are at risk for being evaluated in negative ways, which can indirectly affect how they are viewed in all aspects of their education. Intervention can help them, as well as significant adults around them, understand the effects of this inappropriate behavior upon academic achievement.
4. Many occupations demand efficient and pleasant vocal communication skills. Habits and inappropriate compensations are more difficult to change later in life.

Intervention Models

A variety of intervention strategies can be employed to remediate voice disorders:

1. Consultation
2. Collaborative programs (e.g., with music teachers)
3. Classroom lessons for the entire class
4. Science and health projects associated with voice
5. Voice treatment programs, with small groups or in peer dyads, or one on one
6. Materials that parents can use to teach vocal awareness at home
7. Inservice programs for teachers to encourage innovative "voice lessons" in the classroom
8. Use of amplification in classrooms to help children focus on auditory information

The Singing or Acting Child: A Speech–Language Pathologist's Perspective[1]

The child who engages in singing and acting activities on a regular basis and who derives some success and appreciation from vocal performance usually has a significant emotional investment in voice. Children who perform learn not only a number of skills and enlarge their experience, but their voice becomes a part of their overall identity. Their vocal image is different from that of their peers who do not invest in vocal performance and who are generally unaware of the impact of voice use in their daily lives. Vocal problems have great impact on the lives of performance-oriented children and intervention approaches must be carefully designed to meet their special needs.

There are undoubtedly many factors that contribute to the development of the vocal image of the performance-oriented child. Exposure to and the enjoyment of music and theater, role models, reinforcement, available resources, and opportunities undoubtedly play a part. Additionally, melodic accuracy, auditory memory, pleasing voice quality, and certain personality characteristics may also predispose and maintain children's awareness that voice is a valuable part of themselves. Thus, it is important for clinicians to examine each child's special strengths, backgrounds, and training. A comprehensive interview with the parents, reports from the physician and teacher, and in-depth discussions with the child are critical. The history should include not only the medical and educational aspects but also the psychosocial dimensions.

[1]Reprinted with permission of The Voice Foundation from "The Singing or Acting Child: A Speech–Language Pathologist's Perspective" by Moya L. Andrews, 1998. *Journal of Voice, 11,* 130–134.

Profiles of Children at Risk

Some children receive private voice lessons or training in choirs or children's theater programs at school or in the community. Appropriate training from a teacher or coach who is knowledgeable about the developing voice and who assigns suitable practice activities and repertoire, is of course, optimal. Not all performance-oriented children enjoy this benefit, however. One group of children who are at risk of the development of vocal problems are typically those who have received inadequate training to meet an increased number of vocal demands. Demands may be extrinsic or intrinsic, but the response pattern is often the same. A young performer who lacks the technique necessary to adapt to challenging tasks or conditions adopts inappropriate compensations that are injurious to the vocal mechanism. The use of maladaptive techniques during singing or speaking probably first occurs as an occasional or situation-based response. For example, it may arise in the presence of environmental constraints, such as noise, or it may result from attempts to perform when there are physiologic constraints due to swelling of the vocal folds. Whatever the initial impetus or its cause, the unskilled performer invariably increases tension and effort. In a misguided attempt to improve vocal power and endurance, the vocally naive young performer adopts short-term compensations that then become habituated and deleterious across time. A misguided short-term solution can exacerbate an initial problem and have a snowballing effect. For instance, when tension and effort are increased, so is the vulnerability of the structures. Motivated children try harder. When they try harder in the face of vocal constraints, they rapidly become accustomed to using hyperfunctional behavioral patterns. As the hyperfunctional patterns become ingrained, they begin to feel normal and necessary. Vocal self-perception (Haskell, 1987) is altered. Unaware that such techniques are destructive, the young performer incorporates them, believes in them, and valiantly continues to use them as the voice itself invariably worsens. Speech–language pathologists may be consulted when the child's ability to perform is drastically impaired or when total voice breakdown has occurred.

Careful assessment is needed to identify all aspects of a problem. A team approach to treatment is the approach of choice and ideally the team includes an otolaryngologist and singing or acting specialist in addition to the speech–language pathologist. It is always important to identify lifestyle factors and nonspeech abusive practices (such as throat clearing, coughing, and fillers) in addition to voice production during projected and conversational speech. Table E-1 lists some examples of some areas commonly addressed during retraining of the hyperfunctional voice. Explanations concerning vocal physiology and hygiene and identification of behaviors that inhibit the production of a natural, relaxed voice usually precede direct vocal production activities. It is self-evident that knowledge and insight are prerequisites for the acquisition of new skills (Andrews & Summer, 1991).

The team approach to intervention with young performers who lack appropriate information and training is especially critical when a hyperfunctional pattern is apparent in both the singing and the speaking voice. There are, however, some children who enjoy the care of competent voice teachers and produce their singing or stage voices well but who use inappropriate conversational speech habits. This group of children is also at risk of voice problems but the precipitating factors are related not to their performing but to other lifestyle endeavors. They have not generalized the voice production knowledge and skills they use on stage to their recreational voice use. Some engage in activities such as cheerleading, some are involved in vocally strenuous group activities of other kinds, and most seem to place a high priority on being perceived as outgoing and vivacious. Some of the personality characteristics that serve them well on stage seem to cause them to feel they must also be "on stage" in most other areas of their lives. For example, they frequently are individuals who do not excel at conversational turn taking and question asking and who feel the need to be the center of attention and the life of the party. Most excel as story tellers and mimics and enjoy their ability to entertain their friends. In conversation, they frequently use more self-referenced than other-referenced statements. It often appears that their self-expression skills are highly developed, whereas skills related to attending to the messages of others are less well-honed.

The speech–language pathologist is faced with the task of helping these young people to analyze and gain insight into their overall communication style. Most students will be wary if they feel voice therapy is going to change their personality. One approach that can be used with this group is for the clinician to begin by helping them review their strengths. It will be apparent that in many respects these young people are good communicators. They enjoy communicating and have notable expressive skills. Once this has been established, the clinician can then help them to begin to analyze their receptive skills. The following questions may be raised. "What do you learn from really listening to other people? How can you draw other people out? What nonverbal cues can

Table E-1. Retraining the hyperfunctional voice.

Speech breathing

- Type of inhalation
- Depth of inhalation
- Length and control of exhalation
- Number of replenishing breaths
- Location of replenishing breaths

Posture and body alignment

- Head, neck, thorax
- Jaw, extrinsic laryngeal musculature
- Relaxed stance, unlocked knees

Articulation

- Relaxed articulatory musculature
- Appropriate tongue carriage
- Easy voice onset
- Continuity of voicing on continuant consonants
- Adequate mouth opening
- Improved intelligibility and diction

Resonance

- Tone focus
- Balance of oral–nasal resonance
- Minimize assimilated nasality
- Pharyngeal relaxation

Phonation

- Appropriate vocal fold closure
- Elimination of "pressed" phonation
- Improved airflow
- Elimination of hard onsets
- Relaxed laryngeal posture and movement
- Appropriate variation and prosody

help you to really understand a speaker's true feelings?" If the goal of enriching the existing communication style can be the focus of discussion and analysis, the student may see a personally beneficial rationale for changing some behaviors. New strategies may then be presented as ways to build on existing strengths and defensiveness is minimized. Table E-2 lists some examples of activities that may be effective. Materials that may be used with clients of different ages are described elsewhere (Andrews, 1988, 1991; Andrews & Summers, 1988; Flynn, Andrews, & Cabot, 1990; Sataloff, 1991).

With all young performers who are anxious and frustrated by the threat of restrictions on voice use, it is imperative that the clinician build a trusting therapeutic relationship. The therapeutic relationship may be viewed as a separate part of a treatment program, or it may be seen mainly as a framework to promote behavior modification or to channel information, feedback, and expertise. Naturally, professional orientation and training, the clinician's personal characteristics and preferences, and the chemistry between the client and clinician affect the nature of the clinical relationship, and each relationship established with each individual client is unique. Some clinicians consciously define goals for the client that are relationship based. Goals that address cognitive restructuring are examples of this type of approach. Whether the goals are consciously specified or not, certain effects occur within treatment relationships that are the direct result of the interaction. These effects are not the result of the procedures but rather of the interaction. The advantage for the clinician who consciously considers psychosocial goals is that this aspect of the treatment can be better controlled, and appropriate referrals and team support may be judiciously incorporated early in the treatment protocol, if needed.

The Psychosocial Aspects of Treatment

Treatment programs for young professionals often provide dramatic examples of the way the psychosocial dimensions of a voice disorder may be addressed in the context of the therapeutic relationship. As was noted earlier, the vocal symptoms of young performers often arise as a direct result of the tensions created by competing needs. The acquisition of information and new vocal practices is intimately related to insight development, as well as to physical and emotional development. For example, as children approach puberty, both physical and emotional developmental issues are obviously important to case management.

The speech–language pathologist considers how the young performers' aspirations relate to life stage, role and responsibility within the family, educational and career structure, and identifies stressors. Interaction patterns, social and cultural influences, feelings of self-worth, and signs of compliance/rebellion, as well as defense mechanisms and problem solving, may be pertinent to the elimination of nonproductive vocal behaviors.

One of the major considerations for clinicians is how the psychological and emotional changes have an impact on vocal behavior. Anatomic and physiologic constraints may conflict with performance demands. Has the client completed laryngeal maturation? Is the mechanism more vulnerable because it is not yet mature? Has there been a meshing or a dissonance between the developmental and the training or performance needs? The family system is also of prime importance in assessment and treatment. The dynamics within the family, the way the young performer uses the voice to meet personal as well as family needs, solve problems, and maintain family equilibrium may need to be addressed. This is particularly important

Table E-2. Activities and examples for therapy with the performance-oriented child.

Receptive communication skills

1. Increase percentage of listening versus talking time
2. Identify nonverbal cues that signal meaning and feeling
3. Increase use of questions and attempts to encourage others to talk
4. Analyze the communication strategies used by people with whom you like to talk (e.g., Uncle George's active listening)
5. Discuss turn taking and topic maintenance strategies
6. Read assigned materials on effective interpersonal communication
7. Describe all of the purposes of communication and provide examples of each
8. List examples of reflecting statements
9. Role play an interview where you try to find out as much as you can about a reticent friend

Vocal expressiveness (without increased tension)

1. Practice pitch changes as ways to get and hold attention
2. Explore rate changes to express different meanings and feelings
3. List words and phrases that are most effective when spoken softly
4. Speak in a soothing manner to calm a frightened friend or pet
5. Role play telling the same anecdote to indicate a variety of purposes
   - to entertain
   - to involve others
   - to express empathy
   - to motivate action
6. Read the following sentences, letting the pictures in your mind be reflected in your voice:
   (a) The music swelled to fill the concert hall and then faded away.
   (b) The party was in full swing and the music was blaring when John heard his parent's car in the driveway.
   (c) The runner slowly kept pace until the last lap, sprinted feverishly to the finish line, then collapsed from sheer exhaustion.
   (d) She had waited patiently for hours, but the abrupt tap on her shoulder frightened her.
   (e) The talented actor at the peak of his career became despondent and withdrawn.
   (f) That woman sings soprano, but her husband sings bass.
   (g) She was happy and carefree until she was told of her boyfriend's accident.
   (h) The man crawled down into a deep dark cavern.
   (i) This morning is a downer, but last night was fantastic.
   (j) The movie was long and boring, but the ending was exciting.

when the clinician considers how much family members should be involved in practice and carryover activities. For example, some children benefit from family support. Others, particularly teenagers, need help in practicing autonomy and self-empowerment.

Tension between the educational versus career demands on the young performer may also be a key element. Is the career being emphasized at the expense of the education? Is the young performer missing the critical social and emotional learning that occurs within the peer group and participation in varied extracurricular activities? Has the young performer fast-forwarded through the typical school-age experiences and become a pseudoadult who is then isolated by a type of experiential deprivation? An example is the teenager who is deprived of time to complete the tasks of adolescence and enjoy important peer group activities. Young performers, especially those who are also dealing with the emotional challenges of adolescence, are especially vulnerable to the impact of vocal problems and the threat to their emerging identity. Their voice problems may cause excessive anxiety and depression and threaten their future goals and study plans.

Few young performers are impervious to the genuine undivided attention of an adult who really listens to them. The role of the speech–language pathologist is to build the type of relationship that allows the client to develop his or her own problem-solving and action-planning skills. The speech–language pathologist can provide both support and guidance to ensure that the young performer is empowered. Often, the hardest part for the professional is to resist the urge to give direct advice, and yet the performer must develop his or her own personal commitment to relinquish old patterns in favor of new ones. Although direct advice giving is frequently seen as time saving, it rarely is as effective as guided problem solving.

The conscious planning and use of reinforcement by the speech–language pathologist is also essential. Performers are often applauded for what they do rather than for who they are. The clinician can use reinforcement to undergird the emergence of a realistic sense of self. Specific reinforcement can also aid the development of skills in confronting, analyzing, and solving problems. Examples of this are verbal praise such as, "I like the way you are tackling this problem," "You are good at analyzing why your voice sounds so tight," and "Give yourself a pat on the back." The therapeutic relationship can provide a safe space where a young performer can learn to appreciate the satisfaction of recognizing and applauding one's own efforts to grow and change. If insight into the reasons underlying changes in vocal behavior is developed, the young performer is armed with coping skills, information, and self-knowledge. This provides a foundation for the continued reappraisal and self-evaluation of voice use across a lifetime.

Conclusions

The performance-oriented child who consults a speech–language pathologist is different from other children in some significant ways. This child has a history of receiving important reinforcement and appreciation that is directly tied to vocal expertise. The sense of self includes the perception of superior vocal abilities. Thus, the threat that their voice may be chronically impaired jeopardizes highly valued aspirations and undermines the self-concept. Although the voice symptoms that need to be addressed are often similar to those addressed with other clients, the approach to intervention must be tailored to the unique needs of this population. Treatment involves addressing the psychosocial aspects of the problem that may precipitate and maintain inappropriate vocal practices.

References

1. Haskell JA. Vocal self-perception: the other side of the equation. *Voice* 1987;1:172–9.
2. Andrews ML, Summer AC. The awareness phase of voice therapy: providing a knowledge base for the adolescent. *Language, Speech and Hearing Services in Schools.* 1991; 22:156–7.
3. Andrews ML, Summers AC. *Voice therapy for adolescents.* San Diego: Singular Publishing Group, 1988.
4. Andrews ML. *Your best voice.* Tucson: Communication Skill Builders, 1993.
5. Flynn P, Andrews ML, Cabot B. *Using your voice wisely and well.* Tucson: Communication Skills Builders, 1990.
6. Andrews ML. *Voice therapy for children: the elementary school years.* San Diego: Singular Publishing Group, 1991.
7. Sataloff RT. *Professional voice: The Science and Art of Clinical Care.* New York: Raven Press, 1991.

The "Singing-Acting" Child: The Laryngologist's Perspective—1995[1]

Introduction

A survey of pediatric otolaryngologists about voice disorders in children suggests that ~1% of children examined were noted to have voice problems, and in only one fifth of these children (0.2%) were the voice problems related to professional use of the voice, such as singing. Direct flexible laryngoscopy was the sole method of examination for 80% of the children examined by these pediatric specialists. Voice therapy for 6 months was generally recommended (88%). The survey represents an estimated clinical experience of > 160,000 children per year, and it achieved a response rate of 40% of pediatric otolaryngologists (48/120). Results suggest that the use of video and stroboscopy for examination of the pediatric voice would enhance understanding and assure correct diagnosis and treatment.

The role of the physician, particularly the laryngologist who is responsible for the care of the young child's larynx, has been primarily focused on the treatment of airway obstruction and possible death in the young child. Antibiotics and vaccines have eradicated the scourges of diphtheria and, more recently, epiglottitis (Senior et al., 1994). We now must strive for a better understanding of the child's voice.

We must ask if our present techniques of evaluating young children with voice abnormalities are satisfactory. Some of the questions to be answered include: (a) What are the methods of examination of the child's larynx? (b) What methods of treatment are offered? (c) Are these appropriate methods of therapy? (d) What similarities or differences exist between the child and the adult's larynx, particularly for children with voice disorders? (e) What do pediatric laryngologists know about the young child's voice?

To answer these concerns, a questionnaire was sent to all members of the American Society of Pediatric Otolaryngology (ASPO), laryngologists exclusively devoted to the care of children and primarily representing physicians based at tertiary care children's hospitals and their clinics.

Materials and Methods

A questionnaire was sent to 120 ASPO members (Table E-3). This 13-question form was completed by 48 individuals and returned by mail. Results were compiled and percentages calculated for all questions if answers were provided. Some questions permitted multiple options, and all answers were counted.

Results

Forty-eight physicians completed the survey, and 98% (47/48) stated that they see young children with voice problems. The physicians in this survey are clinicians who examine a large number of children each year (average 3,400 children/year). This reflects a clinical experience total of >160,000 child visits in a 12-month period.

[1]Reprinted with permission of The Voice Foundation from "The 'Singing-Acting' Child: The Laryngologist's Perspective—1995," by J. S. Reilly, 1997. *Journal of Voice, 11,* 126–129.

Table E-3. Questionnaire and responses about pediatric voice problems; survey of American Society of Pediatric Otolaryngology (ASPO) members.

1. Do you see children (less than 12 years) with voice problems? Yes (47/98)[a] No (1/02)
2. The number of children seen with voice problems per year in my practice are: 10 or less (5/11) 20 (22/49) 50 (16/36) 75 (2/4) 100 (0/0) NR = 3
3. The number of children with voice problems caused by singing per year are: 5 or less (21/49) 10 (20/47) 20 (2/5) 50 (0/0) NR = 5
4. The total number of children seen per year are: 500 (1) 1,000 (4) 2,000 (5) 3,000 (10) 4,000 (9) 5,000 (12)
5. Do you make the diagnosis of "singer nodes" of the vocal cords? Yes (37) No (9) NR = 2
6. Do you believe children's vocal cord nodules are caused by any of the following? screaming (43) singing (28) gastroesophageal reflux (24) allergy (15)
7. What medical treatment do you employ for vocal cord nodules in children? antacids (5/10) H-2 blockers (11/23) prokinetics (6/13) steroids (4/8) antihistamines (4/8) none = (36/75)
8. Do you use voice therapists? Yes (37/77) No (5/10) NR = (6/12)
9. Minimum duration of therapy used is: (in months) 1 (2) 3 (7) 6 (16) 12 (7) 24 (0) NR = 16.
10. Do you inspect the vocal cords with flexible laryngoscopy (40) laryngoscopy with video (14) stroboscope (10) videofluroscopy (2)
11. Do you surgically remove vocal cord nodules in children? Yes (14) No (30) NR = 4
12. The type of surgery that I use for vocal cord nodules is primarily microlaryngoscopy with laser (14/29) microlaryngoscopy with microdisection (8/16)
13. Do you feel knowledgeable about the medical care of the professional child's voice? Yes (24) No (20) NR = 4

[a](number/percentage)
NR, no response.

The total number of children with voice problems seen was estimated at 1,440 for a 12-month period, representing a small percentage (0.9%) of the total population examined. The subset of children with voice abnormalities that were estimated to be caused by or related to singing totaled 327 (327/160,000) or 2 of 1,000 (0.2%).

The diagnostic methods used by the physicians in this survey to evaluate the voice disorders of children varied. The vast majority used direct visualization of the larynx, primarily with flexible laryngoscopy without video documentation (83%). Although more reliable, laryngoscopy *with* video documentation (29%) and stroboscopic evaluation (20%) were both used in less than one third of children with voice abnormalities.

The probable etiologies of vocal fold nodules were ranked by the physicians who completed the questionnaire. The most common attributed causes of laryngeal pathology reported were (a) voice abuse, for example screaming (89%) or, less frequently, singing (58%); (b) gastroesophageal reflux (GER) (50%); and (c) allergies (28%). All diagnoses were clinical judgments; most were not confirmed by laboratory tests.

Although both GER and allergies are treatable, three quarters (36/48) of the physicians do not offer medical treatment for these children. Only about one quarter suggest anti-GER medications (23%) (e.g., antacids or prokinetic agents).

Voice therapy is the most commonly endorsed treatment (77%). The average period of recommended treatment was 6 months. If vocal fold nodules are confirmed and voice therapy has not brought improvement, a limited number of physicians (27%) suggest surgical removal for children. Microlaryngoscopy with carbon dioxide laser was utilized about twice as often as microsurgical removal with traditional instrumentation (14 vs. 8).

Only 50% of the responding pediatric otolaryngologists (24/48) stated that they believed they were particularly knowledgeable about the best treatment of the child's voice. Few (4/48) designated a particular interest or study of the child's voice. Over one half in this group acknowledged that they would benefit from additional insight and continued investigation.

Discussion

Children with voice problems are not commonly seen by pediatric otolaryngologists and represent <1% of visits to these physicians. An even smaller percentage, 0.2%, may have their voice abnormality caused by singing. These two groups of children represent the small portion of the pediatric population whose vocal symptoms are persistent or severe enough to merit referral to a pediatric otolaryngologist.

Physician understanding requires knowledge of the unique aspects of the child's larynx. The infant's vocal folds are short, 6 to 8 mm in length; about one half of the length is cartilage. The epiglottis is omega-shaped in ~50% of young infants. Significant growth over the first 12 years of life causes the vocal folds to lengthen to 12 to 17 mm in the mature teenage girl, and to 17 to 23 mm in the older teenage boy. The vocal ligament has been shown to be unidentifiable in the child's larynx until ~8 years of age (Hirano, 1981). Therefore, the superficial, intermediate, and deep layers of the lamina propria are also not well seen until the child reaches the second decade of life.

The laryngeal framework will descend in the neck (C3 to C7) and elongate the oropharynx and the hypopharynx from a conical shape to a more cylindrical contour, altering the resonating cavity for speech. As this lengthening of the vocal folds progresses rapidly during puberty, the fundamental frequency also lowers, particularly in the male. This probably contributes to but may not fully explain the decrease in the pitch of the male voice. Also, as the pharynx changes from conical to a more cylindrical shape in the adolescent, the laryngeal-pharyngeal widening also occurs with the increased diameter of the cricoid cartilage and the expansion of the alar wings of the thyroid cartilages.

This survey shows that ~1 of 100 children examined have a voice problem and that pediatric otolaryngologists diagnose ~30 children per year with a voice condition. About four of five surveyed physicians labeled the laryngeal abnormalities as the result of voice abuse ("screamer's nodes" or "singer's nodes"). The diagnosis is made by flexible laryngoscopy, done without video review ~83% of the time. Mirror examination of the larynx is no longer reported or recommended in young children.

The frequency of vocal fold nodules (<1%) suggests this condition is not commonly diagnosed. Previous reports have suggested that a much higher percentage of all children have voice problems (6–17%) (Senturia & Wilson, 1968). Silverman, in a study of 162 school children, showed that 20% were chronically hoarse and that one half (10%) of these had vocal fold nodules (Silverman & Zimmer, 1975). Investigators estimate that >1,000,000 young children in the United States have vocal fold nodules (Von Leyden, 1985). In young children, they occur more frequently in boys and tend to be more fusiform in shape and less discrete than in adults (MacArthur & Healy, 1995). Many harsh or hoarse voices of children are apparently not referred for direct examination, or pediatric otolaryngologists are not as attentive as they might be to the presence of dysphonia when children are referred for nonvoice problems.

Vocal fold nodules appear to be primarily caused by trauma from the vocal folds through increased intensity, as well as increased duration of phonation. Patients with vocal fold nodules have been shown to speak over three times as long as control subjects with normal voices. Moreover, those with vocal fold nodules speak over one half the time at high intensity (Masuda et al., 1993). Experts now believe that intensity of vocal phonation combines with fundamental frequency to cause localized damage to the vocal folds.

Recent studies have shown that vocal fold nodules in children are probably similar to those in adults despite the anatomic differences. Nodules are similar in composition and structure both by electron microscopy and immunohistologic stains. There is basement membrane duplication and a disorder in rudimentary anchoring fibers if vocal fold nodules occur (Gray, Hammond, & Hanson, 1995).

Repetitive injury appears to result in basement membrane zone disruption and injury to the superficial lamina propria. Aberrant healing leads to fibronectin deposition; efficient tissue vibration is lost. A second kind of injury without basement membrane generally does not include fibronectin or elastin deposition: There is lamina propria injury only, which may be associated with Reinke edema.

The possibility that the proteoglycan, hyaluronic acid, is more common in the intermediate layer of the lamina propria has been raised by investigators at the University of Utah. This protein-carbohydrate complex may serve as a protective factor because hyaluronic acid is able to bind water and may be critical as a volume expander and thus cushion the trauma of vocal fold vibration (S. D. Gray, personal communication, 1995).

Most of the surveyed physicians suggest that chronic voice abuse is the primary problem and that gastroesophageal reflux and allergies are less common. More than three fourths of physicians surveyed do not initiate any medical treatment for possible causes. About 85% use speech therapy regardless of suspected etiology or physical findings. Duration of speech therapy is a minimum of 6 months. When surgery is considered in children, this is limited to significant lesions such as polyps and only rarely used for vocal fold nodules.

Clinical experience supports the observation that benign vocal fold lesions in children will resolve with age as the child enters adolescence. The fundamental frequency of the adolescent child will decrease as the vocal cords lengthen. Surgery is generally not indicated. Continued growth with reduction in fundamental frequency favors resolution. For children who have complied with voice therapy and are bothered socially or professionally (singers, actors) by persistent mass lesions, however, surgery may be appropriate. GER is an unproven but suspicious cause in certain cases.

Conclusion

It is clear that additional research is necessary to clarify the prevalence of voice disorders in the pediatric population. The discrepancy between the high incidence of voice disorders in the previously published surveys and the small percentage of voice disorders seen or recognized by pediatric otolaryngologists requires clarification. In addition, it appears that pediatric otolaryngology has not taken full advantage of the advances in voice science and technology now established for the care of adult patients with voice disorders. Additional clinical expertise should be acquired, pediatric voice research should be encouraged, and pediatric otolaryngology fellowship programs should consider developing greater expertise in state-of-the-art diagnosis and treatment of voice disorders in children.

References

1. Senior BA, Radkowski D, MacArthur CJ, et al. Changing patterns of supraglottitis. *Otolaryngol Head Neck Surg* 1994;110:203–10.
2. Hirano M. Structure of the vocal fold in normal and disease states. Anatomical and physical study. *ASHA* 1981.
3. Senturia BH, Wilson FB. Otorhinolaryngologic findings in children with voice deviation. *Ann Otol Rhinol Laryngol* 1968;77:1027–41.
4. Silverman EM, Zimmer CH. Incidence of chronic hoarseness among school age children. *J Speech Hear Disord* 1975; 40:211–15.
5. Von Leyden H. Vocal cord nodules in children. *ENT J* 1985;64:473–80.
6. MacArthur CJ, Healy GB. Acquired voice disorders in the pediatric population. In: Rubin JS, Sataloff RT, Korovin GS, Gould WJ, eds. *Diagnosis and treatment of voice disorders.* New York: Igaku-Shoin, 1995.
7. Masuda T, Ikeda Y, Manako H, et al. Analysis of vocal abuse: fluctuations in phonation time and intensity in 4 groups of speakers. *Acta Otolaryngol* 1993;113:547–52.
8. Gray SD, Hammond E, Hanson DF. Benign pathologic responses of the larynx. *Ann Otol Rhinol Laryngol* 1995;104:13–18.

The Role of the Speech–Language Pathologist in the NICU

Risa Krupoff

"Why does my baby need a speech pathologist? He's 35 weeks gestation and won't be talking for quite some time . . . ."

This is one of the most frequently asked questions when I first introduce myself to a family of a premature baby in the neonatal intensive care unit. Most are surprised at the role a speech pathologist plays in the care of their infant. A speech–language pathologist is a person who works with people of any age who demonstrate speech, language, swallowing, cognitive, oral motor, or feeding deficits. He or she must have completed a master's degree in speech–language pathology and be certified both nationally and at the state level.

Usually a speech pathologist is contacted anytime after 32 weeks gestation when an infant's sucking and swallowing skills are beginning to develop. In premature and medically compromised infants, feeding can be a complicated skill to acquire. Feeding issues often prolong a child's hospital stay.

Speech–language pathologists provide the following services:

- develop appropriate sucking skills, either with the pacifier, breast feeding, and/or bottle feeding.
- develop swallowing skills
- develop coordination of sucking and swallowing skills
- increase endurance with feedings
- aid the transition between oral feedings and NG/G-tube feedings
- decrease oral aversions
- increase positive feeding experiences between the caregiver and the infant
- implement early intervention for speech and language skills
- stimulate receptive voice learning and vocal play
- help parents develop emotional and vocal connections with their baby

How do we accomplish this?

Usually, oral stimulation exercises are introduced as well as family education concerning the infant's needs. Occasionally it is necessary to complete a videofluoroscopic swallow study. This is a test in which the child swallows barium under an X ray so the process of swallowing can be observed. The speech–language pathologist and the radiologist complete the study together. The results are immediately available and can be reviewed with the family. The speech–language pathologist can answer questions about conditions affecting the respiratory/digestive systems and how these conditions are treated. Suggestions concerning ways to stimulate developmentally appropriate behaviors to support feeding and communication are presented.

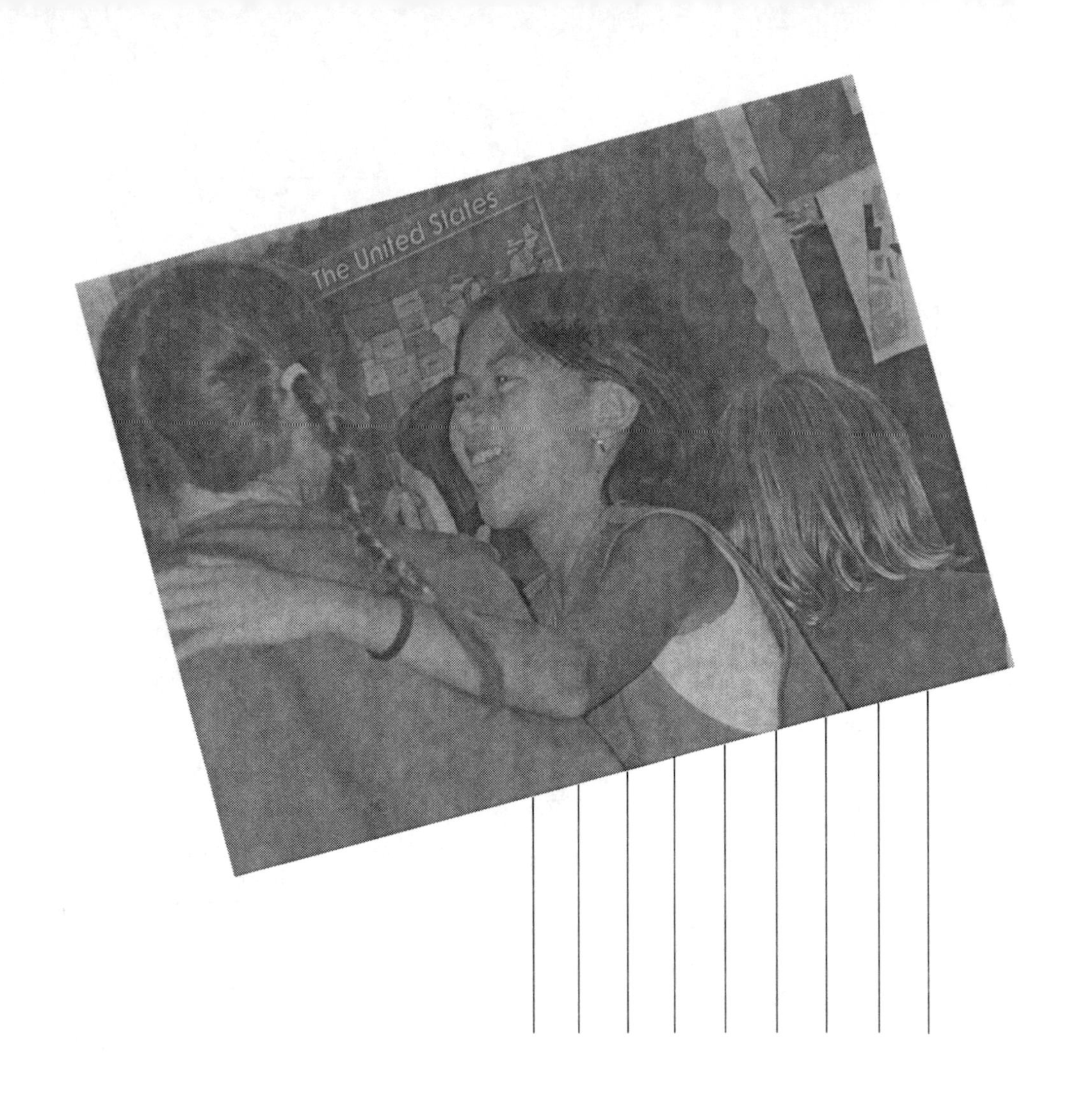

Subject Index

A

B

C

H

I

R

S

T

U

V

W

CPSIA information can be obtained
at www.ICGtesting.com
Printed in the USA
FFOW01n1313191113
2415FF

9 780769 301075